BONES AND JOINTS

INTERNATIONAL ACADEMY OF PATHOLOGY

MONOGRAPHS IN PATHOLOGY

SERIES EDITOR, **Murray R. Abell, M.D.**

Professor, Department of Pathology,
University of Michigan Medical School, Ann Arbor, Michigan

No. 1. **The Lymphocyte and Lymphocytic Tissue**
John W. Rebuck *and* Robert E. Stowell, *Editors*

No. 2. **The Adrenal Cortex**
Henry D. Moon *and* Robert E. Stowell, *Editors*

No. 3. **The Ovary**
Hugh G. Grady *and* David E. Smith, *Editors*

No. 4. **The Peripheral Blood Vessels**
J. Lowell Orbison *and* David E. Smith, *Editors*

No. 5. **The Thyroid**
J. Beach Hazard *and* David E. Smith, *Editors*

No. 6. **The Kidney**
F. K. Mostofi *and* David E. Smith, *Editors*

No. 7. **The Connective Tissue**
Bernard M. Wagner *and* David E. Smith, *Editors*

No. 8. **The Lung**
Averill A. Liebow *and* David E. Smith, *Editors*

No. 9. **The Brain**
Orville T. Bailey *and* David E. Smith, *Editors*

No. 10. **The Skin**
Elson B. Helwig *and* F. K. Mostofi, *Editors*

No. 11. **The Platelet**
K. M. Brinkhous, R. W. Shermer, *and* F. K. Mostofi, *Editors*

No. 12. **The Striated Muscle**
Carl M. Pearson *and* F. K. Mostofi, *Editors*

No. 13. **The Liver**
Edward A. Gall *and* F. K. Mostofi, *Editors*

No. 14. **The Uterus**
Henry J. Norris, Arthur T. Hertig *and* Murray R. Abell, *Editors*

No. 15. **The Heart**
Jesse E. Edwards, Maurice Lev, *and* Murray R. Abell, *Editors*

No. 16. **The Reticuloendothelial System**
John W. Rebuck, Costan W. Berard, *and* Murray R. Abell, *Editors*

No. 17. **Bones and Joints**
Lauren V. Ackerman, Harlan J. Spjut, *and* Murray R. Abell, *Editors*

Succeeding Volumes to Be Announced

INTERNATIONAL ACADEMY OF PATHOLOGY MONOGRAPH

BONES AND JOINTS

by 24 authors

EDITED BY **LAUREN V. ACKERMAN, M.D.**

Professor of Pathology, State University of New York
Stony Brook, New York

HARLAN J. SPJUT, M.D.

Professor of Pathology, Baylor College of Medicine
and
Department of Pathology, St. Luke's Episcopal Hospital
Texas Medical Center, Houston, Texas

AND MURRAY R. ABELL, M.D.

Department of Pathology
University of Michigan, Medical School, Ann Arbor, Michigan

The Williams & Wilkins Company
Baltimore, 1976

Made in the United States of America

Library of Congress Cataloging in Publication Data
Main entry under title:

Bones and joints.

(Monographs in pathology; no. 17)
Bibliography: p.
Includes index.
1. Bones—Diseases—Diagnosis—Congresses. 2. Joints—Diseases—Diagnosis—Congresses. I. Ackerman, Lauren Vedder, 1905- II. Spjut, Harlan J., 1922- III. Abell, Murray R. IV. Series: International Academy of Pathology. Monographs in pathology; no. 17. [DNLM: 1. Bone diseases—Pathology—Congresses. 2. Joint diseases—Pathology—Congresses. W1 M0568H no. 17 / WE200 I604b 1975] RC930.5.B67 616.7′1′075 76-6064 ISBN 0-683-00039-X

COMPOSED AND PRINTED AT
WAVERLY PRESS, INC.
Mt. Royal and Guilford Aves.
Baltimore, MD. 21202, U.S.A.

Contents

CONTRIBUTING AUTHORS vii

FOREWORD *by Murray R. Abell* ix

PREFACE *by Lauren V. Ackerman and Harlan J. Spjut* xi

1. THE EMBRYOLOGY OF BONE AND BONES — *Ronan O'Rahilly and Ernest Gardner* 1
2. NORMAL STRUCTURE OF BONE: LIGHT AND ELECTRON MICROSCOPY — *Gerald S. Laros* 16
3. OSTEOPOROSIS AND OSTEOMALACIA . . . . . . *Hubert A. Sissons* 25
4. OSTEOMYELITIS INCLUDING FUNGAL . . . . . . *Walter G. J. Putschar* 39
5. IDIOPATHIC ASEPTIC NECROSIS — *D. S. Springfield and William F. Enneking* 61
6. IMMUNOLOGIC ASPECTS OF ARTHRITIS AS AN AID IN DIAGNOSIS AND PROGNOSIS OF RHEUMATIC DISEASE — *John T. Sharp, Neal G. Sutherland, Martin D. Lidsky, Donald A. Person, Joseph Duffy and Carolyn Leatherwood* 88
7. RADIOLOGIC DIAGNOSIS OF JOINT DISEASE . . . . . . *Jack Edeiken* 98
8. OSTEOARTHRITIS . . . . . . *Leon Sokoloff* 110
9. RHEUMATOID AND RELATED ARTHRITIDES . . . . . . *Howard D. Dorfman* 130
10. PAGET'S DISEASE OF BONE . . . . . . *Hubert A. Sissons* 146
11. NEOPLASMS AND NEOPLASM-LIKE LESIONS OF THE SYNOVIUM — *Robert E. Fechner* 157
12. ETIOLOGY OF HUMAN SKELETAL AND SOFT TISSUE SARCOMAS: A SUMMARY OF IMMUNOLOGIC AND VIROLOGIC STUDIES — *Frederick R. Eilber and Donald L. Morton* 187
13. THE RADIOLOGIC APPROACH TO BONE TUMORS . . . . . . *Alex Norman* 196
14. FIBRO-OSSEOUS LESIONS OF BONE . . . . . . *Louis P. Dehner* 209
15. DIFFERENTIAL DIAGNOSIS OF GIANT CELL LESIONS OF BONE . *C. P. Schwinn* 236
16. CHONDROSARCOMA AND ITS "VARIANTS" . . . . . . *David C. Dahlin* 300
17. SMALL ROUND CELL TUMORS OF BONE . . . . . . *Walter M. Levy* 312

INDEX 321

CONTRIBUTING AUTHORS

David C. Dahlin, M.D.
Professor of Pathology, Mayo Medical School, Rochester, Minnesota

Louis P. Dehner, M.D.
Associate Professor of Laboratory Medicine and Pathology, University of Minnesota Medical School, Minneapolis, Minnesota

Howard D. Dorfman, M.D.
Pathologist-in-Chief, Sinai Hospital of Baltimore; Associate Professor of Pathology and Orthopaedic Surgery, The Johns Hopkins University, School of Medicine, Baltimore, Maryland

Joseph Duffy, M.D.
Assistant Professor of Medicine, Mayo Clinic, Rochester, Minnesota

Jack Edeiken, M.D.
Professor and Chairman, Department of Radiology, Thomas Jefferson University Hospital, Philadelphia, Pennsylvania

Frederick R. Eilber, M.D.
Associate Professor of Surgery, Division of Oncology, University of California School of Medicine, Los Angeles, California

William F. Enneking, M.D.
Professor of Orthopedics and Pathology, The University of Florida, Gainesville, Florida

Robert E. Fechner, M.D.
Associate Professor of Pathology, Baylor College of Medicine; Surgical Pathologist, The Methodist Hospital, Houston, Texas

Ernest Gardner, M.D.
Professor of Neurology, Orthopaedic Surgery and Human Anatomy, University of California, Davis; and Carnegie Institution of Washington, Department of Embryology, Davis Division, Davis, California

Gerald S. Laros, M.D.
Professor of Surgery, and Chairman, Section of Orthopedics, The University of Chicago, Chicago, Illinois

Carolyn Leatherwood, B.S.
Research Assistant, Department of Internal Medicine, Baylor College of Medicine, Houston, Texas

Walter M. Levy, M.D.
Professor of Pathology, Hahnemann Medical College and Hospital of Philadelphia, Philadelphia, Pennsylvania

MARTIN D. LIDSKY, M.D.
Associate Professor of Internal Medicine, Baylor College of Medicine, Houston, Texas

DONALD L. MORTON, M.D.
Professor of Surgery, and Chief, Division of Oncology, University of California School of Medicine, Los Angeles, California

ALEX NORMAN, M.D.
Director of Radiology, Hospital for Joint Diseases and Medical Center, and Professor of Radiology, Mount Sinai School of Medicine, City University of New York, New York, New York

RONAN O'RAHILLY, M.D.
Director of the Carnegie Embryological Collection, and Professor of Human Anatomy, University of California, Davis, California

DONALD A. PERSON, M.D.
Assistant Professor of Internal Medicine, Virology and Epidemiology, Baylor College of Medicine, Houston, Texas

WALTER G. J. PUTSCHAR, M.D.
Consultant in Pathology, Massachusetts General Hospital; Visiting Lecturer, Department of Pathology, Harvard University; Visiting Lecturer in Pathology, Massachusetts Institute of Technology, Boston, Massachusetts; and Research Associate, Smithsonian Institution, Washington, D.C.

CHARLES P. SCHWINN, M.D.
Associate Professor of Pathology, University of Southern California; and Director of Laboratories, Orthopaedic Hospital of Los Angeles, Los Angeles, California

JOHN T. SHARP, M.D.
Professor of Internal Medicine, Chief, Rheumatic Disease Section, Baylor College of Medicine, Houston, Texas

HUBERT A. SISSONS, M.D.
Professor of Morbid Anatomy, Institute of Orthopaedics, University of London; Honorary Consultant, Morbid Anatomist, Royal National Orthopaedic Hospital, London, England

LEON SOKOLOFF, M.D.
Professor, Department of Pathology, State University of New York, Stony Brook, New York

DEMPSEY S. SPRINGFIELD, M.D.
Orthopaedic Resident, Department of Orthopaedics, University of Florida, Gainesville, Florida 32601

NEAL G. SUTHERLAND, M.D.
Oncologist, Tripler Army Medical Center, APO San Francisco, California

PREFACE

Diseases of bones and joints have long been a source of curiosity and interest, but often have been approached with trepidation. Thus it was the hope of the International Academy of Pathology that a Long Course devoted to this subject would fortify the former two and allay the third. Tumors of bone are uncommon with some 2,000 new malignant tumors seen in the U.S.A. per year. Because of this, it is understandable that histologic diagnoses are approached with considerable uneasiness on the part of most pathologists; only a few are fortunate enough to see the quantity of material that engenders assurance in a diagnosis. Yet, if the pathologist were to know of a few bits of information in regard to location of tumor and age distribution and made an effort to review the roentgenograms on each case, he would formulate a reasonable differential diagnosis to serve as a guide to a final diagnosis. The role of the radiologist and orthopedic surgeon in the diagnosis and treatment cannot be ignored by the pathologist. The latter is but one part of the trio necessary for accurate diagnosis.

The same principles apply to non-neoplastic diseases. True, many of them are common *e.g.*, degenerative arthritis (osteoarthritis), and are often given the "ho-hum" approach. From the standpoint of morbidity these diseases are of considerably greater importance than are tumors, but they have not attained the glamorous aura of the tumors. In the area of arthritic diseases, the surgeon has thrust the pathologist into the thick, if not the thickest, of joint disease with total joint replacements and the many correctional procedures done for deformities of the hands. The pathologist is now expected to recognize the differences between osteoarthritis and rheumatoid arthritis and to have an understanding of ischemic necrosis of bone. In addition, there is an expanding interest in the effects of metabolic disorders on bone, of the various infections on bone, and the results of trauma to bone and joints.

It was with these thoughts in mind that we drew up this first Long Course on Disease of Bones and Joints. More than half of the presentations concern non-neoplastic aspects of bones and joints. Embryology, anatomy and the radiologic aspects were emphasized, as these are of basic importance in the understanding and interpretation of all diseases of bones and joints. In addition, the changing concepts, the morphologic variations, and the pathologic diagnostic features were discussed in detail. All were presented by persons expert in the field of diseases of bone and joints.

Harlan J. Spjut, M.D.
Lauren V. Ackerman, M.D.

FOREWORD

The United States-Candian Division of the International Academy of Pathology is pleased to present the monograph, *Bones and Joints*. It is the 17th in the series of *Monographs in Pathology* which was initiated by the Council of the Academy in 1959. The monographs are the product of the Academy's long courses that comprise one of the major facets of its annual educational program. They constitute a permanent reference of information of acknowledged excellence on normal structure, function, and disease of organs and systems. The long courses and their offspring, the monographs, contribute significantly to the Academy's goal in continuing education for pathologists and clinicians.

"Diseases of Bones and Joints" comprised the long course at the 64th annual meeting of the United States-Canadian Division of the International Academy of Pathology in New Orleans in 1975. Dr. Lauren V. Ackerman and Dr. Harlan J. Spjut, directors of the long course, recruited an eminent faculty for the course. Their presentations, which comprise this monograph, encompass a wealth of knowledge and valuable experience which contribute significantly to the understanding of this facet of pathology.

The United States-Canadian Division of the Academy expresses its sincere thanks to Dr. Ackerman and Dr. Spjut and to their distinguished faculty for their valuable contributions to this monograph and to the publishers, The Williams & Wilkins Company, for their continuing support and expert assistance.

MURRAY R. ABELL, M.D., PH.D.
Series Editor

Chapter 1

The Embryology of Bone and Bones*

RONAN O'RAHILLY AND ERNEST GARDNER

The development of bone, both as a tissue and as individual skeletal units, is a highly complicated subject that includes, among other aspects, chondrification and ossification, calcification and matrix deposition and resorption, and structure and growth. A detailed review of osteogenesis has appeared recently.[7]

The account presented here will be confined to the morphologic aspects of the prenatal development of bone and bones in the human.

All bones begin as mesenchymal condensations during the embryonic period. By mesenchyme is meant the early, delicate, loose connective tissue that is derived from the mesoderm, which, in turn, arises from the mesoblast. The mesoblast first appears in an extraembryonic position (stage 5a; 7 or 8 days) and, within a week, within the body of the embryo (stage 6b; 13 days). The stages mentioned throughout this chapter refer to the Carnegie system of staging the human embryo,[28] and the ages given refer to postovulatory days or weeks.

During the initial formation of various organs, including bones, masses of mesenchyme show an increased number of cells or intercellular fibers, or both, and are referred to as condensations. Particularly in the limbs, "a mass of mesenchymal tissue from which organs are to be differentiated . . . before differentiation has commenced" and even "the structures first differentiated in the limb"[1] is referred to as a blastema.

Ossification may occur directly in a predominantly fibrous or membranous environment, and it is then known as intramembranous ossification. Alternatively, an essentially similar ossific process may occur in cartilage, and the term endochondral ossification is then employed.

INTRAMEMBRANOUS OSSIFICATION

Intramembranous ossification takes place in most of the calvaria and in part of the base of the skull, as well as in some portions of the facial skeleton[5, 34] and partly in the clavicle and mandible.

At the sites of intramembranous ossification, a fibrocellular proliferation appears. The cells, termed osteoblasts, synthesize phosphatase, and a calcified organic matrix that cements the fibers together is formed. Formation and

---

* Aided in part by research program Grant HD08656, Institute of Child Health and Human Development, National Institutes of Health.

calcification of bone matrix are generally contemporaneous, but areas of noncalcified bone matrix, known as osteoid, may be found initially. Bone appears first in the form of spicules surrounded by osteoblasts, some of which become embedded in the matrix as osteocytes. The sites where clusters of osteoblasts are first seen are known as ossific centers. The pattern of growth and the orientation of the bony spicules or trabeculae vary with the individual bone. The frontal and parietal bones, for example; are characterized by a radiating bony network (Fig. 10 of Ref. 33). Moreover, the developing vault of the skull presents a number of special features, such as relationship to the underlying meninges and brain, absorption and reconstruction in relation to changing curvatures, formation and growth of sutures, and development of diploë.[7]

The clavicle, which (together with the mandible) is the first skeletal element to show signs of bone formation,[30] undergoes intramembranous ossification (*cf.* cleidocranial dysostosis). Nevertheless, after ossification begins, a peculiar type of ("secondary") cartilage is found in the clavicle and mandible.

ENDOCHONDRAL OSSIFICATION

Skeletal elements that are characterized by endochondral ossification appear first as mesenchymal condensations (Fig. 1). An intercellular matrix then separates the cells, so that the area involved appears more lightly stained. This initial phase of chondrification is often called precartilage. The mesenchymal cells at the periphery of the condensation form a perichondrium which outlines the skeletal blastema. Before the end of the embryonic period proper (8 postovulatory weeks), each skeletal element shows the basic features of its adult form. The cartilaginous model is then gradually replaced by bone.

Endochondral ossification is found in a number of short, flat, and irregular bones, such as the scapula, carpal and tarsal bones, and vertebrae. The time of onset of ossification varies considerably and ranges from the end of the embryonic period proper (in the case of the scapula) to postnatal life (*e.g.*, carpals and most tarsals). In some instances (*e.g.*, scapula, calcaneus, neural arches of vertebrae) the cartilage calcifies and periosteal bone forms, and then vascular invasion and endochondral ossification begin. In other examples (*e.g.*, centra of vertebrae) the calcified cartilage is invaded by blood vessels, and endochondral ossification begins, periosteal bone generally being formed later. Most of these bones develop in a manner similar to that of epiphyses. Ossification spreads to the periphery of the cartilage. On reaching articular cartilage (or the hyaline cartilaginous rings of the vertebral centra), growth zones develop which are similar to the articular zones in epiphyses. Hence, postnatal growth takes place from both periosteum and articular cartilage.

Endochondral ossification is typical of the so-called long or tubular bones, such as the humerus[11] and the femur.[9] The cartilaginous models of such bones are sharply defined by their perichondria. They grow (1) by apposition from perichondrium and from tissue forming the interzones of joints, and (2) by multiplication of cartilage cells already formed and by increase in intercellular matrix. The youngest cells (Figs. 2 and 3) are at the ends of the skeletal element, where most growth occurs, and are small and lack a specific arrangement (phase 1 cartilage).[36] These cells multiply and form rows of flattened, closely packed

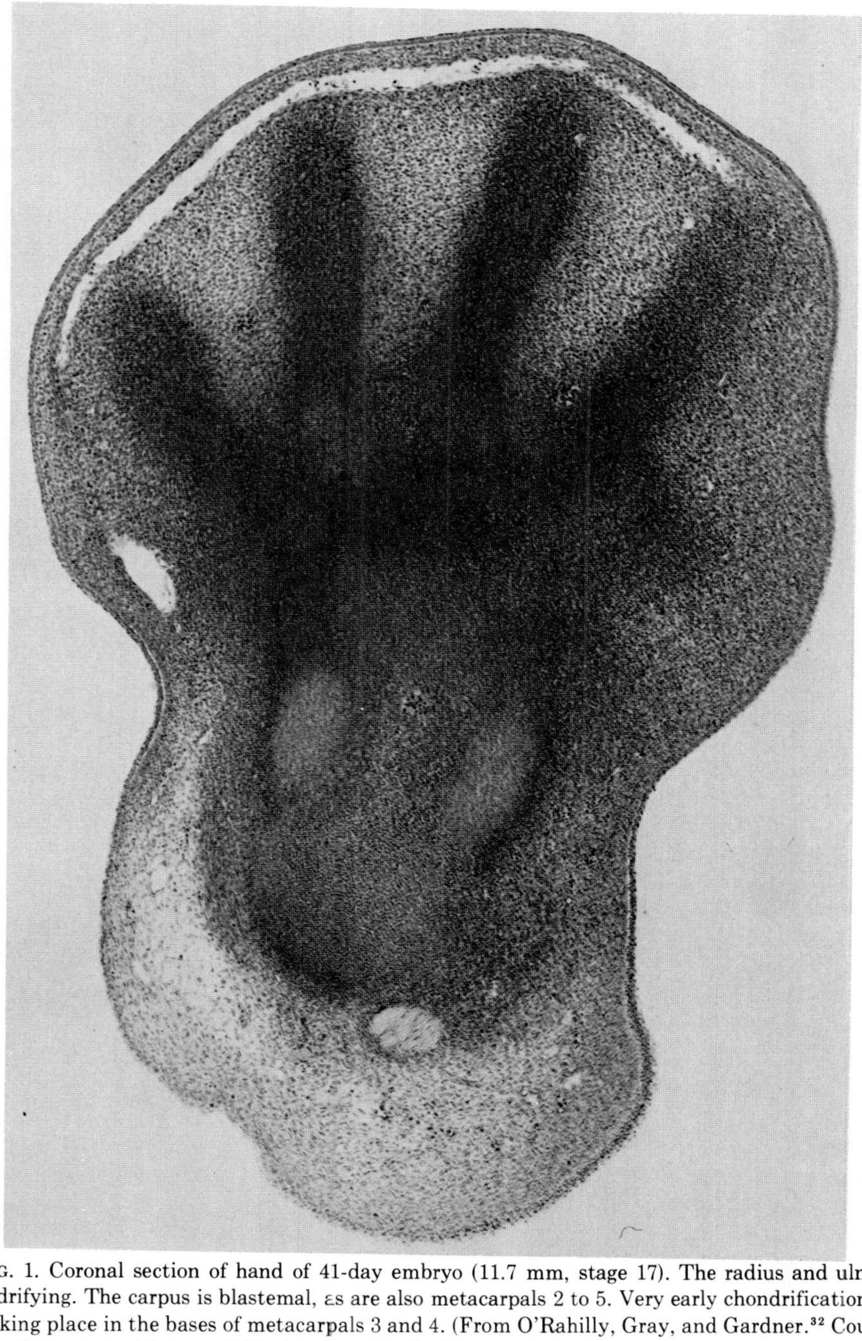

FIG. 1. Coronal section of hand of 41-day embryo (11.7 mm, stage 17). The radius and ulna are chondrifying. The carpus is blastemal, as are also metacarpals 2 to 5. Very early chondrification may be taking place in the bases of metacarpals 3 and 4. (From O'Rahilly, Gray, and Gardner.[32] Courtesy of the Carnegie Institution of Washington. Used with permission.)

cells (phase 2). The intercellular matrix then increases in amount, the cells enlarge, and their cytoplasm becomes vesicular (phase 3). When the cartilage cells reach their maximum size, they undergo pronounced vacuolization (phase 4). Finally, the cells begin to disintegrate and disappear (phase 5). The oldest cartilage cells (phase 4 and 5) are found as a more lightly staining area in the midsection of the shaft (Figs. 3 and 4).

Ossification commences at the middle of the cartilaginous model (Fig. 5). (In the distal phalanges, however, ossification commences at the distal ends, and Fig. 6 shows that the tuberosity that forms at the ends is particularly striking.) A thin layer of osteoid is laid down between the perichondrium and the hypertrophied cartilage cells of the shaft (Fig. 4). The osteoid is rapidly calcified, and the

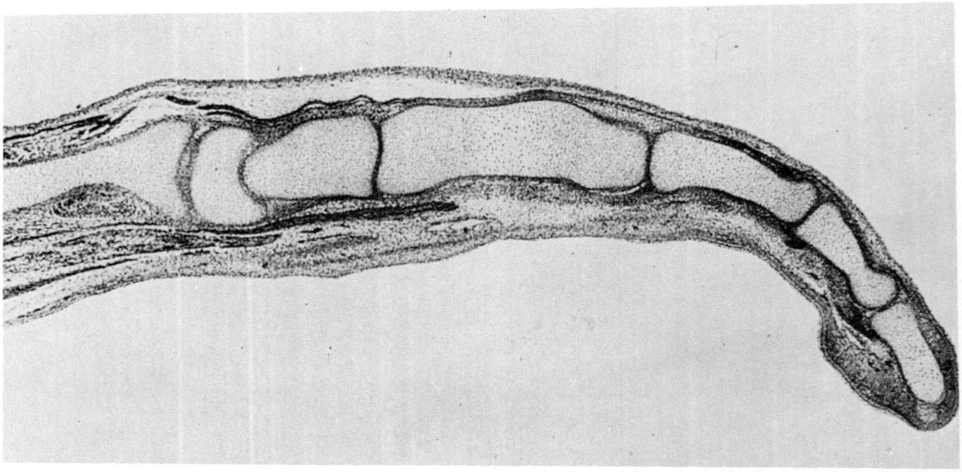

FIG. 2. Sagittal section of the third finger of a 54-day embryo (26 mm C.-R.). The cartilaginous skeletal elements visible are radius, lunate, capitate, third metacarpal, and the three phalanges of the third finger. Ossification is beginning at the tip of the distal phalanx. (From Gray, Gardner, and O'Rahilly, *Am. J. Anat. 101:* 169–223, Fig. 7, 1957. Used with permission.)

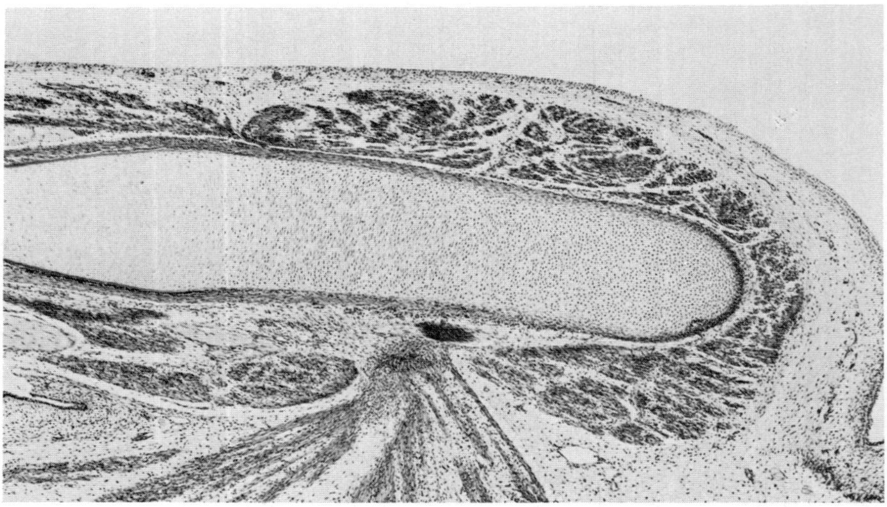

FIG. 3. Longitudinal section of upper end of humerus, not including head, from an 8-week embryo (28 mm, crown-rump), illustrating several developmental phases of cartilage. A thin layer of periosteal bone is situated next to the zone of hypertrophic cartilage. (From Gardner.[7] Used with permission.)

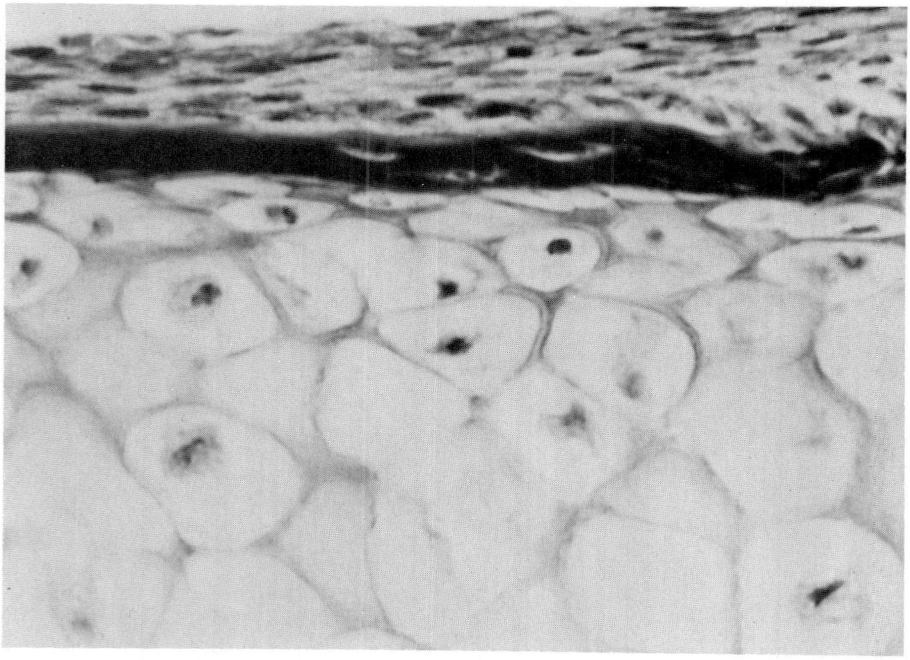

FIG. 4. Longitudinal section of portion of the central area of the shaft of a metacarpal of a 10-week fetus (50 mm, crown-rump). Immediately deep to the periosteum, a very thin layer of osteoid (*i.e.*, noncalcified bone matrix) is present (stained differentially in the actual preparation), followed by a thicker and darker band of bone, which is a portion of the periosteal bone collar. Hypertrophic cartilage cells can be seen internal to the collar.

innermost cells of the perichondrium (which is termed periosteum from now onwards) differentiate into osteoblasts. Trabeculae begin to form in relation to collagenous fibers in a manner similar to that found in intramembranous ossification. The primary (or periosteal) bone collar thereby formed gradually becomes multilayered. The matrix of the zone of hypertrophied cartilage cells becomes calcified.

After a highly variable interval, depending on the individual skeletal element, vascular invasion of the cartilage begins (Figs. 7 and 8). The primary bone collar is penetrated at several points (Fig. 9) by cellular buds derived from the periosteum, and these buds constitute what is termed an ossific center. The buds consist chiefly of undifferentiated cells and of osteoclasts. The cartilage is destroyed and replaced by the cells of the periosteal bud. Blood vessels develop, and a circulation becomes established. Osteoblasts and blood-forming cells develop, and bone begins to be deposited around the remnants of calcified cartilage matrix, that is, endochondral ossification occurs (Fig. 10). The processes of cartilage destruction, marrow formation, and endochondral ossification extend rapidly toward the ends of the skeletal elements. The endochondrally formed trabeculae fuse with those of the periosteal shell. Many of the centrally situated trabeculae, however, are rapidly removed, so that a marrow cavity is formed.

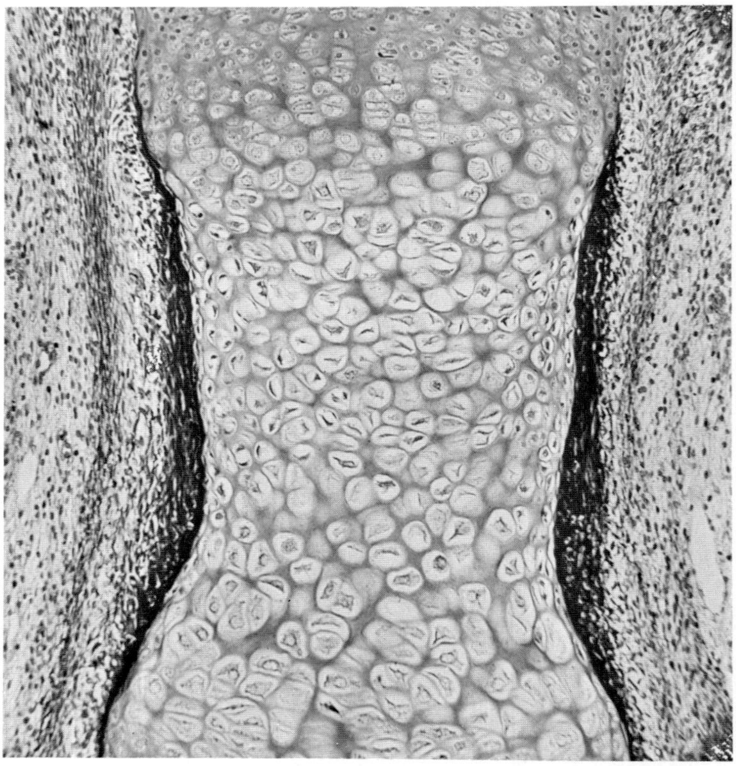

FIG. 5. Coronal section of proximal phalanx of second finger of 11-week fetus (69 mm crown-rump), showing bone collar and hypertrophic cartilage (From Gray, Gardner, and O'Rahilly, *Am. J. Anat. 101:* 169–223, Fig. 41, 1957. Used with permission.)

Before the middle of prenatal life, endochondral ossification reaches the epiphysial regions, and an orderly cellular arrangement is characteristic. Hypertrophic cartilage cells appear in longitudinal columns, separated by thin walls of calcified matrix. As the cells become destroyed by the invasion from the shaft, bars of calcified matrix are exposed, and bone is deposited around them.

Later, generally after birth, one or both ends of many long bones are characterized by the appearance of one or more epiphysial centers of ossification (Fig. 11).

As a bone grows in length, its shape is maintained by reconstruction or remodeling. For example, the wider parts (metaphyses) of the shaft near the epiphysial ends are reduced (by osteoclasts), thereby avoiding the formation of club-shaped ends. Such reconstructions, however, are usually quite selective, so that such complicated shapes as the lower end of the humerus are retained during development. Moreover, local processes related to the development of ridges, grooves, and torsion modify the general processes of reconstruction. Detailed accounts of the nature and principles of skeletal reconstruction are provided by Lacroix,[16] Enlow,[4] and Gardner.[7]

TIMING OF EVENTS IN SKELETAL DEVELOPMENT

In order to determine the precise sequence and timing of developmental events, it is necessary to employ a system of staging. At the present time this is possible, but only within the embryonic period proper, that is, the first 8 postovulatory weeks (the 8 weeks following the ovulation and fertilization that resulted in pregnancy). In the Carnegie system of staging[28] human embryos have been arranged in 23 groups (based primarily on the work of Streeter), which are determined by a number of morphological criteria, such as the appearance of the eyes and the limb buds. The detailed application of the staging system to human embryology has been described in various organs, such as the brain.[29] It should be noted particularly that such expressions as "at the 18-mm stage" should be replaced by "at 18 mm" because embryonic length is a single and variable criterion that is not in itself adequate to establish a stage.

The earliest manifestation of the future skeleton is associated with the vertebrae. The somites begin to appear at 20 postovulatory days (stage 9). Within a week (stage 12; 26 days), they send cellular prolongations ventral and dorsal to the notochord (these form the centra) and also dorsally (the neural processes). Within another few days, the precursors of ribs (stage 13, 28 days) and articular processes (stage 14; 32 days) can be detected.[35] Slightly later, chondrification

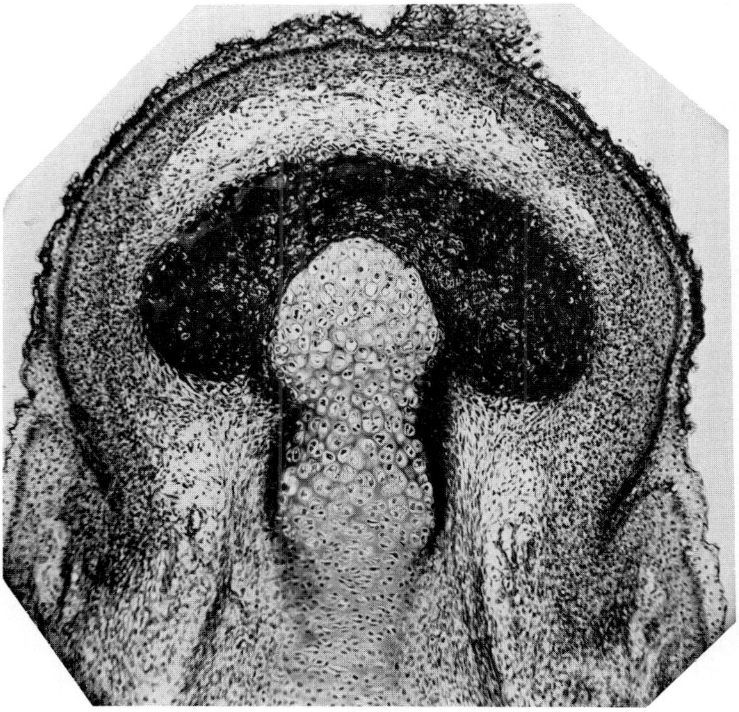

FIG. 6. Coronal section of distal phalanx of second finger of 11-week fetus (69 mm crown-rump), showing characteristic bony formation at tip. (From Gray, Gardner, and O'Rahilly, *Am. J. Anat.* *101:* 169–223, Fig. 44, 1957. Used with permission.)

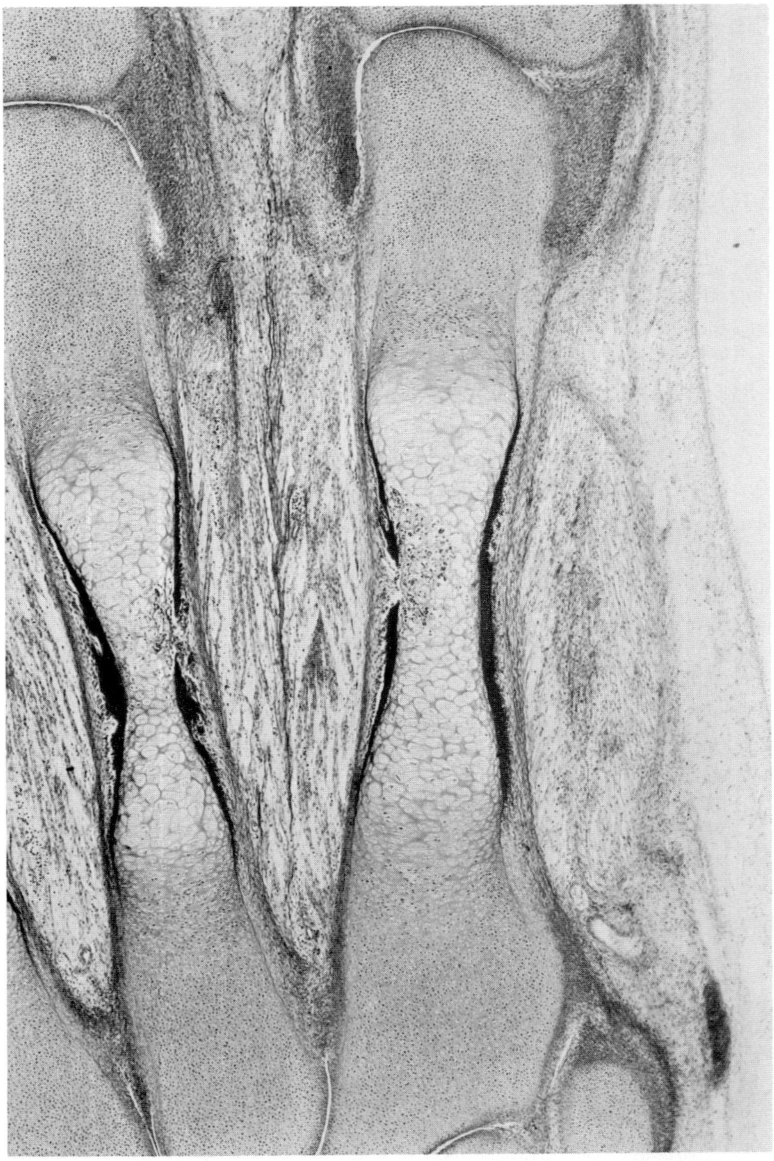

FIG. 7. Coronal section of two metacarpals of 11-week fetus (69 mm crown-rump), showing several developmental phases of cartilage and the penetration of the bone collars by periosteal buds.

begins in the centra (stage 17; 41 days) and, within a week, in the neural processes, laminae, ribs, and articular processes. Ossification may begin in the ribs as early as at the end of the embryonic period proper (29 mm).[22] In the thoracic centra and neural arches, ossification generally commences at about 40 to 60 mm, crown-rump (C.-R.), *i.e.*, early in the fetal period, and the times of initial appearance throughout the vertebral column have been ascertained.[33] Several tables showing the time of onset of ossification in the various regions of the body have been published.[7]

The initial formation of the skull has not yet been studied in adequate detail. It is probable, however, that the chondrocranium is present in the occipital region by 41 days (stage 17),[2, 3] and is perhaps detectable as a condensation even as early as 37 days (stage 16) in the parachordal area (personal observations). Ossification occurs first in the mandible (6 to 7 weeks; stages 18 to 20) and maxilla (7 weeks; stages 19 or 20).[30]

The upper and lower limb buds are first seen as elevations of the body wall at 26 (stage 12) and 28 (stage 13) days, respectively.

Although the skeletal blastemata appear in the depth of the limb, there is reason to believe that (in the mouse) the perichondrium, muscles, and tendons arise by centripetal migration from the superficial mesenchyme.[21] Moreover, it is generally held that a continuous morphogenetic interdependence exists between the apical ectoderm (found at the tip of the limb bud)[14, 31] and the underlying mesoderm. This relationship is believed to be important in the developmental laying down of limb components in proximodistal sequence. As in many other regions, physiological necrosis takes place during the development of the limbs.[20]

The mesenchymal condensations for the skeleton of the limbs appear at 33 days (stage 15) in the upper limb and at 37 days (stage 16) in the lower limb. Within a few days, the major long bones are indicated individually in mesen-

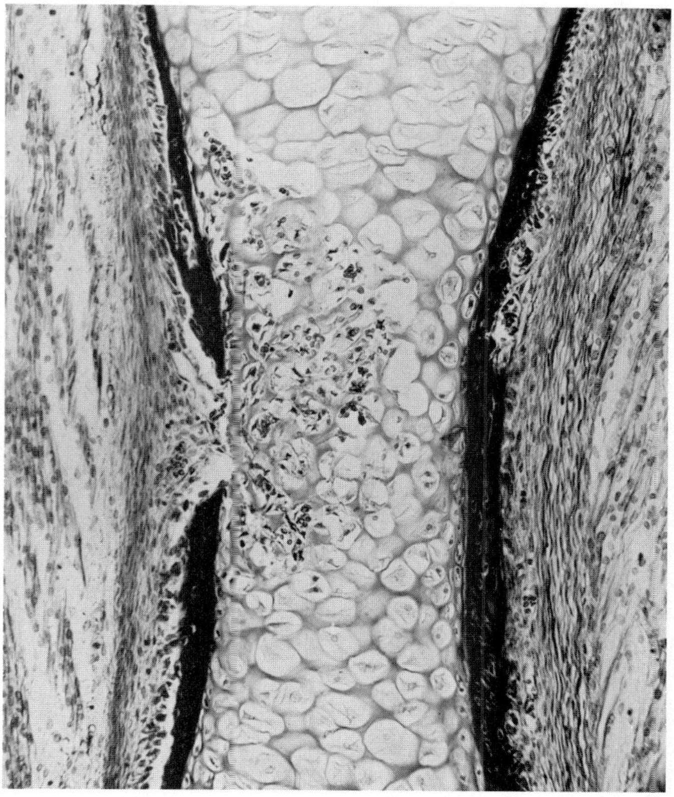

FIG. 8. Coronal section of second metacarpal of 11-week fetus (69 mm crown-rump), showing perforation of bone collar and invasion of hypertrophic cartilage by periosteal bud. (From Gray, Gardner, and O'Rahilly, *Am. J. Anat.* *101:* 169–223, Fig. 40, 1957. Used with permission.)

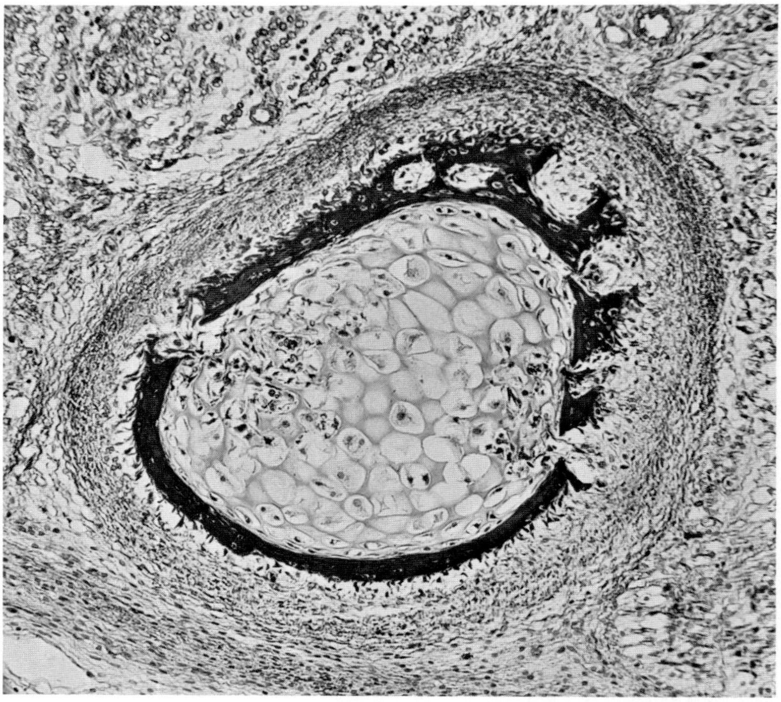

FIG. 9. Transverse section of second metacarpal of 11-week fetus (69 mm crown-rump), showing multiple points of invasion of bone collar and cartilage by periosteal buds. (From Gray, Gardner, and O'Rahilly, *Am. J. Anat. 101:* 169–223, Fig. 43, 1957. Used with permission.)

chyme and then in cartilage (Fig. 12). Ossification begins before the end of the embryonic period proper (Fig. 12). Numerous epiphysial centers appear postnatally.[26]

The development of joints, particularly the synovial joints of the limbs, has been studied extensively and is reviewed briefly elsewhere.[8, 24] By the end of the embryonic period proper, the developing joints resemble closely their adult counterparts, and, in the larger articulations (such as the knee), cavitation has already begun.

Chondrification of the skeletal elements of the hand and foot appears in a definite pattern, beginning at about 6 weeks (Fig. 13). The number of chondrific centers in the hand and foot increases between 6 and 8 weeks (Fig. 14). It has even been possible to arrange the sequence of events into a precise series of stages.[32] More recently, it has been found that, during at least the first 11 postovulatory weeks, male embryos are more advanced (for a given C.-R. length) than female embryos with respect to the development of the skeleton of the hand.[10]

CONGENITAL ANOMALIES

An interesting example of the developmental deviations that may be encountered in the skeleton is the group known as the paraxial hemimelias.[23] These are characterized by a partial or total defect of one side of the forearm and/or hand, or of one side of the leg and/or foot. The pathogenesis of the paraxial hemimelias has been reviewed recently.[6] They may occur as isolated anomalies, or may be found in association with other malformations, and may be a component of a syndrome.[15, 37] Tibial hemimelia, for example, may be found in the thalidomide embryopathy.

The lower limb buds, which, in their early development, are generally a couple of days less advanced than their upper counterparts, appear at 28 days (stage 13).[27] Femoral and crural components, and a foot-plate, are distinguishable by 37 days (stage 16). The tibia and fibula are discernible in mesenchyme at 41 days (stage 17) and begin to chondrify at 41 to 44 days (stages 17 and 18). The tibia commences to ossify at 54 to 57 days (stages 22 to 23). The circumstance that the fibula begins to ossify a little later, namely, 57 days or even in the fetal period, indicates that the two crural elements have slightly different timings and suggests that a teratogen acting at a critical moment might affect one rather than the other.

In the thalidomide syndrome, although slightly different critical or sensitive periods have been recorded in different countries,[13] the teratogen was most damaging between 5 and 7 postmenstrual weeks, or perhaps (the subtraction of 2 weeks involves assumptions that may or may not be justifiable) between 3 and 5 postovulatory weeks of age. It should be understood, however, that intake of thalidomide during the teratogenic period does not necessarily result in malfor-

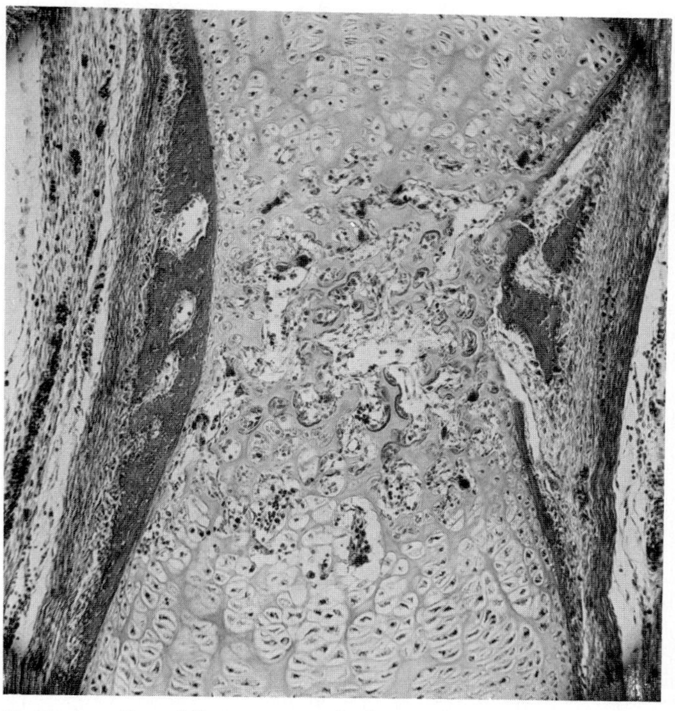

FIG. 10. Longitudinal section of first metacarpal of 12-week fetus (83 mm crown-rump), showing early endochondral ossification. New bone is evident as very thin dark lines on the surface of some of the calcified cartilage matrix.

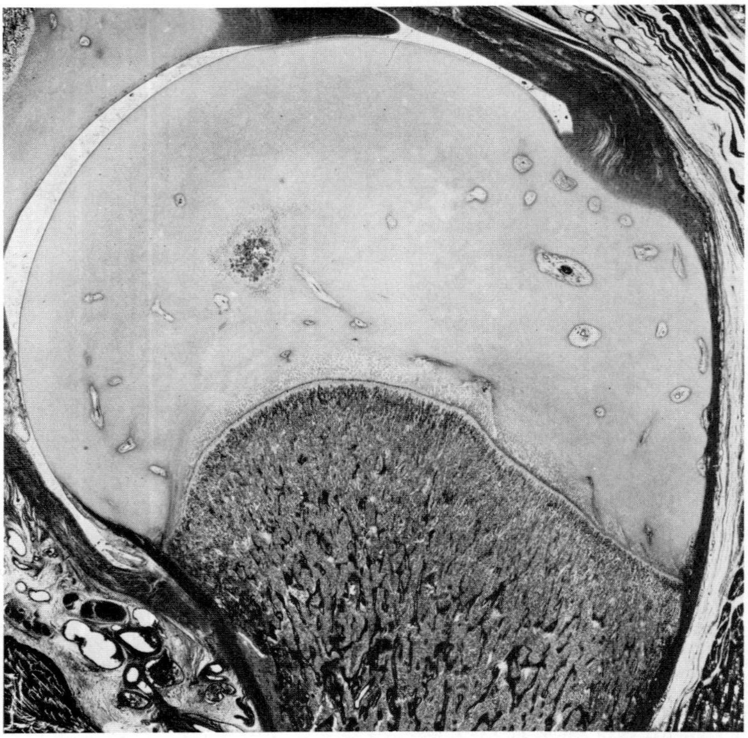

FIG. 11. Coronal section of head of humerus at term (348 mm crown-rump). Numerous cartilage canals are visible in the cartilaginous head, and an epiphysial ossific center is beginning to form. The endochondral growth zone is sharply defined. (From Gardner.[7] Used with permission.)

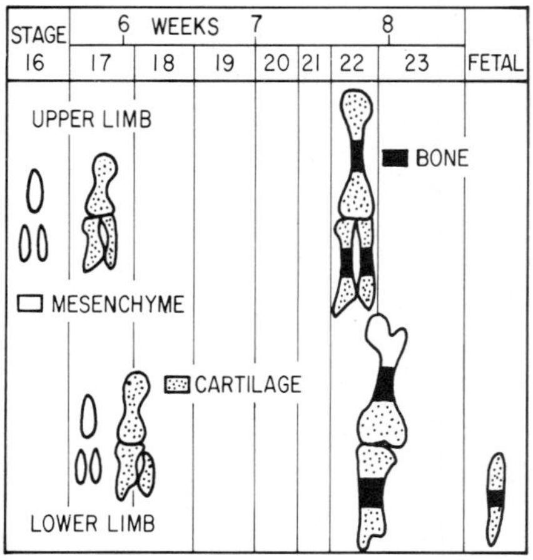

FIG. 12. Diagram showing the stages and times by which individual mesenchymal, cartilaginous, and osseous skeletal elements are first seen in the developing upper and lower limbs. Only the three major elements (the stylopodium and zygopodium) are indicated. Based on data of the authors.

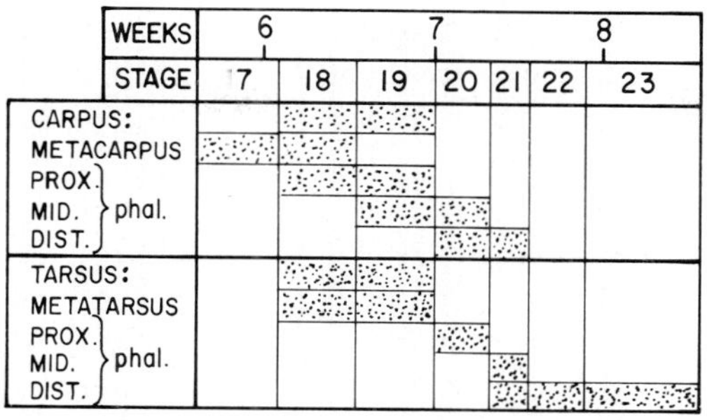

FIG. 13. Diagram showing the stages and times at which chondrification occurs initially in the skeletal elements of the developing hand and foot (autopodium). Based on data of the authors.

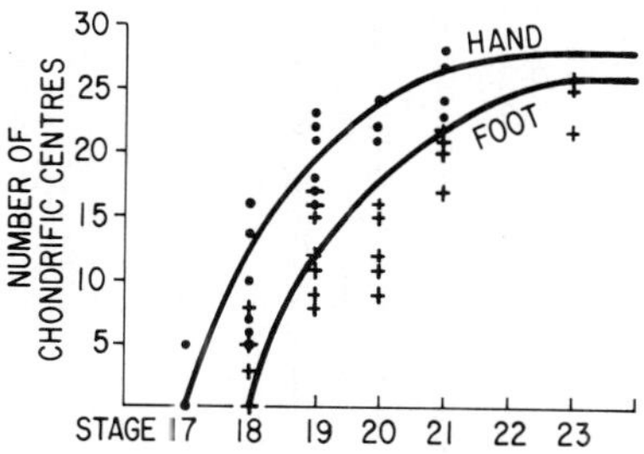

FIG. 14. Graph showing the increasing number of chondrific centers (*ordinate*) with stage (*abscissa*) in the developing hand and foot. Based on data of the authors.

mations: normal infants have been born (thalidomide-resistant pregnancy).[13] In a number of instances of thalidomide-associated tibial hemimelia, the intake ranged from 35 to about 60 postmenstrual days.[18] If this were to correspond to 21 to about 46 postovulatory days, then the embryos would have ranged from stage 9 or 10 (a week before limb buds become visible) to approximately stage 18 or 19 (when the tibia would be beginning to chondrify).

Similarly, in the upper limb, a radiogram of radial hemimelia has been published (Fig. 3b-2 of Ref. 18) from an instance in which thalidomide had been taken on the 46th postmenstrual day. If this were to correspond to approximately 32 postovulatory days, the embryo would have been at about stage 14, at which time the upper limb bud would have been a rounded, curved projection with an apical ectodermal ridge but lacking a visible hand plate. Radial hemimelia is generally, as in the above example, accompanied by a defective or absent thumb, an anomaly which, when isolated, appears to be produced at an earlier time (*e.g.*, thalidomide intake at 38th postmenstrual day)[17] than when combined with radial hemimelia (46th postmenstrual day).

A particularly interesting but rare occurrence is the association of polydactyly with paraxial hemimelia,[6] a paradoxical relationship which may sometimes be of medico-legal importance.[25] In the thalidomide syndrome, duplication of the big toe is associated with intake (37th to 55th postmenstrual days)[18] at approximately the same time as for tibial hemimelia. The metacarpals, metatarsals, and phalanges appear as cartilage between 6 and 7½ weeks (with the exception of some of the distal phalanges of the toes), and hence it may be assumed that polydactyly must be manifested before the end of the embryonic period proper.

Tibial hemimelia appears at a very early time in embryonic life, as is indicated by important observations on a strain of affected mice.[12] In the human, the paraxial hemimelias undoubtedly become visible before the end of the embryonic period proper. A well developed example of unilateral intercalary radial hemimelia has been found in a 50 mm C.-R. fetus by Mall and Meyer,[19] and verified by O'Rahilly, and an instance of unilateral radial hemimelia (with no thumb), unilateral duplication of big toe, and other anomalies has been reported in a 63 mm C.-R. fetus.[38]

The number and arrangement of skeletal elements are determined genetically, and the cells that are going to form these elements may be affected (genetically and/or environmentally) even before limb buds are visible. From studies of the thalidomide syndrome, it is probable that the critical periods extend from about 1½ to approximately 7 postovulatory weeks of age. During this time, the various skeletal elements of the limbs are laid down first in mesenchyme and then in cartilage, and ossification is already commencing in some of them.

REFERENCES

1. Bardeen, C. R.: The development of the thoracic vertebrae in man. *Am. J. Anat. 4:* 163–174, 1905.
2. Blechschmidt, E.: *Der menschliche Embryo, Dokumentationen zur kinetischen Anatomie* Stuttgart, Schattauer, 1963.
3. Blechschmidt, E.: *Die pränatalen Organsysteme des Menschen, Untersucht unter funktionellen Gesichtspunkten.* Stuttgart. Hippokrates Verlag, 1973.
4. Enlow, D. H.: *Principles of Bone Remodeling; An Account of Post-natal Growth and Remodeling Processes in Long Bones and the Mandible.* Springfield, Illinois, Thomas, 1963.
5. Enlow, D. H.: *The Human Face, An Account of the Postnatal Growth and Development of the Craniofacial Skeleton.* New York, Hoeber, Medical Division, Harper and Row, 1968.
6. Frantz, C. H., and O'Rahilly, R.: Ulnar hemimelia. *Artif. Limbs 15:* 25–35, 1971.
7. Gardner, E.: Osteogenesis in the human embryo and fetus. In *The Biochemistry and Physiology of Bone,* Vol III, *Development and Growth,* edited by Bourne, G. H. , 2nd ed., pp. 77–118. New York, Academic Press, 1971.
8. Gardner, E.: The structure and function of joints. In *Arthritis and Allied Conditions,* edited by Hollander, J. L., and McCarty, D. J., Jr., 8th ed., pp. 32–50. Philadelphia, Lea and Febiger, 1972.
9. Gardner, E., and Gray, D. J., The prenatal development of the human femur. *Am. J. Anat. 129:* 121–140, 1970.
10. Garn, S. M., Burdi, A. R., and Babler, W. J.: Male advancement in prenatal hand development. *Am. J. Phys. Anthropol. 41:* 353–359, 1974.
11. Gray, D. J., and Gardner, E.: The prenatal development of the human humerus. *Am. J. Anat. 124:* 431–445, 1969.
12. Hovelacque, A., and Noel, R.: Processus embryologique de l'absence congénitale du tibia. *C. R. Soc. Biol. (Paris) 88:* 577–578, 1923.
13. Kajii, T., Kida, M., and Takahashi, K.: The effect of Thalidomide intake during 113 human pregnancies. *Teratology 8:* 163–166, 1973.
14. Kelley, R. O.: Fine structure of the aspical rim-mesenchyme complex during limb morphogenesis in man. *J. Embryol. Exp. Morphol. 29:* 117–131, 1973.
15. Kühne, D., Lenz, W., Petersen, D., and Schönenberg, H.: Defekt von Femur un Fibula mit Amelie, Peromelie oder ulnaren Strahldefekten der Arme. Ein Syndrom. *Humangenetik 3:* 244–263, 1967.
16. Lacroix, P.: *The Organization of Bones.* Philadelphia, Blakiston, 1951.

17. Lenz, W.: Zur Genese der angeborenen Handfehlbildungen. *Chir. plast. reconstr. 5:* 3–15, 1968.
18. Lenz, W.: Der Zeitplan der menschlichen Organogenese als Maßstab für die Beurteilung teratogener Wirkungen. *Fortschr. Med. 87:* 520–526, 1969.
19. Mall, F. P., and Meyer, A. W.: Studies on abortuses: a survey of pathologic ova in the Carnegie Embryological Collection. *Contr. Embryol. Carneg. Instn. 12:* 1–364, 1921.
20. Menkes, B., Deleanu, M., and Ilieş, A.: Comparative study of some areas of physiological necrosis at the embryo of man, some laboratory mammalians and fowl. *Rev. roum. Embryol. Cytol., Sér Embryol. 2:* 161–171, 1965.
21. Milaire, J.: Aspects of limb morphogenesis in mammals. In *Organogenesis*, ed. by De Haan, R. L., and Ursprung, H., pp. 238–300, New York, Holt, Rinehart and Winston, 1965.
22. Noback, C. R., and Robertson, G. G.: Sequences of appearance of ossification centers in the human skeleton during the first five prenatal months. *Am. J. Anat. 89:* 1–28, 1951.
23. O'Rahilly, R.: Morphological patterns in limb deficiencies and duplications. *Am. J. Anat. 89:* 135–193, 1951.
24. O'Rahilly, R.: The development of joints. *Ir. J. Med. Sci.*., 6th series, No. 382, pp. 456–461, 1957.
25. O'Rahilly, R.: The development and the developmental disturbances of the limbs. *Ir. J. Med. Sci.* 6th series, No. 397, pp. 30–33, 1959.
26. O'Rahilly, R.: The ossification of the skeleton of the limbs. *Ir. J. Med. Sci.* 6th series, No. 434, pp. 78–81, 1962.
27. O'Rahilly, R.: The human foot. Part I: prenatal development. In *Foot Disorders. Medical and Surgical Management*, edited by Giannestras, N. J., 2nd ed., pp. 16–23. Philadelphia, Lea and Febiger, 1973.
28. O'Rahilly, R.: *Developmental Stages in Human Embryos, Including a Survey of the Carnegie Collection. Part A: Embryos of the First Three Weeks (Stages 1 to 9)*. Washington, D.C., Carnegie Institution of Washington (Publication 631), 1973.
29. O'Rahilly, R., and Gardner, E.: The timing and sequence of events in the development of the human nervous system during the embryonic period proper. *Z. Anat. Entwicklungsgesch. 134:* 1–12, 1971.
30. O'Rahilly, R., and Gardner, E.: The initial appearance of ossification in staged human embryos. *Am J. Anat. 134:* 291–307, 1972.
31. O'Rahilly, R., Gardner, E., and Gray, D. J.: The ectodermal thickening and ridge in the limbs of staged human embryos. *J. Embryol. Exp. Morphol. 4:* 254–264, 1956.
32. O'Rahilly, R., Gray, D. J., and Gardner, E.: Chondrification in the hands and feet of staged human embryos. *Contr. Embryol. Carneg. Instn. 36:* 183–192, 1957.
33. O'Rahilly, R., and Meyer, D. B.: Roentgenographic investigation of the human skeleton during early fetal life. *Am. J. Roentgenol. 76:* 455–468, 1956.
34. Scott, J. H.: *Dento-facial Development and Growth.* Oxford, Pergamon Press, 1967.
35. Sensenig, E. C.: The early development of the human vertebral column. *Contr. Embryol. Carneg. Instn. 33:* 21–41, 1949.
36. Streeter, G. L.: Developmental horizons in human embryos (fourth issue). A review of the histogenesis of cartilage and bone. *Contr. Embryol. Carneg. Instn. 33:* 149–167, 1949.
37. Temtamy, S. A.: Genetic Factors in Hand Malformations. Thesis, Johns Hopkins University, 1966.
38. Yasuda, M., and Poland, B. J.: A 63-mm human fetus with radial aplasia, tibial polydactyly, rib and vertebral fusions, and right aortic arch. *Teratology 10:* 119–124, 1974.

Chapter 2

Normal Structure of Bone: Light and Electron Microscopy

GERALD S. LAROS

The skeleton functions to provide structural support and to serve as a mineral reservoir. Both functions are reflected in the structure of bone. Bone cells produce an intercellular matrix composed of mineral-impregnated collagen and protein polysaccharides. Collagen forms at least 96% of unmineralized bone matrix. Soluble tropocollagen molecules, 2800 Å long, are secreted by matrix-producing cells, and these molecules then aggregate into a regular, close-fitting pattern to form fibrils. Molecules line up in parallel fashion, each molecule overlapping the adjacent one by about one-quarter of its length, which is about 700 Å. Actually the overlap is less, coming to about 640 to 670 Å. This leaves a gap at the end of one molecule before the next molecule begins, which is designated the "hole zone" (Fig. 1). Side chains on adjacent tropocollagen molecules align to form visible bands on the aggregated collagen fibril when viewed through the electron microscope. A pattern of five major bands repeats at 640 to 670 Å intervals to produce alternating light and dark segments on each fibril. These bands are designated by the letters A through E. Bands E through B form the dark portion of each segment, and bands C and D are included in the light portion (Fig. 2).

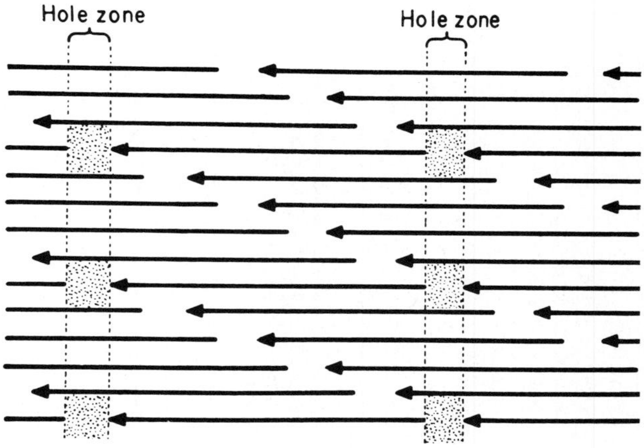

FIG. 1. *Arrows* represent tropocollagen molecules aligned into fibrils, with a gap between molecules in their long axes which is the "hole zone." (From Glimcher, M. J.[4] Used with permission.)

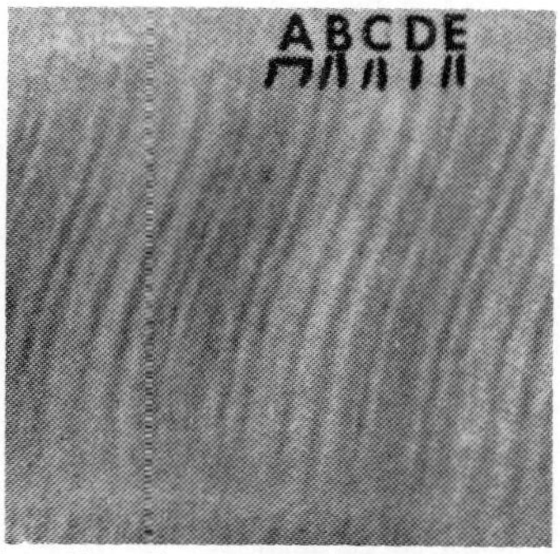

FIG. 2. Collagen fibril cross-banding showing bands A through E, which measures 640 to 670 Å. (From Cooper, R. R., and Misol, S.[2] Used with permission.)

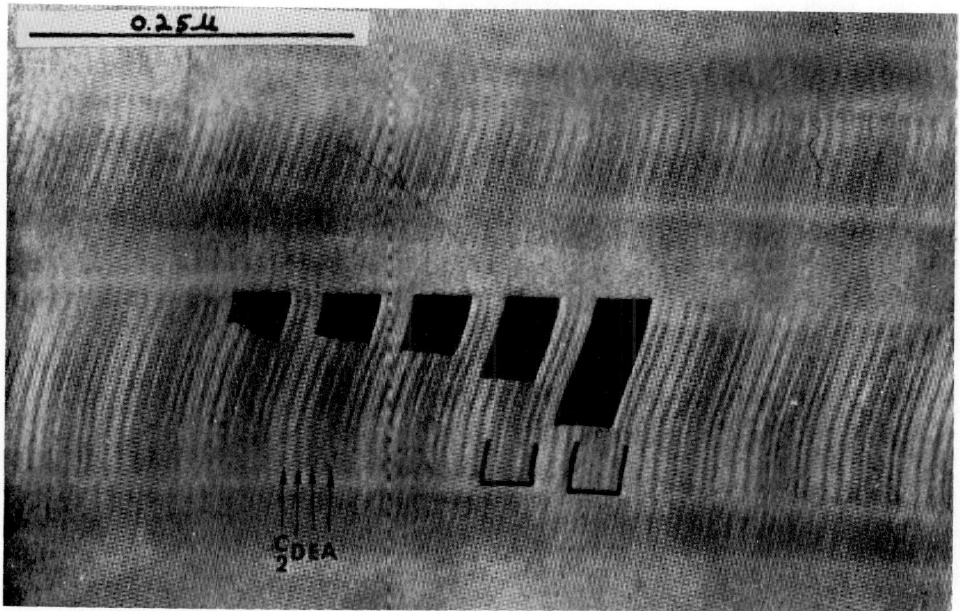

FIG. 3. Site of mineral deposition in collagen fibrils. *Brackets* indicate dark segments of unmineralized fibrils, which include bands *E*, *A*, and *B*. *Light segments* in between include bands *C* and *D*. *Shaded areas* show dark segments of mineralized fibrils, where mineral is deposited. The mineralized *dark segment* includes bands C_2, *D*, *E*, and *A*, which is also the hole zone. (From Cooper, R. R., and Misol, S.[2] Used with permission.)

From 35 to 65% of the dry weight of bone is mineral composed primarily of calcium phosphate. About 45% of the total mineral content is amorphous calcium phosphate, while most of the remainder is in the form of hydroxyapatite crystals. Mineral is deposited both between and within the collagen fibrils to produce a material more rigid than collagen alone and stronger and more flexible than the hydroxyapatite crystal. Within fibrils, mineral is deposited first in the "hole zone" located between bands C and A. Although mineralized collagen has a 640 to 670 Å light-dark periodicity, the light-dark segments are not the same ones seen in nonmineralized fibrils. In mineralized fibrils, the dark segment bridges bands C, D, E, and A, while for unmineralized fibrils, bands E, A, and B compose the dark segment (Fig. 3).

Protein polysaccharides make up a very small proportion of matrix by weight. Ruthenium red staining reveals these macromolecules to be attached at regular intervals to collagen fibrils between bands D and E in relation to hole zones. These macromolecules appear to participate in the organization of fibrils along lines of stress and may also have a role in the control of mineralization (Fig. 4).

Three basic types of cells populate bone tissue: the osteoblast, the osteocyte, and the osteoclast.

Osteoblasts are the primary producers of bone matrix. They range from 20 to 30 μ in maximum diameter and are best seen along the surface of bone in developing areas where new bone matrix is being formed. They are polarized to the extent that the nucleus is at the end of the cell opposite the bone surface and the basophilic cytoplasm is near the bone surface (Fig. 5).

The reason for the basophilic staining of the cytoplasm becomes apparent when the cell is viewed with the electron microscope. The cytoplasm is packed with well developed endoplasmic reticulum having numerous basophlic ribosomes attached to its membrane as well as numerous free ribosomes. There is a wide Golgi zone made up primarily of vesicles. The mitochondria are small and round and in close proximity to the membrane surfaces of the endoplasmic reticulum. The osteoblasts lay down collagen without mineral, which is designated as osteoid. Long cytoplasmic processes from the cell penetrate this osteoid on the side of the cell adjacent to the matrix. The osteoblast nucleus is not distinctive.

Osteocytes are those cells embedded in bone matrix and concerned more with bone maintenance than with new bone production. The mature osteocyte has an endoplasmic reticulum which is less abundant than in the osteoblast, has less tendency for lamellar arrangement of the membrane, and has a wide cisterna and a diminished number of ribosomes on its surface. The Golgi apparatus of the osteocyte tends to be more lamellar with stacks of membranes and some minute

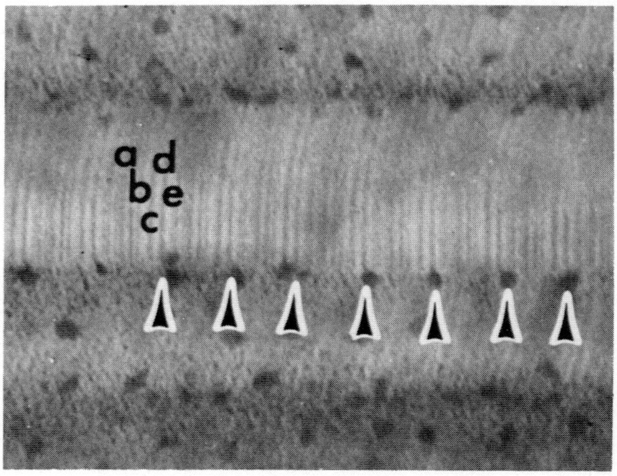

FIG. 4. In fibrocartilage which subsequently converts to bone as well as in bone itself, polysaccharides (stained by ruthenium red and designated by *arrows*) are seen attached to collagen fibrils between *d* and *e* bands. This is within the "hole zone" region. Bands identified by letters. (From Laros, G. S., and Cooper, R. R.[5] Used with permission.)

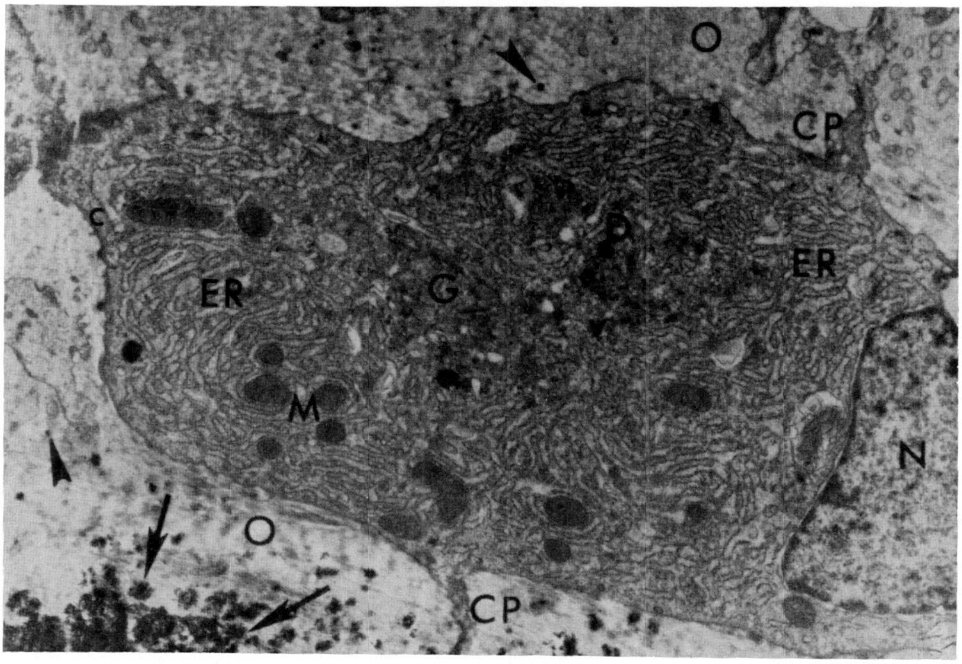

FIG. 5. Osteoblast. Cytoplasm contains abundant endoplasmic reticulum (*ER*), dense bodies (*D*), Golgi apparatus (*G*) with vesicles (*v*) and rounded mitochondria (*M*). A cortical zone (*c*) separates organelles and plasma membrane. The nucleus (*N*) is not distinctive. Cytoplasmic processes (*CP*) extend into osteoid (*O*) where initial foci of mineralization (*short arrows*) and subsequent expansion of mineral deposits (*long arrows*) are seen. (From Fetter, A. W., and Capen, C. C.[3] Used with permission.)

vesicles. The mitochondria are often rodlike rather than round and sometimes they contain electron-dense granules in the cristae. Osteocytes have a sufficient concentration of ribosomes to make their cytoplasm basophilic, though less so than osteoblasts. The cisternae of the endoplasmic reticulum indicate active and continuous synthesization of protein but at a slower rate than for the osteoblast. The mature osteocyte has a greater nucleus to cytoplasm ratio than the osteoblast.

In addition to retaining a capacity to produce matrix, the osteocyte also has a capacity for osteolysis. When the osteocyte is in an osteolytic phase of activity, its organelles bear a similarity to those of an osteoclast. Following a period of osteolysis, perilacunar matrix formation or osteoplasis can occur which leaves a well defined perilacunar region with calcified matrix visibly differing in its orientation from the adjoining matrix (Fig. 6). In this osteoplastic phase, osteocyte organelles more closely resemble those of an osteoblast.

Osteocytes have numerous processes which extend out from the lacunae into canaliculi and contact processes from other ostoecytes. The canalicular and lacunar surfaces add tremendously to the surface area of mineral available for exchange with tissue fluids and adjacent cells.

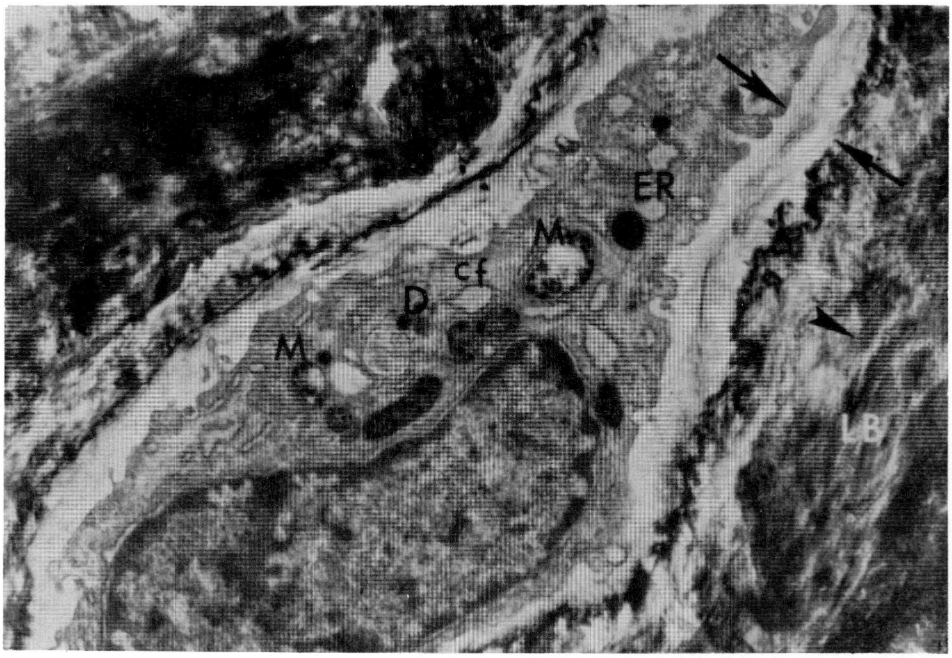

FIG. 6. Osteocyte. Cytoplasm contains endoplasmic reticulum (*ER*), but it has more dilated cisternae and fewer ribosomes than osteoblasts. Mitochondria (*M*) contain electrondense granules. Dense bodies (*D*) and cytoplasmic filaments (*cf*) may be seen. There is a perilacunar space (between *long arrows*) and partially mineralized collagen with crossbanding patterns (*short arrow*). (From Fetter, A. W., and Capen, C. C.[3] Used with permission.)

The osteoclast is a large multinucleated cell which participates actively in bone resorption. Osteoclasts have some rather specific structural features in relation to this function. The many nuclei have no distinctive individual features. They are generally located in the part of the cell away from the bone surface. Mitochondria are numerous, especially in the parts of the cell nearest the bone (Fig. 7). They are globular to ovoid in shape. Many contain electron-dense granules similar to those seen in osteocytes. The cytoplasm has numerous non-membrane-associated ribosomes, but little granular endoplasmic reticulum. The part of the cell adjacent to the bone surface in resorption lacunae shows multiple infoldings of plasma membrane, producing the brush border characteristic of an active osteoclast (Fig. 8). The infoldings of plasma membrane form numerous channels which often contain mineral crystals. Motion pictures of the brush border in the living active osteoclast show the cytoplasmic folds to be actively beating at the surface of the matrix as though physically shaking loose mineral and subsequently collagen. Ringing the brush border is a modified zone of cytoplasm with increased density and few organelles. This zone appears to function as a seal around a resorption compartment. Presumably this sealed compartment could contain an altered microenvironment which could chemically and/or enzymatically aid resorption.

Primary bone tissue, which is the first to appear embryologically, is nonlamellar or woven bone. It is torn down and replaced by bone arranged in alternating

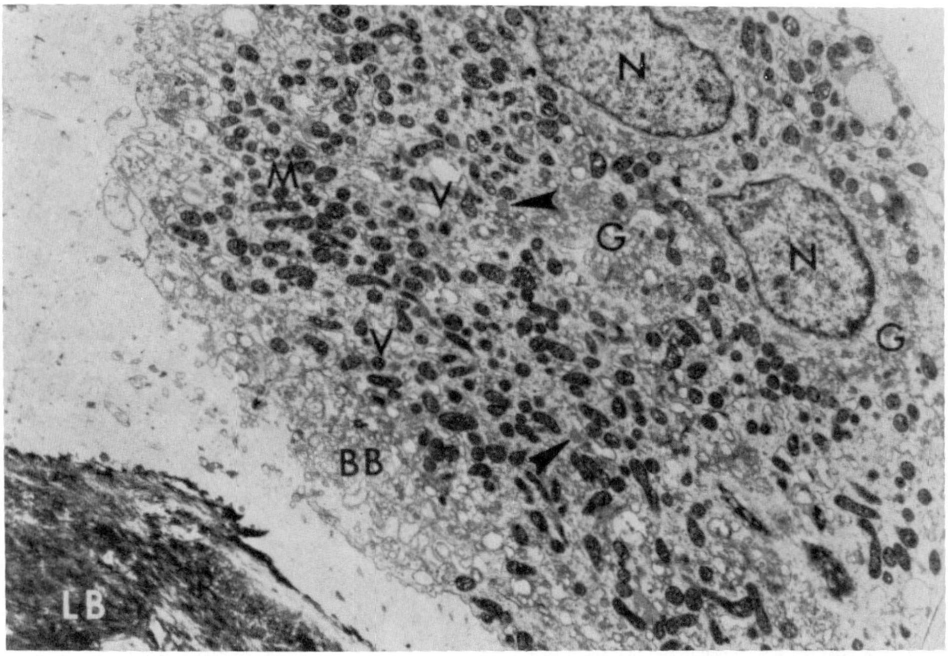

FIG. 7. Osteoclast. Several nondescript nuclei (*N*) are present with Golgi apparatus (*G*) nearby. Vacuoles (*V*) and dense bodies (*short arrows*) are numerous, as are mitochondria (*M*). The brush border (*BB*) is facing the bone surface. (From Fetter, A. W., and Capen, C. C.[3] Used with permission.)

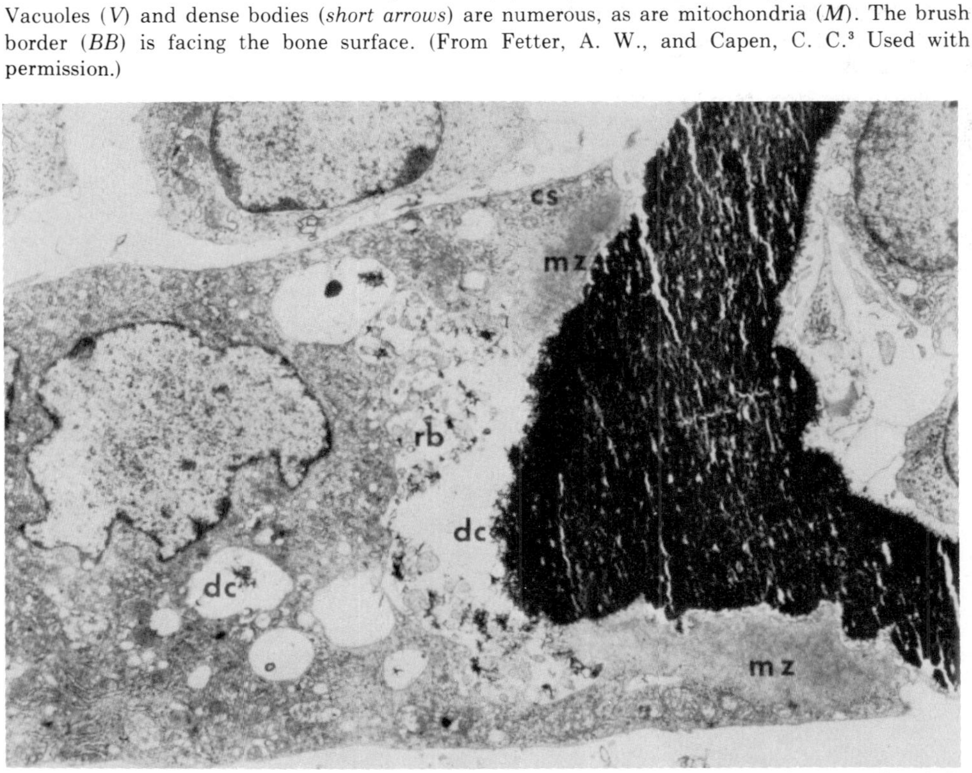

FIG. 8. Osteoclast with resorption compartment. A cytoplasmic strip (*cs*) lies outside of the modified cytoplasmic zones (*mz*). The ruffled border (*rb*) faces the bone surface, and dissociated crystals of mineral (*dc*) are seen in the resorption compartment and within vesicles. (From Malkani, K., Luxembourger, M-M., and Rebel, A.[6] Used with permission.)

layers of matrix and designated as secondary or lamellar bone. Woven bone has less co-orientation of the long axes of collagen than lamellar bone, less dense packing of the collagen fibrils, a larger bone-cell population relative to matrix, and a more variable mineral content. Within each layer of lamellar bone, collagen fibrils tend to be parallel with each other, but fibrils of adjacent lamellae are oriented in different directions.

The process of replacing woven primary bone with lamellar secondary bone is associated with the development of a unit of bone called the osteon or Haversian system. The osteon is an irregular branching and anastomosing tubular structure with a central neurovascular canal surrounded by concentric lamellae of bone matrix. Osteons are oriented within the cortex of bone so as to enhance the strength of the bone. Osteocytes lie in lacunae oriented parallel to the bone lamellae. The system of canaliculi links lacunae with each other and with the extracellular extravascular space of the central canal. In each canal there are one or two vessels with the ultrastructural characteristics of capillaries. If two

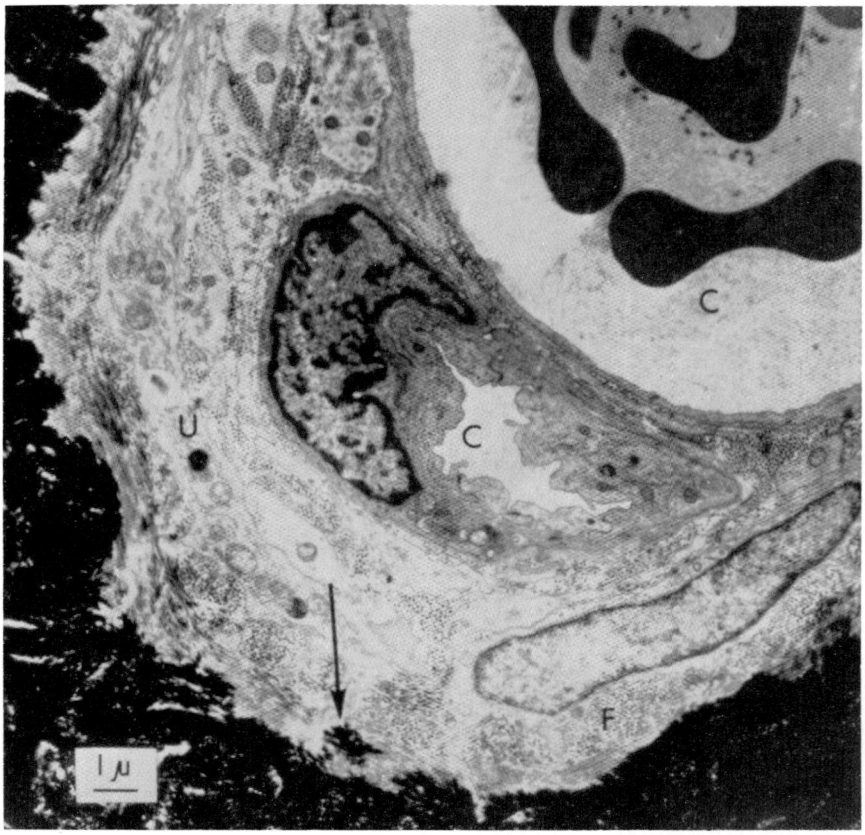

FIG. 9. Developing osteon. Two capillaries (*C*) are seen, one thick-walled and one thin-walled. Undifferentiated mesenchymal cells (*U*) lie between the capillaries and the bone surface. Collagen fibrils surround the undifferentiated mesenchymal cells. Irregular deposits of mineral (*arrow*) are seen in the collagen. (From Cooper, R. R., Milgram, J. W., and Robinson, R. A.[1] Used with permission.)

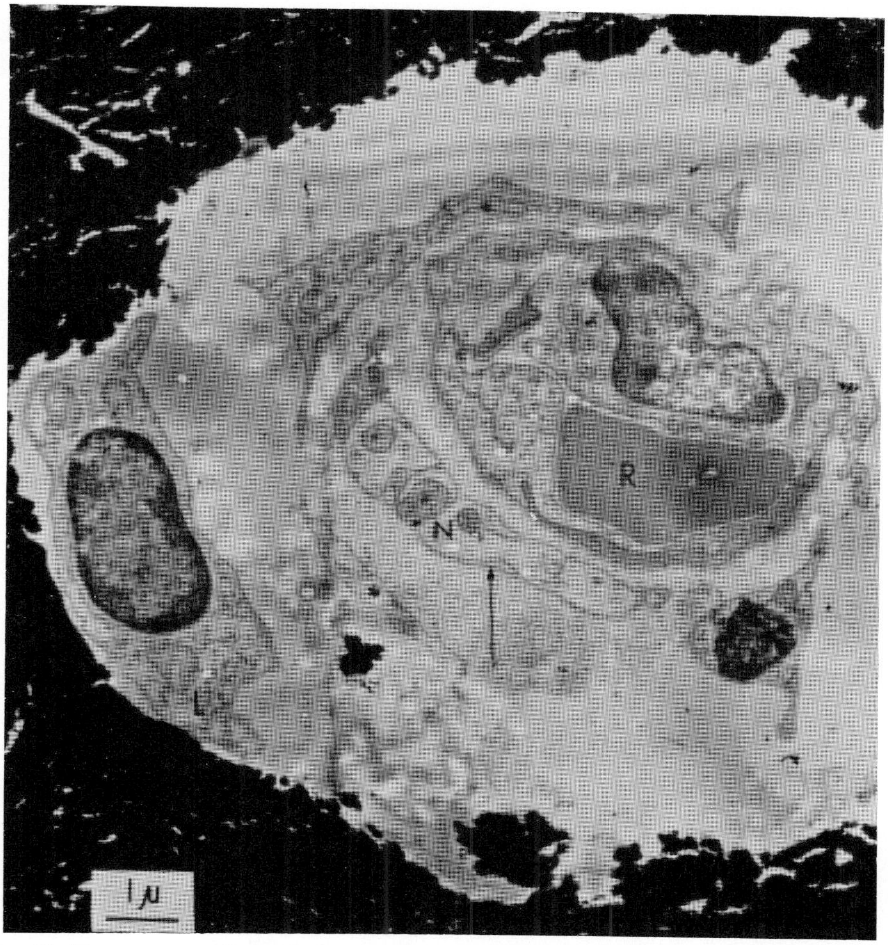

FIG. 10. Mature osteon. Red cell (*R*) seen in capillary. An unmyelinated nerve (*N*) is enclosed in the capillary's basement membrane (*arrow*). A lining cell (*L*) lies against a bone surface. (From Cooper, R. R., Milgram, J. W., and Robinson, R. A.[1] Used with permission.)

capillaries are present together, one will tend to be thick-walled and the other thin. No smooth muscle cells have been identified within the osteon, but other cells (pericytes) may be seen. Nerves may be found in many canals.

Osteons may be classified into three types, reflecting the active and changing nature of bone tissue. The types are: developing, mature, and resorbing.

In developing canals, lining cells are present adjacent to the matrix. These cells are often rather nondescript, having minimal endoplasmic reticulum and ribosomes and appearing to be relatively inactive. Other lining cells may lie adjacent to a well developed layer of osteoid and have the ultrastructural characteristics of osteoblasts (Fig. 9). In the mature osteon, the lining cells have fewer organelles and appear to be more like osteocytes or undifferentiated mesenchymal cells, but there is still the small layer of unmineralized osteoid several microns thick (Fig. 10). The resorption canal is a new vascular canal which cuts through existing lamellae with a cone of osteoclasts leading a capillary bud and with osteoblasts following to fill the widened canal with new lamellae.

REFERENCES

1. Cooper, R. R., Milgram, J. W., and Robinson, R. A.: Morphology of the osteon. An electron microscopic study. *J. Bone Joint Surg. 48A:* 1239–1271, 1966.
2. Cooper, R. R., and Misol, S.: Tendon and ligament insertion. A light and electron microscopic study. *J. Bone Joint Surg. 52A:* 1–20, 1970.
3. Fetter, A. W., and Capen, C. C. The fine structure of bone in the nasal tubinates of young pigs. *Anat. Rec. 171:* 329–345, 1971.
4. Glimcher, M. J. A basic architectural principle in the organization of mineralized tissues. *Clin. Orthop. 61:* 16–36, 1968.
5. Laros, G. S., and Cooper, R. R. Electron microscopic visualization of proteinpolysaccharides. *Clin. Orthop. 84:* 179–192, 1972.
6. Malkani, K., Luxembourger, M.-M, and Rebel, A. Cytoplasmic modifications at the contact zone of osteoclasts and calcified tissue in diaphyseal growing plate of foetal guinea-pig tibia. *Calcif. Tissue Res., 11:* 258–264, 1973.

Chapter 3

Osteoporosis and Osteomalacia

H. A. SISSONS

Although the general pathologist is not often concerned with problems relating to osteoporosis and osteomalacia, they represent two of the most frequent generalized abnormalities of the skeleton, and neither is rare. Their pathology is basically different: this, and a reminder of the special techniques needed for the recognition of osteomalacia, are the central themes of this brief review.

OSTEOPOROSIS

This term is properly applied to any condition in which there is a reduction in the amount of bone tissue. But the bone tissue that is present shows a normal degree of calcification, and this is the essential difference from osteomalacia. Osteoporosis can be either local or general, and can result from a variety of causes. On the histologic level, osteoporosis is always due to an interference with the normal balance between osteoblastic bone formation and osteoclastic bone resorption, the two processes concerned in the maintenance of skeletal mass and bone structure.[28]

Disuse osteoporosis

Immobilization of a limb results in local osteoporosis, which can be regarded as disuse atrophy of bone. Bony rarefaction can be recognized radiologically within a few weeks of the commencement of immobilization: at this stage the change consists of focal osteoporosis of cancellous bone, particularly in the subchondral situation (Fig. 1).[27] With more prolonged immobilization or disuse, as in a paralyzed limb in poliomyelitis, bone changes become more diffuse and involve cortical as well as cancellous bone.

Relatively little information is available on the histologic mechanism of disuse osteoporosis. In an experimental study using tetracycline labeling, Landry and Fleisch[17] found that increased bone resorption and decreased bone formation were both involved.

General immobilization results in more widespread osteoporosis, and balance studies have shown losses of up to 9% of total body calcium, sometimes accompained by hypercalcemia.[33] The condition of weightlessness associated with space flight is accompained by a similar loss of calcium.[20]

Idiopathic osteoporosis

Generalized loss of bone is most commonly seen after middle age, and occurs more frequently in women than in men. Loss of bone is not, by itself, a cause of symptoms: these follow some complication, usually fracture or collapse of the involved bone. Information on the amount of bone tissue present in different parts of the skeleton, either in health or disease, can be obtained by a variety of methods. Histologic study,[11, 22, 23, 30] weighing of individual bones,[32] measure-

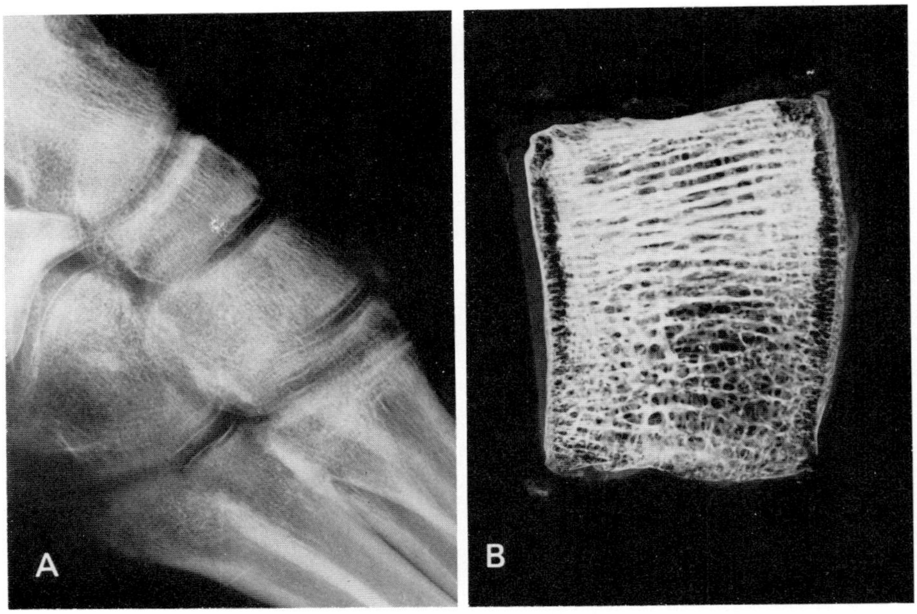

FIG. 1. Disuse osteoporosis, the result of three months' immobilization. *Left*, Radiograph of the bones of the foot. *Right*, radiograph of a slab of tissue from the same leg after amputation showing thinning of bone trabeculae deep to subchondral plate. (From Sissons, H. A.[27] Used with permission.)

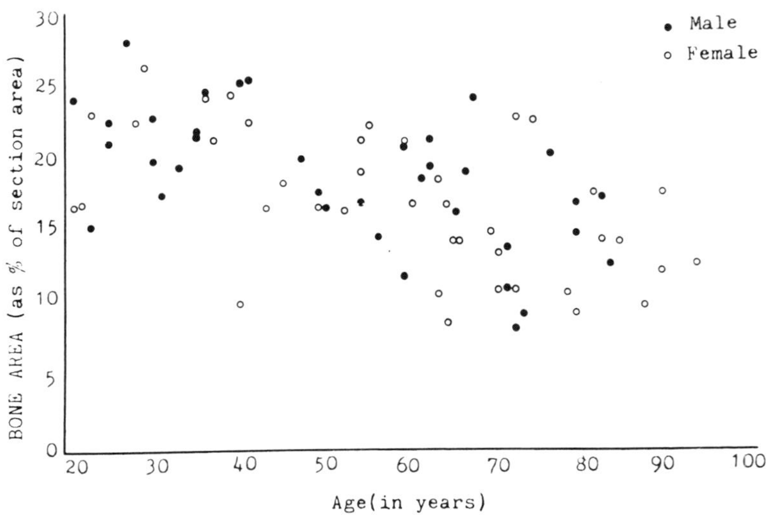

FIG. 2. Iliac crest (cancellous bone). Results for bone area plotted against age for 80 normal individuals. (From Sissons, H. A., Holley, K. J., and Heighway, J.[30] Used with permission.)

ment of cortical thickness,[4, 10, 13] determination of radiographic density and measurement of physical density[18] have all been employed.

The decrease in the amount of cancellous bone in the iliac crest with increasing age, from area measurements on histologic sections from normal subjects at autopsy is shown in Figure 2.[30] No obvious sex difference is apparent, and values fall from approximately 25% of the section area at the age of 20 years to approximately 15% at 80 years: this represents a loss of about 40% of the amount of bone originally present.

The comparable changes in cortical bone, as seen from measurements of cortical thickness and total diameter in radiographs of the 2nd metacarpal bone in a large series of normal subjects is shown in Figures 3 and 4. A marked difference between the rate of bone loss in males and females is apparent. Despite the reduction in cortical thickness, calculation of the "bending moment" of the

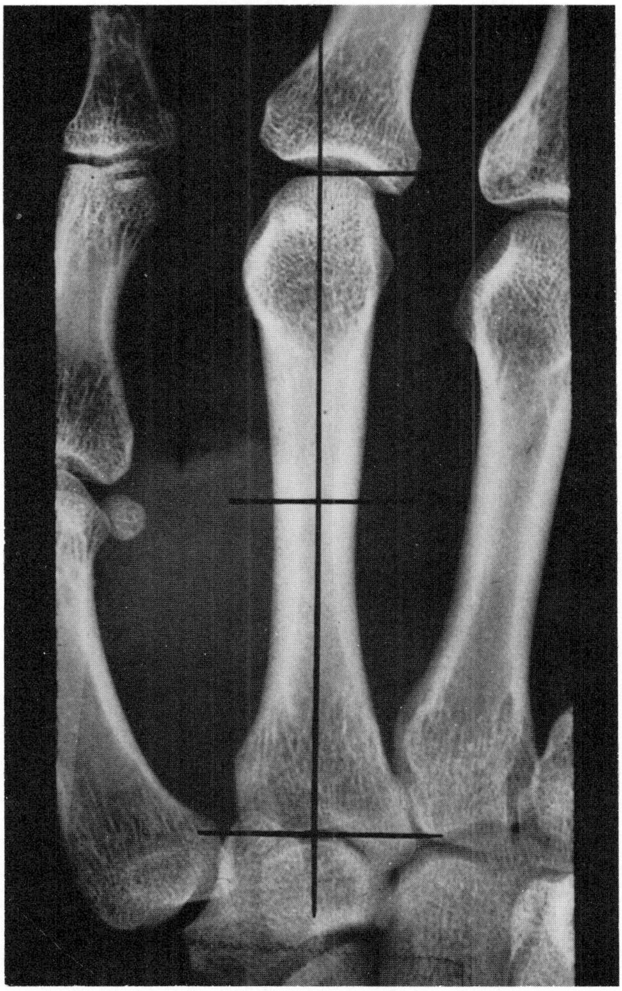

FIG. 3. Radiograph of 2nd metacarpal, showing measurement of total diameter and cortical thickness at midpoint of bone.

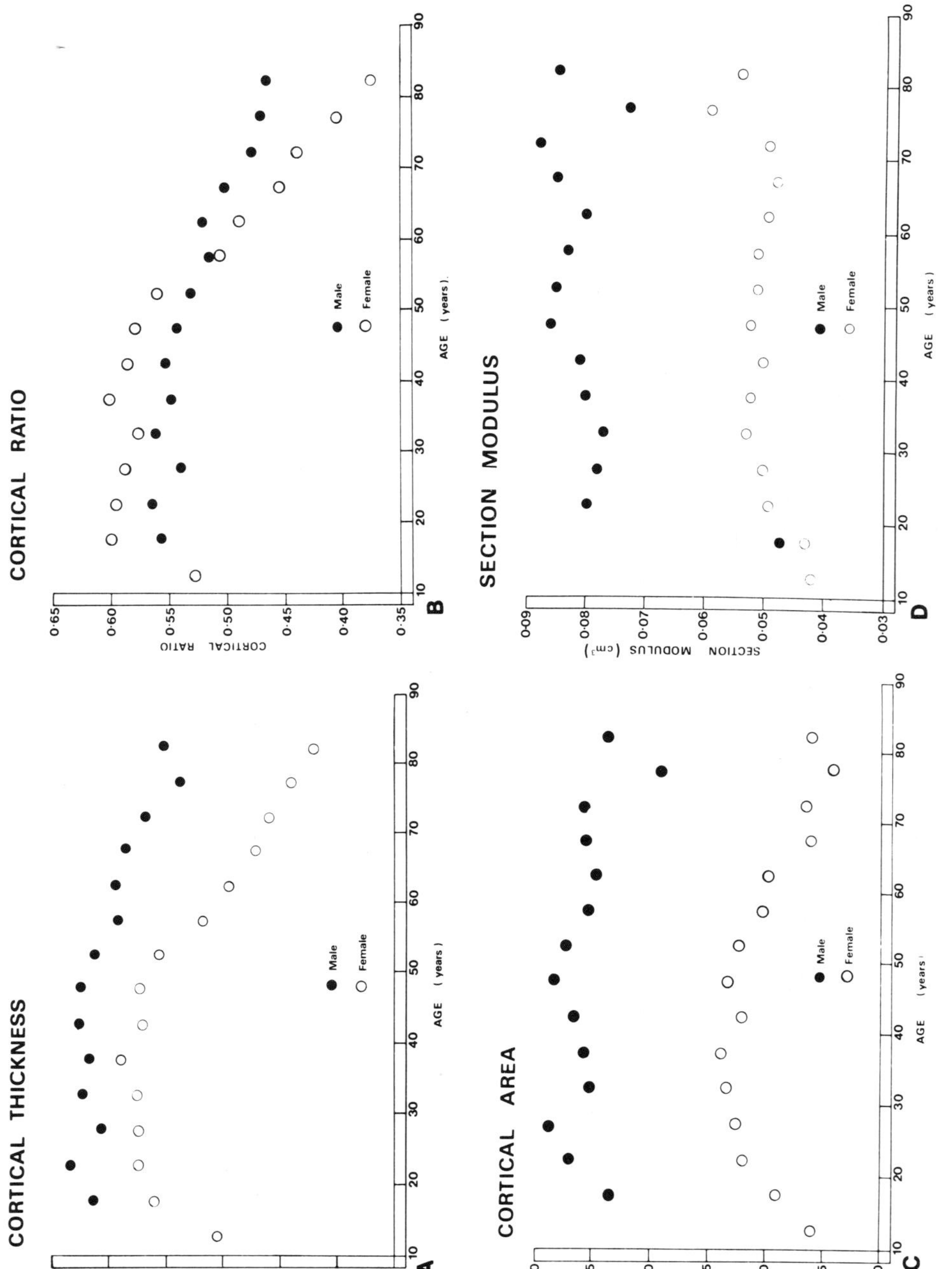

FIG. 4. 2nd metacarpal bone. Mean values for cortical thickness, cortical ratio, cortical area, and bending moment, plotted against age.

bone, the engineer's measurement of the resistance of a structure to bending, fails to show much change. This is perhaps why old people fail to suffer from metacarpal fractures, whereas loss of bone from the femoral neck or the vertebral bodies in old people is associated with significant loss of strength and liability to fracture.[8]

It is difficult, and perhaps impossible, to distinguish between this "normal" loss of bone with increasing age, and "idiopathic osteoporosis," which can be regarded as an exaggeration of it. The bone changes are not accompanied by any abnormalities of blood biochemistry: in particular the values for calcium, phosphorus, and alkaline phosphatase are normal. Loss of estrogens or other hormonal abnormalities, calcium deficiency, and many other factors have been discussed in connection with the etiology of idiopathic osteoporosis, but this is still obscure. The loss of bone mainly affects the spine and pelvis. The trabeculae of the cancellous bone of the vertebral bodies become thin, and collapse (fracture) of vertebrae occurs. The cortex of the shafts of the long bones shows less change, but here, too, there is a reduction in the amount of bone by enlargement of the vascular canals. Osteoporosis is an important predisposing cause of fractures in elderly people, particularly fractures of the femoral neck.[6]

Relatively little histologic information is available with regard to the dynamic cellular aspects of idopathic osteoporosis, but recent studies indicate that both reduced bone formation, and exaggerated resorption may be concerned.[22, 23, 26]

OSTEOMALACIA

This condition, in adults, in common with rickets in children, is characterized by failure of calcification of bone tissue. This is apparent, histologically, from the presence of abnormally large amounts of uncalcified bone matrix, or osteoid tissue. In the past, rickets and osteomalacia usually resulted from a deficient intake of vitamin D, but dietary rickets and osteomalacia are now rare in most civilized countries, and other causes, such as interference with intestinal absorption, renal tubular disorders, renal failure, and the rare genetic condition hypophosphatasia, are now more often concerned. Osteomalacia occurs in a significant proportion of patients after gastrectomy or other gastric surgery, presumably as a result of intestinal malabsorption of calcium:[16, 24] it is also relatively common in elderly people, particularly women, and in patients with femoral neck fractures.[1, 7]

Skeletal pain and muscle weakness are the characteristic clinical features of severe osteomalacia. Radiographs of the skeleton may show decreased density of bone: a characteristic feature are the Looser zones or "umbauzonen" which appear as translucent bands of decreased density (Fig. 7).[19] In contrast to osteoporosis, osteomalacia is usually associated with abnormal biochemical findings, in the form of low values for serum calcium and inorganic phosphorus and high values for serum alkaline phosphatase.

The histologic diagnosis of osteomalacia depends on the identification of osteoid tissue. This is best done using sections of undecalcified bone after embedding in paraffin or plastic material.[3, 21, 26, 29] A variety of staining methods can be used, including hematoxylin and eosin, solochrome cyanin, and the von

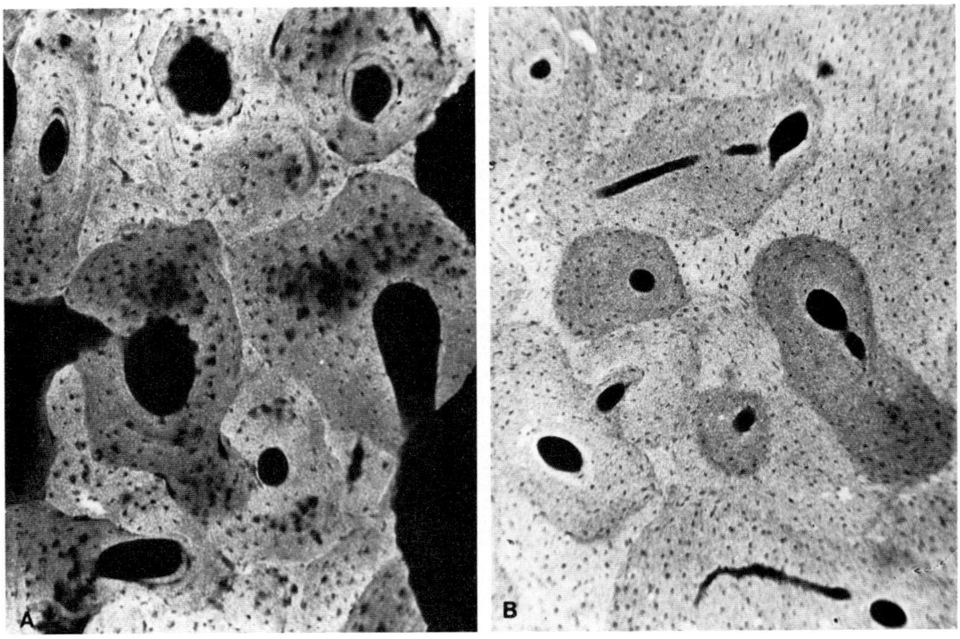

FIG. 5. Vitamin D-resistant rickets. *Left*, microradiograph showing poor mineralization with apparent enlargement of osteocyte lacunae. *Right*, microradiograph of normal bone for comparison (× 65).

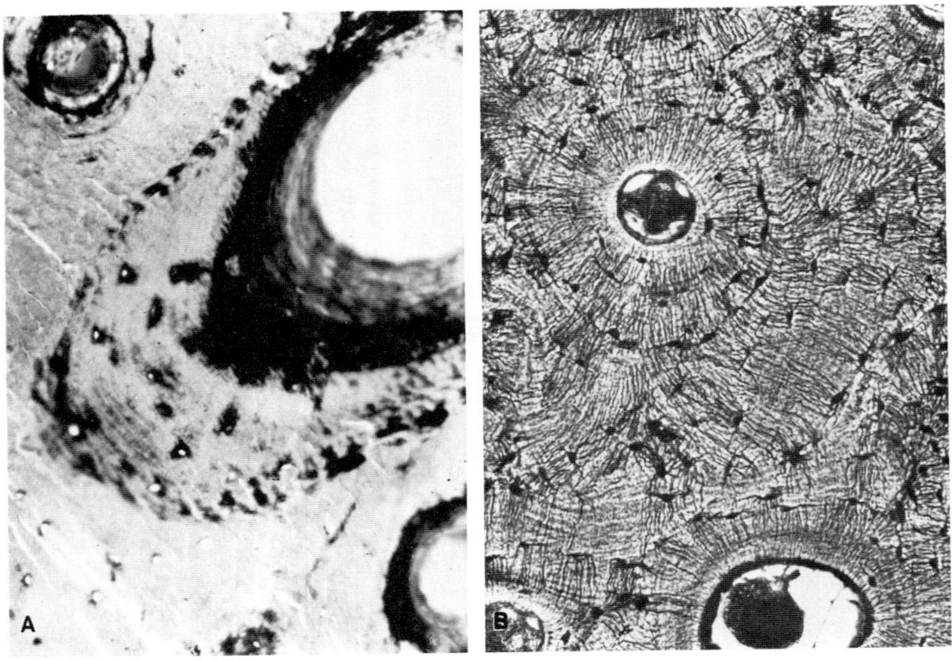

FIG. 6. Vitamin D-resistant rickets: same case as Fig. 5. *Left*, stained section of undecalcified bone showing osteoid tissue (staining darkly, in this preparation) surrounding osteocyte lacunae (Masson stain × 165). *Right*, decalcified section stained with Schmorl's picrothionin to show osteocyte lacunae and canaliculi (× 165).

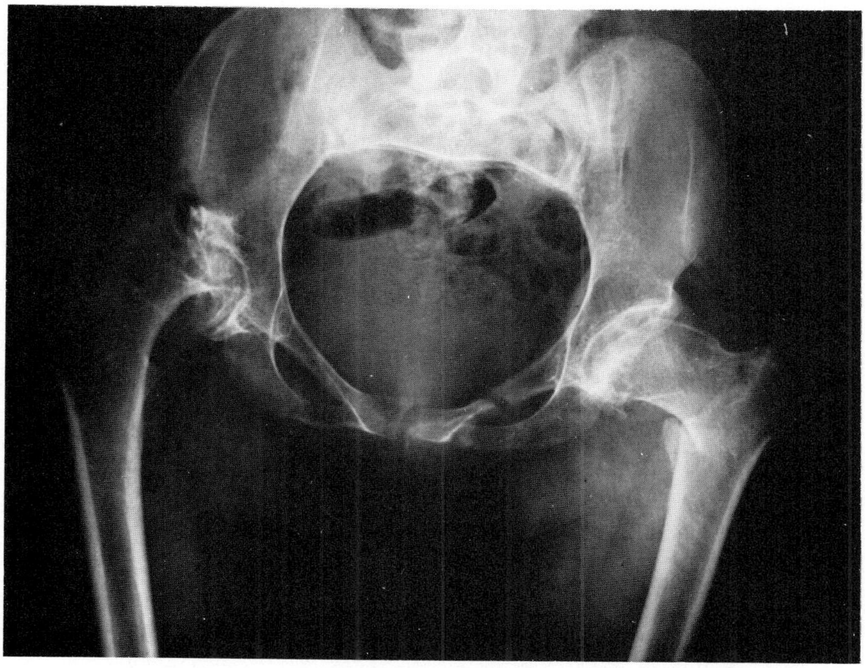

FIG. 7. Case 1. Radiograph of pelvis showing gross fracture of neck of femur. Note also the pseudofracture (Looser zone, "umbauzone") of one pubic ramus.

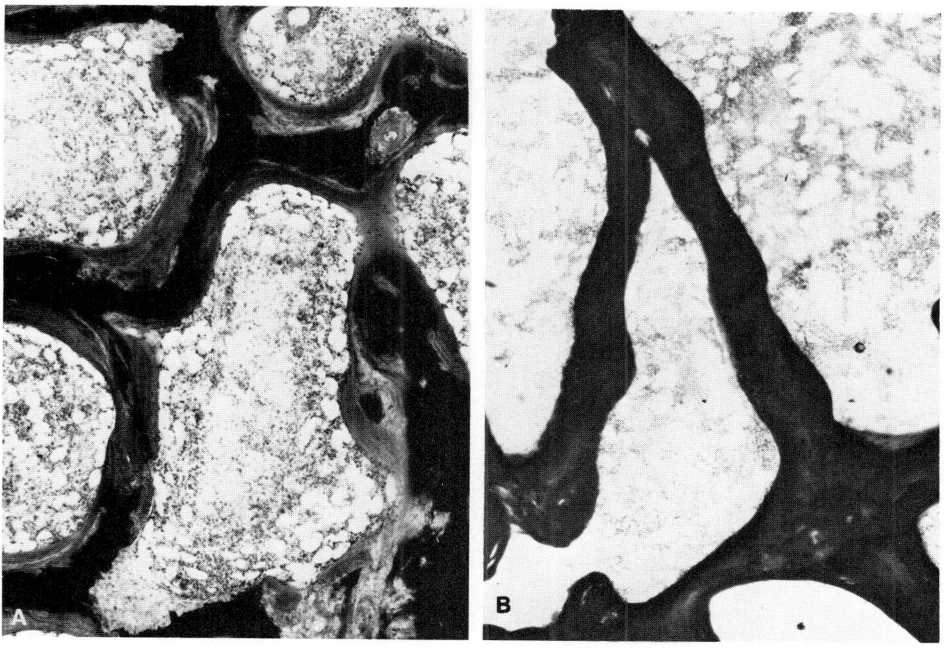

FIG. 8. Case 1. *Left*, undecalcified section of iliac crest biopsy showing a large amount of pale-staining osteoid tissue on the surface of bone trabeculae. *Right*, section fron normal iliac crest for comparison. Hematoxylin and eosin stain; × 45.

Kossa reaction. An iliac crest biopsy is a convenient diagnostic procedure. Quantitative information is accumulating on the amount of osteoid tissue in normal bone.[5, 15, 22, 23, 30] In most cases of osteomalacia (Fig. 8), however, a very large amount of osteoid tissue is present, while in normal bone there is very little. Care must be taken, of course, to distinguish between osteomalacia and other conditions—fracture callus, Paget's disease, etc.—where an increased amount of osteoid tissue may also be found. Attention has been directed to the partial or complete disappearance, in osteomalacia, of the "calcification front," which in normal bone marks the interface between osteoid tissue and calcified bone.[5]

The low serum calcium in osteomalacia is a stimulus to parathyroid overactivity, and histologic changes of secondary hyperparathyroidism are not infrequently seen (Fig. 11).

Another type of structural abnormality seen in osteomalacia, particularly in the vitamin D-resistant osteomalacia of certain renal tubular conditions such as Fanconi's disease, is the apparent enlargement of osteocyte lacunae in microradiographs (Fig. 5). This results from the presence of zones of osteoid tissue around individual osteocytes and not from any increase in size of lacunae themselves (Fig. 6).

Most types of osteomalacia respond dramatically to the administration of

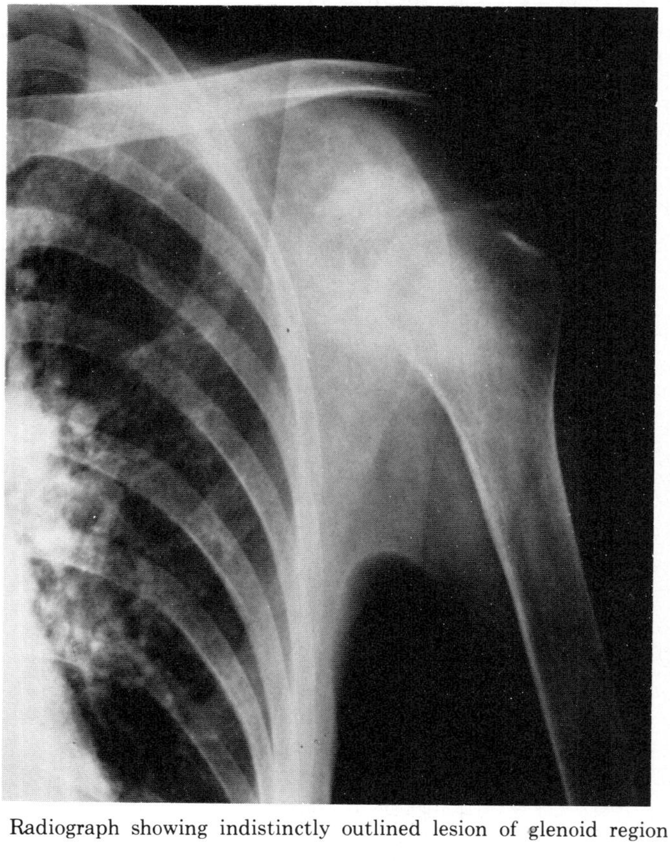

FIG. 9. Case 2. Radiograph showing indistinctly outlined lesion of glenoid region of scapula.

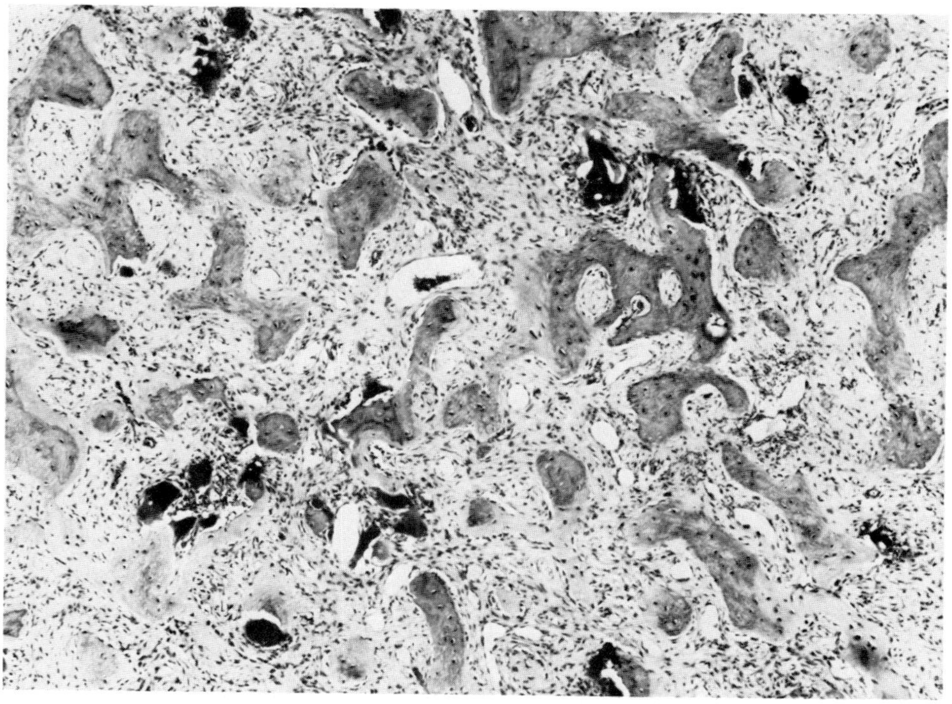

FIG. 10. Case 2. Biopsy from lesion of scapula. Hematoxylin and eosin stain; × 60.

vitamin D: exceptions are the vitamin D-resistant osteomalacia of certain renal tubular disorders, and the osteomalacia component of renal osteodystrophy. The biochemical and metabolic aspects of osteomalacia are reviewed by Fourman and Royer[14] and by Dent.[9]

ILLUSTRATIVE CASES

The following 3 cases illustrate some of the diagnostic problems which can be encountered with osteomalacia.

Case 1. A female 47 years of age was admitted to the hospital because of a fracture of the neck of the femur. X-ray examination showed thin bones with Looser zones of the pubic ramus and ribs in addition to the fracture of the neck of the femur (Fig. 7). There was a past history of long standing arthritis and epilepsy, and the patient lived a very restricted life without normal exposure to sunlight.

Biochemical investigations gave the following results: serum calcium, 2.0 mmol/liter (8.0 mg/100 ml); serum phosphorus, 0.7 mmol/liter (2.2 mg/100 ml); serum alkaline phosphatase, 213 IU/liter (30 King-Armstrong (KA) units/100 ml); and blood urea, 4.0 mmol/liter (24.0 mg/100 ml).

An iliac crest biopsy showed an abnormally large amount of osteoid tissue (Fig. 8).

The patient responded well to treatment with vitamin D.

A number of etiologic factors appear to be involved in this case. The absence of normal exposure to sunlight has already been mentioned. In addition, she had a

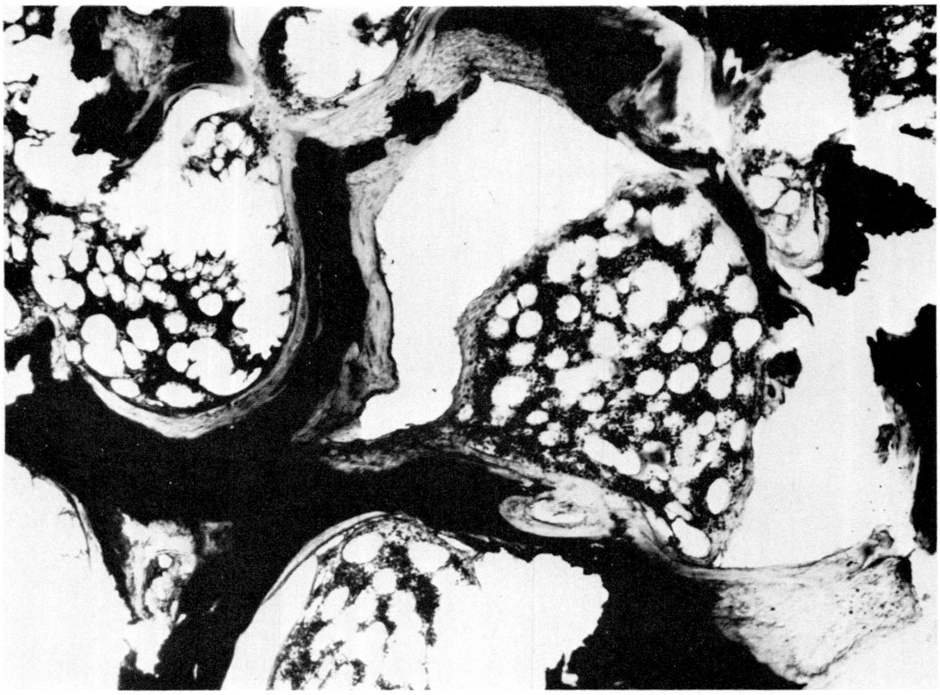

FIG. 11. Case 2. Biopsy from iliac crest (Hematoxylin and eosin stain of undecalcified section × 80).

poor dietary intake of vitamin D; a further factor was heavy dosage of phenobarbitone for her epilepsy, which has been reported to predispose to the development of osteomalacia.

Case 2. A female 56 years of age gave a history of pain in the left shoulder with progressive loss of movement. X-ray examination showed an ill-defined lesion of the glenoid part of the scapula with involvement of the coracoid and spinous processes (Fig. 9).

Biochemical investigation gave the following results: serum calcium, 2.4 mmol/liter (8.8 mg/100 mg); serum phosphorus, 0.8 mmol/liter (2.5 mg/100 mg); and serum alkaline phosphatase, 550 IU/liter (77 KA units/100 ml).

The lesion was regarded, clinically, as a bone tumor. A biopsy suggested a diagnosis of hyperparathyroidism, fibrous dysplasia, or Paget's disease (Fig. 10): the first of these was regarded as excluded because of the absence of an elevated serum calcium, and by the absence of evidence of renal failure.

Two years later the patient still complained of pain in the shoulder. Pain was also present in the hips and thighs, and she found walking difficult. A further x-ray suggested extension of the lesion of the scapula, and this was surgically resected, still being regarded as a tumor. At this stage, more careful clinical, biochemical, and radiologic study established a diagnosis of osteomalacia, and this was confirmed by iliac crest biopsy (Fig. 11). The low serum calcium is consistent with this, and there was evidence of generalized thinning of bone with a pseudofracture (Looser zone) of the femoral neck. A careful medical history revealed a gastrojejunostomy for duodenal ulcer at the age of 28 years and a more recent history of loose stools. The diagnosis was further confirmed by a good response to treatment with vitamin D: the patient's bone pain disappeared, and she was able to walk normally for the first time in many years.

This case provides a number of salutary lessons for the clinician, the radiologist, the biochemist, and the pathologist, all of whom missed clear pointers to a diagnosis of osteomalacia. In retrospect, it is clear that the appearance in the original bone biopsy is that of hyperparathyroidism secondary to osteomalacia. The lesion of the scapula is, in fact, a "brown tumor."

Case 3. A female 48 years of age gave a history of pain in the right leg. X-ray examination showed an osteolytic lesion involving the lower part of the tibia (Fig. 12 *left*). Three years before, the patient had been investigated for pain in the same part of the leg: an x-ray (Fig. 12 *right*) had shown what was regarded as a "stress fracture," and a diagnosis of osteomalacia was made on the following biochemical evidence: serum calcium, 2.3 mmol/liter (9.6 mg/100 ml); serum

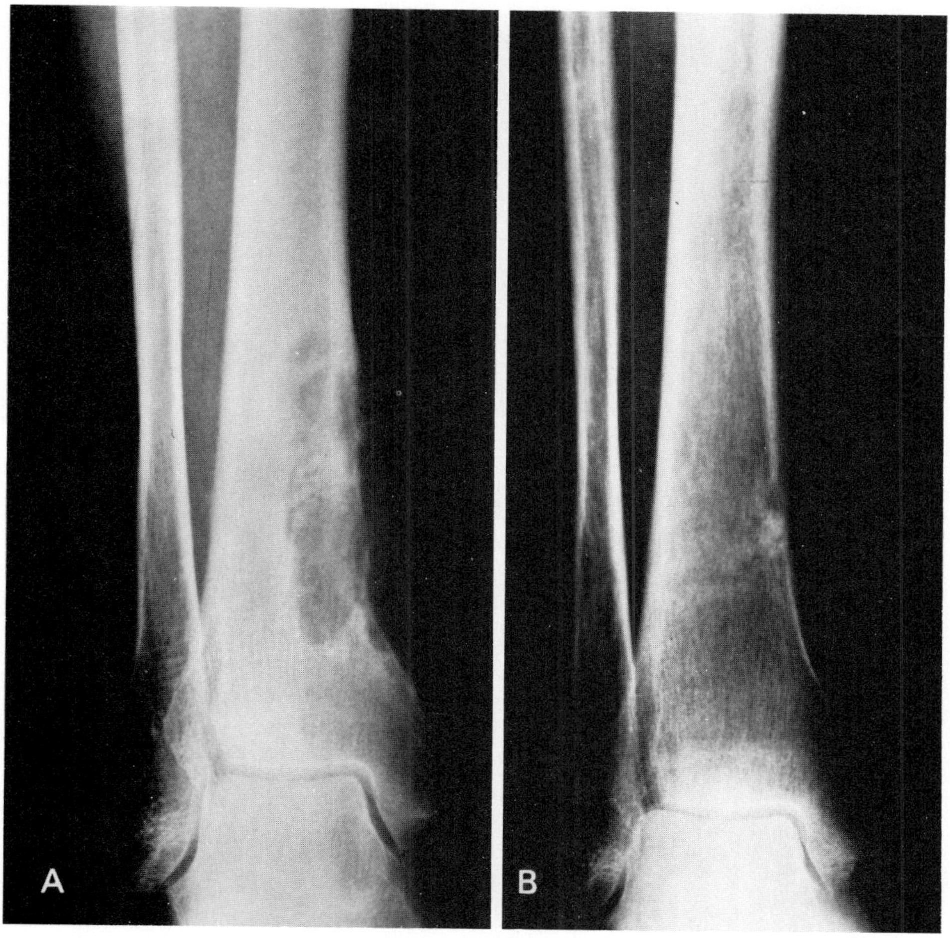

FIG. 12. Case 3. *Left*, radiograph showing osteolytic lesion involving lower part of tibia. *Right*, radiograph taken 3 years previously.

phosphorus, 0.2 mmol/liter (0.8 mg/100 ml); and serum alklaine phosphatase, 120 IU/liter (17 KA units/100 ml).

The diagnosis was confirmed by iliac crest biopsy, and the patient was treated by vitamin D.

Following presentation of the patient 3 years later, a biopsy of the large lesion of the tibia was carried out. The lesion was a relatively undifferentiated sarcoma (Fig. 13): it is not altogether clear whether the neoplasm originated in bone or soft tissues, although it appeared to be in about the same position as the original

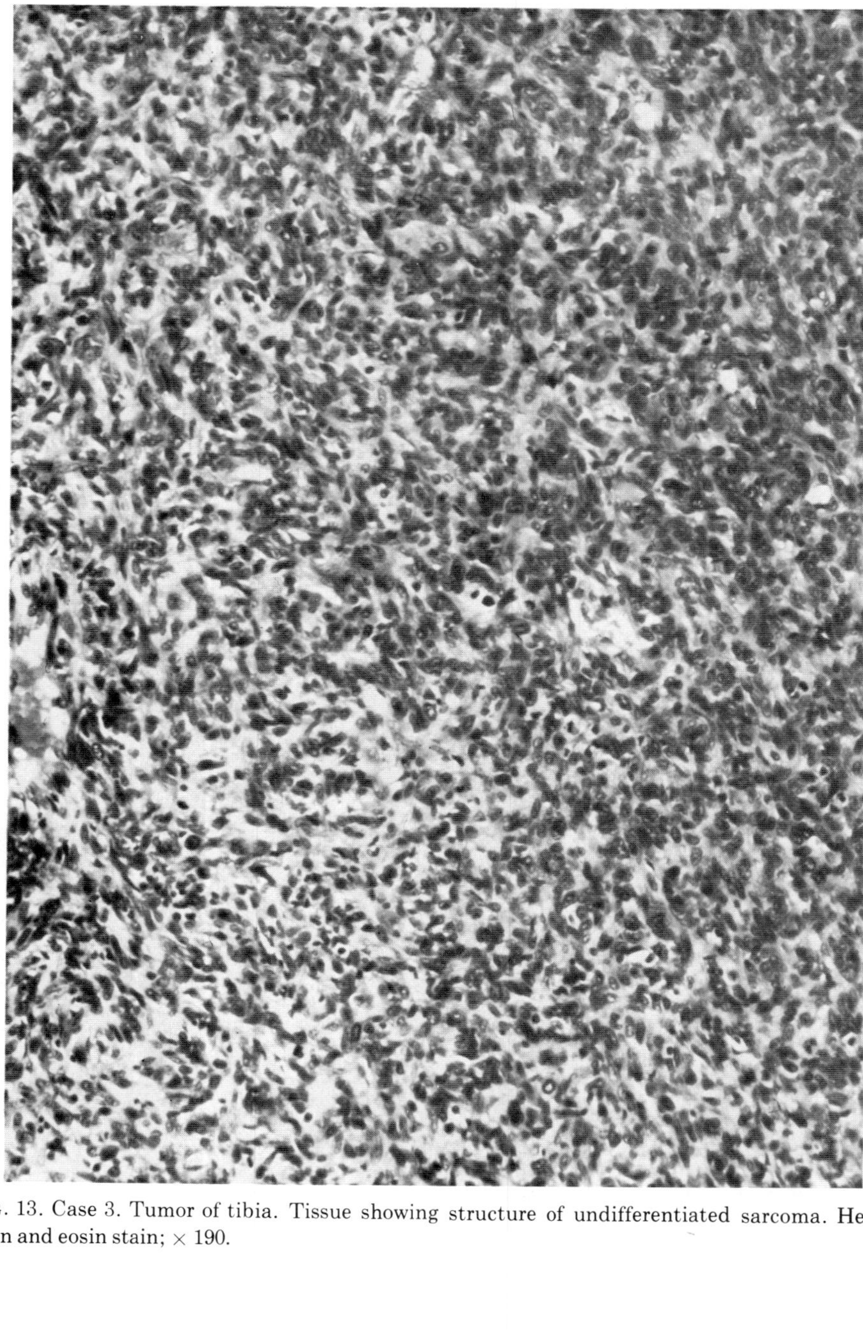

FIG. 13. Case 3. Tumor of tibia. Tissue showing structure of undifferentiated sarcoma. Hematoxylin and eosin stain; × 190.

"stress fracture." Reexamination of the earlier films showed an interesting area of erosion of the cortical surface. Biochemical evidence of osteomalacia is still present, despite continued treatment with vitamin D.

The tumor was treated by amputation. Vitamin D treatment was discontinued, and an increase in the serum calcium to 2.85 mmol/liter (11.4 mg/100 ml) after 3 months suggests that, as observed in other cases of this kind, the osteomalacia had responded to the removal of the tumor.[12, 25]

REFERENCES

1. Aaron, J. E., Gallagher, J. C., and Nordin, B. E. C.: Seasonal variation of histological osteomalacia in femoral neck fractures. *Lancet 2:* 84–85, (1974).
2. Anderson, J. B., Shimmins, J., and Smith, D. A.: A new technique for the measurement of metacarpal density. *Brit. J. Radiol. 39:* 443–450, (1966).
3. Ball, J.: A simple method of defining osteoid in undecalcified sections. *J. Clin. Pathol. 10:* 281–282, (1957).
4. Barnett, E., and Nordin, B. E. C.: The radiological diagnosis of osteoporosis: a new approach. *Clin Radiol. 11:* 166–174 (1960).
5. Bordier, P. J., and Tun Chot, S.: Quantitative histology of metabolic bone disease. *Clin. Endocrinol. Metabol. 1:* 197–215, (1972).
6. Buhr, A. J., and Cooke, A. M.: Fracture patterns. *Lancet, 1,* 531–536, (1959).
7. Chalmers, J., Conacher, W. D. H., Gardner, D. L., and Scott, P. J.: Osteomalacia; a common disease in elderly women. *J. Bone Joint Surg. 49B:* 403–423, (1967).
8. Chalmers, J., and Weaver, J. K. Cancellous bone; its strength and changes with aging and an evaluation of some methods for measuring its mineral content. *J. Bone Joint Surg. 48A:* 299–308, (1966).
9. Dent, C. E.: Rickets (and osteomalacia), nutritional and metabolic (1919–69). *Proc R. Soc. Med. 63:* 401–408, (1970).
10. Dequeker, J.: Bone Loss in Normal and Pathological Conditions. Leuven, Leuven University Press, 1972.
11. Ellis, H. A., and Peart, K. M.: Quantitative observations on mineralized and non-mineralized bone in the iliac crest. *J. Clin. Pathol. 25:* 277–286, (1972).
12. Evans, D. J., and Azzopardi, J. G.: Distinctive tumours of bone and soft tissue causing acquired vitamin D-resistant osteomalacia. *Lancet 1:* 353–354, (1972).
13. Exton-Smith, A. N., Millard, P. H., Payne, P. R., and Wheeler, E.: A method of measuring quantity of bone. *Lancet 2:* 1153, (1966).
14. Fourman, P., and Royer, P.: *Calcium Metabolism and the Bone.* 2nd ed., Blackwell Scientific Publications, Oxford, 1970.
15. Garner, A., and Ball, J.: Quantitative observations on mineralised and unmineralised bone in chronic renal azotaemia and intestinal malabsorption syndrome. *J. Pathol. Bacteriol. 91:* 545–561, (1966).
16. Garrick, R., Ireland, A. W., and Posen, S.: Bone abnormalities after gastric surgery; a prospective histological study. *Ann. Intern. Med. 75:* 221–225, (1971).
17. Landry, M., and Fleisch, H.: The influence of immobilisation on bone formation as evaluated by osseous incorporation of tetracyclines. *J. Bone Joint Surg. 46B:* 764–771, (1964).
18. Lindahl, O., and Lindgren, A. G. H.: Grading of osteoporosis in autopsy specimens; a new method. *Acta orthop. Scand. 32:* 85–100, (1962).
19. Looser, E.: Uber Spätrachitis und Osteomalacie; klinishe röntgenologische und pathologischanatomische Untersuchungen. *Dtsch. Z. Chir. 152:* 210–357, (1920).
20. Lutwak, L., Whedon, G. D., Lachance, R. A., Reid, J. M., and Lipscomb, H. S.: Mineral, electrolyte, and nitrogen balance studies of the Gemini-VII fourteen-day orbital space flight. *J. Clin. Endocrinol. 29:* 1140–1156, (1969).
21. Matrajt, H., and Hioco, D.: Solochrome cyanine R as an indicator dye of bone morphology. *Stain technol. 41:* 97–100, (1966).
22. Merz, W. A., and Schenk, R. K.: Quantitative structural analysis of human cancellous bone. *Acta anat. 75:* 54–66, (1970).

23. Merz, W. A., and Schenk, R. K.: A quantitative histological study on bone formation in human cancellous bone. *Acta anat. 76:* 1–15, (1970).
24. Morgan, D. B., Paterson, C. R., Woods, C. G., Pulvertaft, C. N., and Fourman, P.: Search for osteomalacia in 1228 patients after gastrectomy and other operations on the stomach. *Lancet 2:* 1085–1088, (1965).
25. Salassa, R. M., Jowsey, J., and Arnaud, C. D.: Hypophosphataemic osteomalacia associated with "nonendocrine" tumors. *New Engl. J. Med. 283:* 65–70, (1970).
26. Schenk, R. K., Merz, W. A., and Müller, J.: A quantitative histological study on bone resorption in human cancellous bone. *Acta anat. 74:* 44–53, (1969).
27. Sissons, H. A.: Osteoporosis and epiphysial arrest in joint tuberculosis; an account of the histological changes in involved tissues. *J. Bone Joint Surg. 34B:* 275–290, (1952).
28. Sissons, H. A.: Osteoporosis of Cushing's Syndrome. In *Bone as a Tissue*, edited by Rodahl, K., Nicholson, J. T., and Brown, E. M., pp. 3–17. New York, McGraw-Hill Book Co., Inc., 1960.
29. Sissons, H. A.: Preparation of undecalcified bone sections. Association of Clinical Pathologists, Broadsheet No. 62, 1968.
30. Sissons, H. A., Holley, K. J., and Heighway, J.: Normal bone structure in relation to osteomalacia. In *l'Ostéomalacie*, edited by Hioco, Paris, 1967.
31. Sorenson, J. A., and Cameron, J. R.: Measurements of bone mineral content, *in vivo*, by monochromatic radiation absorption. In *Symposium Ossium*, ed. by Jelliffe, A. M., and Strickland, B. Edinburgh, Livingstone, 1970.
32. Trotter, M., Broman, G. E., and Peterson, R. R.: Densities of bones of white and negro skeletons. *J. Bone Joint Surg. 42A:* 50, 1960.
33. Whedon, G. D.: Osteoporosis; atrophy of disuse. In *Bone as a Tissue*, edited by Rodahl, K., Nicholson, J. T., and Brown, E. M., pp. 67–82. New York, McGraw-Hill Book Co., Inc., 1960.

Chapter 4

Osteomyelitis including Fungal*

WALTER G. J. PUTSCHAR

The changed clinical[1, 2] and pathologic[3, 4] spectrum of osteomyelitis justifies a review of the subject. The mortality has decreased from about 20[5] to 2%[2] since the introduction of antibiotics, but the morbidity remains high.[6, 7] In a large necropsy statistic, acute and chronic osteomyelitis have decreased from 0.5% in the preantibiotic era to 0.16%.[4] This decrease is mainly due to the diminished frequency and mortality of septic hematogenous osteomyelitis. The decrease is marked in childhood and adolescence, while there is an actual increase in infants and adults.

Hematogenous osteomyelitis now presents in a milder form and more often takes a subacute course.[8] Increasingly frequent vertebral osteomyelitis poses a diagnostic problem, especially in the older age groups. Patients with chronic renal disease on hemodialysis[9, 10] and heroin addicts[11, 12] have also contributed to the number of cases, especially of thoracic and spinal osteomyelitis. Subacute focal and spinal osteomyelitis have with increasing frequency come into the realm of surgical pathology in the differential diagnosis of bone biopsies. While 278 cases of osteomyelitis were clinically observed from 1963 to 1966 at the Massachusetts General Hospital,[2] 210 specimens have been diagnosed histopathologically.

Direct bone infection has increased due to the marked rise in the number of traumatic accidents and to the use of more extensive orthopedic procedures such as: open reductions, nailing, insertion of intramedullary rods, and prosthetic replacement of bones and joints.[2] More extensive thoracic surgery and splitting of the sternum during cardiac surgery have occasionally led to osteomyelitis of sternum and ribs.[13] Osteomyelitis of the lower extremities in peripheral vascular disease, mostly of older diabetic patients, accounts for 34% of cases in the Massachusetts General Hospital series.[2]

BACTERIOLOGY

The etiologic agent in all types of osteomyelitis still is overwhelmingly the coagulase-positive staphylococcus (60 to 90%).[2, 14] The second most common

* By request, mycobacterial (tuberculosis and leprosy) and spirochetal infections (syphilis and yaws) are omitted in this chapter.

organism, especially in infants, was the streptococcus,[5, 14] but with the appearance of more and more penicillin-resistant strains of staphylococci and their ubiquitous presence, resistant staphylococci have been found in as many as 80% of the cases.[15] In the Massachusetts General Hospital series of hematogenous osteomyelitis, *Pneumococcus*, *Escherichia coli*, *Klebsiella*, *Aerobacter*, *Salmonella*, and *Bacteroides* have been occasionally isolated. Five cases showed more than one organism. In postoperative and contiguous infections, in addition to staphylococci, streptococci, pseudomonas, proteus, and *E. coli* were isolated with significant frequency. These are nosocomial organisms with varying antibiotic resistance. Osteomyelitis secondary to peripheral vascular disease showed a variety of multiple infections.[2] In patients receiving steroid and/or immunosuppressive therapy, a variety of opportunistic invaders have been found.

OSTEOMYELITIS AS A PROBLEM OF SURGICAL PATHOLOGY

Insidious subacute hematogenous osteomyelitis presents, in the majority of cases, an unsolved clinical problem.[15, 2] Characteristic signs and symptoms are often lacking. A preceding illness or portal of entry usually remains obscure. If there is a radiologically demonstrable lesion, biopsy with culture and histologic examination have to provide the diagnosis. Prebiopsy antibiotic therapy not uncommonly obscures the picture by suppression of the inflammatory reaction and prevention of the growth of the cultures. This requires, on the part of the pathologist, a full understanding of the clinical and radiologic findings, a satisfactory technique for preparing bone sections, and an adequate knowledge of the structure of different portions of bones in different age groups. The evaluation of an infectious bone lesion may require more extensive sampling of the material than that of an obvious primary or metastatic neoplasm. The question concerning infection after surgical procedures, especially with implantation of plastic and metal prostheses or bone grafting, is often difficult to answer because scarring, macrophages with hemosiderin, bone dust, giant cells, and accumulations of lymphocytes are usually present even without infection. Similarly, in peripheral vascular disease of diabetics, the differentiation between ischemic necrosis or gangrene and superimposed infection can be difficult to decide. Direct, postoperative and contiguous infections usually remain local.

The microscopic picture of purulent osteomyelitis is essentially the same as that of acute and chronic inflammation elsewhere, modified by the local environment and peculiar reactivity of bone. In the acute phase, necrosis and abscess formation in the marrow lead to focal necrosis or extensive ischemic infarction of bone. The dead bone has to be either removed by osteoclastic resorption (Fig. 1) or mechanically eliminated. Small pieces of dead bone can serve as scaffolding for reparative new bone formation. Large sequestra, if allowed to remain for long periods, are capable of harboring residual bacteria which may precipitate a recurrence after long dormancy if host resistance is decreased. The periosteum, if attacked by infection, trauma, or neoplasm is mainly capable of one response: the formation of reactive bone. Since bone, in contrast to other organs, is principally completely renewable, the sequelae of healed osteomyelitis may completely disappear without residual scar, especially

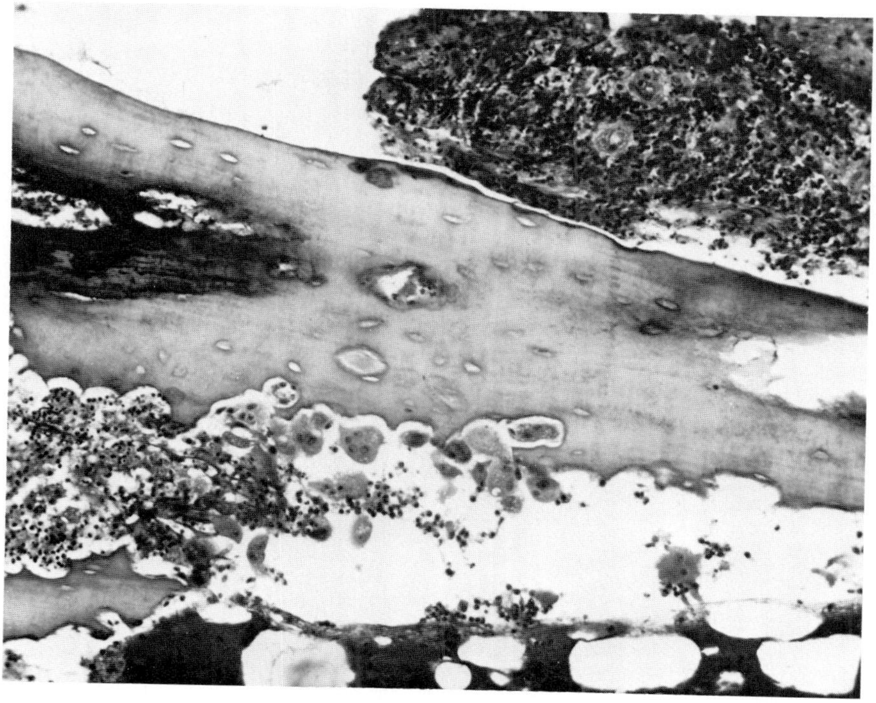

FIG. 1. Small sequestrum surrounded by purulent exudate, showing active osteoclastic resorption; × 160.

in young individuals. In older individuals, fibrous scarring of the marrow or residual abscess cavities lined by fibrotic granulation tissue may remain permanently.

HEMATOGENOUS OSTEOMYELITIS

The patterns of hematogenous osteomyelitis differ significantly with age. Trueta, in his extensive studies concerning the vascular architecture of bones at different ages, has largely clarified the patterns of infantile, childhood, and adult osteomyelitis.[16, 17] In his series of 202 cases of acute hematogenous osteomyelitis, 7% were infants, 80% children and 13% adults.[14]

INFANTILE OSTEOMYELITIS

At neonatal and infant age, the cortex is thin and loose, consisting mainly of woven bone with wide spaces filled by osteogenic mesenchyme, permitting rapid extension of the medullary infection into the subperiosteal area. The periosteum shows a very active inner osteogenic layer which is easily detached from the cortical surface, permitting rapid formation of a subperiosteal abscess. The detached osteogenic periosteum responds with marked formation of reactive woven bone (involucrum). The porous cortex, permitting the escape of the intra-osseous exudate, usually is spared massive necrosis, and large sequestrum formation is usually not observed (Fig. 2). Since, at this age, metaphysial blood

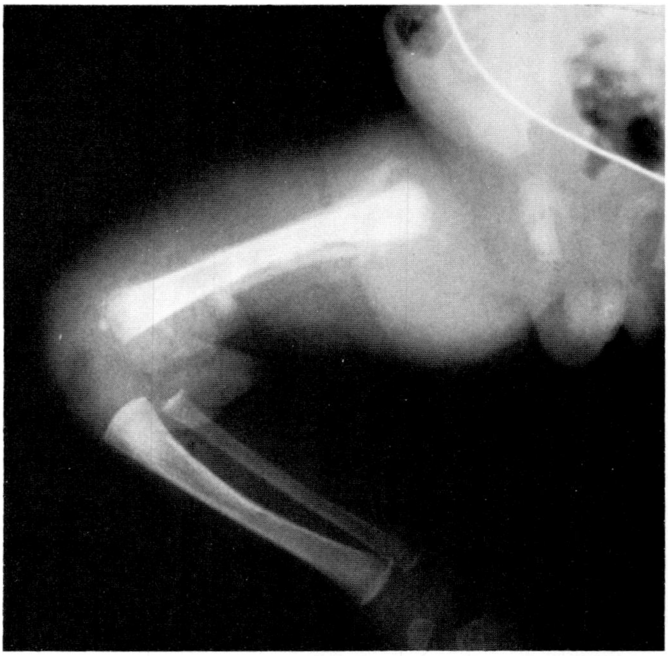

FIG. 2. Acute hematogenous staphylococcic osteomyelitis of right femur and pyarthrosis of hip joint: female infant, 3 weeks old. Notice marked involucrum and absence of sequestrum.

vessels extend into the cartilaginous epiphysis and its secondary ossification center (if present), the metaphysial infection easily extends into the epiphysis and the adjacent joint, causing epiphysial necrosis and pyarthrosis. This may result in sequestration of the necrotic ossification center[18] but, in less severe cases, repair of the epiphysis occurs.[19, 20] It is the epiphysial and articular involvement in infantile osteomyelitis that leaves the most permanent sequelae in the form of inhibited growth and joint deformity or ankylosis. The infection also easily spreads into the short diaphysis but, since massive sequestration is rare, the continued periosteal bone apposition accompanied by endosteal resorption restores the diaphysial configuration. The infantile cortex as well as the involucrum disappear in the remodeling process.

Infantile and neonatal osteomyelitis is increasing in frequency because neonatal sepsis is more often survived under present antibiotic treatment. Eighty to ninety per cent of the cases are presently caused by coagulase-positive staphylococci which are mostly penicillin-resistant.[21, 22] There is no significant sex difference in this age group.[5]

CHILDHOOD OSTEOMYELITIS

The classical hematogenous osteomyelitis occurs in the growing age and localizes, primarily, in the metaphysis of long bones. The correlation of the localization with the growth activity is so great that the fastest growing metaphyses are most commonly involved in the following order of frequency[3]: distal femur, proximal and distal tibia, proximal femur, and proximal and distal humerus. The detached periosteum usually responds with the formation of an involucrum. The bacteria lodge in the metaphysial sinusoids and elicit edema and purulent exudate. The spread of the infection is influenced by the structural peculiarity and vascular architecture of this age group. During the growing period the metaphysial cortex is very thin, due to periosteal osteoclastic remodeling, permitting easy extension of the exudate beneath the periosteum (Fig. 3). The active cambium layer is easily stripped by the accumulation of purulent exudate, resulting in a large subperiosteal abscess, disrupting the periosteal blood supply of the cortex. The pressure of the intramedullary exudate permits spread of the infection into the diaphysis and leads to ischemic necrosis of the compact diaphysial cortex, with or without thrombosis of nutrient vessels, resulting in massive sequestration. This used to be a common event in preantibiotic days, leading to chronic osteomyelitis of long duration. Presently, massive sequestration and its sequelae are mostly prevented by antibiotic therapy. Extension of the metaphysial infection into the epiphysis and from there into the joint is usually prevented by the presence of the cartilaginous growth plate separating the

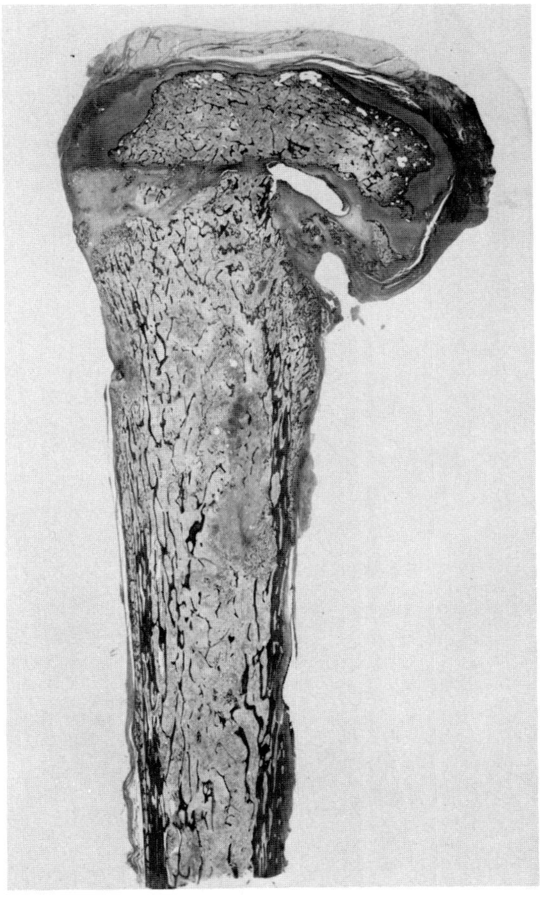

FIG. 3. Hematogenous osteomyelitis of proximal tibia. Notice metaphysial location with subperiosteal abscess and secondary extension into diaphysis; 14-year-old male, preantibiotic period.

epiphysial blood supply from the metaphysis. Only in the hip join and to a lesser extent in the shoulder, where a portion of the proximal metaphysis is within the synovial space, a complicating septic arthritis is not uncommon. Partial or complete destruction of the growth plate (Fig. 4) with slipping of the epiphysis may occur and lead to growth asymmetry and retardation. More common is accelerated growth and earlier epiphysial closure in the area of venous congestion after the infectious focus has been shifted away from the growth plate by new enchondral bone (Fig. 5). In Trueta's series, accelerated growth occurred in 30% of the cases.[14] In this age group the male-female ratio is about 3:1.

ADULT OSTEOMYELITIS

Acute hematogenous osteomyelitis of the long bones in the adult is uncommon. However, its peculiarities deserve consideration. The infection is often diaphysial with secondary extension to the epiphysial area (Fig. 6). Since vascular connections between metaphysis and epiphysis are reestablished to some extent after the disappearance of the growth plate, involvement of the epiphysis and of the adjacent joint by this route is possible. The firm attachment of the resting adult periosteum prevents extensive periosteal stripping and, therefore, a massive subperiosteal abscess and large cortical sequestra are usually not formed.[23] Local subperiosteal and adjacent soft tissue abscesses (Fig. 7) with the formation of fistulae are frequent. The continued resorption of the viable cortex may lead to pathologic fracture.

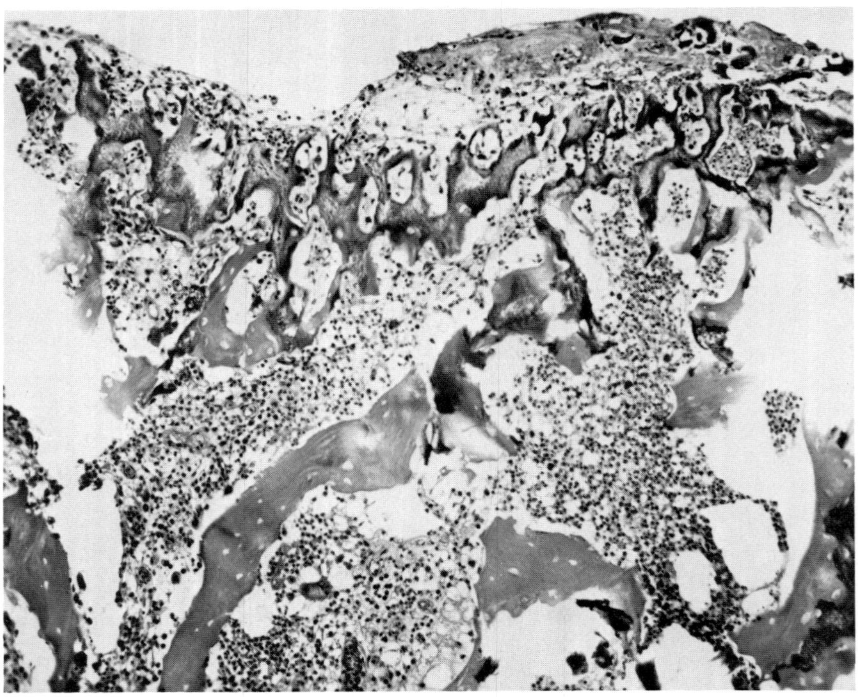

FIG. 4. Destruction of growth plate by purulent exudate, acute hematogenous osteomyelitis of tibia; 12-year-old female; × 100.

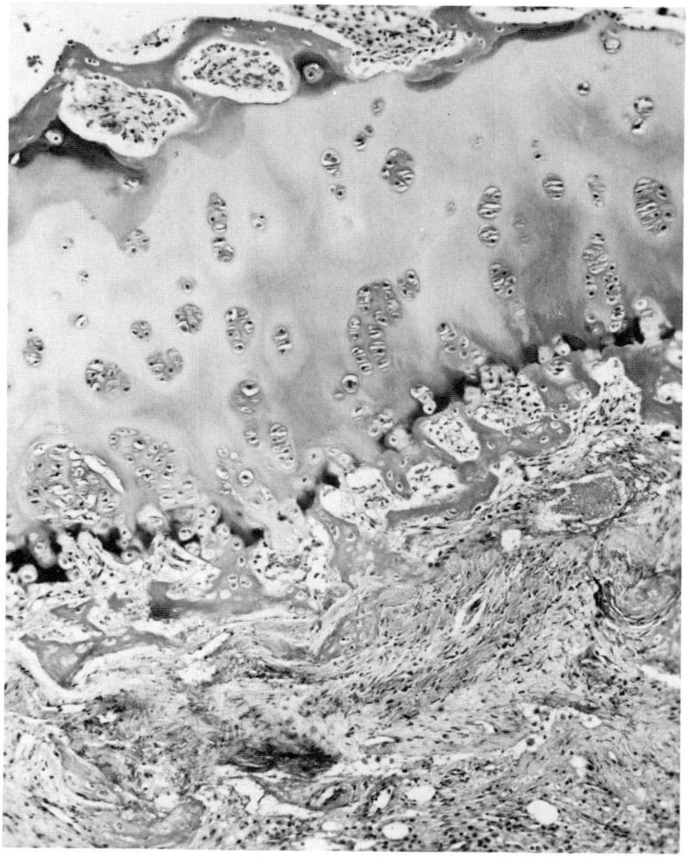

FIG. 5. Resumption of enchondral growth, acute hematogenous osteomyelitis of tibia; 12-year-old female; × 100.

VERTEBRAL OSTEOMYELITIS

Adult osteomyelitis localizes in the cancellous bones, particularly the spine, in about 50% of the cases.[24] The process, as in tuberculosis, often starts in the vertebral body near an intervertebral disc which becomes involved and radiologically narrowed. From the disc the infection extends into the next vertebra. But, in contrast to tuberculosis, involvement of the neural arches and transverse processes is not uncommon.[25] Paravertebral abscess occurs less often than in tuberculosis. The lumbar and lower thoracic vertebrae are most often affected.[25, 26]

Although the venous route of infection has been postulated, especially for the spread of urinary tract and pelvic infections, the arterial route is probably more important,[24] since the majority of cases of spinal osteomyelitis are not secondary to pelvic disease. Direct infection of the spine can occur after intervertebral disc surgery.[2]

Vertebral osteomyelitis has more frequently become a problem of surgical pathology in the form of needle, trocar, and even open biopsy.[26] The differential diagnosis from tuberculous or neoplastic disease is the main consideration.

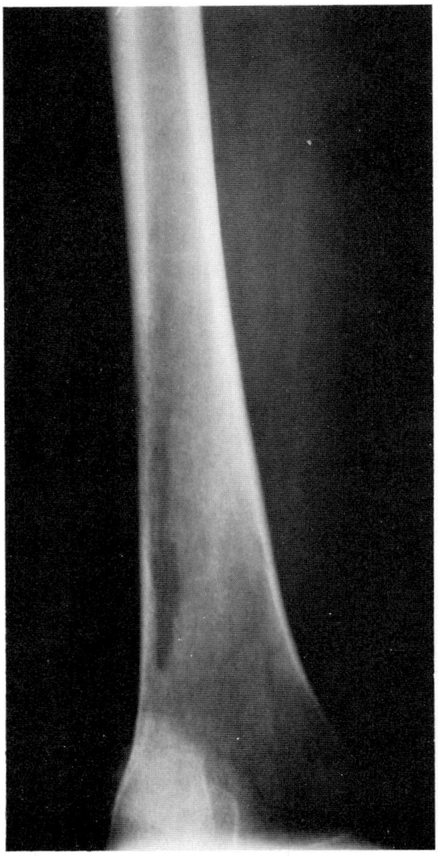

FIG. 6. Subacute hematogenous streptococcic osteomyelitis of femur, oblique view; 38-year-old male.

Culture, in addition to the histologic study, is an absolute necessity since, besides the usual coagulase positive staphylococci, Gram-negative rods (from enteric and urinary tract infections)[27] as well as brucellosis and some fungi are prone to locate in the vertebral column. In adults, the male predominance is even greater than in children.

OSTEITIS PUBIS

This is an acute, very painful spottily lytic bone change on both sides of the pubic symphysis developing weeks or months after retropubic surgery (mostly prostatectomy). The lesion is self-limiting and has been interpreted by some as a neurovascular disturbance secondary to the adjacent surgical intervention.[28] Other investigators consider it to be a true osteomyelitis and report positive cultures of pseudomonas and proteus.[29, 30]

SUBACUTE OR PRIMARY CHRONIC OSTEOMYELITIS

Osteomyelitis of insidious onset and protracted course has become more frequent than the acute septic form.[8] This may be in part due to lowered virulence or better host resistance but also to a large extent is undoubtedly the

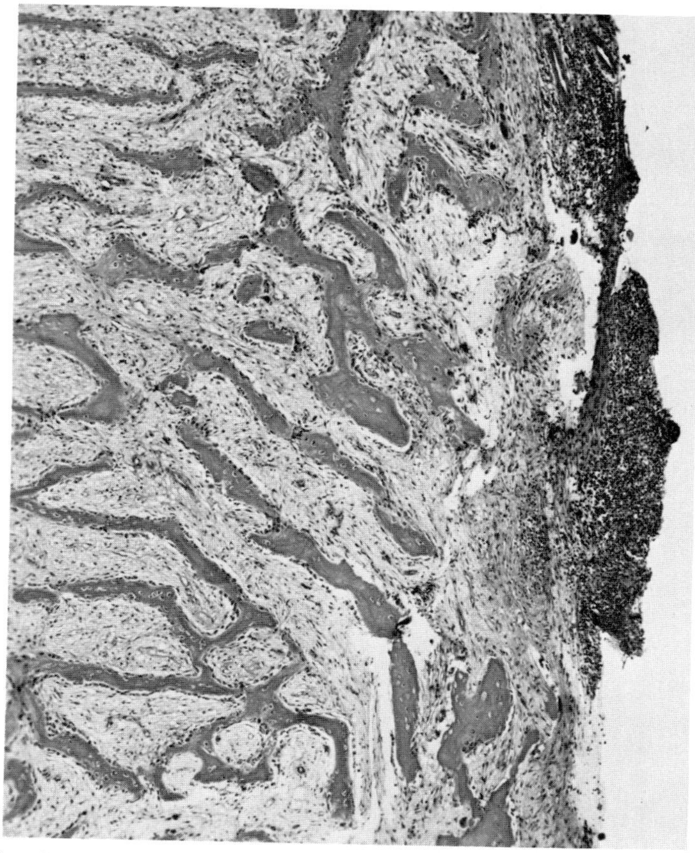

FIG. 7. Subperiosteal abscess with reactive woven bone (*left*), femur; 38-year-old male; × 56.

result of the effect of antibiotics. These infections present, radiologically and anatomically, either as a focal, usually metaphysial, destructive lesion (Brodie's abscess) or as marked periosteal and endosteal new formation of bone (sclerosing osteomyelitis of Garré). The less circumscribed foci, usually of metaphysial location, are microscopically characterized by the presence of numerous plasma cells (so-called plasma cell osteomyelitis).[31] Sequestra are usually not observed; fistulae can occur.

The focal lesion of a Brodie's abscess often exhibits a pronounced perifocal, mostly endosteal, bony sclerosis. The abscess cavity usually contains some residual purulent exudate and exhibits a fibrous wall with granulation tissue, leukocytes and plasma cells.[32]

The purely sclerosing form of osteomyelitis is uncommon (Fig. 8). Undoubtedly in the past it has often been confused with osteoid osteoma. It sometimes requires examination of many areas of the specimen before the inflammatory nature of this reactive bony sclerosis is revealed, because most areas merely show apposition of lamellar bone and fibrous marrow. Inflammations with a predominantly osteosclerotic reaction occur not uncommonly in the jaw after dental infections.[33, 34]

In the so-called plasma cell osteomyelitis little bone destruction is observed.

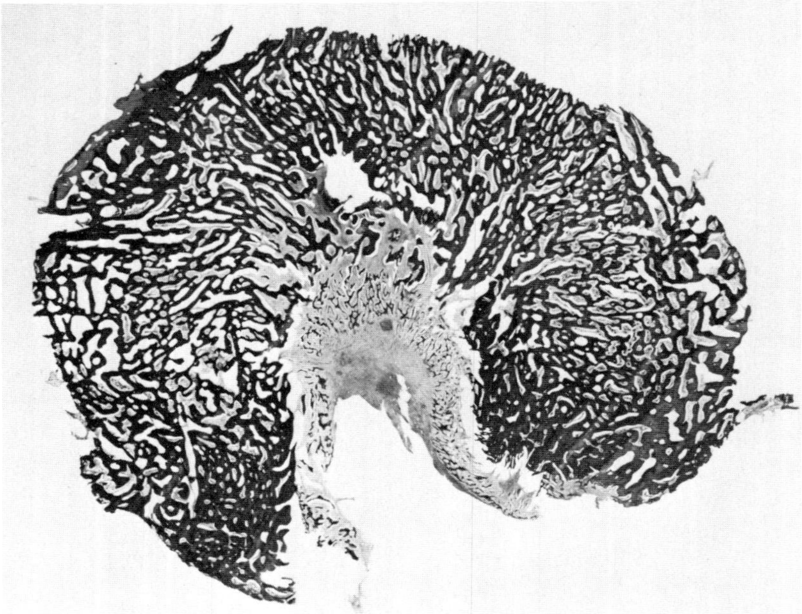

FIG. 8. Sclerosing osteomyelitis, cross-section; 8-year-old boy. (Courtesy of Dr. E. Uehlinger, Zurich.)

The marrow spaces are permeated by a proteinaceous exudate containing loosely scattered plasma cells as the predominant cell.[31] The periphery of the lesion usually shows a border of granulation tissue and perifocal fibrosis. Since the onset of these infections can not be precisely timed, it may be that one is merely observing a late phase of a low grade process.

Secondary chronic osteomyelitis as a continuation of childhood septic osteomyelitis with continued fistulous drainage has become rather rare. Concomitantly, late complications of protracted bone infection, such as fistula-carcinoma and amyloidosis, have almost disappeared.

SALMONELLA OSTEOMYELITIS

In typhoid fever, osteomyelitis occurs in slightly less than 1% of patients, sometimes a considerable period after the acute intestinal disease (164 cases in 18,840 typhoid infections).[35] The most frequent location is in ribs and rib cartilages (perichondritis), closely followed in frequency by the tibia and the lumbar spine. The tibial lesion is often a diaphysial abscess close to the periosteum, yielding *S. typhosa* on culture of the exudate. The spinal lesion often involves two adjacent vertebral bodies and the disc between them. The course is chronic and elicits perifocal sclerosis with narrowing of the disc. All other bones are less often involved.

In other salmonella infections in the hematologically normal patients, osteomyelitis is much less common (about 0.2%).[35] The long bones, especially femur and humerus, as well as the costochondral junctions are frequently involved, and in 15% of cases multiple bones are affected.[36-39] The disease develops insidiously, and diaphysial involvement is not uncommon; sequestra usually do not develop. In infants epiphysial involvement and pyarthrosis also occur.[40]

The most important association exists between the hemoglobinopathies and salmonella osteomyelitis.[41-43] In sickle cell anemia, focal necrosis and infarction of bone is common after sickling crises. Close to 90% of osteomyelitis in patients with sickle cell disease is due to salmonella; staphylococci are the cause in only a small percentage.[43] The organisms most frequently present are *Salmonella typhimurium*, paratyphoid B, and *Salmonella cholerasuis* (in about two-thirds of the cases).

Multiple bone involvement is found in about two-thirds of the cases, and the male-female sex ratio is 3:1. Long bones are frequently involved, but in about 25% of the cases, the bones of the hands and feet are also affected. Even heterozygotes with various combinations of abnormal hemoglobins have a high incidence of salmonella osteomyelitis, which may be the only clinical manifestation.[44] The lesion is radiologically difficult to differentiate from cortical infarction and aseptic necrosis, and the periosteal reactive bone is sparse (Fig. 9). The reason for the frequency of salmonella bacteremia in these patients is not clear. Undoubtedly the presence of necrotic bone serves as a nidus for infection, and the frequent fibrotic atrophy of the spleen lowers the host resistance.[45] It also has been shown experimentally that hemolysis lowers the resistance of mice to *S. typhimurium* infection.[46]

BRUCELLA OSTEOMYELITIS

Skeletal involvement in brucellosis is not uncommon. Spink reported bone and joint lesions in 10% of his patients in Minnesota.[47] Of 300 reported cases of Brucella osteomyelitis, three-fourths show lesions located in the spine, especially in the lumbar vertebral bodies.[48, 49] Most cases of Brucella osteomyelitis are caused by *Brucella melitensis*, but *Brucella abortus* and *Brucella suis* are also found. The lesion begins with an abscess causing a local lytic area in one or several vertebral bodies. The destruction may involve the intervertebral disc and so extend into adjacent vertebrae. The chronic abscess contains inspissated necrotic exudate bordered by granulation tissue with epithelioid histiocytes, lymphocytes, and plasma cells. There is microsequestration of necrotic trabeculae and perifocal fibrosis. In the late phases, sclerotic bony reaction can occur. Long bones are much less often affected, but here also the formation of local abscesses dominates the picture. The vertebral lesion resembles tuberculosis radiologically and grossly, but paravertebral abscesses are uncommon. Histologically distinct tuberculoid granulomas are usually not seen, although Langhans' giant cells do occur. Staphylococcus establishes itself occasionally as a secondary invader. After healing, a narrowed disc bridged by marginal exostoses remains.[49]

VIRAL OSTEOMYELITIS

In smallpox epidemics, 2 to 5% of children and adolescents develop osteomyelitis and arthritis, usually 2 to 3 weeks after the appearance of the skin lesions.[50]

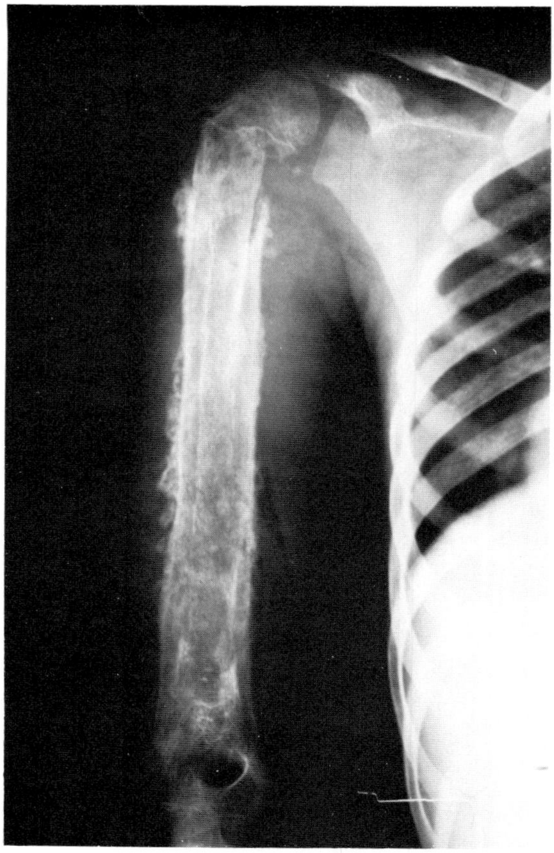

FIG. 9. Salmonella osteomyelitis in sickle cell anemia. (Courtesy of Dr. Stanley Bohrer, Ibadan, Nigeria.)

There is no sex difference. The most common location is around the elbow; proximal radius and ulna and distal humerus. The lesions are frequently bilateral (Fig. 10). The bones of the ankle and foot are the second most common site of involvement.[51] The lesions are restricted to the extremities and are often multifocal.[52] Aspiration of the moderate joint effusion reveals a sterile nonpurulent exudate from which elementary bodies of variola virus can be recovered. Radiologically, a transverse metaphysial porotic band in contact with the growth plate is observed. Involucrum formation can be quite marked but diaphysial sequestra usually are not formed. Complete detachment of the epiphysis with marked displacement is characteristic for this disease. Sinuses can occur. The disease is self-limiting, if not secondarily infected with staphylococci, and cortical remodeling is accomplished in a year. Growth retardation is common, and occasionally ankylosis occurs.

Vaccinial osteomyelitis has been occasionally observed several weeks after vaccination against smallpox, also predilecting the upper extremities.[53, 54] Mandibular and scapular involvement resembling Caffey's disease have been reported.[54, 55] Biopsy shows nonpurulent chronic inflammation and fibrosis.

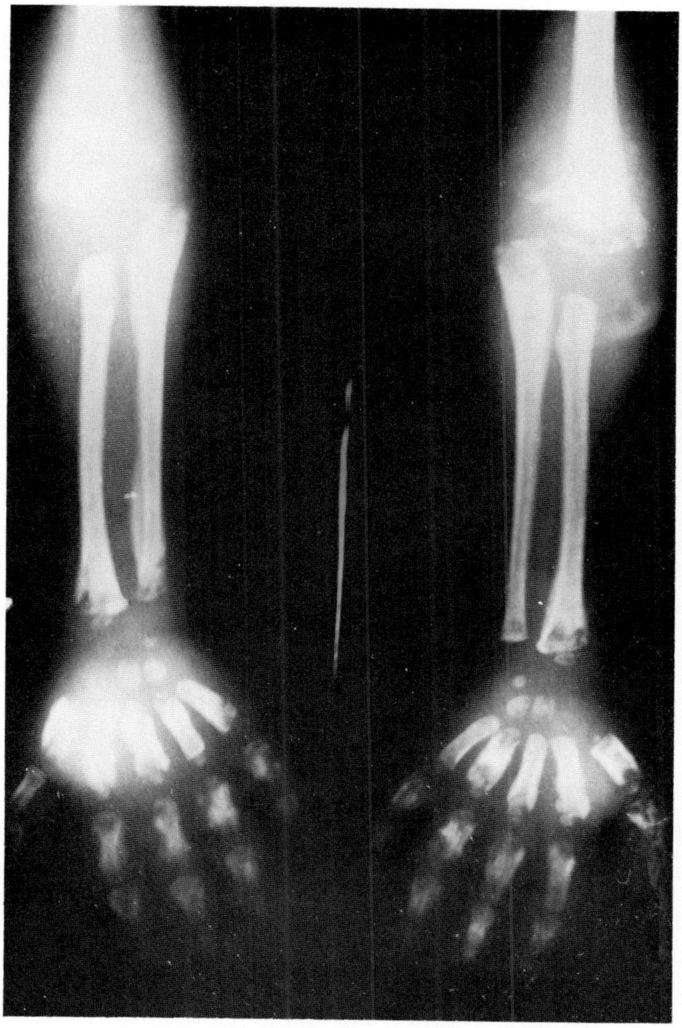

FIG. 10. Variola osteomyelitis and arthritis; 2-year-old female. (Courtesy of Dr. L. A. Tamaela, Djakarta.)

Vaccinia virus has been cultured (on embryonated eggs) from aspirated material.[53]

Two cases of questionable viral osteomyelitis of the pubic area have been described in women with lymphogranuloma venereum.[56]

FUNGAL OSTEOMYELITIS

Compared with bacterial osteomyelitis, all types of fungal bone infection are rare. However, in systemic dissemination of true fungus infections, the skeleton is not uncommonly involved. Marked male predominance is noted. The portal of entry is usually the respiratory tract, and the organisms reach the bone by the hematogenous route. Any bone may be involved but certain locations, especially small bones, are predilected (Fig. 11). The bone lesions are mostly circumscribed

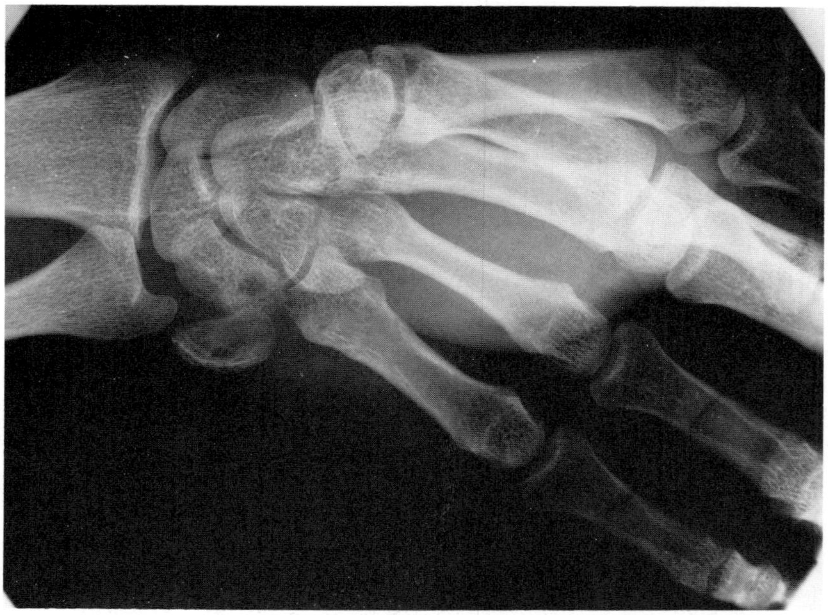

FIG. 11. Coccidioidomycosis of os pisiforme and os triquetrum; 38-year-old male.

on x-ray and mainly osteolytic with little perifocal bone reaction, simulating neoplastic lesions. Multiple bone involvement is not uncommon. Soft tissue abscesses, fistulae, and extension of the inflammatory process into adjacent joints are often observed. The tissue response is a chronic suppurative inflammation assuming a definite granulomatous character as in tuberculosis (Fig. 12). Microscopically, distinct granulomas with epithelioid cells and giant cells, in addition to neutrophilic leukocytes, lymphocytes, and plasma cells, are often seen. The organisms are usually present in their yeast form in the exudate and are often found in the giant cells (Fig. 13). They can be seen in hematoxylin and eosin sections but are better demonstrated by the periodic acid Schiff reaction and the methenamine silver stain. Although the morphology of the fungi is often diagnostic, this is not always the case. Since the granulomatous reaction is not specific, identification of the organism by any means is essential for diagnosis and therapy.

COCCIDIOIDOMYCOSIS

Infections with *Coccidioides immitis* seldom progress to systemic dissemination. However, if they do, single or multiple bone involvement is not uncommon.[57, 58] Areas beneath insertions of tendons and ligaments are predilected.[59] The lesions are most often found in the small bones of the hands and feet (carpals and metacarpals, tarsals and metatarsals and phalanges).[58] Second in frequency is spinal and rib involvement.[60] In vertebral lesions the intervertebral discs are usually spared.[59] Facial bones may be affected in children.[57] Lesions of the cranial vault occur.[61] These are larger on the outer than on the inner table.[62] The long bones of the extremities are usually spared.[60] Although subcutaneous abscesses and fistulae often develop, the lesions ulti-

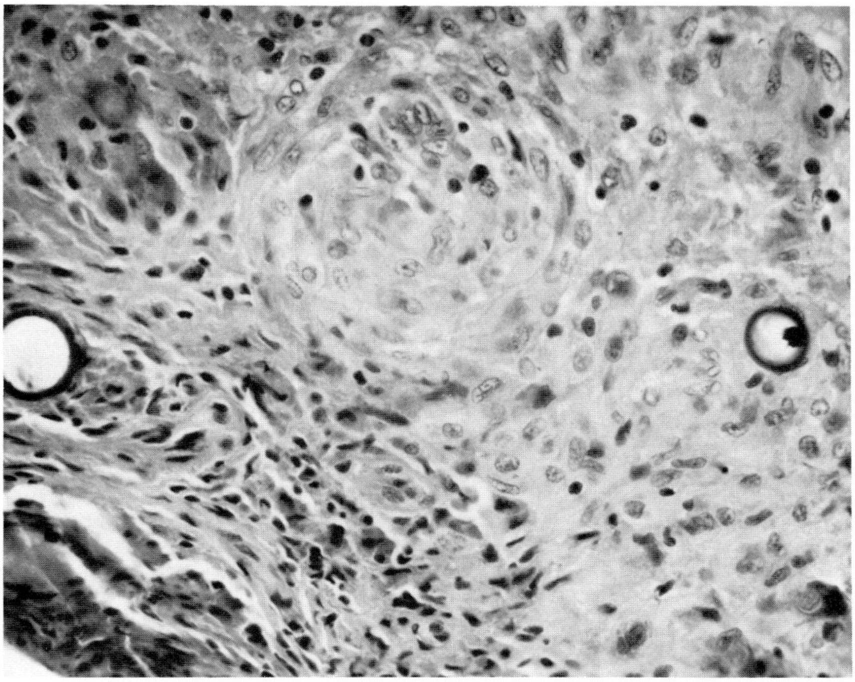

FIG. 12. Coccidioidal granulomas in carpal synovium, fungi stained with periodic acid Schiff reaction; 38-year-old male; × 400.

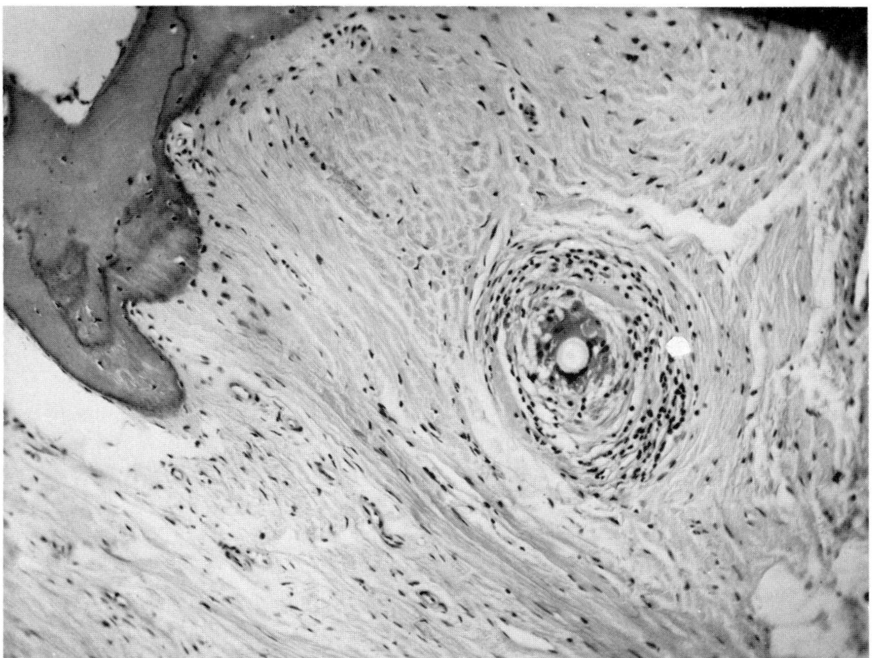

FIG. 13. Coccidioidal granuloma in ligamentous attachment of os pisiforme. Note fungus in giant cell. Hematoxylin and eosin stain; × 160.

mately heal, leaving permanent lytic foci, presumably cystic cavities.[58] The mortality is low and not caused by the bone lesions. A survey of Miller and Birsner[60] in California revealed that the majority of systemic infections with bone lesions concerned Negroes, Mexicans, and Filipinos.

BLASTOMYCOSIS

Multifocal osteomyelitis in systemic infections with *Blastomyces dermatitidis* is found in about 25% of the cases.[63, 64] The predilected sites are, again, spine, skull, and the bones of the hands, lower legs and feet. Radiologically and microscopically, the lesions are not different from coccidioidomycosis.[65] Soft tissue abscesses, fistulae, and joint involvement are common.[59]

PARACOCCIDIOIDOMYCOSIS

Paracoccidioides brasiliensis, which usually localizes in the nasal or oral cavity, may occasionally, in systemic infections, cause lytic caseating bone lesions. They are similar to those seen in blastomycosis except for the different morphology of the fungus.[61]

CRYPTOCOCCOSIS

About 10% of infections with *Cryptococcus neoformans* show hematogenous lesions in the skeleton, usually multiple.[61] The lesions are mostly circumscribed and osteolytic on x-ray.[66] The microscopic appearance, however, is different from the other systemic fungus infections. The usual response of inflammatory cells is sparse or lacking. The predominating cell reaction is histiocytic and may simulate a neoplasm. The organisms are frequently present in large numbers, mostly intracellular, but may not be readily recognized in routine hematoxylin- and eosin-stained sections. Cryptococcus infection is not uncommonly found as a complication of lymphoma, especially Hodgkin's disease.[67, 68]

HISTOPLASMOSIS

Systemic infections with *Histoplasma capsulatum* rarely involve bone.[69] However, the African species of *Histoplasma duboisii* often causes multiple lytic bone lesions, especially in the skull and in the small bones of the hands and feet (Fig. 14). The tissue response is mainly a histiocytic, tumor-like granuloma. Other than histiocytes there is very little inflammatory cell reaction.[70]

PHYCOMYCOSIS

Mucor and similar opportunistic invaders may cause infections, most commonly of the paranasal sinuses, which occasionally extend into bone. The majority of the patients are diabetics.[71] The author has seen progressive destruction of the cranial vault in an Iranian boy due to a mixed staphylococcal and mucor osteomyelitis.

SPOROTRICHOSIS

Infection with *Sporothrix schenckii* rarely disseminates; however, about 10% of systemic sporotrichosis show focal osteomyelitis[72] and often joint involvement.[73]

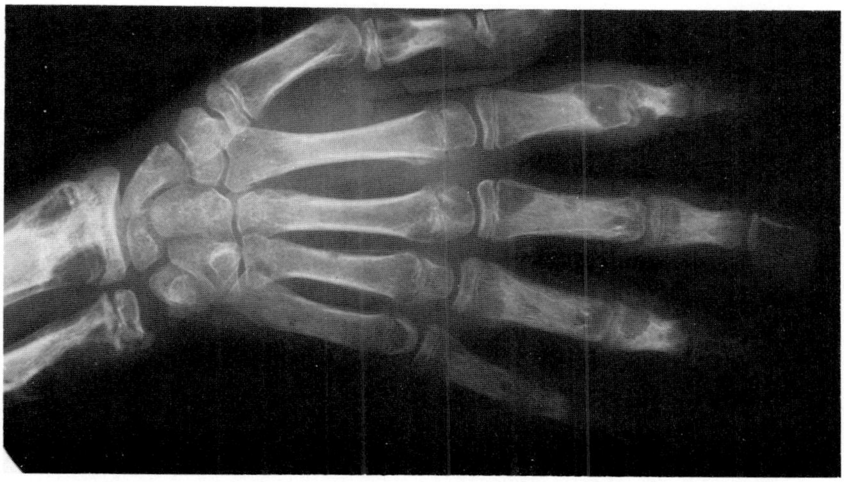

FIG. 14. Disseminated lytic bone lesions in *Histoplasma duboisii* infection. (Courtesy of Dr. Stanley Bohrer, Ibadan, Nigeria.)

The abscesses consist of a granuloma-like border containing giant cells surrounded by a wall of lymphocytes and plasma cells. Extensive necrosis is uncommon. The organisms, with the rare exception of eosinophilic asteroid bodies containing fungus cells, are usually not demonstrable in human lesions but can be recovered in culture. The bone lesions are mostly lytic, but marked periosteal bone formation is observed if the process involves the periosteum. The bones most commonly involved are the tibia, skull (especially the frontal bone), and the tubular bones of the feet. The diagnosis depends mainly on obtaining a positive culture. The staphylococcus is often a secondary invader.[73]

ACTINOMYCOSIS

Actinomyces israelii is a higher branching bacteria and not a true fungus. Although it is frequently present in the oral cavity and in tonsillar crypts, it seldom causes infection. If it does, it is almost always accompanied by one or several other bacteria from the beginning.[61] It reaches the bone, usually, by direct extension from an adjacent lesion rather than by the hematogenous route. The most common locations are mandible, maxilla, spine, and ribs.[74, 75] The extremities are rarely involved.[76, 77] The spine and ribs are affected by extension of pulmonary and pleural actinomycosis causing periostitis and osteomyelitis of several adjacent vertebrae and ribs. The transverse processes and neural arches are often more affected than the vertebral bodies. The process is mainly lytic except for reactive periosteal bone formation. The mandible or, less commonly, the maxilla are directly infected through carious teeth and infected tooth sockets. In the jaws, sclerotic reactive bone around the abscesses is more marked than in other fungus infections. The actinomycotic tissue is often grossly yellow. The abscesses show a border of abundant lipid macrophages and contain floating colonies of the organism surrounded by an eosinophilic material (sulphur granules) which can be seen with the naked eye as yellow particles (Fig. 15). In

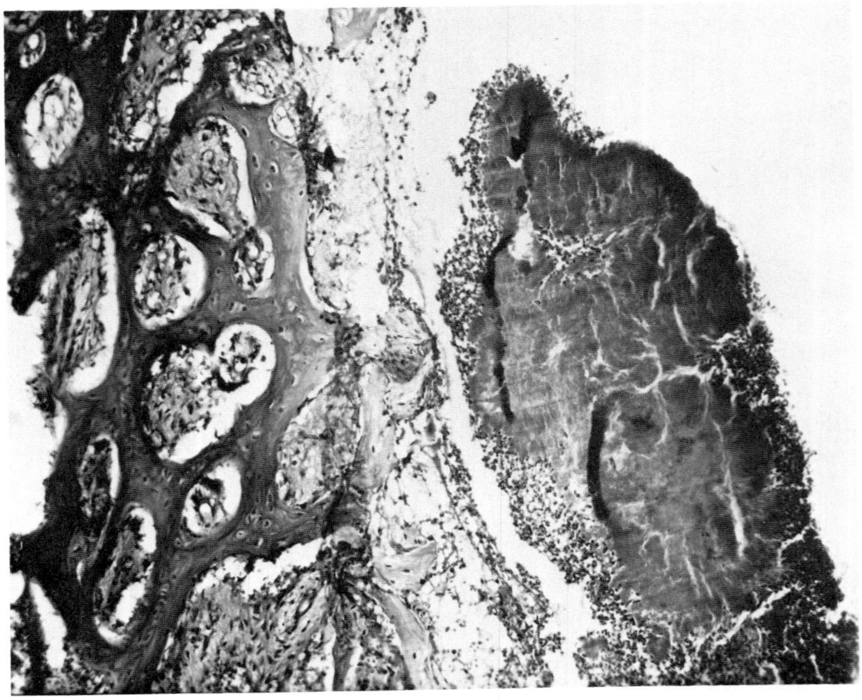

FIG. 15. Actinomycotic abscess of mandible with sulphur granule surrounded by purulent exudate; 14-year-old male; × 100.

chronic cases with marked fibrosis, sulphur granules may be very scarce. Tubercle-like granulomas and giant cells are usually not found. Anaerobic culture is important in suspected cases. Extensive fistula formation is common, but larger sequestra are usually not found.

NOCARDIOSIS

Nocardia asteroides can occasionally cause focal bone lesions, secondary to pulmonary disease (Fig. 16). The organism is not seen in routine hematoxylin and eosin stains, and granules are usually absent.

MADUROMYCOSIS

This is an infection caused by a variety of actinomycetes and true fungi, occurring in tropical and subtropical areas. At least 6 species of actinomycetes and 16 different fungi have been identified as etiologic agents.[61] The lesions usually involve the foot[78] in barefoot going populations, and rarely the upper extremity[79] or other areas.[80] The disease is much more common in males. The organisms reach the deeper tissue and bones from skin lacerations. The bone lesion is characterized by a multifocal lytic osteomyelitis with multiple skin fistulae, progressively involving most of the tarsal and adjacent bones. Microscopically, it appears as a chronic purulent osteomyelitis with very little, if any, reactive bone formation. The colonies of organisms are usually abundantly present in the purulent exudate, forming grossly visible granules of various colors (black, red, pink, white, and yellow). The color of the granules allows one to

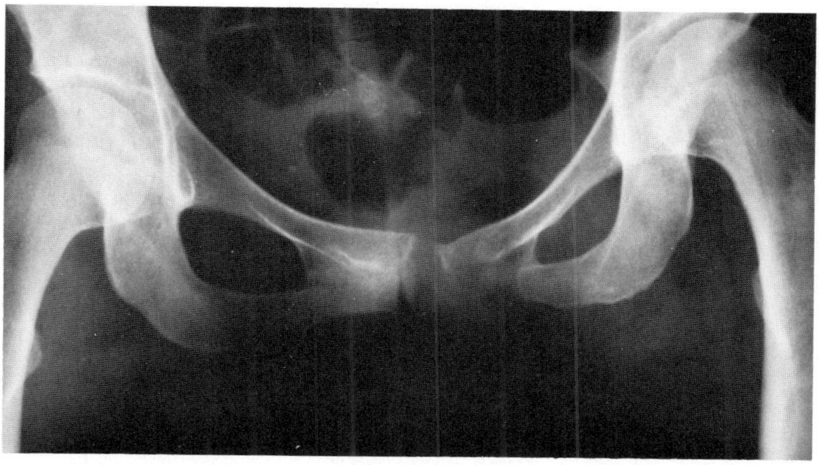

FIG. 16. Nocardia osteomyelitis of pubic bone. The organism was recovered from fistula drainage; 27-year-old female.

narrow down the choice to a smaller group of organisms producing the same pigment. The granules, as in actinomycosis, consist of a central core of filamentous or mycelial organisms and a peripheral zone of eosinophilic material, similar in all granule-forming infections and possibly of host origin. The use of the immunofluorescence technique might clarify this point.[81]

REFERENCES

1. Wilensky, A. O.: *Osteomyelitis: Its Pathogenesis, Symptomatology, and Treatment*. New York, Macmillan Co., 1934.
2. Waldvogel, F. A., Medoff, G., and Swartz, M. N.: Osteomyelitis; clinical features, therapeutic considerations and unusual aspects. Springfield, Ill., Charles C. Thomas, 1971.
3. Lauche, A.: 1. Die unspezifischen Entzündungen der Knochen. In *Handbuch der speziellen pathologischen Anatomie und Histologie*. IX/4, pp. 1–80, Berlin, J. Springer, 1939.
4. Lennert, K.: Pathologische Anatomie der Osteomyelitis, *Verh. Dtsch. Orthop. Ges. 51:* 27–64, 1965.
5. Green, W. T., and Shannon, J. G.: Osteomyelitis of infants; a disease different from osteomyelitis of older children. *Arch. Surg. 32:* 462–493, 1936.
6. Winters, J. L., and Cahen, I.: Acute hematogenous osteomyelitis; a review of sixty-six cases. *J. Bone Joint Surg. 42A:* 691–704, 1960.
7. Gilmour, W. N.: Acute haematogenous osteomyelitis. *J. Bone Joint Surg. 44B:* 841–853, 1962.
8. Harris, N. H., and Kirkaldy-Willis, W. H.: Primary subacute pyogenic osteomyelitis. *J. Bone Joint Surg. 47B:* 526–532, 1965.
9. Leonard, A., Comty, C. M., Shapiro, F. L., and Raij, L.: Osteomyelitis in hemodialysis patients. *Ann. Intern. Med. 78:* 651–658, 1973.
10. Krempien, B., and Ritz, E.: Osteomyelitis of both femora in a patient on maintenance hemodialysis with severe uremic osteopathy. *Virchows Arch. (Pathol. Anat.) 356:* 119–126, 1972.
11. Holzman, R. S., and Bishko, F.: Osteomyelitis in heroin addicts. *Ann. Intern. Med. 75:* 693–696, 1971.
12. Selby, R. C., and Pillay, K. V.: Osteomyelitis and disc infection secondary to Pseudomonas aeruginosa in heroin addiction. Case Report. *J. Neurosurg. 37:* 463–466, 1972.
13. Wray, T. M., Bryant, R. E., and Killen, D. A.: Sternal osteomyelitis and costochondritis after median sternotomy. *J. Thorac. Cardiovasc. Surg. 65:* 227–233, 1973.
14. Trueta, J.: The three types of acute haematogenous osteomyelitis; a clinical and vascular study. *J. Bone Joint Surg. 41B:* 671–680, 1959.

15. Harris, N. H.: Some problems in the diagnosis and treatment of acute osteomyelitis. *J. Bone Joint Surg. 42B:* 535–541, 1960.
16. Trueta, J., and Harrison, M. H. M.: The normal vascular anatomy of the femoral head in adult man. *J. Bone Joint Surg. 35B:* 442–461, 1953.
17. Trueta, J.: The normal vascular anatomy of the human femoral head during growth. *J. Bone Joint Surg. 39B:* 358–394, 1957.
18. Spurrier, E.: Joint sequestra of osteomyelitis. *J. Bone Joint Surg. 11:* 747–753, 1929.
19. Banks, S. W., Krigsten, W., and Compere, E. L.: Regeneration of epiphyseal centers of ossification. *J. A. M. A. 114 2:* 23–27, 1940.
20. Halbstein, B. M.: Bone regeneration in infantile osteomyelitis; report of a case with fourteen year follow-up. *J. Bone Joint Surg. 49A:* 149–152, 1967.
21. Blanche, D. W.: Osteomyelitis of infants. *J. Bone Joint Surg. 34A:* 71–85, 1952.
22. Dennison, W. M.: Haematogenous osteitis in the newborn. *Lancet 2:* 474–476, 1955.
23. Zadek, I.: Acute osteomyelitis of the long bones of adults. *Arch. Surg. 37:* 531–545, 1938.
24. Wiley, A. M., and Trueta, J.: The vascular anatomy of the spine and its relationship to pyogenic vertebral osteomyelitis. *J. Bone Joint Surg. 41B:* 796–809, 1959.
25. Kulowski, J.: Pyogenic osteomyelitis of the spine; an analysis and discussion of 102 cases. *J. Bone Joint Surg. 18:* 343–364, 1936.
26. Bruno, M. S., Silverberg, T. N., and Goldstein, D. H.: Embolic osteomyelitis of the spine as a complication of infection of the urinary tract. *Am. J. Med. 29:* 865–878, 1960.
27. Griffiths, H. E. D., and Jones, D. M.: Pyogenic infection of the spine; a review of twenty-eight cases. *J. Bone Joint Surg. 53B:* 383–391, 1971.
28. Barnes, W. C., and Malament, M.: Osteitis pubis. *Surg. Gynecol. Obstet. 117:* 277–284, 1963.
29. Lavalle, L. L., and Hamm, F. C.: Osteitis pubis; its etiology and pathology. *J. Urol. 66:* 418–423, 1951.
30. Mortensen, H.: Osteitis pubis. *J. Urol. 66:* 412–417, 1951.
31. Exner, G. U.: Die plasmacelluläre Osteomyelitis. *Langenbecks Arch. Chir. 326:* 165–185, 1970.
32. Freund, E.: Über Osteomyelitis und Gelenkseiterung. *Virchows Arch. (Pathol. Anat.) 283:* 325–353, 1932.
33. Kinnman, J. E. G., and Lee, H. S.: Chronic osteomyelitis of the mandible; clinical study of thirteen cases. *Oral Surg. 25:* 6–11, 1968.
34. Panders, A. K., and Hadders, H. N.: Chronic sclerosing inflammations of the jaw; osteomyelitis sicca (Garré), chronic sclerosing osteomyelitis with fine-meshed trabecular structure, and very dense sclerosing osteomyelitis. *Oral Surg. 30:* 396–412, 1970.
35. Murphy, J. B.: Bone and joint disease in relation to typhoid fever. *Surg. Gynecol. Obstet. 23:* 119–143, 1916.
36. Giaccia, L., and Idriss, H.: Osteomyelitis due to salmonella infection. *J. Pediatr. 41:* 73–78, 1952.
37. Saphra, I., and Winter, J. W.: Clinical manifestations of Salmonellosis in man; an evaluation of 7779 human infections identified at the New York Salmonella Center. *N. Engl. J. Med. 256:* 1128–1134, 1957.
38. Black, P. H., Kunz, L. J., and Swartz, M. N.: Salmonellosis; a review of some unusual aspects. *N. Engl. J. Med. 262:* 811–817, 1960.
39. Ebrahim, G. J., and Grech, P.: Salmonella osteomyelitis in infants. *J. Bone Joint Surg. 48B:* 350–353, 1966.
40. Weaver, J. B., and Sherwood, L.: Hematogenous osteomyelitis and pyarthrosis due to salmonella suipestifer. *J. A. M. A. 105:* 1188–1189, 1935.
41. Hook, E. W., Campbell, C. G., Weens, H. S., and Cooper, G. R.: Salmonella osteomyelitis in patients with sickle-cell anemia. *N. Engl. J. Med. 257:* 403–407, 1957.
42. Golding, J. S. R., MacIver, J. E., and Went, L. N.: The bone changes in sickle cell anaemia and its genetic variants. *J. Bone Joint Surg. 41B:* 711–718, 1959.
43. Diggs, L. W.: Bone and joint lesions in sickle cell disease. *Clin. Orthop. 52:* 119–143, 1967.
44. Widen, A. L., and Cardon, L.: Salmonella typhimurium osteomyelitis with sickle cell-hemoglobin C disease; a review and case report. *Ann. Intern. Med. 54:* 510–521, 1961.
45. Hook, E. W.: Salmonellosis; certain factors influencing the interaction of *Salmonella* and the human host. *N. Y. Acad. Med. Bull. 37:* 499–512, 1961.

46. Kaye, D., and Hook, E. W.: The influence of hemolysis on susceptibility to Salmonella infection; additional observations. *J. Immunol. 91:* 518–527, 1963.
47. Spink, W. W.: *The Nature of Brucellosis.* Minneapolis, University of Minnesota Press, 1956.
48. Lowbeer, L.: Brucellotic osteomyelitis of the spinal column in man. *Am. J. Pathol. 24:* 723–724, 1948.
49. Kelly, P. J., Martin, W. J., Schirger, A., and Weed, L. A.: Brucellosis of the bones and joints. Experience with thirty-six patients. *J. A. M. A. 174:* 347–353, 1960.
50. Cockshott, P., and MacGregor, M.: The natural history of osteomyelitis variolosa. *J. Fac. Radiologists, London. 10:* 57–63, 1959.
51. Cockshott, P., and MacGregor, M.: Osteomyelitis variolosa. *Quart. J. Med. 51:* 369–387, 1958.
52. Davidson, J. C., and Palmer, P. E. S.: Osteomyelitis variolosa. *J. Bone Joint Surg. 45B:* 687–693, 1963.
53. Sewall, S.: Vaccinia osteomyelitis; report of case with isolation of vaccinia virus. *Bull. Hosp. Joint Dis. 10:* 59–63, 1949.
54. Elliott, W. D.: Vaccinial osteomyelitis. *Lancet 2,* 1053–1055, 1959.
55. Cochran, W., Connolly, J. H., and Thompson, I. D.: Bone involvement after vaccination against smallpox. *Brit. Med. J. 2:* 285–287, 1963.
56. Wright, L. T., and Logan, M.: Osseous changes associated with lymphogranuloma venereum. *Arch. Surg. 39:* 108–121, 1939.
57. Dykes, J., Segesman, J. K., and Birsner, J. W.: Coccidioidomycosis of bone in children. *Am. J. Dis. Child. 85:* 34–42, 1953.
58. Birsner, J. W., and Smart, S.: Osseous coccidioidomycosis; a chronic form of dissemination. *Am. J. Roentgenol. 76:* 1052–1060, 1956.
59. Wilson, J. W., and Plunkett, O. A.: The fungous diseases of man. Berkeley, Univ. of California Press, 1965.
60. Miller, D., and Birsner, J. W.: Coccidioidal granuloma of bone. *Am. J. Roentgenol. 62:* 229–236, 1949.
61. Emmons, C. W., Binford, C. H., and Utz, J. P.: Medical Mycology, 2nd ed., Philadelphia, Lea and Febiger, 1970.
62. Carter, R. A.: Infectious granulomas of bones and joints, with special reference to coccidioidal granuloma. *Radiology 23:* 1–16, 1934.
63. Witorsch, P., and Utz, J. P.: North American blastomycosis; a study of 40 patients. *Medicine 47:* 169–200, 1968.
64. Cushard, W. G., Jr., Kohanim. M., and Lantis, L. R.: Blastomycosis of bone; treatment with intramedullary amphotericin-B. *J. Bone Joint Surg. 51A:* 704–712, 1969.
65. Boswell, W. L.: Roentgen aspects of blastomycosis. *Am. J. Roentgenol. 81:* 224–230, 1959.
66. Collins, V. P.: Bone involvement in cryptococcosis (torulosis). *Am. J. Roentgenol. 63:* 102–112, 1950.
67. Collins, V. P., Gellhorn, A., and Trimble, J. R.: The coincidence of cryptococcosis and disease of the reticulo-endothelial and lymphatic systems. *Cancer 4:* 883–889, 1951.
68. Littman, M. L., and Walter, J. E.: Cryptococcosis; current status. *Am. J. Med. 45:* 922–932, 1968.
69. Schwartz, J.: Histoplasmosis in *Human Infections with Fungi, Actinomycetes and Algae,* edited by Baker, R. D., pp. 67–130. Berlin and New York, J. Springer-Verlag, 1971.
70. Cockshott, W. P., and Lucas, A. O.: Radiological findings in histoplasma duboisii infections. *Brit. J. Radiol. 37:* 653–660, 1964.
71. Straatsma, B. R., Zimmerman, L. E., and Gass, J. D. M.: Phycomycosis; a clinicopathologic study of fifty-one cases. *Lab. Invest. 11:* 963–985, 1962.
72. Beitzke, H.: 11. Aktinomykose der Gelenke, pp. 563–567; 15. Seltene Mykosen der Knochen und Gelenke I. Sporotrichose, pp. 612–623. In *Handbuch der speziellen pathologischen Anatomie und Histologie.* IX/2, *Gelenke und Knochen.* Berlin, J. Springer, 1939.
73. Altner, P. C., and Turner, R. R.: Sporotrichosis of bones and joints; review of the literature and report of six cases. *Clin. Orthop. 68:* 138–148, 1970.
74. Nathan, M. H., Radman, W. P., and Barton, H. L.: Osseous actinomycosis of the head and neck. *Am. J. Roentgenol. 87:* 1048–1053, 1962.
75. Young, W. B.: Actinomycosis with involvement of the vertebral column; case report and review of

the literature. *Clin. Radiol. (London). 11:* 175–182, 1960.

76. Martinelli, B., and Tagliapietra, E. A.: Actinomycosis of the arm. *Bull. Hosp. Joint Dis. 31:* 31–42, 1970.
77. Mendelsohn, B. G.: Actinomycosis of a metacarpal bone; report of a case. *J. Bone Joint Surg. 47B:* 739–742, 1965.
78. Oyston, J. K.: Madura Foot; a study of twenty cases. *J. Bone Joint Surg. 43B:* 259–267, 1961.
79. Symmers, D., and Sporer, A.: Maduromycosis of the hand; with special reference to heretofore undescribed foreign body granulomas formed around disintegrated chlamydospores. *Arch. Pathol. 37:* 309–318, 1944.
80. Majid, M. A., Mathias, P. F., Seth, H. N., and Thirumalachar, M. J.: Primary mycetoma of the patella. *J. Bone Joint Surg. 46A:* 1283–1286, 1964.
81. Winslow, D. J., and Steen, F. G.: Considerations in the histologic diagnosis of mycetoma. *Am. J. Clin. Pathol. 42:* 164–169, 1964.

Chapter 5

Idiopathic Aseptic Necrosis

D. S. SPRINGFIELD AND W. F. ENNEKING

Aseptic necrosis (osteonecrosis) of the bone occurs in multiple clinical settings. Trauma damages local vessels, leading to bone necrosis along the opposing surfaces of all fractures. In selected anatomic locations this vascular damage may lead to necrosis of significant portions of bone, *i.e.*, femoral head, carpal navicular bone, and talar body.

Aseptic necrosis of bone, in the absence of trauma, is also well recognized. The ossific nucleus of the femoral head prior to epiphyseal plate closure (Legg-Calvé-Perthes disease), humeral capitulum (Panner's disease), tarsal navicular (Köhler's disease), carpal lunate (Kienböck's disease), and second metatarsal head (Freiberg's disease) are common sites of bone infarction not associated with trauma. Osteochondritis dissecans includes both traumatic and nontraumatic lesions. The large majority of these lesions occur prior to epiphyseal closure.

In the adult, nontraumatic aseptic necrosis is associated with several systemic diseases. However, the majority of nontraumatic aseptic necrosis of bone occurring after epiphyseal closure has no known cause and is appropriately termed idiopathic aseptic necrosis (IAN). The common site of this lesion is the femoral head, and the resultant damage to this major weight-bearing joint is a significant cause of disability. The need for early treatment, when the clinical signs are occult, the roentgenographic findings are subtle, and the histopathologic changes are limited, adds to the need for a clear understanding of this disorder.

The gross and microscopic findings in traumatic aseptic necrosis of the femoral head have been well described.[6, 7, 33] These consist essentially of necrosis of the marrow elements, marrow infiltration with histiocytes, loss of osteocytes, invasion of the marrow spaces by reparative granulation tissue, osteoblastic deposition of reparative new bone upon the scaffold of the necrotic matrix, osteoclastic resorption of necrotic matrix, and, when this process of "creeping substitution" is complete, repopulation of the marrow spaces with hemopoietic or fatty marrow elements. Though similar reparative events occur, the atraumatic lesion has several significant gross and histologic differences. In addition, an underlying associated systemic disease may be discerned in some instances of atraumatic lesions.

In this chapter the clinical, roentgenographic, gross, histologic, and microradiographic findings in IAN will be correlated. In addition, the differences between

IAN and post-traumatic aseptic necrosis and nontraumatic aseptic necrosis of the femoral head associated with certain systemic diseases will be discussed.

HISTORICAL BACKGROUND

Ernst Freund's description of nontraumatic aseptic necrosis of the adult femoral head in 1926 is credited as the original.[14, 15] In 1939, Chandler, with a simile to myocardial infarction, called IAN "coronary disease of the hip,"[8] and his name is occasionally used as an eponym. These early reports established the now familiar clinical syndrome. Atraumatic necrosis was etiologically associated with SS hemoglobinopathy in 1937 and later.[9, 10, 37] Following the first reported association, other systemic diseases have also been associated with an increased incidence of aseptic necrosis: Gaucher's disease,[1, 2] caisson disease,[24] corticosteroid therapy,[11-13, 39] alcoholism,[22] gout,[20] altered hemostasis,[3] and others.[30] Despite these associations, the pathogenesis of nontraumatic aseptic necrosis remains obscure, and the term "idiopathic" is appropriate. The reported incidence of bilaterality has steadily increased over the years and now approaches 80% with prolonged follow-up.[28]

ANATOMIC CONSIDERATIONS

Although the etiology remains obscure, the vascular anatomy of the femoral head makes it peculiarly vulnerable to ischemia. An appreciation of the femoral head's blood supply leads to an understanding of why it is a predominant site of either traumatic or nontraumatic aseptic necrosis.

The head of the femur is an irregular sphere covered almost entirely by avascular articular cartilage. An intra-articular ligament (ligamentum teres) crosses the cavity of the joint and connects the femoral head to the acetabulum. The base of the femoral head lies at about the rim of the acetabulum and marks the insertion of the joint capsule at the junction of the articular cartilage and the neck of the femur. This insertion lies just proximal to the cartilaginous epiphyseal plate in childhood.

The pattern of the vessels leading to, and within, the femoral head has been extensively described.[18, 23, 31, 36, 42-44] In the adult, the obturator and profunda femoris arteries are the major vessels from which the femoral head vasculature arises. The medial femoral circumflex (MFC), the major vessel to the femoral head, arises posteriorly from the profunda femoris and courses to a lateral posterior position at the base of the femoral neck. Here, at the trochanteric fossa, a branch penetrates the femoral neck and gives rise to the inferior metaphyseal vessels. The terminal branches of the MFC are the more proximal superior metaphyseal, the lateral epiphyseal vessels, and an anastomosis with the lateral femoral circumflex. (LFC). The LFC, also from the profunda femoris, courses anteriorly to the base of the femoral neck and the greater trochanter. The terminal branches are the lateral epiphyseal vessels and the anastomosis with the MFC. Thus the anastomosis of the two circumflex vessels forms a ring about the base of the femoral neck from which the epiphyseal vessels enter the joint capsule distally, run within its reflection about the femoral neck, and enter the femoral head at the base of the articular cartilage. The obturator artery gives rise to the vessel within the ligamentum teres called the medial epiphyseal artery.

Within the femoral head the terminal branches of the epiphyseal and metaphyseal arteries form varying patterns of anastomoses. There is no constant pattern which results in a particular segment of the femoral head being supplied by a particular vessel or set of vessels. In contrast, the vascular supply of the femoral head changes with growth and development. At birth the femoral head has three distinct arterial supplies: 1) medial epiphyseal artery coursing through the ligamentum teres, 2) lateral epiphyseal vessels pass within the capsule, penetrate the femoral head at the capsular insertion, and run extraosseously and horizontally into the cartilaginous femoral head, and 3) metaphyseal vessels, which arise intraosseously, pass up the femoral neck, cross the epiphyseal mechanism, and enter vertically into the femoral head. These three systems have little or no functional anastomosis. The vessel within the ligamentum teres supplies the inferior medial portion of the head about the fovea. The lateral epiphyseal vessels and the metaphyseal vessels are randomly intermixed and do not supply distinct portions of the developing head. During the first 4 years the metaphyseal vessels are the major blood supply to the femoral head, and, save for severe trauma, aseptic necrosis is rare. The medial epiphyseal vessels become progressively less important during this period. The maturing transverse epiphyseal plate becomes an apparent barrier to the metaphyseal vessels by 4 years of age and although the medial epiphyseal vessels can occasionally supply a significant portion of the femoral head by 9 years of age, the lateral epiphyseal vessels are the significant blood supply to the femoral head from 4 to 9 years of age. Thus the femoral head is vulnerable to intra-articular pressure, and Legg-Perthes disease is seen during these years. During early adolescense the medial and lateral epiphyseal vessels establish anastomoses, and with epiphyseal plate closure the metaphyseal vessels cross into the femoral head providing additional anastomoses. With skeletal maturity the lateral epiphyseal vessels continue to furnish the majority of blood supply to the femoral head (Fig. 1). The particular vascular pattern established within the femoral head after epiphyseal plate closure remains constant throughout life.

PATHOLOGIC CONSIDERATIONS

IAN of the femoral head in the adult is the result of segmental infarction of a portion of the femoral head. At its onset the infarct involves a greater portion of the femoral head than the anterior-superior-lateral cone that subsequently becomes delineated by roentgenographs. It is puzzling that the pattern of infarction does not correspond to the anatomic distribution of any single major vessel. The medial portion of the femoral head, supplied by the medial epiphyseal vessel of the ligamentum teres, is spared from infarction.

The consequences of the infarct in this anatomic location are pathologic fracture through the infarct, progressive collapse of the infarct with loss of head contour, and finally, superimposed degenerative arthritis. These gross changes are reflected by clinical and roentgenographic findings of increasing severity during the evolution of the lesion. Previously reported histologic findings during the course of IAN include: articular cartilage invasion by reparative granulation tissue,[26, 32] inadequate creeping substitution,[19, 32] subchondral fracture,[29, 38] marrow necrosis with calcification,[27, 32] synovitis,[32] and trabecular collapse.[16, 38] A

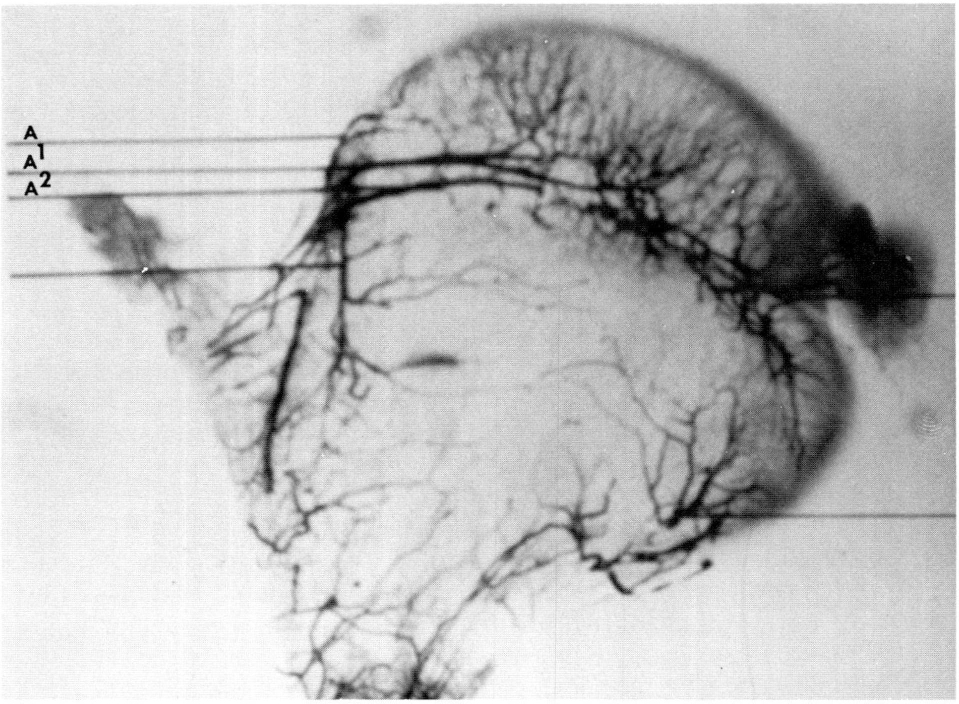

FIG. 1. A coronal section of a normal adult femoral head demonstrating the intraosseous blood supply. Note the abundant anastomoses within the area of the secondary ossification center. The vessels A, A^1, and A^2 are branches of the lateral epiphyseal arteries from the medical femoral circumflex artery. (From Harrison, H. M., and Trueta, J.: *J. Bone Joint Surg. 35-B:* 445. Used with permission.)

previous correlative study of these and other micropathologic observations with the clinical findings and roentgenographic changes led us to a description of six stages in the course of IAN of the femoral head.[28] These are supplemented in this report by additional microradiographic observations of material labeled with tetracycline, and the correlative radioscanning. This correlative data is presented in the six stages previously delineated.

Stage I. The involved hip is asymptomatic, and the patient presents with a normal gait and full range of motion. The early lesion is usually first suspected because of more advanced IAN in the contralateral hip. The diagnosis is suggested by irregular mottled densities within the femoral head on the roentgenogram without clear definition of the infarct (Fig. 2, *A* and *B*). Increased uptake of a bone isotope is seen in Stage I with sufficiently sensitive techniques. This increased radioactivity has been reported up to 18 months prior to identifiable roentgenographic changes.[5] If an arthrotomy of the hip is done at this point, the articular surface appears normal in color, texture, and consistency. Core biopsies of the infarct and the overlying articular cartilage show well advanced creeping substitution about the periphery of the infarct. Seams of viable bone are annealed on necrotic preexisting trabeculae (Fig. 2*C*). These thickened trabeculae account for the mottled densities seen on the roentgenogram. The seam of new bone lining the edges bind the radioisotopes and account for the increased scan activity. If the patient is given tetracycline prior to biopsy, this new bone can be identified macro- and microscopically in undecalcified sections by its characteristic yellow fluorescence when exposed to ultraviolet light (Fig. 2*D*). In these peripheral areas of early repair the marrow spaces are filled with vascular granulation tissue.

The more central and subchondral areas of the infarct contain acellular trabeculae with occasional repair trabeculae which are tetracycline-positive (Fig. 2*E*). The marrow spaces are filled with histiocytes, monocytes, and ghost cells of adipose tissue. There is no calcification of the necrotic fat on microradiographs made on Stage I. The deep layer of the articular cartilage below the osteochondral junction is acellular. This is the portion of the articular cartilage that is dependent upon the subchondral capillaries for nutritional support. The more superficial layers (circa 60%) of the articular cartilage contain viable chondrocytes. This portion receives its nutrition from the synovial fluid.

Stage II. The patient remains asymptomatic in Stage II. The cardinal distinction that marks the gradual transition from Stages I to II is the clear demarcation of the infarct by a thick rim of radiodensity about its periphery. This rim, seen on anterior-posterior (AP) and lateral roentgenograms, invariably demonstrates the lesion to lie in the antero-superior-lateral portion of the femoral head (Fig. 3*A*). Careful inspection of the roentgenograms including laminograms shows no change in the contour of the femoral head, no narrowing of the articular cartilage, and no pathologic fracture beneath the subchondral plate. This is reflected in the normal appearance of the articulating surface and the absence of clinical symptoms.

Core biopsies through Stage II infarcts demonstrate the outer portion of the radiodense rim to be thick reactive viable trabeculae surrounding the infarct. The inner portion of this rim is composed of areas of well advanced creeping substitution (Fig. 3*B*). In some of these trabeculae, multiple cement lines within the trabeculae suggest that the infarction may be a repetitive phenomenon. These areas are positive on radio scintimetry and are tetracycline-positive on fluorescent microscopy. The more central portion of the infarct is filled with necrotic fat and acellular unrepaired trabeculae. The peripheral area of creeping substitution makes surprisingly little inroads on the unrepaired areas over rather prolonged periods of time. The transition from Stage I through Stage II, as measured by roentgenograms, has been shown to vary from 6 months to 5 years with an average of 15 months. Here and there in the unrepaired tetracycline negative, scan negative, portions of the infarct, the necrotic fat is replaced by a dense eosinophilic amorphous material that has a fibrillar pattern when observed with polarizing lenses (Fig. 3*C*). Microradiographs from undecalcified sections demonstrate mineralization within the eosinophilic amorphous material (Fig. 3*D*). This mineralization is in the form of scattered macroscopic punctate masses rather than ground off bits of necrotic trabeculae as previously supposed. These areas of mineralization are tetracycline-negative indicating that this process is one of avascular deposition of minerals from tissue fluids rather than the result of repair following revascularization. These areas are seen from one to two

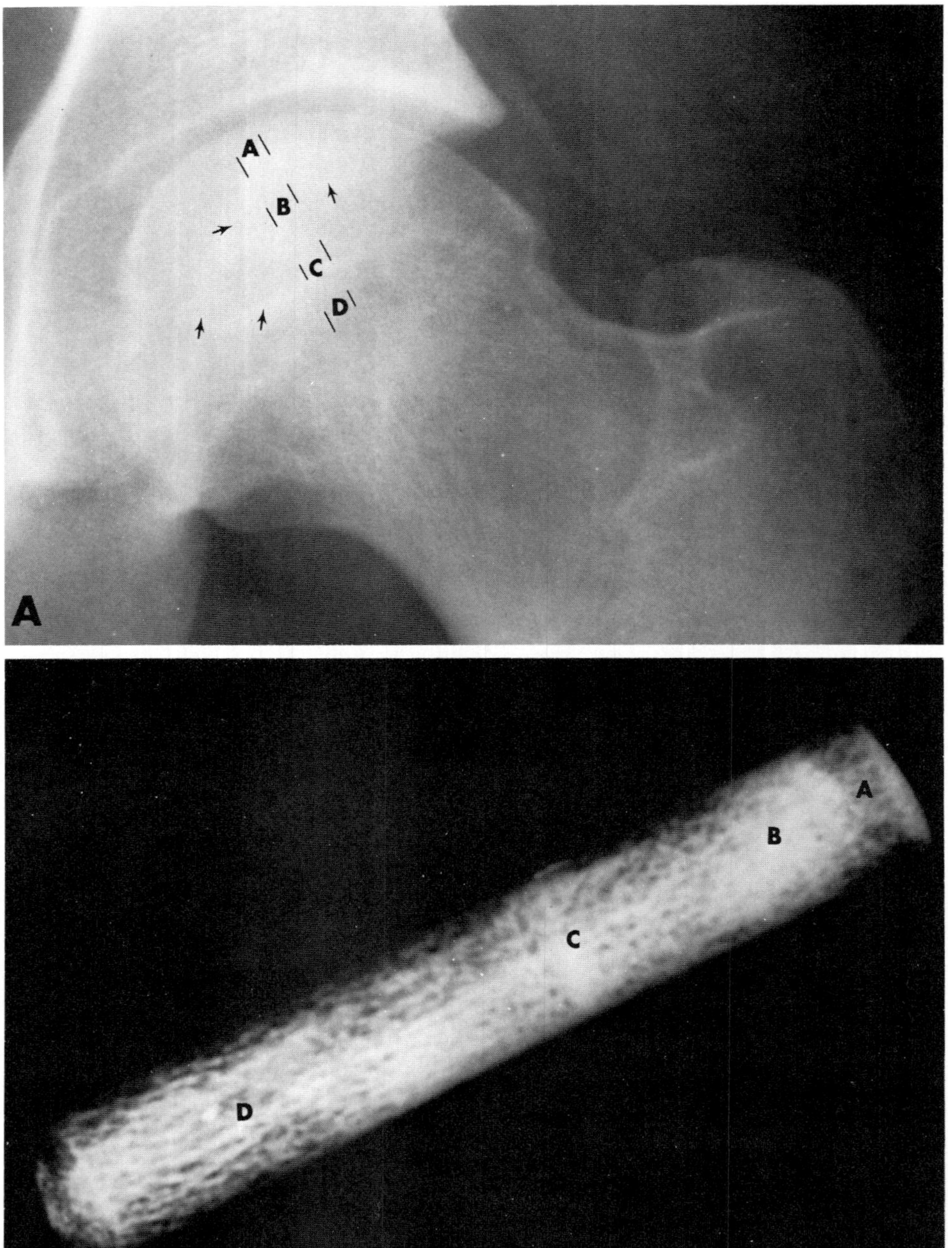

FIG. 2. The illustrations are from a 26-year-old male with bilateral idiopathic aseptic necrosis. They demonstrate the typical findings in Stage I. *A*, Anterior-posterior (A-P) roentgenogram. Note the mottled radiodensities within the femoral head (*arrows*). The broken lines outline the position of the core biopsy. *A* is over the subchondral portion; *B* is over the infarct; *C* is over the junction of infarct and viable bone; and *D* is over a normal portion of the femoral head. The remainder of the roentgenogram appears normal. *B*, roentgenogram of core biopsy (× 5). The letters correspond to those in Figure 2*A*. The subchondral bone (*A*) is of normal density. The area within the infarct (*B*)

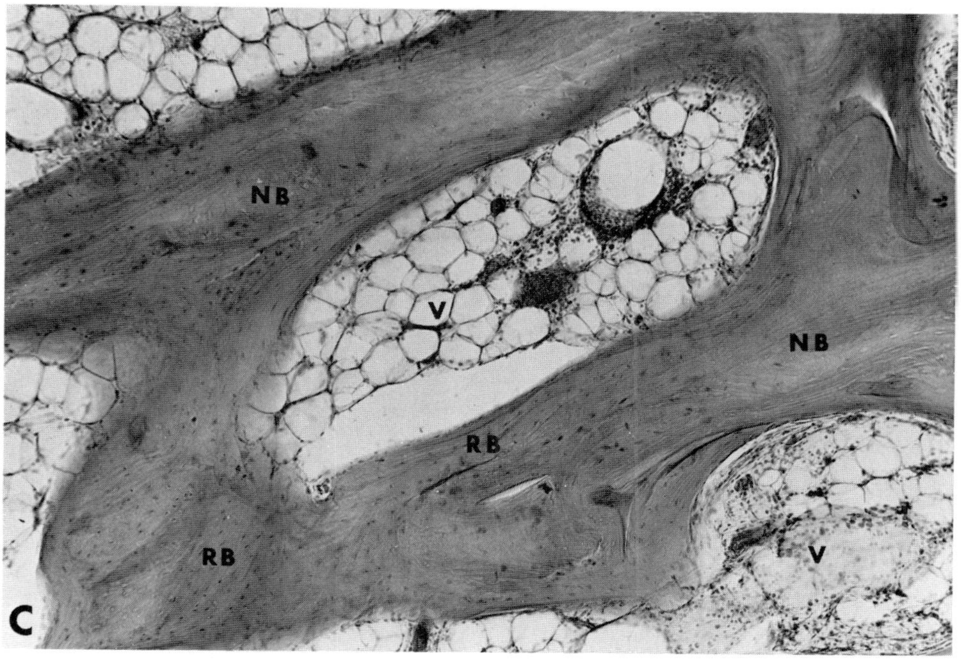

centimeters below the articular surface but at this stage are so scattered as to not contribute appreciably to the overall radiodensity of the infarct.

The deep layer of the articular cartilage and the underlying subchondral plate remain intact and acellular, save at the periphery of the infarct. At this junction the vascular reaction about the infarct penetrates the subchondral plate and invades the deep portion of the articular cartilage. These penetrations are so small that they are not apparent on roentgenograms or gross inspection.

The principal significance in distinguishing Stage I from Stage II lies in the certainty of the diagnosis. In many instances, the subtle changes in Stage I

---

is more radiodense than normal. This increased radiodensity accounts for the mottling seen on the roentgenogram of the Stage I femoral head. A reactive rim (*C*) can be seen marking the edge of the infarct. The reactive rim is not seen on the plain roentgenogram until Stage II. A portion of the femoral head (*D*) outside the infarcted cone demonstrates the "normal" density. *C*, photomicrograph (× 100). This is a representative histologic section within the infarct marked *B* in Figure 2*B*. The marrow is viable (*V*). Repair bone (*RB*) is annealed to necrotic bone (*NB*) as creeping substitution occurs. The increased thickness of the trabeculae account for the increased radiodensity identified by the *arrows* on the A-P roentgenogram in Figure 2*A*. *D*, photograph (× 5). This is the core biopsy as outlined in Figure 2*A*. The letters mark the portion of the biopsy as described in Figure 2*A*. The photograph was made under ultraviolet light. The patient had received 250 mg of tetracycline for 10 days preoperatively. Within the infarct (*B*) areas of fluorescence (*arrows*) are seen. The fluorescence within the infarct supports the thesis that there was active bone production when the patient received the tetracycline. *E*, photomicrograph (× 100). This is a section of the subchondral bone marked by *A* in the preceding illustrations. Viable articular cartilage (*VC*) is present. The subchondral bone is necrotic (*NB*), and there is no evidence of creeping substitution. The radiodensity of this area is unchanged as the trabeculae are of normal thickness.

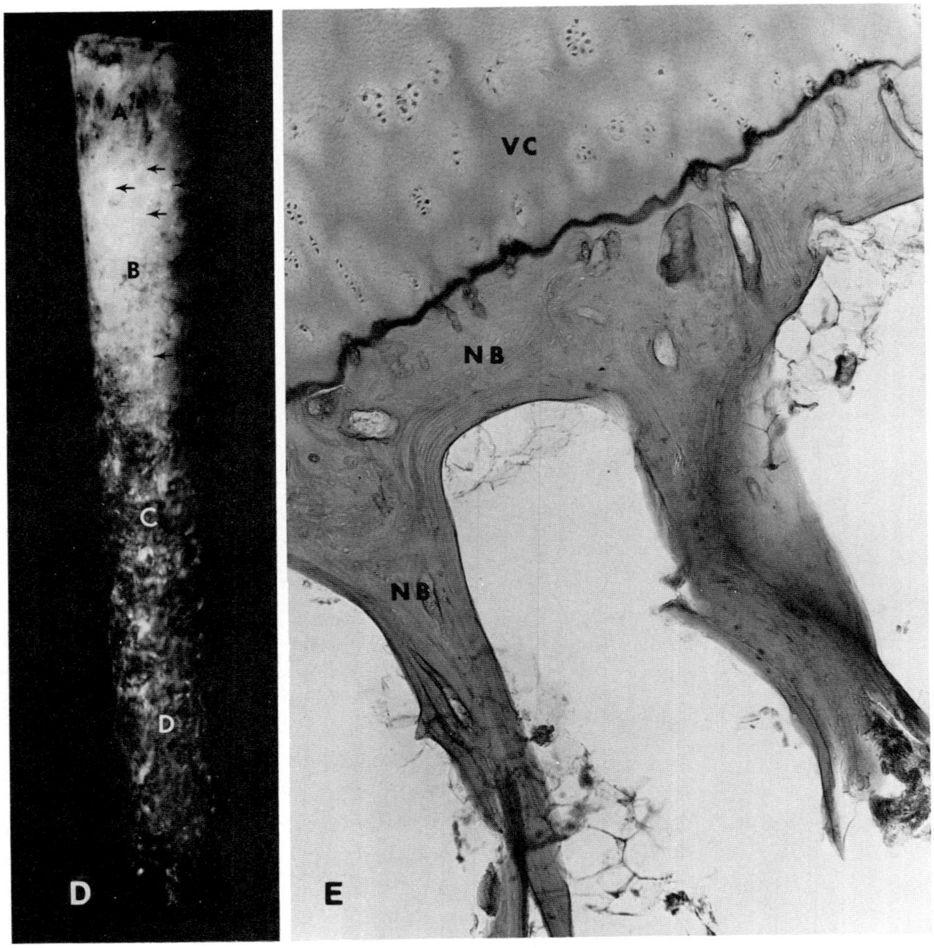

require confirmatory core biopsy with tetracycline labeling prior to therapeutic decision, while in Stage II the roentgenographic findings are generally so distinctive that, when accompanied by the appropriate clinical signs, biopsy is usually unnecessary.

Stage III. The sudden onset of hip pain and the roentgenographic appearance of a pathologic subchondral fracture are the hallmarks of Stage III. The patient complains of mild, intermittent pain in the groin which radiates down the medial thigh. The gait and range of hip motion remain normal although the extremes of motion are painful. Core biopsies of symptomatic infarcts have disclosed roentgenographically occult subchondral fractures. In general, the symptoms are more reliable than the roentgenogram in announcing the occurrence of a fracture. The subchondral fracture is first seen on the lateral view (Fig. 4*A*). In the A-P view, the head maintains a normal contour, and the articular cartilage appears intact. This so-called "crescent sign" is not seen on the A-P view because it is in the anterior quadrant and appears in profile only when viewed laterally. The infarcted cone remains well outlined on both views by a dense border of reactive and reparative new bone. The entire infarct now appears homogeneous and more radiodense than in the earlier stages. There continues to be increased activity on radioscan.

The gross examination of the femoral head is now abnormal. The articular cartilage covering the anterior-superior-lateral portion of the femoral head is "ballottable" due to the underlying fracture, having the feel of a tennis ball. Early in Stage III this ballottement is the only abnormal gross finding, while later, although the cartilage is intact, a distinct wrinkle in the articular cartilage outlines the anterolateral portion of the underlying infarct (Fig. 4*B*). Coronal sections show the central unrepaired portion as a chalky ivory white necrotic area. The subchondral fracture is seen just beneath the articular cartilage and its subchondral plate (Fig. 4*C*). Coronal sections through the posterior portion usually demonstrate the underlying infarct to be more posterior in extent than the subchondral fracture would indicate. Study of many specimens show that generally the cap of articulating cartilage with its 1 to 2-mm-thick rim of subchondral bone covers the anterior 75% of the infarct. The more posterior 25% of the infarct has an intact overlying articular cartilage. The radiodense rim of reaction remains and appears as reddish-tan dense cancellous bone.

Microscopic examination of the coronal sections show more inactive reparative bone than Stage II. The intratrabecular granulation tissue is less vascular and has much more dense fibrous connective tissue (Fig. 4*D*). Creeping substitution has not penetrated the infarct to any great extent. On the inner border of the reparative zone occasional osteoclasts are seen resorbing acellular unrepaired trabeculae. Granulation tissue at the subchondral periphery of the infarct continues to invade the deeper layers of the articular cartilage and produces clefts which dissect towards the surface. These underlie the wrinkle seen from the surface. The subchondral fracture occurs through unrepaired bone and is bordered on either side by necrotic bone and marrow. Within the cleft are seen bits of ground-off trabecular debris and fibrin. Small fragments of necrotic trabeculae are seen within the marrow spaces abutting the subchondral fracture. In the central, grossly evident, unrepaired area there is no reparative-bone or evidence of revascularization, and the marrow is replaced by calcified debris (Fig. 4*C*). Microradiographs demonstrate calcified debris within the marrow spaces and distinguish the debris from the fragmented necrotic trabeculae. The calcified debris has no organization on the microradiograph, while the fragmented necrotic trabeculae maintain their lamellar pattern. Tetracycline does not label the center of the infarct confirming the histologic picture of avascularity. The periphery of the infarct is, however, heavily labeled with tetracycline suggesting increased bone formation bordering the infarct as did the dense border seen on the roentgenogram.

Determination of the pathologic fracture on core biopsy in the symptomatic patient prior to its appearance on the roentgenogram and the tetracycline labeling of the reactive reparative rim (now so heavy that it is readily apparent grossly) are helpful diagnostic procedures in Stage III. These gross observations may be quickly and easily complemented by a roentgenogram of the core

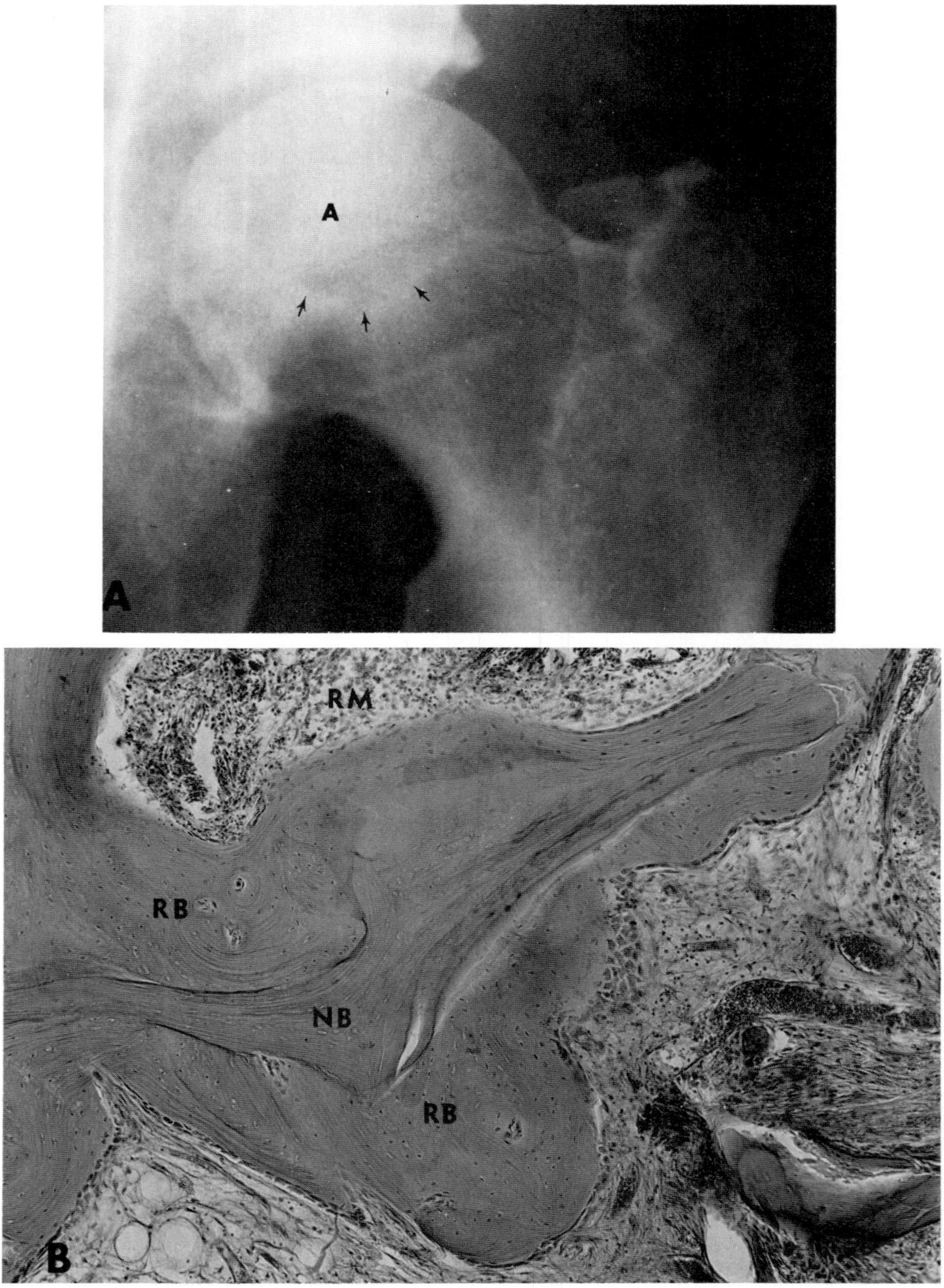

FIG. 3. The illustrations are from a 40-year-old male with bilateral idiopathic aseptic necrosis demonstrating the typical findings in Stage II. *A*, anterior-posterior roentgenogram. The infarcted cone (*A*) has become a homogeneous radiodensity. The border of the infarcted cone is marked by a reactive rim (*arrows*). The articular cartilage appears of normal thickness. There is no abnormality of the femoral head configuration. *B*, photomicrograph (× 100). This histologic section is typical of the reactive rim (*arrows* in Fig. 3*A*). At the periphery of the infarcted cone creeping substitution continues. Thick bars of repair bone (*RB*) are annealed to old necrotic trabecular bone (*NB*). The

specimen and macroscopic inspection of the unembedded fluorescent core with a dissecting microscope.

Stage IV. This stage is marked by substantial increase in disability and beginning collapse of the femoral head. These changes generally ensue within a few months after the onset of Stage III. Episodes of "locking" of the hip in flexion are experienced when patients arise. Pain is more severe and constant. The gait becomes antalgic, the Trendelenburg sign positive, the range of motion decreases, and occasionally an audible click can be produced by external rotation of the flexed and abducted hip ("figure 4" sign). The A-P roentgenogram now shows distinct flattening of the dome of the femoral head, and there is a "step-off" at the lateral margin of the acetabulum (Fig. 5*A*). The density is more apparent within the infarct. This is due in part to the continuing mineralization of the unrepaired necrotic fat and in part to the increasing osteoporosis in the viable portions of the femoral head and neck adjacent to the infarct. This porosity is due to the disuse occasioned by pain. Between the peripheral rim and the inner "wedge"-shaped infarct a radiolucent zone begins to emerge that may appear to be a second more major fracture. Radioactive scans become increasingly positive secondary to the thickening reactive bone surrounding the infarct and the reactive bone of early degenerative arthritis about the acetabular side of the joint (Fig. 5*B*).

On inspection, the femoral head appears deformed with depression of the anterosuperiolateral quadrant (Fig. 5*C*). With this depression the articular cartilage fractures where it was previously wrinkled and this cleft forms a loose flap of articular cartilage. The flap when curled up, produces the locking of the hip. Extruding from under the flap is creamy, chalky, gritty debris which irritates the synovium causing a secondary painful synovitis. On the cut surface the infarct is seen as a chalky yellowish triangle beneath the cleft. It is surrounded by dense reactive trabeculae. The differences between the unrepaired central infarct and the combination of the repairing periphery and reaction are well brought out by tetracycline labeling. Studying coronal sections demonstrates that the deep infarct extends considerably more posterior than the loose flap.

Microscopically the reparative bone at the periphery is much more mature. Heavy seams of new, fluorescent bone are much more prominent than the acellular central cores. Osteoclastic activity is also more prominent. A broad dense layer of mature fibrous tissue is present between the now stalled repair and the central infarct. This zone accounts for the radiolucency seen on the A-P

---

marrow appears reactive (*RM*) suggesting continued biologic activity. *C*, photomicrograph (× 100). This histologic section is from the roentgenographic homogeneous density (*A* in Fig. 3*A*) within the infarcted cone. The marrow is necrotic and calcifying (*CM*). The trabeculae are necrotic (*NB*), and no evidence of actively creeping substitution exists. The calcifying debris within the marrow spaces appears to block the advancing granulation tissue and to impede creeping substitution. *D*, microradiograph (× 100). This is a roentgenogram made of a histology section from a 100 micron thick undecalcified section of bone embedded in epoxy. This section is from an area similar to that shown in Figure 3*C*. Necrotic trabeculae (*NB*) surround the calcifying marrow (*CM*). The punctate calcifications (*arrows*) within the marrow are evidence that the necrotic marrow is calcifying. The homogeneous radiodensity of the infarct on the roentgenogram is secondary to the even distribution of these punctate calcifications.

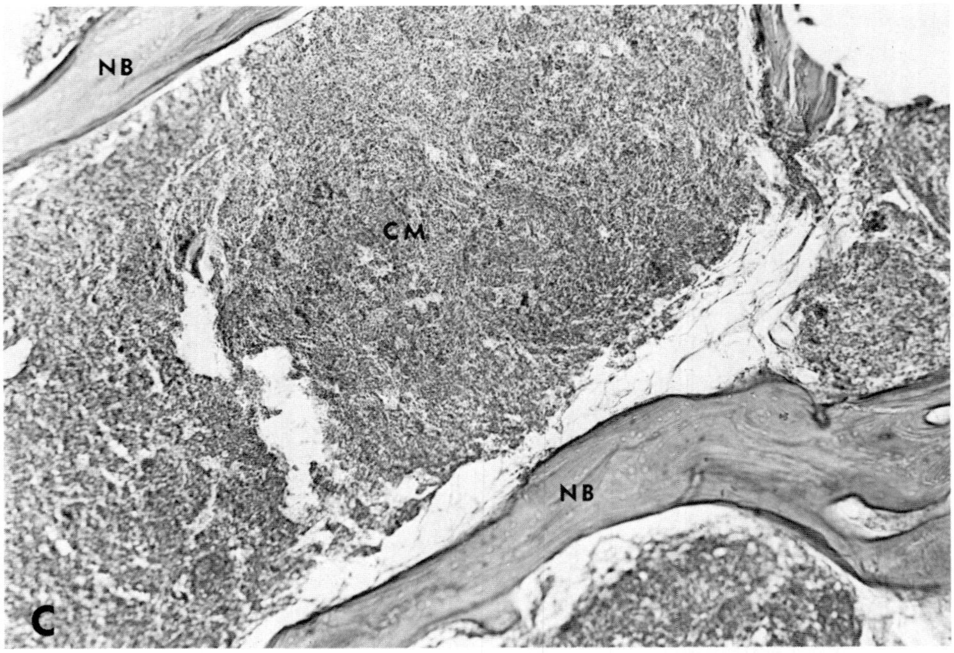

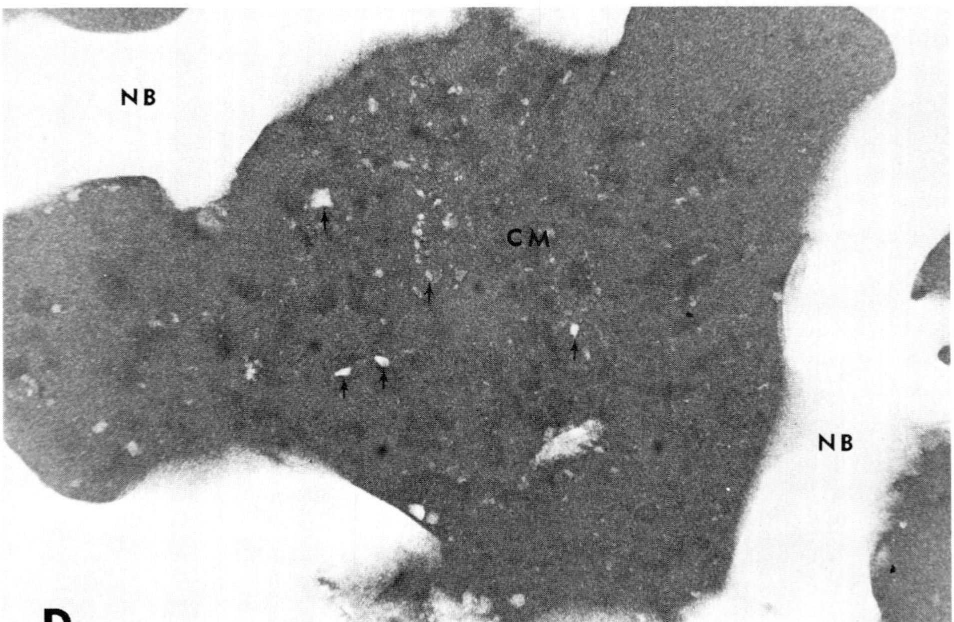

roentgenogram separating the reactive peripheral rim and the inner "wedge"-shaped infarct. The fibrous tissue is quite poorly vascularized and may show scattered minor clefts and/or nests of fibrocartilage. The central unrepaired area of the infarct continues to show no evidence of revascularization, calcified necrotic debris in the marrow spaces, and acellular trabeculae without evidence of creeping substitution. Calcified necrotic debris is a prominent feature in the marrow spaces on the microradiograph.

From the periphery of the subchondral fracture granulation tissue invades the cleft and slowly covers the infarct. With time these granulations mature and, stimulated by the motion of the loose flap, islands of fibrocartilage and bone develop in the pannus-like granulation tissue. The tetracycline label may now be seen lightly bordering the fracture as a result of this reparative tissue as well as heavily marking the mature reparative peripheral rim.

Stage V. The continuous pain is now, months after the onset of collapse, so severe that the patient voluntarily uses external support. A "crunchy" sound may be appreciated at each attempt to bear weight. Marked limitation of motion is quite frequent. The A-P roentgenogram shows progressive flattening, degenerative arthritic changes in the acetabulum, and fragmentation of the infarcted segment (Fig. 6*A*). The infarct itself appears not only fragmented but nearly opaque. Radioscanning continues to be markedly positive with dual activity of aborted repair and arthritic changes.

On gross examination the articular surface is quite irregular. The cartilage overlying the subchondral fracture may be entirely separated from its bed. Frequently this flap is more normal in appearance than the remaining articular cartilage of the femoral head and acetabulum. The weight-bearing surfaces are thin, yellowish, and frayed.

Grossly on the cut surface the depressed, fragmented infarct is mottled by invading granulation tissue. This is reflected by tetracycline fluorescence in these areas. The disintegrating infarct may move slightly, when pushed, through the grayish white fleshy zone of fibrous tissue and fibrocartilage that separates it from the rim of repair (Fig. 6*B*).

Histologic examination of the coronal sections shows completion of repair of the peripheral margin (Fig. 6*C*). Only occasional acellular trabecular cores remain to mark the edge of the infarct. Deep to the loose flap of articular cartilage is an admixture of fibrocartilage, fibrous connective tissue, and new bone produced by reparative enchondral ossification of this reparative fibrocartilage. In the central fragmented area fibrous or granulation tissue has now invaded the areas of amorphous mineralization. The acellular trabeculae in some areas are being resorbed by osteoclasts while in other areas thin seams of new bone show a continuing feeble reparative effort.

Stage VI. Clinically the "end stage" of IAN is pain and restricted motion which incapacitates the patient. Ambulation generally requires two crutches or a wheelchair. Roentgenographically, the severity of the degenerative changes are such that it may be difficult to recognize the underlying cause (Fig. 7*A*). Lateral displacement of the femoral head by large osteophytes, severe flattening, loss of articular cartilage, and large juxta-articular cysts are common to both Stage VI IAN and late degenerative arthritis. Radioscans remain quite positive. The gross appearance of the femoral head is that of degenerative arthritis save in the area of the previous infarct. Here the head is irregularly depressed and covered by wisps of scar of fibrocartilage (Fig. 7*B*). Loose bodies are commonly found within the

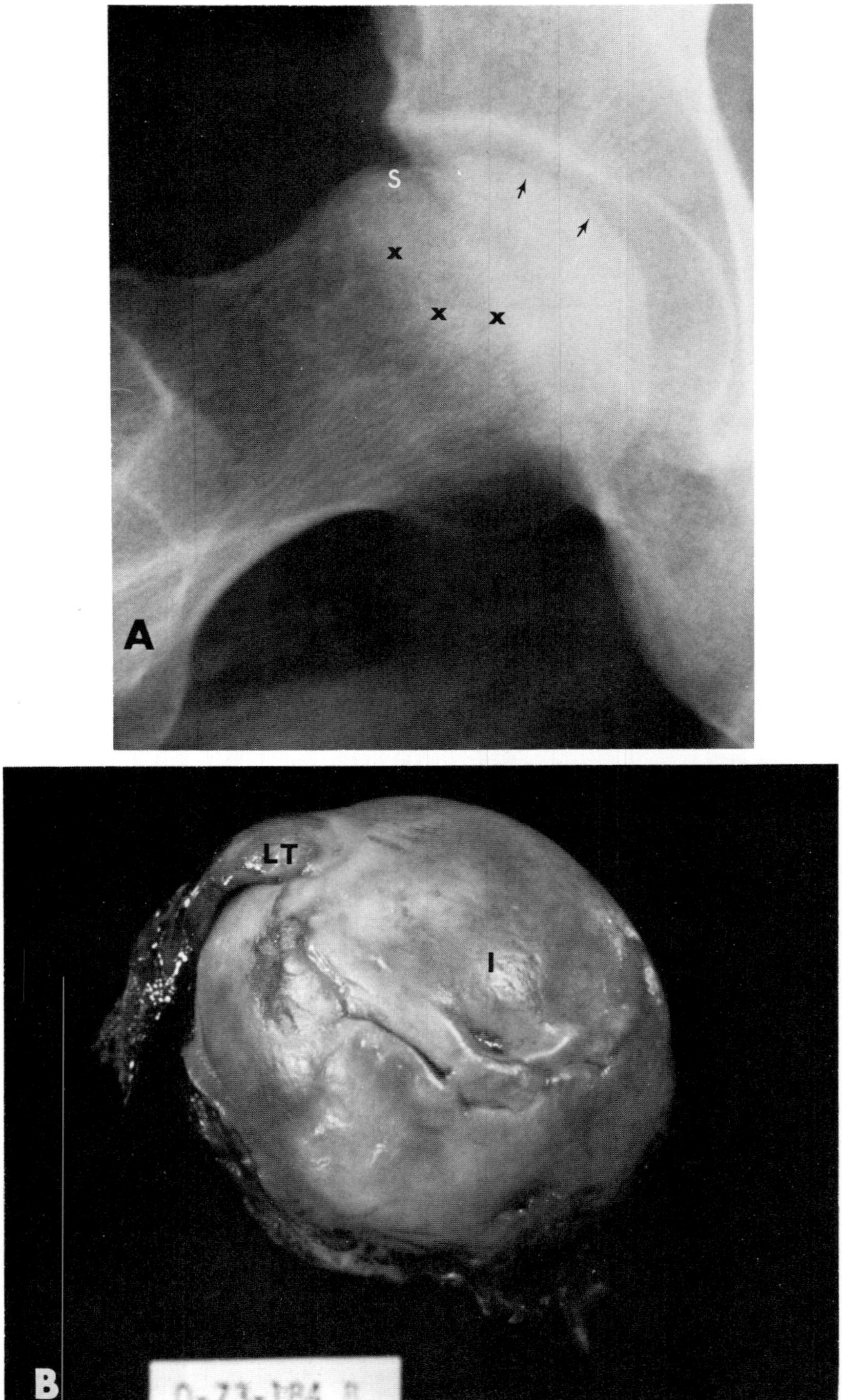
S
x
x
x
A
LT
I
B
0-73-184 B

joint. On coronal section through the infarct the necrotic area may be quite obscure, and a combination of fragmentation and repair makes identification of the necrotic cone difficult. However, under uv light the infarct may now be identified by its increase in fluorescence. At this stage the repair process has finally permeated the central infarct. This is reflected microscopically by revascularized marrow spaces and osteoid-coated trabeculae in the remaining disorganized infarct. This repair seems to penetrate from the subchondral cleft area rather than from the surrounding femoral head. Incomplete repair of isolated acellular trabeculae is still in progress. In fact complete repair may take several years to be accomplished.

It is of some importance to distinguish the severely degenerative hip of IAN from the more common osteoarthritis—particularly when it is unilateral. Identification of IAN leads to a high degree of suspicion that the opposite asymptomatic hip may be involved with an early stage. There may be, in bilateral cases, a long time period between the involvement of both hips as the incidence of bilaterality steadily rises from 40 to 80% when clinical observation is extended from 2 to 10 years.[28]

DIFFERENTIAL DIAGNOSIS

In the majority of instances, the clinical setting associated with aseptic necrosis will indicate the presence or absense of known underlying causes or associations. In some circumstances, however, the clinical presentation is only that of unilateral aseptic necrosis and the associated findings are subtle. In such situations the differential diagnosis may be aided by the gross findings as shown by roentgenograms and by the microscopic examination.

Trauma. Aseptic necrosis following trauma is caused by either fracture of the femoral neck or dislocation of the hip. The fracture is almost always intracapsu-

---

FIG. 4. The illustrations are from a 28-year-old male with bilateral idiopathic aseptic necrosis demonstrating the findings in Stage III. *A*, lateral roentgenogram. This roentgenogram demonstrates the subtle subchondral fraction (*arrows*) referred to as the "crescent sign." The crescent sign is the hallmark of Stage III. Usually the subchondral fracture cannot be seen on the standard anterior-posterior roentgenogram during Stage III. Occasionally, the fracture cannot be demonstrated roentgenographically, but is clinically suspected because of groin pain. A small "step off" (*S*) in the subchondral plate is seen. The reactive rim (*X*'s) continues to be present as in Stage II. *B*, Photograph (× 3). This is a photograph of the gross specimen from Figure 4*A*, The anterior-superior portion is in the foreground, and the ligamentum teres (*LT*) is labeled. The wrinkle in the articular cartilage outlines the underlying subchondral fracture which is present over the anterior-lateral portion of the infarcted cone. The articular cartilage covering the infarct (*I*) does not appear significantly abnormal. There is no cleft in the articular cartilage at this stage, and the subchondral fracture does not communicate with the joint. *C*, histologic section (× 3). This is a coronal section of a Stage III femoral head. The wrinkle in the articular cartilage (*arrow*) is shown to mark the extent of the subchondral fracture (*A*). Beneath the subchondral fracture, an area of necrotic trabeculae with calcifying marrow (*B*) is present. The histologic appearance of this area is similar to that shown in Figure 3*C*. A zone of necrotic fibrous tissue yet to calcify (*C*) is located between the reactive rim (*D*) and the area of calcified marrow and necrotic bone (*B*). *D*, photomicrograph (× 100). This histologic section is representative of area *C* in Figure 4*C*. The trabeculae are necrotic (*NB*) with no evidence of creeping substitution. The marrow spaces are filled with dense avascular fibrillar tissue (*FT*). This appearance is representative of "stalled repair" and is in marked contrast to the picture of active creeping substitution as shown in Figures 2*C* and 3*B*.

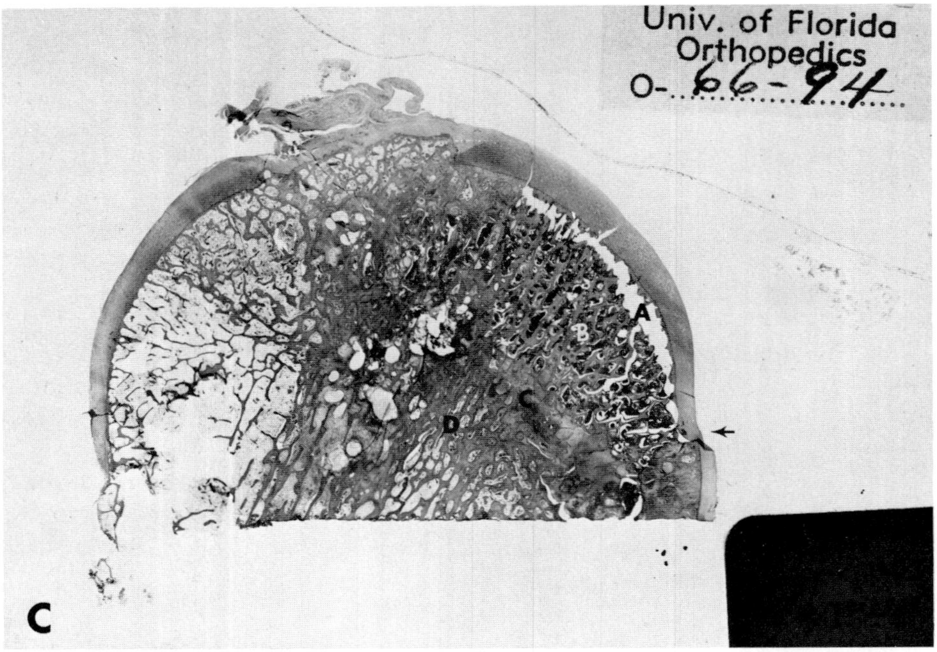

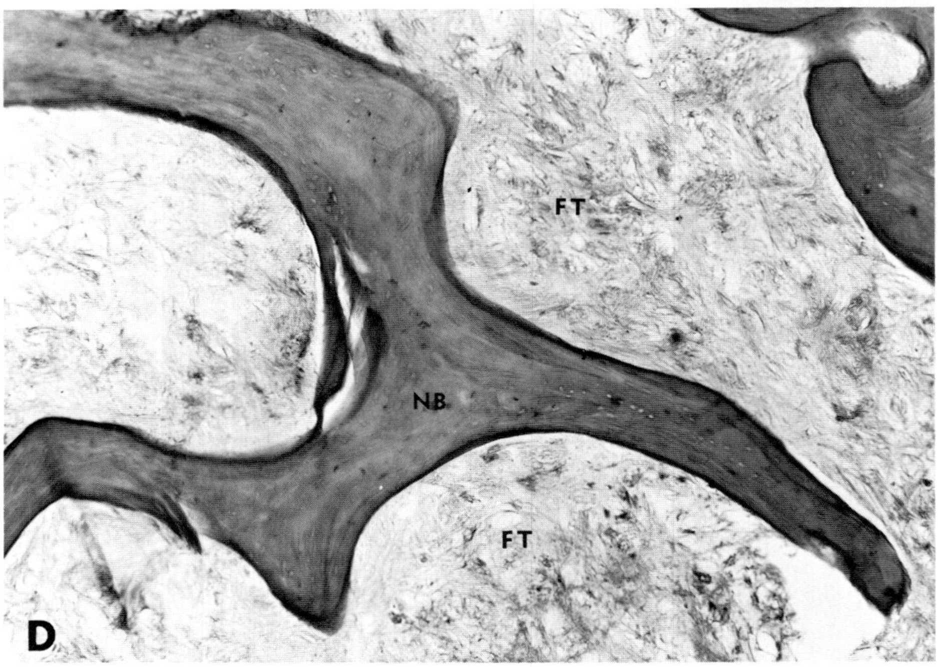

lar, and the incidence rises with the proximity of the fracture line to the base of the femoral head. The roentgenographic and histologic appearance of aseptic necrosis following a femoral neck fracture is dependent upon whether the fracture unites. The ununited femoral neck fracture with a necrotic femoral head is

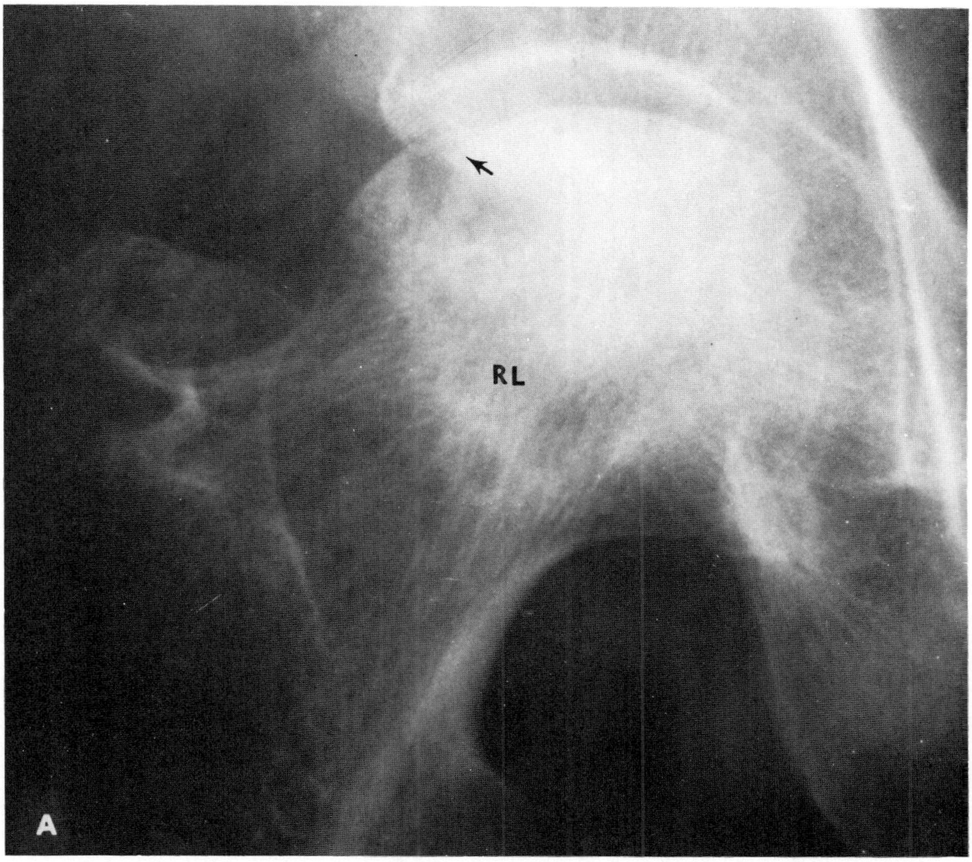

FIG. 5. These illustrations are composite from patients with Stage IV idiopathic aseptic necrosis. *A*, anterior-posterior roentgenogram. The femoral head is more misshapen than in Stage III. The "step off" (*arrow*) is obvious, and flattening of the femoral head apparent. The radiolucency (*RL*) about the base of the infarct is an area of "stalled repair" without calcification as demonstrated in Figure 4*D*. This has occasionally been mistaken for a fracture. The acetabulum appears normal roentgenographically at this stage. *B*, technetium 99 radioactive scan. The left hip (*arrow*), with marked increase in reactivity, is consistent with this patient's diagnosis of unilateral idiopathic necrosis, Stage IV. The increased reactivity results from the combination of persistent creeping substitution and concomitant degenerative arthritis. Sensitive radioscanning techniques are capable of demonstrating increased activity in a necrotic femoral head prior to changes on the plain roentgenogram. *C*, photograph ($\times$ 1). A sagittal section of a Stage IV femoral head demonstrates the loose "flap" (*arrow*) of articular cartilage and attached subchondral plate. This flap may cause "locking" of the hip and accounts for the positive "Figure 4" sign.

easily distinguished from IAN. The nonunion is easily recognised, the entire femoral head is necrotic, and it is extremely rare for collapse of the head to occur.

Aseptic necrosis following a united femoral neck fracture often is difficult to distinguish from IAN. Once the fracture is united, the patient may be asymptomatic for years with a revascularizing femoral head. The anterosuperior-lateral portion of the femoral head is the last to revascularize.[12] Occasionally this area will revascularize, and the patient will remain asymptomatic and without collapse, but more frequently creeping substitution does not occur in this area

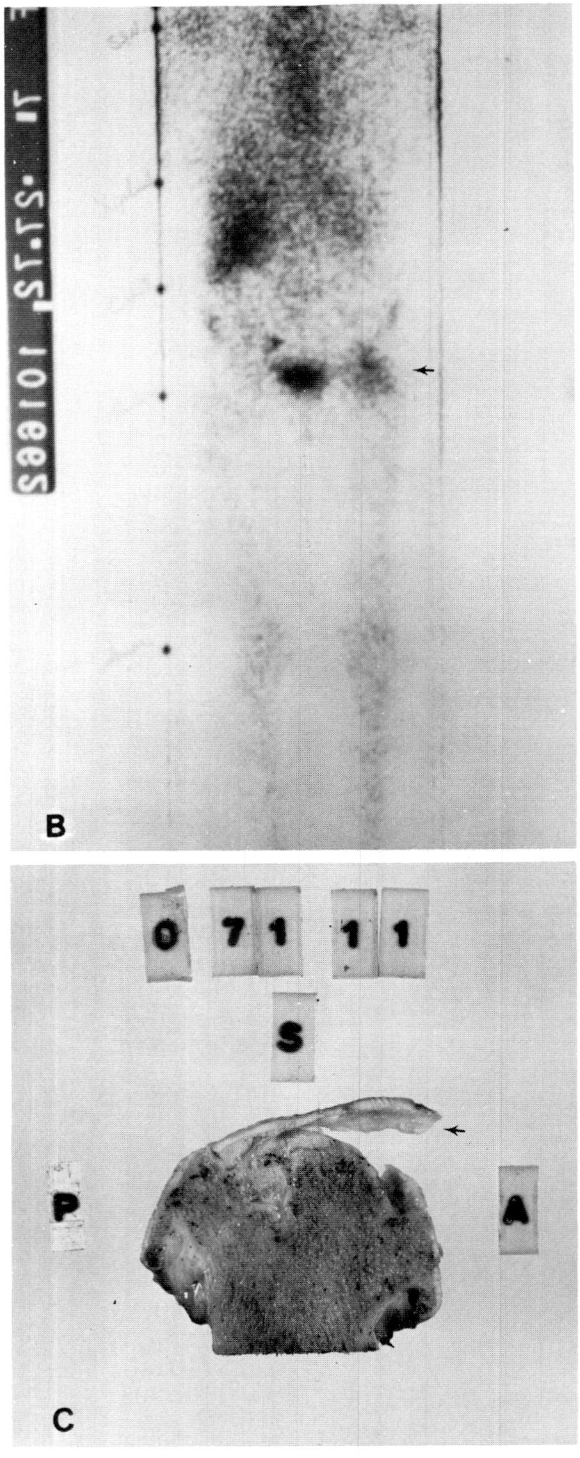
B
0 7 1 1 1
S
P
A
C

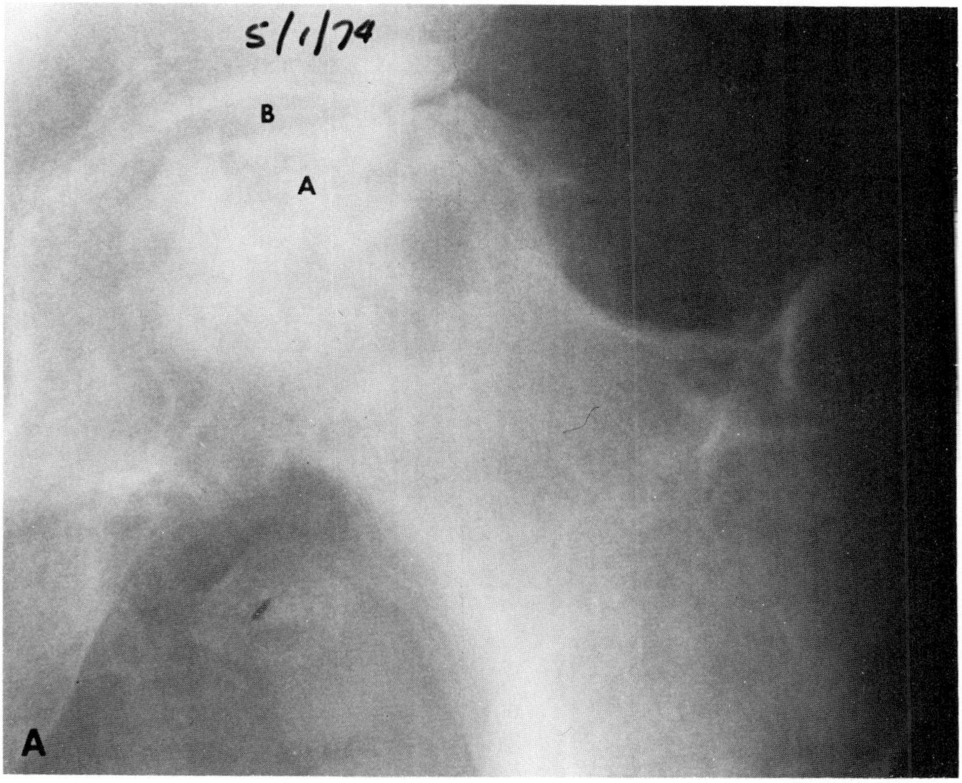

FIG. 6. The illustrations are from a 32-year-old male with unilateral idiopathic aseptic necrosis demonstrating the characteristics of Stage V. *A*, anterior-posterior roentgenogram. The marked deformity of the femoral head with secondary acetabular changes is present. This roentgenographic presentation may easily be mistaken for primary degenerative arthritis. The increase in density within the femoral head (*A*) and preservation of articular cartilage (*B*) should lead to the diagnosis of underlying aseptic necrosis. *B*, histologic section (× 2). This is a coronal section of the femoral head shown in Figure 6*A*. Thick bars of repair bone (*RB*) surround the residual necrotic trabeculae (*NB*). Zones of fibrous tissue (*FT*) are present and indicate that motion occurs between the necrotic bone and repair bone. A loose fragment of articular cartilage is present (*AC*). *C*, photomicrograph (× 100). This histologic picture is typical of *RB* in Figure 6*B*. This advanced repair with thick trabeculae accounts for the increased radiodensity seen within the femoral head in Stage V.

before a deep fracture occurs with collapse of the infarct. Two distinguishing points are present between this "late segmental" collapse after femoral neck fracture and IAN: (1) The necrotic portion of the femoral head at the time of collapse is large (about 50%) compared to that of IAN (about 25%), and the fracture is much deeper or at the periphery of the infarct. (2) Amorphous calcification of necrotic material in the intertrabecular marrow spaces is usually absent. This leads to a more mottled appearance of the infarct on roentgenograms.

Aseptic necrosis following dislocation may resemble IAN quite closely. The onset of symptoms is usually 18 to 21 months after injury. Roentgenogram at this time reveals infarction of the same conelike segment of the femoral head. The evolution is that of aborted repair followed by subchondral fracture leading to severe degenerative arthritis. Only the lack of marrow mineralization is a

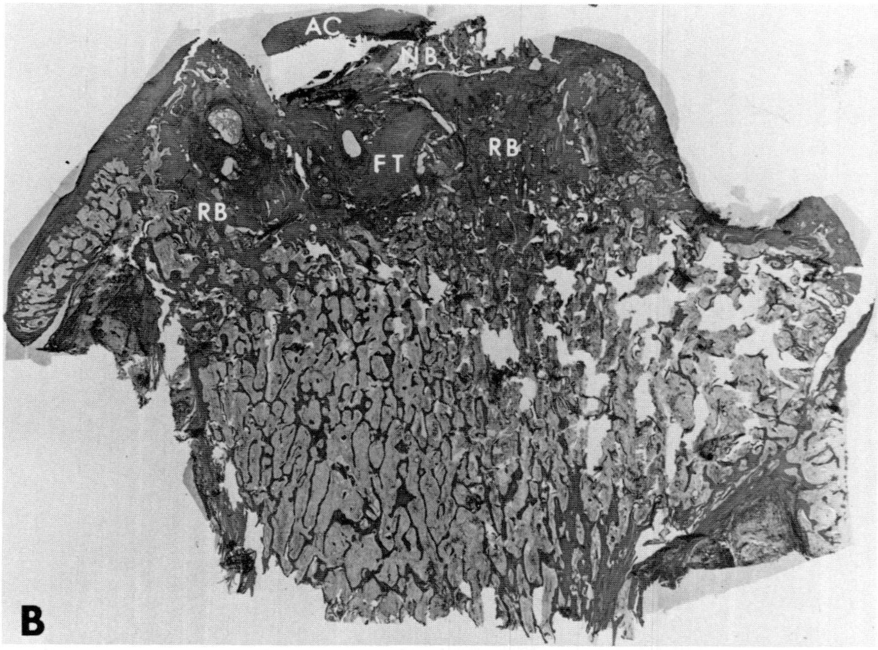

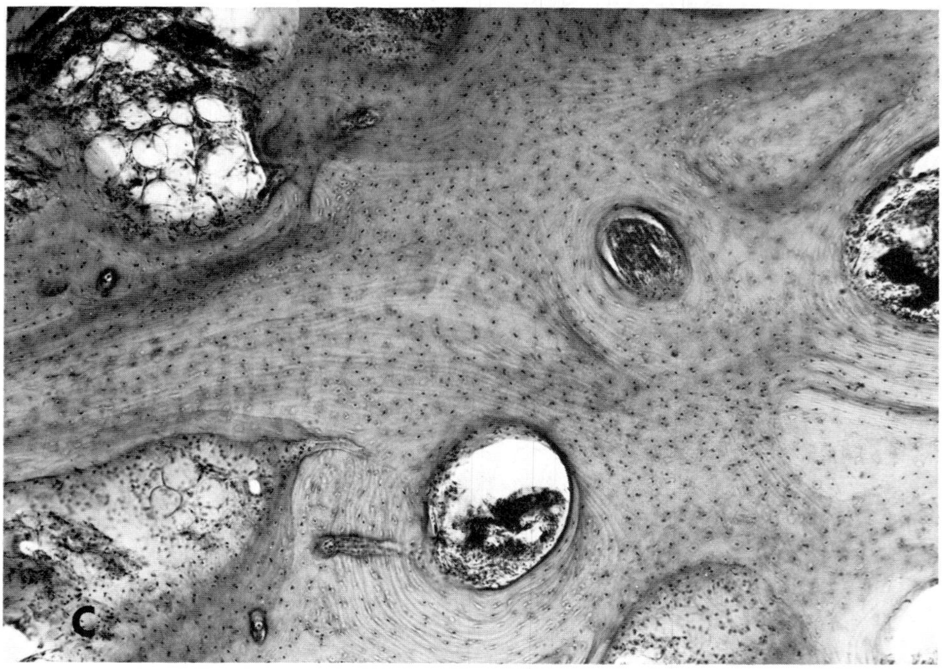

distinguishing feature, and even this finding may be present in long-standing cases.

Sickle cell anemia and related hemoglobinopathies. The skeletal infarcts associated with these conditions, while most common in the femoral head, also

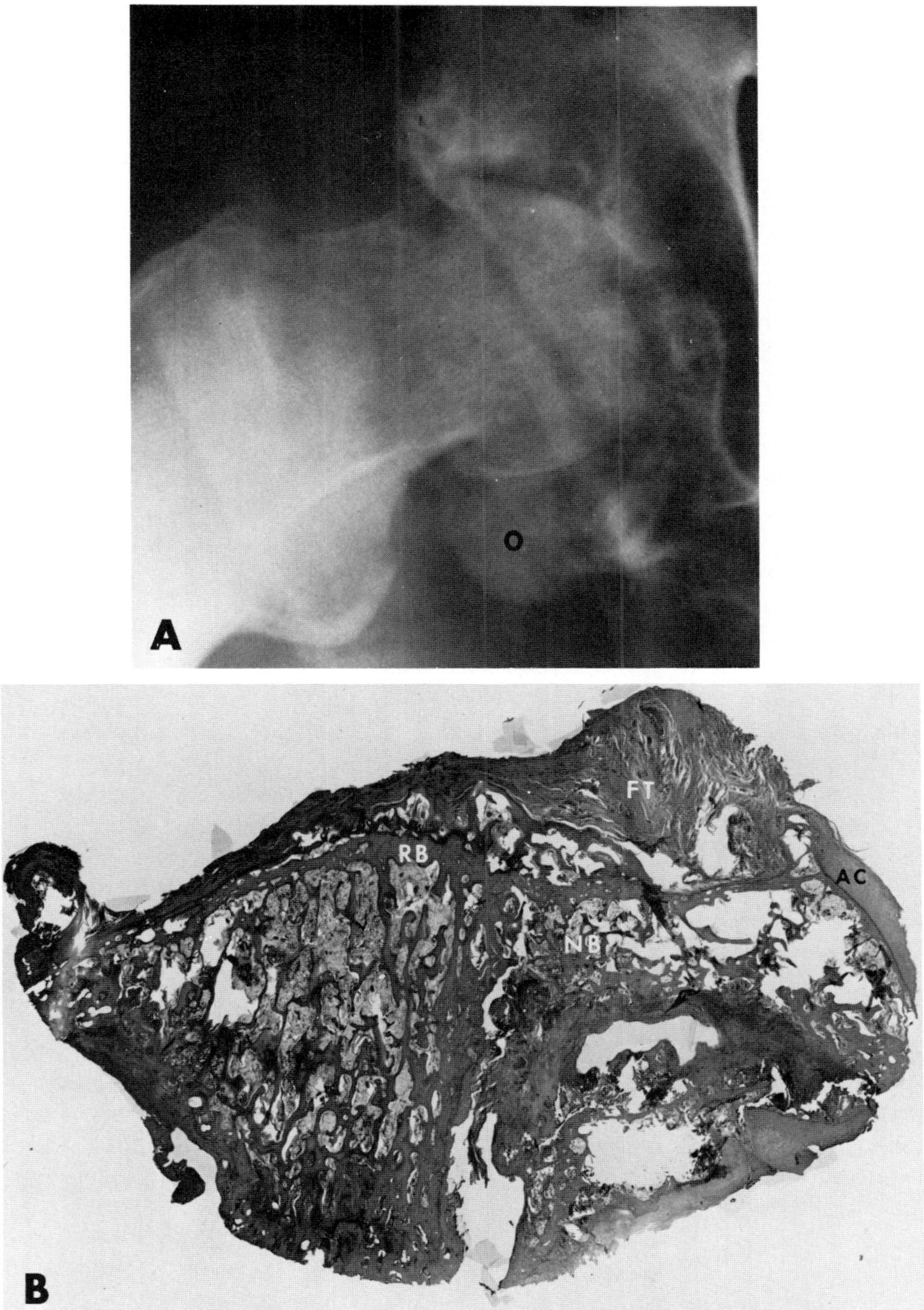

FIG. 7. The illustrations are from an 80-year-old male with bilateral idiopathic aseptic necrosis and demonstrates the findings of Stage VI. *A*, anterior-posterior roentgenogram. Marked destruction of the femoral head, acetabular irregularities, and the medial osteophyte (*O*) are nonspecific roentgenographic changes of "end-stage" degeneration of the hip joint. The irregular density within the femoral head represents the combination of late repair, osteoporosis, and persistent necrotic trabeculae. *B*, histologic section (× 2). This coronal section of the Stage V femoral head shows the marked destruction of articular cartilage (*AC*). Repair bone (*RB*) surrounds the necrotic bone (*NB*) while fibrous tissue (*FT*) covers the major portion of the surface of the femoral head.

and regularly appear simultaneously in the metaphyseal-epiphyseal regions of multiple long bones. When they appear as a lesion of the femoral head the following points are helpful in separating them from IAN: (1) The infarct involves the head in a patchy fashion and extends well down into the femoral neck. (2) The infarcted areas appear ivory-like in their density and with time undergo less mottling and fragmentation. There is frequently a marked discrepancy between the severity of the changes on x-ray and the relatively minor clinical symptoms. (3) Subchondral fracture is unusual. (4) On cut surface the infarct appears as dense white islands of vascular bone surrounded by reddish purple cancellous bone. This reflects the lack of reparative revascularization and the presence of hyperplastic hematopoietic marrow in areas usually filled with fatty marrow. On uv light examination there is relatively little fluorescence in comparison with extensive infarct. (5) Histologically the acellular trabeculae are markedly thickened. They contain multiple parallel cement lines denoting the cyclic reinfarction that may follow each attempt at repair. The marrow spaces contain ghosts of previously thrombosed vessels and dense fibrous connective tissue. Invasion of the subchondral plate and the deep zones of the articular cartilage is much less common than in IAN.

In sum, such changes paint a picture of an infarct in which repair is initiated but with subsequent reinfarction leading to a gradual increase in trabecular size and forestalling collapse for long periods of time. It is noteworthy that such infarcts are frequently contaminated with *Escherichia coli*, and these show superimposed inflammatory changes.

Hypercortisonism. Although the principal skeletal manifestation of prolonged hypercortisonism is severe osteoporosis, aseptic necrosis of the femoral head is quite common. It is most frequently seen as the result of steroid therapy for rheumatoid arthritis, lupus erythematosus, or when used as an immunosuppressant after renal transplantation. The distinguishing features of such infarcts are: (1) Marked osteoporosis of the area of cancellous bone about the infarct. (2) The infarct usually involves the weight-bearing superior dome of the femoral head and is less dense than IAN. (3) Subchondral fracture occurs but is much less common than a gentle sinking of the entire infarct. (4) Histologically the infarct consists of slender acellular trabeculae with little or no annealed repair seams seen. The marrow spaces are sparsely revascularized and contain mostly wispy immature fibrous connective tissue. (5) The bone peripheral to the infarct shows little reaction. The trabeculae are quite slender, and the marrow is hypervascular.

Caisson disease. Infarcts of bone associated with working in compressed air environment, be it deep sea diving or in a caisson, are more common in the humeral head than in the femoral head. The etiology of these infarcts remains obscure. When present in the hip they mimic IAN in all respects, and there are no apparent gross or histologic clues as to their distinctive etiology.

Gaucher's disease. Infarction of the femoral head is a frequent finding in patients afflicted with this peculiar aberration in lipoid storage. The infarcted areas themselves resemble IAN in all respects. The presence of large lipoid-filled macrophages in the marrow spaces of the viable cancellous bone about the infarct is diagnostic. These so-called Gaucher cells are not seen within the infarcted segment itself.

Gout. Patients who present with primary hip pain and who have the picture of IAN are occasionally hyperuricemic. In such instances the synovium of the affected joint may show the histologic reflection of gout. The infarct and surrounding bone of the femoral head, however, show no evidence of gouty tissue. Although the hyperuricemic patient may have subtle alterations in hemostasis leading to aseptic necrosis there is no obvious direct invasion and/or infarction caused by the gouty inflammation *per se*.

Chronic alcoholism. There is a high incidence (0ver 50%) of chronic alcoholism in patients with IAN. Although there have been many speculative discussions of cause and effect there is no documentation of an etiologic relationship. There are no distinguishing gross or microscopic features that permit separation of the alcoholic from the nonalcoholic IAN. The same general situation pertains to the subtle alterations in hemostasis. Although the group at Iowa[3] have shown many different laboratory alterations in coagulation in patients with IAN, no firm etiologic relationship of pathogenesis has been established. These patients have no distinguishing features in their infarcts that might shed light in this regard.

DISCUSSION

The natural history of traumatic aseptic necrosis (TAN) is revascularization, the creeping substitution of living for dead bone, and remodeling of the repaired bone to meet the functional demands placed upon it. This occurs in the TAN seen to some degree at the surfaces of all fractures. TAN of the femoral head does not routinely collapse—in fact spontaneous healing has been well documented.[6] When pathologic fractures and/or collapse occur in TAN they are attendant upon the mechanical weakening produced by the invasive revascularizing granulation tissue that removes the necrotic trabeculae or osteons prior to their repair by new bone. If, however, this pathologic fracture is guarded against by protective devices or supplemented by gratifying procedures, collapse may be averted until sufficient repair has taken place. Similar situations occur in nontraumatic aseptic necrosis particularly in childhood. Spontaneous healing of Legg-Perthes disease without deformity is the rule in young children, and although deformity occurs in older children, it can be to some extent avoided by protection during the reparative and remodeling phases. Spontaneous healing of osteochondritis dissecans about the knee is well known when the condition is recognized prior to pathologic fracture, and adequate steps are taken to prevent it.

In IAN spontaneous healing is rarely observed. In contrast to TAN, the pathologic fracture in IAN occurs through the subchondral area in the absence of weakening by resorption of the acellular trabeculae. It appears rather as a "stress" fracture of the cap of bone and cartilage over the main portion of the infarct. The direction and location of the fracture indicates that the cap is sheared off by a rotary stress—much like twisting off the lid of a jar—rather than impacted by compressive stress. Whether this is due to an alteration in the viscoelastic property of bone by the mineralized marrow as seems possible—or whether it is the result of weakening about the cap due to subtle changes in strength and contour from the early subchondral invasion at its periphery—is a matter of speculation. The biomechanical thesis is supported by the observation that the area of fracture not only does not encompass the entire infarct but that it corresponds to the area of stress concentration. This is evident from both the experimental work of Rydell[34] and the observation that the location of the crack corresponds to the principal area of cartilage loss in primary osteoarthritis.

Stress fractures within the normal femoral head have been reported and do heal.[41] However, when they occur in IAN, there is no capacity within the infarct for healing. Clearly both the calcification and peripheral vascular invasion occur in and about the infarcted segment prior to the fracture.

The "stalling" of the repair of the infarct in IAN occurs at the zone of fibrous connective tissue that separates the repairing rim and the more central area of marrow calcification. When experimental aseptic necrosis is produced in animals by charcoal embolization,[25] lipoidal embolization,[21] or surgical trauma,[4, 40] the subsequent lesion heals spontaneously without "stalling" or collapse. However, when Sanchis, Zahir, and Freeman developed an experimental model in puppies to simulate the deformity of Legg-Perthes disease in humans they found it necessary to reinfarct the capital femoral epiphysis a second time to produce collapse.[35] Freeman also states that marrow calcification occurs only after a second infarcting maneuver. The frequent appearance of multiple cement lines in the repairing zone of IAN—and the more striking appearance of such findings in sickle cell lesions where reinfarction is quite likely—suggests that "stalling" in IAN may be due to more than one episode of infarction.

Another puzzling aspect of IAN is the location of the infarct. There simply is no evidence to suggest that the many anastomoses of the three sets of terminal vessels provide a single source where vascular obstruction could produce such an infarct. This is substantiated to a certain extent by the anatomy of the post-traumatic lesions. It is, however, difficult to understand how diseases that produce infarction by intravascular sludging or thrombosis could so regularly pick out such an area. Although quite obviously the anatomic site has a connotation that bears on pathogenesis its meaning remains an enigma to date.

Still another question is why the pain so reliably heralds the onset of the subchondral fracture. It, not infrequently, is felt by the patient weeks before the crescent sign is apparent on the roentgenogram. Although such a situation is not unknown in "stress" fractures of the long bones it is generally held that such pain is perceived by the nerve endings in the enveloping periosteum and soft tissues. In IAN, however, there are no intraosseous nerve receptors within the infarct, and pain is thought of as being secondary to the synovitis of the hip that occurs in the later stages of the disease.

A final comment about the diagnostic maneuvers is in order. The correlation of the roentgenographic and pathologic findings have made clear the biologic significance of the roentgenogram findings at various stages of the lesion. Radioscans and/or scintimetry are, as yet, of little value in evaluating the stage of the lesion. While they hold promise for the early detection of a roentgenographically normal lesion this has yet to become a reliable tool. Certainly once the process has produced enough reaction-repair density to be seen by roentgenogram the radio scans are so nonspecific as to be interesting rather than useful. Prebiopsy labeling with tetracycline is of some practical value. After one becomes familiar with the techniques the rapid evaluation of the biologic activity in and about the infarct is helpful in making therapeutic decisions. This information is best gotten by core biopsies done under roentgenogram control. The rapid information so gained frequently permits a decision as to the stage of the lesion *viz-a-viz* supplemental grafting *versus* prosthetic joint implants. Such cores also permit accurate estimation of whether or not a roentgenographically occult fracture is present. Good quality diagnostic roentgenograms remain the most helpful tool in studying the gross pathology in clinical material.

SUMMARY

The gross and microscopic changes in idiopathic aseptic necrosis of the femoral head during the evolution of the lesion have been correlated with the clinical and roentgenographic findings. These have been supplemented by radio scans, tetracycline labeling, and microradiography. These observations make possible the distinction of IAN from the traumatic and systemic disease lesions. Their interpretation also enhances rational therapeutic decisions.

REFERENCES

1. Amstutz, H. C., and Carey, E. J.: Skeletal manifestations and treatment of Gaucher's disease; review of twenty cases. *J. Bone Joint Surg., 48-A:* 670–701, 1966.
2. Arkin, A. M., and Schein, A. J.: Aseptic necrosis in Gaucher's disease. *J. Bone Joint Surg. 30-A:* 631–641, 1948.
3. Boettcher, W. G., Bonfiglio, M., Hamilton, H. H., Shects, R. F. and Smith, K.: Non-traumatic necrosis of the femoral head. I. Relation of altered hemostasis to etiology. *J. Bone Joint Surg. 52-A:* 312–321, 1970.
4. Bonfiglio, M.: Aseptic necrosis of the femoral head in dogs; Effect of drilling and bone grafting *Surg. Gynecol. Obstet. 98:* 591–599, 1954.
5. Cameron, R. B.: Strontium-85 scintimetry in nontraumatic necrosis of the femoral head. *Clin. Ortho. 65:* 243–261, 1969.
6. Catto, M.: A histological study of avascular necrosis of the femoral head after transcervical fracture. *J. Bone Joint Surg. 47-B:* 749–776, 1965.
7. Catto, M.: The histological appearances of late segmental collapse of the femoral head after transcervical fracture. *J. Bone Joint Surg. 47-B:* 777–791, 1965.
8. Chandler, F. A.: Coronary disease of the hip. *J. Int. Coll. Surg. 11:* 34–36, 1948.
9. Chung, S. M. K., and Ralston, E. L.: Necrosis of the femoral head associated with sickle cell anemia and its genetic variants, a review of the literature and study of thirteen cases. *J. Bone Joint Surg. 51-A:* 33–58, 1969.
10. Diggs, L. W., Pulliam, H. N., and King, J. C.: The bone changes in sickel cell anemia. *South. Med. J. 30:* 249–259, 1937.
11. Evarts, C. M., and Phalen, G. S.: Osseous avascular necrosis associated with renal transplantation. *Clin. Orthop. 78:* 330–335, 1971.
12. Fisher, D. E., and Bickel, W. H.: Corticosteroid induced avascular necrosis; a clinical study of seventy-seven patients. *J. Bone Joint Surg. 53-A:* 859–873, 1971.
13. Fisher, D. E., Bickel, W. H., and Halley, K. E.: Histologic demonstration of fat emboli in aseptic necrosis associated with hypercortisonism. *Mayo Clin. Proc. 44:* 252–259, 1969.
14. Freund, E.: Bilateral aseptic necrosis of the femoral head; problems arising in a compensation case. *Ann. Surg. 104:* 100–106, 1936.
15. Freund, E.: Zur Trage der aseptischer Knochennekrose. *Virchows Arch. (Pathol. Anat.) 261:* 287–314, 1926.

16. Hastins, D. E., and MacNab, W. B.: Spontaneous avascular necrosis of the femoral head; a clinical and pathological review. *Can. J. Surg., 8:* 68–83, 1965.
17. Herndon, J. H., and Aufranc, O. E.: Avascular necrosis of the femoral head in the adult; a review of its incidence in a variety of conditions. *Clin. Orthop. 86:* 43–62, 1972.
18. Howe, W. W., Lacey, T., II, and Schwartz, R. P.: A Study of the gross anatomy of the arteries supplying the proximal portion of the femur and the acetabulum. *J. Bone Joint Surg. 32-A:* 856–866, 1950.
19. Hulth. A.: Necrosis of the head of the femur; a roentgenological microradiographic and histological study. *Acta Chir. Scand. 122:* 75–84, 1961.
20. Hunder, G. G., Worthington, J. W., and Bickel, W. H.: Avascular necrosis of the femoral head in a patient with gout. J. A. M. A. 203: 47–49, 1968.
21. Jones, J. P., Englemen, E. P., Steinbach, H. L., Murray, W. R., and Rambo, O. N.: Fat embolization as a possible mechanism producing a vascular necrosis (abstract). *Arthritis Rheum. 8:* 449, 1965.
22. Jones, J. P., Jameson, R. M., and Engleman, E. P.: Alcoholism, fat embolism, and avascular necrosis (abstract). *J. Bone Joint Surg. 50-A:* 1065, 1968.
23. Judet, J., Judet, R., Lagrange, J., and Dunoyer, J.: A study of the arterial vascularization of the femoral neck in the adult. *J. Bone Joint Surg. 37-A:* 663–680, 1955.
24. Kahlstrom, S. C., Burton, C. C., and Phemister, D. B.: Aseptic necrosis of bone I. Infarction of bones in caisson disease resulting in encapsulated and calcified areas in diaphysis and in arthritis deformans. *Surg. Gynecol. Obstet. 68:* 129–146, 1939.
25. Kistler, G. H.: Sequences of experimental infarction of the femur in rabbits. *Arch. Surg. 29:* 589–611, 1934.
26. Malka, S.: Idiopathic aseptic necrosis of the head of the femur in adults. *Surg. Gynecol. Obstet. 123:* 1057–1065, 1966.
27. Mankin, H. J. and Brower, T. D.: Bilateral idiopathic aseptic necrosis of the femur in adults; "Chandler's disease." *Bull. Hosp. Joint. Dis. 23:* 42–57, 1962.
28. Marcus, N. D., Enneking, W. F. and Massam, R. A.: The Silent hip in idopathic aseptic necrosis., treatment by bonegrafting. *J. Bone Joint Surg. 55-A:* 1351–1366, 1973.
29. McCallum, R. I., and Walder, D. N.: Bone lesions in compressed air workers. with special reference to men who worked on the Clyde tunnels 1958 to 1963. Report of decompression sickness panel, Medical Research Council. *J. Bone Joint Surg. 48-B:* 207–235, 1966.
30. Merle, d'Aubigné, R., Postel, M., Mazabrand, A., Mossias, P., and Quequer, J.: Chronic ischemia at the upper end of the femur. *Ann. Rheum. Dis. 29:* 688, 1970.
31. Müssbichler, H.: Arteriographic investigation of the hip in the adult human subjects. A clinical study of the arteries in the healthy hip, in neck and pertrochanteric fractures, and in necrosis of the femoral head. *Acta Orthop. Scand. Suppl. 132:* 1–39, 1970.
32. Patterson, R. J., Bickel, W. H., and Dahlin, D. C.: Idiopathic avascular necrosis of the head of the femur. a study of fifty-two cases. *J. Bone Joint Surg. 46-A:* 267–282, 1964.
33. Phemister, D. B.: Changes in bones and joints resulting from interruption of circulation. I. General considerations and changes resulting from injuries. *Arch. Surg. 41:* 436–472, 1940.
34. Rydell, N. W.: Forces acting on the femoral head prosthesis. a study on strain guage supplied prothesis in living persons. *Acta. Orthop. Scand. Suppl. 88:* 1–132, 1966.
35. Sanchis, M., Zahir, A., and Freeman, M. A. R.: The experimental stimulation of Perthes disease by consecutive interruptions of the blood supply to the capital femoral epiphysis in the puppy. *J. Bone Joint Surg. 55-A:* 335–342, 1973.
36. Sevitt, S. and Thompson, R. G.: The distribution and anastomoses of arteries supplying the head and neck of the femur. *J. Bone Joint Surg. 47-B:* 560–573, 1965.
37. Sherman, M.: Pathogenesis of disintegration of the hip in sickel cell anemia. *South. Med. J. 52:* 632–637, 1959.
38. Sherman, M. S., and Phemister, D. B.: The Pathology of ununited fractures of the neck of the femur. *J. Bone Joint Surg. 29:* 19–40, 1947.
39. Smyth, C. J., and Leidholt, J. D.: Steroid arthropathy of the hip. *Clin. Orthop. 90:* 50–56, 1973.
40. Stewart, W. J.: Aseptic necrosis of the head of the femur following traumatic dislocation of the hip joint, case report and experimental studies. *J. Bone Joint Surg. 15:* 413–438, 1933.

41. Todd, R. C., Freeman, M. A. R., and Pririe, C. J.: Isolated trabecular fatigue fractures in the femoral head. *J. Bone Joint Surg. 54-B:* 723–728, 1972.
42. Trueta, J.: The normal vascular anatomy of the human femoral head during growth. *J. Bone Joint Surg. 39-B:* 358–394, 1957.
43. Trueta, J., and Harrison, M. H. M.: The normal vascular anatomy of the femoral head in adult man. *J. Bone Joint Surg. 35-B:* 442–461, 1953.
44. Woods, C. B., Greenwald, A. S., and Haynes, D. W.: Subchondral vascularity in the human femoral head. *Ann. Rheum. Dis. 29:* 138–142, 1970.

Chapter 6

Immunologic Aspects of Arthritis as an Aid in Diagnosis and Prognosis of Rheumatic Disease*

John T. Sharp, M.D., Neal G. Sutherland, M.D., Martin D. Lidsky, M.D., Donald A. Person, M.D., Joseph Duffy, M.D., and Carolyn Leatherwood, B.S.

Immunologic reactions have been shown to underly the pathogenesis of a number of rheumatic diseases, and studies on immunologic reactivity are being intensively pursued in most of the other inflammatory connective tissue disorders. It is manifestly impossible to cover in any meaningful way this entire field. We have therefore choosen to review a limited number of reactions that provide the basis for laboratory aids in establishing the diagnosis and prognosis in various rheumatic diseases, giving special attention to those laboratory procedures which it is believed that the modern hospital should provide. In addition, comments will be made about tests that have undergone extensive clinical investigation in specialty clinics and that in our view are ready for general application in clinical medicine. Finally, a few comments are offered about developments that are foreseen in the relatively near future but which as yet are not quite ready for general application.

ANTISTREPTOCOCCAL ANTIBODIES IN RHEUMATIC FEVER

It has been more than a decade since studies established that rheumatic fever is always preceeded by an infection with a group A streptococcus. Furthermore it was shown in the 1950's that the simultaneous measurement of antibodies to four or more streptococcal antigens permits the detection of more than 95% of recent infections.[5, 30] This information is invaluable in evaluating the possibility of rheumatic fever in patients with acute polyarthritis of recent onset. For example, a combination of four negative tests will furnish convincing evidence that the patient has been free of a streptococcal infection within recent weeks and almost excludes rheumatic fever from consideration. On the other hand, a positive test, while not providing strong evidence for acute rheumatic fever, since only about 3% of individuals recently infected with a group A streptococcus develop acute

* Aided by grants from the National Institute of Arthritis, Metabolic and Digestive Diseases, the Arthritis Foundation, the Paul Kayser Foundation, and the Veterans Administration.

rheumatic fever, alerts the physician to that possibility. Tests which incorporate multiple streptococcal antigens in the same system recently have been introduced in the hope of accomplishing the same efficiency in detecting a recent infection as the multiple, separate tests, but the single test with multiple antigens is open to major theoretical objections and cannot be accepted until thorough clinical and serologic correlations have established its validity. When one considers the large number of laboratory tests which provide at best only obliquely inferential information it seems extraordinary that we have not utilized the full potential of the clinical laboratory in this situation where we have the opportunity to provide quite definitive information.

IMMUNOLOGIC REACTIONS IN SYSTEMIC LUPUS ERYTHEMATOSUS

Shortly after the discovery of the lupus erythematosus (LE) cell, it was demonstrated that one crucial factor in its production was an antibody in the patient's serum which reacted to one or more antigens in the nucleus of damaged or killed white blood cells. Since many other factors which are not unique to the systemic lupus erythematous (SLE) blood are necessary for production of the LE cell phenomenon, such as viable phagocytes, biologically active complement, and other phagocytosis-promoting factors, clinical investigators in the early and middle 1950's began looking for a more direct measure of the autoantibodies peculiar to the SLE patient. Most widely utilized has been the so-called fluorescence antinuclear antibody (ANA) test. In this system, a cellular substrate, either whole cells or sections which include nuclei, is reacted with the patient's serum, and after an appropriate period of incubation and washing, the reaction of antibodies with nuclear components is detected by the use of fluorescein-conjugated anti-human globulin. The substrate used for the antigen has varied widely and includes leukocytes, cultured cells, and sections of tissue. Evidence that the antigenic specificity of the nuclear constituents varies with the type of cell used was presented by Elling,[8] who reported a higher frequency of ANA detected in rheumatoid sera when human polymorphonuclear granulocytes were used as antigen. However, antigenic differences between tissues have not been characterized fully, since most laboratories have used a single substrate which generally has been mouse or rat liver sections. With regard to the class of immunoglobulin, ANA may be IgG, IgM or IgA.[3, 10, 15] In SLE sera ANA's most often are IgG, and furthermore the frequency of IgG ANA relative to IgM and IgA ANA is higher in SLE sera than in several other connective tissue diseases. For this reason some laboratories determine only IgG ANA.

A sample of our experience with the antinuclear antibody test, performed with mouse liver sections and fluorescein-conjugated anti-human IgG as detector, is given in Table 1. The data make several points. First, although antinuclear antibodies were present almost universally in the patients with SLE, these antibodies were not specific for that disease. Almost half of the patients with rheumatoid arthritis, most of whom had multiple tests, had a positive antinuclear antibody test on at least one occasion, and patients with scleroderma had positive tests even more often. The other rheumatic diseases were associated with

TABLE 1. IGG ANTINUCLEAR ANTIBODY IN RHEUMATIC DISEASES

	No. Patients	Any Test		First Test	
		≧1:4	≧1:64	≧1:4	≧1:64
Systemic lupus erythematosus	91	91	84	88	74
Rheumatoid arthritis	110	53	34	32	13
Scleroderma	18	15	15	15	15
Dermatomyositis	20	10	8	9	7
Rheumatic fever	25	0	0	0	0
Periarteritis	14	3	1	2	1
Reiter's syndrome	12	0	0	0	0
Adult males	56	1	1	1	1

positive tests less frequently. Somewhat greater discrimination between SLE and rheumatoid arthritis but not between SLE and scleroderma was achieved at the expense of a slight reduction in sensitivity by taking into consideration the titer of antinuclear antibodies, *e.g.*, using titer of 1:64 or greater as a dividing line. Another feature that stands out is that patients with SLE usually had persistently positive tests, which is reflected by the data relating to the first test performed. Taking into account the ANA titer, when applied to the first test, was even more discriminating in terms of excluding patients with rheumatoid arthritis. These data are generally comparable to those reported by others.

Soon after the fluorescence antinuclear antibody test was developed, different nuclear staining patterns were observed and these were correlated with antibodies to specific antigens.[7, 10, 22] Thus a peripheral or rim staining pattern was attributed to antibodies to deoxyribonucleic acid (DNA). A diffuse staining pattern was associated with antibodies to deoxyribonucleoprotein, and a speckled pattern was observed with antibodies to either ribonucleoprotein (RNP) or a soluble antigen that was called Sm. Nucleolar staining in some preparations was distinguished from the finer, speckled pattern and was associated with antibodies to ribonucleic acid or a precusor of ribonucleic acid. Clinical correlations with staining patterns suggested significant associations. For example, a peripheral staining pattern generally was seen only with SLE and usually in the presence of active disease.[7, 10, 15] A speckled pattern was seen with moderate frequency in SLE but with high frequency in scleroderma. [20, 21] Although these associations were highly significant statistically they were not universally present. It soon became clear from observing mixed staining patterns and from studies on isolated antigens that a majority of patients with SLE had more than one ANA.

In order to permit more precise evaluation of the clinical significance of antibodies directed against a given antigen, studies were carried out on antibodies to several specific antigens. First the clinical significance of antibodies to DNA is considered. Data that we have obtained using radiolabeled DNA from T_2 phage in the Farr technique are shown in Table 2. One hundred and sixty sera from 38 patients with SLE and 65 patients with other diseases were tested. Thirty-three serum samples were considered positive, namely they bound more than 20% of the antigen. Thirty-two were from patients with SLE; one was from a patient with discoid lupus erythematosus. The relationship of anti-DNA binding to disease activity is shown in Table 3. Twenty-eight of 32 positive sera were obtained at a time when the patients were judged to be in an active stage of illness. Two sera from patients with inactive disease were obtained during the first few months following a flare, the disease activity having been suppressed by ongoing treatment. This close association of anti-DNA antibodies to disease activity is in contrast to ANA's, which are unrelated to disease activity. Even after prolonged remission many patients continue to have positive tests for ANA as shown in Table 4. Of greater interest is the relationship of anti-DNA antibodies to the presence of renal disease. As shown in Table 5 a majority of

TABLE 2. ANTI-DEOXYRIBONUCLEIC ACID BINDING (FARR TECHNIQUE)

	No. Tested	No. Positive
SLE sera[a]	94	32
SLE patients	38	18
Other diseases—sera	66	1
Other diseases—patients	65	1

[a] SLE, systemic lupus erythematosus.

TABLE 3. ANTI-DEOXYRIBONUCLEIC ACID BINDING (FARR TECHNIQUE)

	No. Sera	Mean	No. >20%
Active SLE[a]	47	47%	28
Inactive SLE	42	−3.3%	2
Other diseases[b]	66	−10%	1

[a] SLE, systemic lupus erythematosus.
[b] Rheumatoid arthritis, slceroderma, polymyositis, rheumatic fever, periarteritis, gout, etc.

TABLE 4. IGG ANTINUCLEAR ANTIBODY (ANA) AND REMISSION IN SYSTEMIC LUPUS ERYTHEMATOSUS

	No. Patients
Clinical remission, off drugs 1 year or more	8
ANA converted positive to negative, 1 month to 3 years	3
ANA continued positive 1 to 5 years	5

TABLE 5. SYSTEMIC LUPUS ERYTHEMATOSUS, ANTI-DEOXYRIBONUCLEIC ACID (DNA) BINDING, AND RENAL DISEASE

	Anti-DNA	
	Positive	Negative
Active renal disease	16	12[a]
No renal disease	14	46
No data	2	4

[a] Renal disease subsiding in 6.

patients with active renal disease had anti-DNA antibody, but this type of immunologic reactivity was not present exclusively in patients with active renal disease. Our findings are in agreement with others who have found anti-DNA antibodies to be relatively specific for active SLE and more frequently positive in the presence of active renal disease, but not limited to patients with renal involvement.[12, 13, 19, 25, 27, 31]

Several techniques have been utilized to measure anti-DNA antibodies. Some require specialized equipment, and others utilize methods that are not performed in most clinical laboratories. Furthermore, recent studies have indicated that the physical and antigenic properties of DNA solutions are not particularly stable.[31] Evidence has been presented that storage and gentle manipulation may result in the DNA molecule unraveling to some extent, exposing a varying amount of single-stranded DNA. Since antibodies to single-stranded DNA do not have the same clinical significance as do antibodies to native or double-stranded DNA, our concern is with developing a simple method that will permit the accurate measurement of the latter. Recently a technique that appears to be practical for any laboratory that is capable of performing the fluorescence ANA was reported by Aarden and De Groot[1] and by Feltkamp.[9] These investigators took advantage of the large kinetoplast of the trypanosome, *Crithidia luciliae*, which apparently contains DNA without histone,[4] and, utilizing a fluorescein-conjugated antihuman globulin, developed a test comparable to that used for detecting ANA. Our experience, although still quite preliminary, suggests that this technique may be reliable for measuring anti-DNA antibodies. Table 6 compares the results of tests on the same sera using T_2 phage antigen in the Farr technique and the crithidia fluorescence test. The correlation of the two test systems is quite good. If these results stand up to more rigorous clinical testing it is believed that the method can be adapted readily to the routine clinical laboratory and will be a significant aid to the clinician in evaluating patients with SLE.

MIXED CONNECTIVE TISSUE DISEASE

Gordon Sharp and his colleagues[25, 26] have carried out a number of studies that relate antibodies to RNP to clinical manifestations of an illness similar to scleroderma and dermatomyositis, the so-called "mixed connective tissue disease." This group of patients was characterized by sclerodactyly, Raynaud's phenomenon, dysphagia, muscle weakness, arthralgia, and a low incidence of renal disease. Sharp et al.[25, 26] extracted nuclear antigens with phosphate buffer and performed a hemagglutination test using sheep cells coated with the extracted antigen. They found that patients with mixed connective tissue disease

TABLE 6. CORRELATION OF FARR AND CRITHIDIA ANTI-DEOXYRIBONUCLEIC ACID TECHNIQUES

Farr Binding	Crithidia	
	Positive	Negative
>60%	16	2
>20%, <60%	2	8
<20%	0	30

had very high titers of antibody to this antigen. They subsequently examined the sera of patients from several other clinics, the clinical diagnoses not being known to them, and successfully identified most patients with the combination of clinical disorders described above. These observations, if confirmed in other laboratories, will establish a specific relationship of a clinical picture to anti-RNP antibodies and emphasize the importance of studying specific antigens in determining the pathogenetic significance of a given immune reaction. Although the test is not yet developed to a stage that is ready for general application, it is predicted that measurement of antibodies to RNP will be a routine procedure as soon as a stable antigen preparation becomes available.

In summary, the immunologic services that a well run clinical laboratory should provide for the study of the patient with SLE should include both the ANA test, performed with fluorescein-conjugated anti-human IgG and some form of anti-DNA determination. If further studies confirm the specificity of the *Crithidia luciliae* anti-DNA test its use is recommended. If these tests can be performed accurately and reproducibly, there may be no need for performing the LE cell test. Although the LE phenomenon is of great historical significance, the test is time-consuming and expensive, depends on multiple, complex reactions, and by modern standards provides inadequate information.

COMPLEMENT IN SYNOVIAL FLUID

Our laboratory has measured the third component of complement (C3) in synovial fluid on a regular basis for several years utilizing the radial immunodiffusion technique. Analysis of our data indicates, that this measurement provides diagnostic assistance in many instances comparable to that obtained by measurement of whole complement or complement component activities.[6, 11, 16, 23, 24, 29] Normal joint fluid contains complement in a concentration that appears to be related to (1) the concentration of complement in serum and (2) the concentration of protein in the joint fluid. In disease states, both of these factors may be altered. We have therefore analyzed the relationship of C3 content to protein for 299 synovial fluids. Protein and C3 values were plotted for individual fluids from patients with all conditions excluding SLE, rheumatoid arthritis, and hepatitis-associated arthritis. We then drew a line above which 90% of these values fell. Nearly half of the fluids from patients with SLE and rheumatoid arthritis fell below this line as shown in Figure 1. Based on this empirical analysis, we believe that determination of C3 content as related to protein concentration, in synovial fluid frequently will provide diagnostically useful information. Furthermore the SLE and rheumatoid fluids often can be differentiated, since in a majority of instances SLE patients with low synovial fluid complement had low serum complement, whereas rheumatoid patients with low synovial fluid complement usually had normal serum complement.

CELL-MEDIATED IMMUNE REACTIONS IN THE RHEUMATIC DISEASES

The dissection of the mechanisms responsible for delayed hypersensitivity into its component parts has been initiated during the last 1 or 2 decades. At present

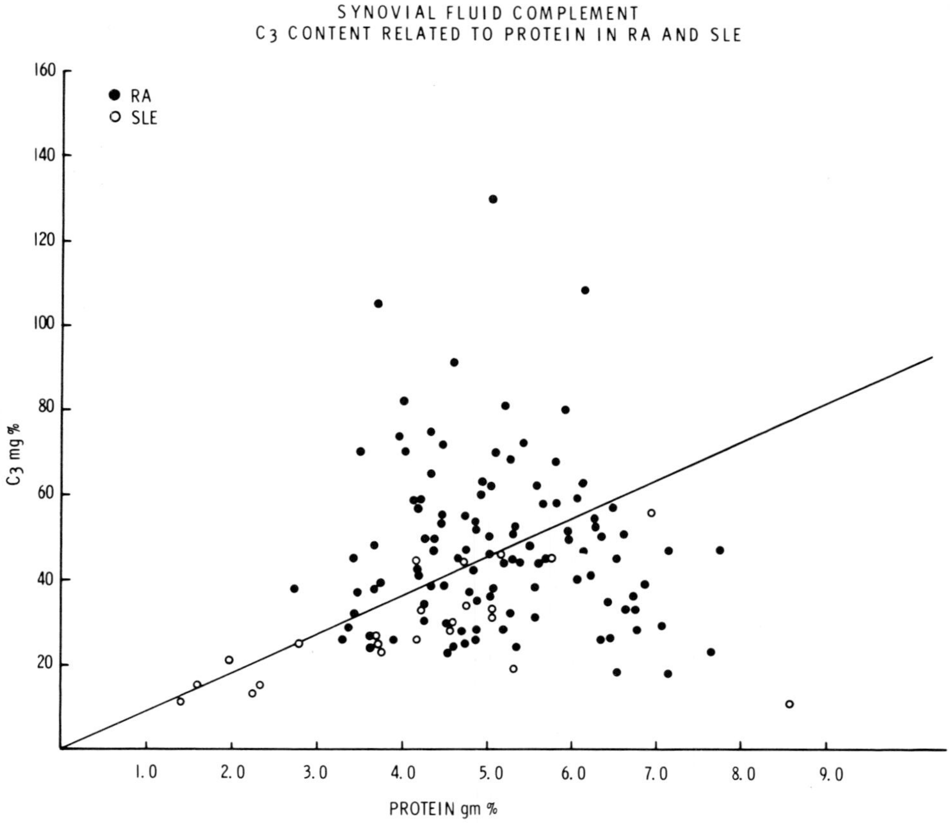

FIG. 1. Content of the third component of complement as related to protein fell above the line for 121 of 135 synovial fluids from patients with various forms of arthritis excluding rheumatoid arthritis, systemic lupus erythematosus, and hepatitis-associated arthritis. These include gout (34 fluids), pseudogout (10), degenerative joint disease (10), acute rheumatic fever (13), septic arthritis (16), suspected septic arthritis (7), Charcot arthropathy (4), Reiter's syndrome (4), and undiagnosed arthritis patients whose fluids contained fewer than 2000 white blood cells per cubic millimeter (28). Fluids from patients with rheumatoid arthritis (●) and systemic lupus erythematosus (○) whose individual C_3, protein values are plotted in this chart fell below the line for 57 of 107 rheumatoid fluids and 18 of 23 SLE fluids.

exciting work is being done on cellular immunity in many research laboratories, and some of this work is directly related to the various rheumatic diseases. Although the full implications of some of these studies are not yet clear, it is predicted that within the next decade many of the advances in our understanding of the pathogenesis of rheumatic diseases and in the development of satisfactory diagnostic tests and procedures for evaluating the course and prognosis of these diseases will come in the area of cellular immunity.

Systemic lupus erythematosus is characterized by a multiplicity of abnormal antibodies found in the serum, many autoantibodies having been described in addition to those discussed earlier. Clearly patients with this disease are subjected either to an extraordinary variety and intensity of immunization with self-antigens, or something has gone awry with their mechanism for controlling antibody production. In the last few years, studies in animals have established that T cells, or a subclass of T cells, play a regulatory role in the humoral immune system. This has led immunologists to propose that the central problem in the immune aberrations of patients with SLE is a deficiency in T cell suppressor activity.[2, 28] Perhaps this is a deficiency in thymosin, or perhaps there is some other defect inherent in the T cell system which accounts for this abnormal function. Whatever it is, if this hypothesis proves to be correct, a simple test which measures this function will provide a definitive diagnostic tool and a guide for the treatment of this disease.

In our laboratory Person, Sharp, and Lidsky[17, 18] have discovered an important new immune abnormality in patients with rheumatoid arthritis. In a search for a unique antigen in the synovial cells of patients with rheumatoid arthritis, they have shown that lymphocytes from the peripheral blood of affected patients killed rheumatoid synovial cells cultured *in vitro* in about one third of the mixtures tested. Cytotoxic reactions were observed infrequently with lymphocytes from healthy individuals, and killing was seen much less frequently when rheumatoid lymphocytes were mixed with normal synovial cells. In other words these cytotoxic tests have demonstrated highly significant differences between rheumatoid and nonrheumatoid lymphocytes and between rheumatoid and nonrheumatoid synovial cells cultured *in vitro*, but the test is not universally positive. It is not yet clear whether tests are negative in two-thirds of the mixtures because the technique is not sufficiently sensitive to detect all of the reactions or whether there are other explanations. For example rheumatoid arthritis, as we now define it, may well be more than one disease. At any rate, if the antigen which was detected in this system can be isolated and characterized it may be possible to develop a simple and highly specific test for rheumatoid arthritis as well as to advance our understanding of this disease.

Johnson, Fink, and Ziff[14] demonstrated the production of lymphotoxin by lymphocytes of the peripheral blood from patients with dermatomyositis when these cells were mixed with autochthonous muscle tissue. The role of cellular immunity in causing tissue destruction was not established, but these studies hold promise for providing new insights into the pathogenesis of dermatomyositis.

Although these comments on cell-mediated immune reactions are quite limited, touching on only a few areas, they illustrate the likelihood that cell-mediated immune reactions may be central to the pathogenesis of many of the rheumatic diseases. If this proves to be the case we are confident that tests suitable for the routine laboratory will be developed to aid in establishing the diagnosis and prognosis of these disorders.

REFERENCES

1. Aarden, L. A., and de Groot, E. R.: Crithidia luciliae, simple substrate for the anti-ds-DNA determination by the immunofluorescence technique. *Trans. N. Y. Acad. Sci. 36:* 703, 1974.
2. Allison, A. C., Denman, A. M., and Barnes, R. D.: Cooperating and controlling functions of thymus-derived lymphocytes in relation to autoimmunity. *Lancet 2:* 135–140, 1971.
3. Barnett, E. V., North, A. F., Jr., Condemi, J. J., Jacox, R. F., and Vaughan, J. H.: Antinuclear

factors in systemic lupus erythematosus and rheumatoid arthritis. *Ann Intern. Med. 63:* 100–108, 1965.

4. Beck, J. S., and Walker, P. J.: Antigenicity of trypanosome nuclei: Evidence that DNA is not coupled to histone in these protozoa. *Nature 204:* 194–195, 1964.
5. Bernhard, G. C., and Stollerman, G. H.: Serum inhibition of streptococcal diphosphopyridine nucleotidase in uncomplicated streptococcal pharyngitis and in rheumatic fever. *J. Clin. Invest. 38:* 1942–1949, 1959.
6. Bunch, T. W., Hunder, G. G., McDuffie, F. C., O'Brien, P. C., and Markowitz, H.: Synovial fluid complement determination as a diagnostic aid in inflammatory joint disease. *Mayo Clin. Proc.* 49: 715–720, 1974.
7. Casals, S. P., Friou, G. J., and Teague, P. O.: Specific nuclear reaction pattern of antibody to DNA in lupus erythematosus sera. *J. Lab. Clin. Med. 62:* 625–631, 1963.
8. Elling, P.: On the incidence of antinuclear factors in rheumatoid arthritis; *Acta Rheum. Scand. 13:* 101–112, 1967.
9. Feltkamp, T. E. W.: In *Progress in Immunology II*, edited by Brent, L., and Holborow, J., vol. 5. Amsterdam, North-Holland Publishing Co., p. 304, 1974.
10. Gonzalez, E. N., and Rothfield, N. F.: Immunoglobulin class and pattern of nuclear fluorescence in systemic lupus erythematosus. *N. Engl. J. Med. 274:* 1333–1338, 1966.
11. Hedberg, H.: Studies on synovial fluid in arthritis. *Acta. Med. Scand. (Suppl.) 479:* 1–137, 1967.
12. Hughes, G. R. V., Cohen, S. A., and Christian, C. L.: Anti-DNA activity in systemic lupus erythematosus: A diagnostic and therapeutic guide. *Ann. Rheum. Dis. 30:* 259–264, 1971.
13. Johnson, G. D., Edmonds, J. P., and Holborow, E. J.: Precipitating antibody to D.N.A. detected by two-stage electroimmunodiffusion; study in systemic lupus erythematosus and rheumatoid arthritis. *Lancet 2:* 883–885, 1973.
14. Johnson, R. L., Fink, C. W., and Ziff, M.: Lymphotoxin formation by lymphocytes and muscle in polymyositis. *J. Clin. Invest 51:* 2435–2449, 1972.
15. Parker, M. D., and Kerby, G. P.: Combined titre and fluorescent pattern of IgG antinuclear antibodies using cultured cell monolayers in evaluating connective tissue diseases. *Ann. Rheum. Dis. 33:* 465–472, 1974.
16. Pekin, T. J., Jr., and Zvaifler, N. J.: Hemolytic complement in synovial fluid. *J. Clin. Invest. 43:* 1372–1382, 1964.
17. Person, D. A., Sharp, J. T., and Lidsky, M. D.: Cytotoxicity of rheumatoid arthritis leukocytes for synovial cells. *J. Rheumatol. (Suppl.) 1:* 61, 1974.
18. Person, D. A., Sharp, J. T., and Lidsky, M. D.: Cytotoxicity of rheumatoid mononuclear cells for synovial cells. *Clin. Res. 23:* 24A, 1975.
19. Pincus, T., Schur, P. H., Rose, J. A., Decker, J. L., and Talal, N.: Measurement of serum DNA-binding activity in systemic lupus erythematosus. *N. Engl. J. Med. 281:* 701–705, 1969.
20. Ritchie, R.: Antinuclear antibodies, their frequency and diagnostic association. *N. Engl. J. Med. 282:* 1174–1178, 1970.
21. Rothfield, N. F., and Rodnan, G. P.: Serum antinuclear antibodies in progressive systemic sclerosis (scleroderma). *Arthritis Rheum. 11:* 606–617, 1968.
22. Rothfield, N. F., and Stollar, B. D.: The relation of immunoglobulin class, pattern of antinuclear antibody, and complement-fixing antibodies to DNA in sera from patients with systemic erythematosus. *J. Clin. Invest. 46:* 1785–1794, 1967.
23. Ruddy, S., and Austen, K. F.: The complement system in rheumatoid synovitis. I. An analysis of complement activities in rheumatoid synovial fluids. *Arthritis Rheum. 13:* 713–723, 1970.
24. Ruddy, S., and Austen, K. F.: Activation of the complement system in rheumatoid synovitis. *Fed. Proc. 32:* 134–137, 1973.
25. Sharp, G. C., Irvin, W. S., LaRoque, R. L., Velez, C., Daly, V., Kaiser, A. D., and Holman, H. R.: Association of autoantibodies to different nuclear antigens with clinical patterns of rheumatic disease and responsiveness to therapy. *J. Clin. Invest. 50:* 350–359, 1971.
26. Sharp, G. C., Irvin, W. S., Tan, E. M., Gould, R. G., and Holman, H. R.: Mixed connective tissue disease; an apparently distinct rheumatic disease syndrome associated with a specific antibody to an extractable nuclear antigen (ENA). *Am. J. Med. 52:* 148–159, 1972.
27. Schur, P. H., and Sandson, J.: Immunologic factors and clinical activity in systemic lupus erythematosus. *N. Engl. J. Med. 278:* 533–538, 1968.

28. Talal, N.: Lymphocyte heterogeneity and function. *Arthritis Rheum. 16:* 422–425, 1973.
29. Townes, A. S., and Sowa, J. M.: Complement in synovial fluid. *Johns Hopkins Med. J. 127:* 23–37, 1970.
30. Wannamaker, L. W., and Ayoub, E. M.: Antibody titers in acute rheumatic fever. *Circulation 21.* 598–614, 1960.
31. Winfield, J. B., and Davis, J. S., IV.: Anti-DNA antibody in procainamide-induced lupus erythematosus. Determinations using DNA fractionated by methylated albumin-Kieselguhr chromatography. *Arthritis Rheum. 17:* 97–110, 1974.

Chapter 7

Radiologic Diagnosis of Joint Disease

JACK EDEIKEN

The radiologic approach to arthritis is simplified if one constantly bears in mind that there are two types—the clinical and the radiologic. Indeed, the roentgen study may only confirm the clinical fact that a patient with a specific disease now has joint manifestations of that disease. In contrast, the radiologic type occurs in patients with complaints referable only to a joint, or joints, and without other clinical findings. In the latter, roentgen changes are the first tangible manifestations of the disease and the first clues for the clinician. In the evaluation of the latter group of diseases, it is the radiologist who first makes the diagnosis and it is his prime responsibility to report the diagnosis to the clinician.

Whenever the roentgenogram of a patient with arthritis is considered, the clinical arthritides must be ruled out. By history alone, the diagnosis may have been established long before the patient arrives for roentgen study. However, there are times when patients with one of the clinical arthritides do arrive without the diagnosis having been made. This is usually in early rheumatoid arthritis and perhaps in long-standing psoriatic arthritis. It is then up to the radiologist to unearth a history that establishes the disease (Table 1).

The arthritides that appear clinically before a roentgenographic change takes place include bacterial, advanced rheumatoid, psoriatic, hemophiliac, gouty, and neurotrophic arthropathy. With these diseases, the radiologist evaluates the nature and degree of involvement that does not assist in the diagnosis. Although subtle differences may make roentgenographic distinction possible early in the course of the arthritis, it must be emphasized that the diagnosis is initially made by the clinician. Bone changes tend to occur later in these diseases, are dramatic, and are diagnostic, but little credit can be given to the radiologist for his diagnosis, as it has already been made by the referring physician.

Occasionally, bacterial arthritis is confused with other arthritides. The roentgenographic distinction may be useful and depends on the appearance of the articular cortex which may be destroyed early in bacterial arthritis, but is maintained later in the other types.

Confusion between tuberculous and nontuberculous infections may occur because, although the radiographic manifestations may be distinctive, the two frequently cannot be differentiated on roentgenographic evidence alone. Tuberculous arthritis smolders for months and years; its symptoms are mild and

TABLE 1. ARTHRITIDES

Clinical Erosive Arthritis	Radiologic Arthritis
Pyogenic (nontuberculous) arthritis	Tuberculous arthritis
Advanced rheumatoid disease	Ankylosing spondylitis
Psoriasis	Chondrocalcinosis (pseudogout)
Hemophilia	Osteoarthritis
Gout	Pigmented villonodular synovitis
Reiter's disease	Ochronosis
Neurotrophic arthropathy	Early rheumatoid arthritis
Boeck's sarcoid	Reiter's disease (diagnosis may be suggested by history)
Rheumatic fever	

protracted, and initial roentgenographic study reveals advanced abnormalities. On the other hand, pyogenic or nontuberculous arthritis causes early severe complaints and roentgenographic bone changes are often not seen on the initial study.

The erosions of psoriatic and rheumatoid arthritis are similar and may not always be sufficiently characteristic for separation. The presence of the rheumatoid factor in the blood aids in their differentiation, but is not present in all patients with rheumatoid disease. The presence of psoriatic skin lesions, although helpful, is not conclusive evidence, since psoriasis and rheumatoid arthritis may exist concurrently in the same joint. Also, psoriatic arthritis occasionally precedes the skin lesions by as long as 7 years.

The radiologist is often requested to exclude gout in a patient whose foot pain is of short duration. Gout does not produce roentgen changes until 6 to 8 years after its onset and early symptoms are so severe that the diagnosis is established long before the roentgen changes are present.

The roentgen manifestations of hemophiliac arthritis are dramatic, but the history and clinical evaluation unmask hemophilia long before joint and bone changes develop.

The arthritides for which the radiologist bears prime responsibility for the diagnosis include chondrocalcinosis (pseudogout), ankylosing spondylitis, early rheumatoid arthritis, ochronosis, degenerative arthritis, especially erosive osteoarthritis, and pigmented villonodular synovitis. These arthritides show distinctive roentgen changes early. Characteristics of each should be well known for most are pathognomonic roentgenographically and are often the first clues to the identity of the disease. The patient's history and laboratory findings are important only in excluding other conditions.

CLINICAL ARTHRITIDES

Pyogenic arthritis. Pyogenic or nontuberculous arthritis is usually an acute fulminating disease, and the most common offender is the staphylococcus. The patient is usually studied within 48 hr after the onset of the disease because of the severe symptoms and the high fever. No roentgenographic changes will be found, except for swelling of the joint (Fig. 1), and the clinician should be warned that roentgenographic changes will not appear for approximately 10 days.

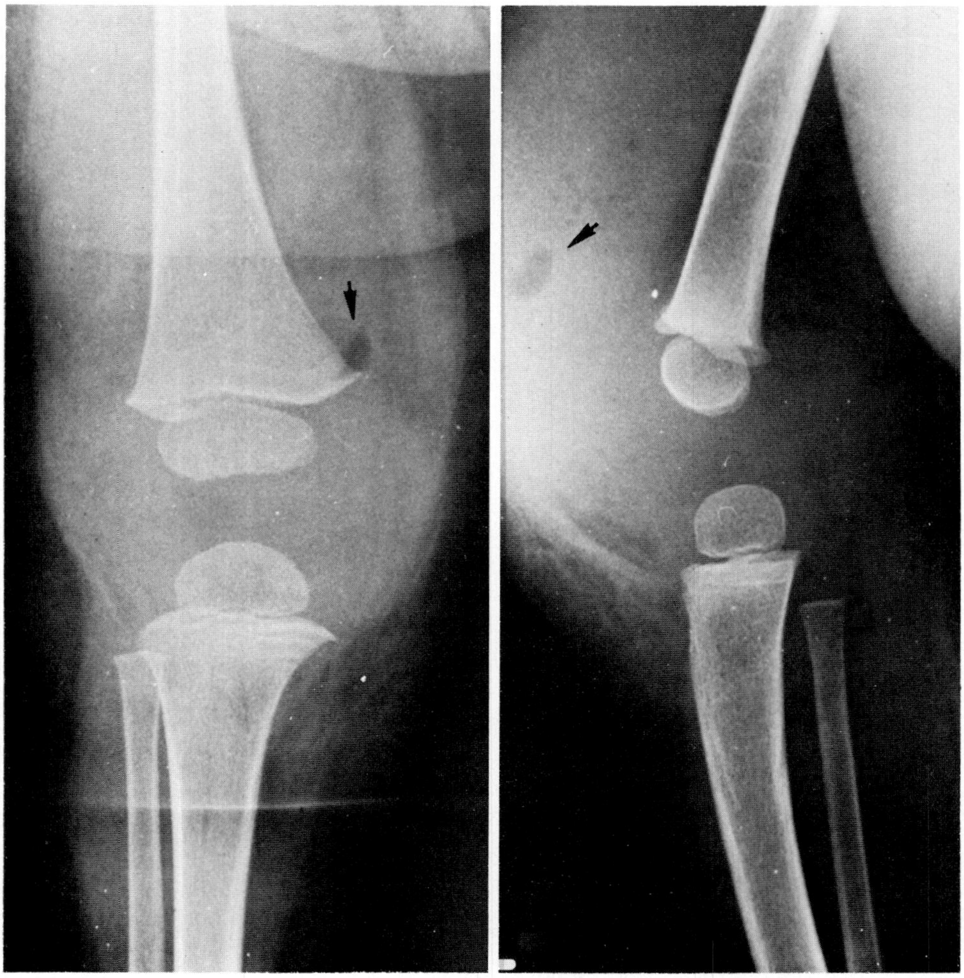

FIG. 1. Staphylococcus arthritis. There is extensive soft tissue swelling and a small air pocket resulting from joint fluid aspiration. Symptoms were severe for 12 hr and included fever, leukocytosis, and chills. There are no bone changes.

Tuberculous arthritis. Patients with tuberculous arthritis usually have mild pain for a few months to more than 2 years before they are studied. The first roentgenograms have extensive bone changes, joint space narrowing, and loss of the articular cortex (Fig. 2). Deossification of the bones distal and proximal to the joints is usually dramatic.

Advanced rheumatoid arthritis. Patients with advanced rheumatoid arthritis have had a diagnosis for years, and the characteristics are symmetrical arthritis of both hands. The wrist joints and the metacarpophalangeal joints (Fig. 3) are most severely involved, and ulnar deviation of the rays may be prominent. Erosive changes are almost always present and are most marked at the second and third metacarpophalangeal joints. At times, a large mass forms with rheumatoid arthritis, especially in the region of the gastrocnemius muscle (Fig.

4). This is most likely due to a giant rheumatoid cyst. The patients are usually believed to have a fibrosarcoma or thrombophlebitis.

Hemophiliac arthritis. The arthritic changes in hemophilia occur after repeated hemorrhages into a joint, and the characteristic findings are present from childhood. The knee is most often involved, and the epiphysis is enlarged, and the intracondylar notch is widened. There may be erosive changes. The synovium is bulky, and an intra-articular soft tissue mass is demonstrated.

Gout. A patient is often referred for roentgenographic examination with pain of the foot for a few days or weeks. It is certain that if the symptoms are of short duration, gouty bone changes will not be present. If there are erosive changes, they are not due to gout.

The changes in gout are due to the tophaceous deposits near the joint which cause large erosions usually extending away from the joint and not at the

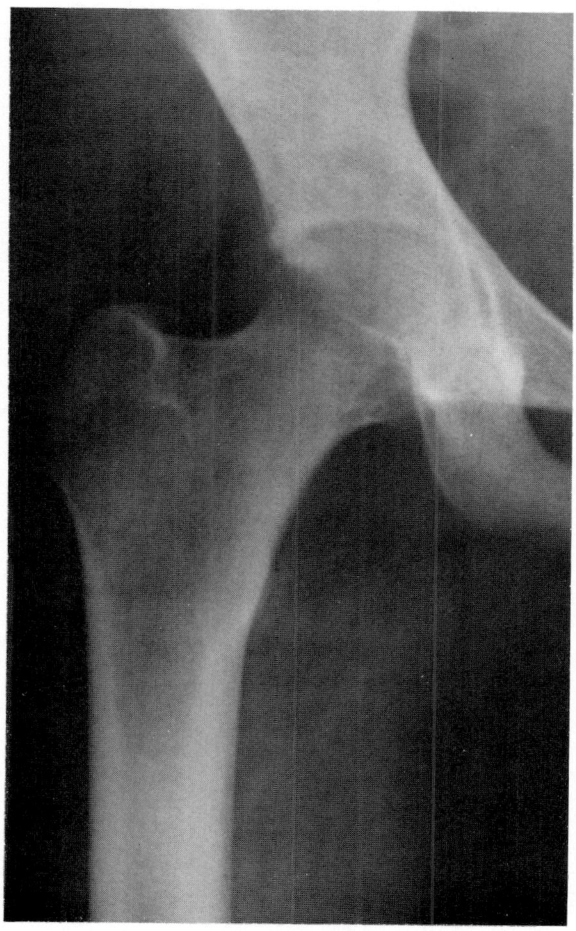

FIG. 2. Tuberculous arthritis. This is the first examination on a 15-year-old male who had minor joint pain for 13 months. There is deossification of the neck of the femur, narrowing of the joint space, and a loss of the articular cortex of the femur.

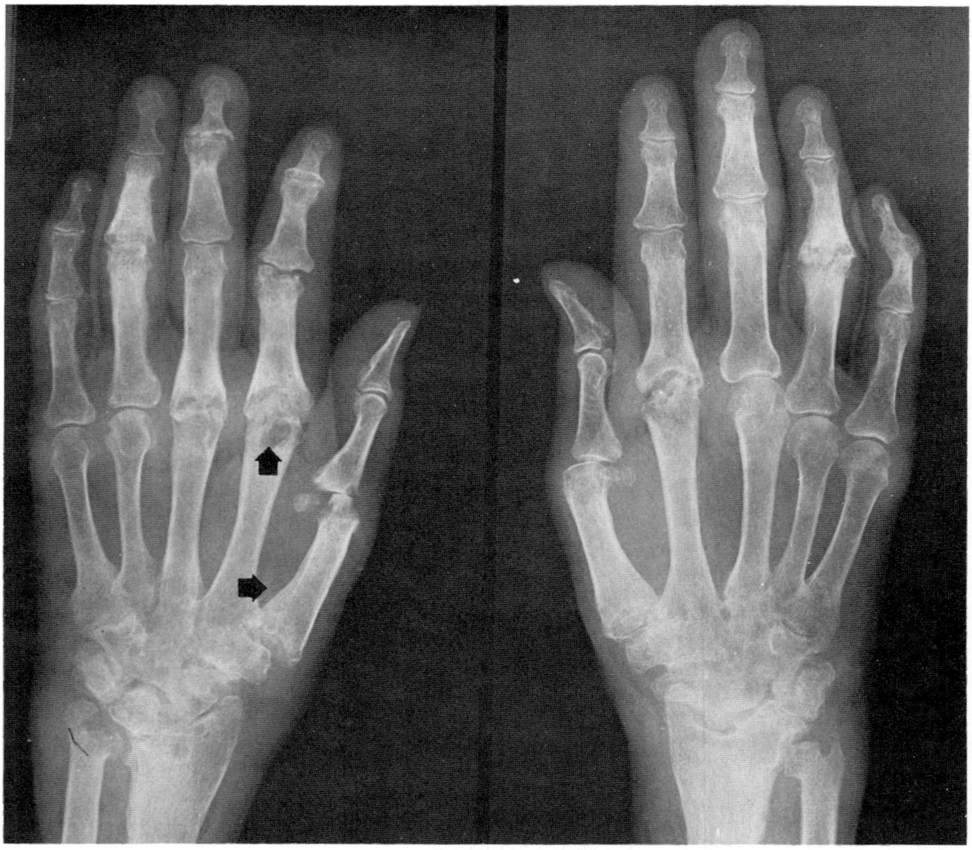

FIG. 3. Advanced rheumatoid arthritis. The most severe erosive changes are in the wrist and metacarpophalangeal joints. A rheumatoid cyst is present in the second metacarpal (*vertical arrow*), and periosteal reaction is present on the first metacarpal (*horizontal arrow*).

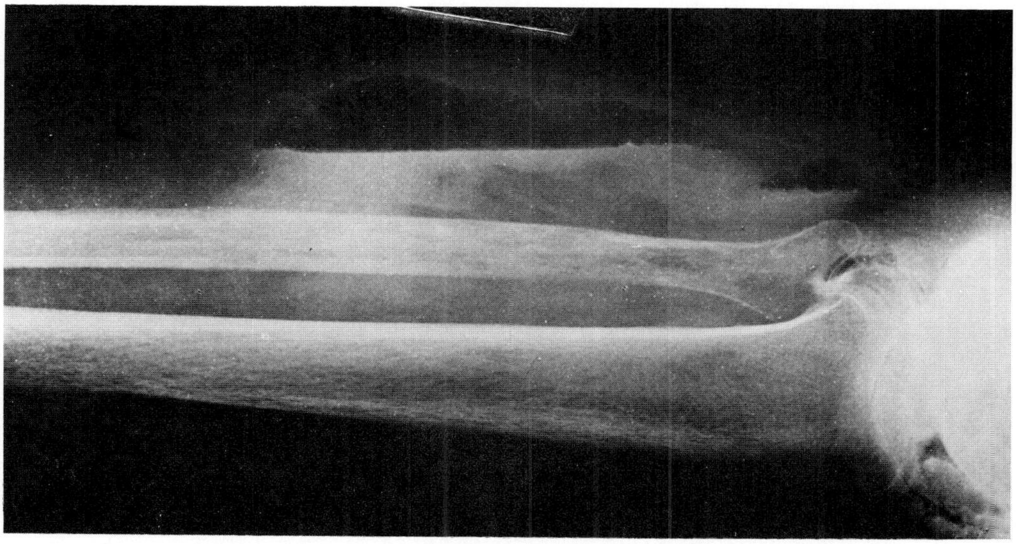

FIG. 4. Giant rheumatoid cyst. Opaque medium and air were injected into the knee joint. In the prone-lateral position an air-fluid level is noted in the region of the gastrocnemius muscle. These lesions are often mistaken for malignant tumors or thrombophlebitis.

articular surfaces. Late in the course of the disease, the joints are also destroyed at the articular surfaces (Fig. 5).

Reiter's disease. This disease should be suspected in any young man who has pain in one or both feet. The most common finding is a periarticular deossification at the metatarsophalangeal joints of one or both feet. Periosteal reactions may be present. Later in the disease, severe erosive change may occur and may be indistinguishable from the other erosive arthritides. Patients with Reiter's disease usually are sent to the radiologist without a diagnosis, and on questioning, it is usually evident that a mild urethritis and conjunctivitis are present or have occurred. A mild rash occurs in the acute phase.

Neurotrophic arthropathies. These arthropathies may be unsuspected, and historically they are usually painless. When pain occurs it is a confusing finding and often misleads the diagnostician. One must remember that neurotrophic arthropathy is a severe degenerative arthritis. In the shoulders and hips, it is a destructive lesion and resorption of bone and debris are present. In the spine and some other joints, it is a productive type of arthritis. In the spine, there is disc involvement with narrowing, large spur formations, and increase in density of the vertebral bodies.

RADIOLOGIC ARTHRITIDES

Tuberculous arthritis. Tuberculous arthritis occurs frequently in the shoulder or hip of a young person. The symptoms are usually mild pain for more than 1 year, and the roentgenographic features are dramatic. There is marked joint space narrowing, loss of the articular cortex, and varying degrees of deossification (Fig. 2). If, on the initial roentgen examination, these findings are present, the diagnosis of tuberculous arthritis is almost assured.

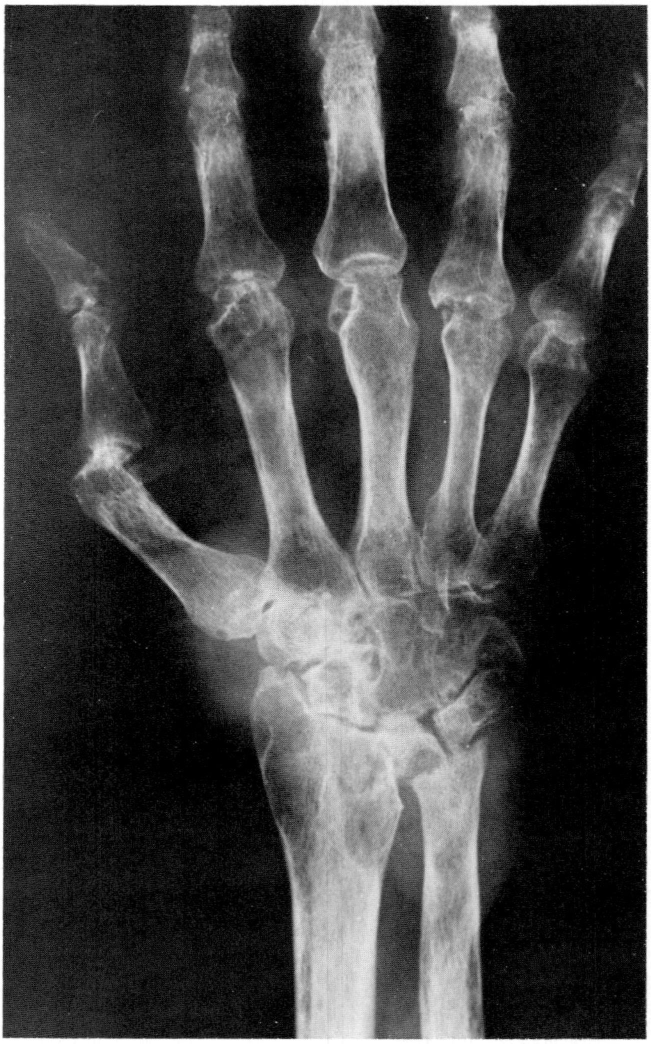

FIG. 5. Gout. This patient had symptoms for 23 years. There are erosive changes of most of the joints of the wrist and hand. Soft tissue masses representing tophi are noted in the wrist.

Ankylosing spondylitis. This condition is characterized by sacroiliac joint involvement bilaterally and symmetrically (Fig. 6) and usually by spinal changes consisting of loss or straightening of the anterior portion of the body of the vertebra and later calcification producing a bamboo spine. Other conditions which may cause sacroiliac arthritis bilaterally are psoriasis and Reiter's disease. They may be indistinguishable radiographically, but if syndesmophytes are present, they may be distinguished. The syndesmophytes of ankylosing spondylitis are symmetrical and extensive and usually are very delicate. They are attached to the middle of the body, crossing the joint, and are parallel to the long axis of the spine. The syndesmophytes of psoriasis and Reiter's disease have a wide base, are usually asymmetrical, and extend slightly further laterally than those of ankylosing spondylitis.

Any inflammatory condition such as hemophilia or old tuberculous abscess may cause a syndesmophyte. An osteophyte originates at the level of a disc or joint surface and extends laterally with its axis perpendicular to the long axis of the spine or limb. An osteophyte is invariably due to degenerative change and may occur in neuropathic arthritis, because this is a severe degenerative change.

Erosive osteoarthritis. This disease is often mistaken for rheumatoid arthritis, but it has several features, especially in the hands, which all radiologists should know. The erosions occur along the articular surface, usually at the distal interphalangeal joints and sometimes in the proximal interphalangeal joints. There is usually subchondral sclerosis, which is rare in other conditions except for psoriasis. The bones of the hands are well mineralized. There may be narrowing

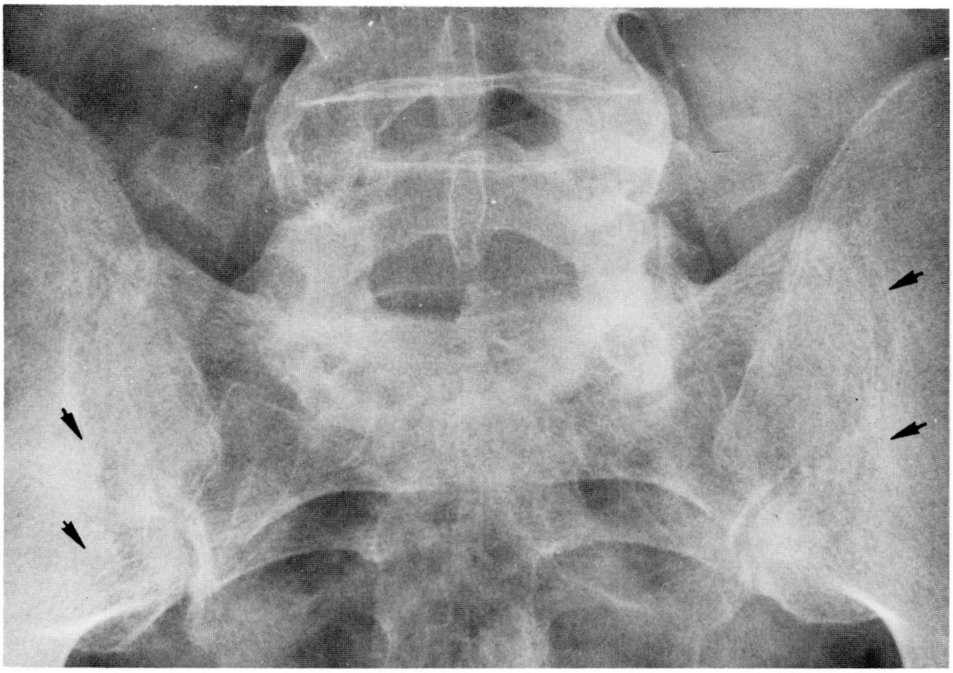

FIG. 6. Ankylosing spondylitis. There is increased density of both sacroiliac bones (*arrows*) and bambooing of the lower spine.

of the metacarpophalangeal joints without erosions. There is often hypertrophic arthritis of the first carpometacarpal joint (Fig. 7). The distribution, presence of subchondral sclerosis, and the involvement of the first carpometacarpal joint are usually characteristic.

Pigmented villonodular synovitis. Bone changes are not often present, but usually there are masses in the joint space. When there is bone erosion, it is regular with a sclerotic margin and usually bridges the joint, being found in at least two of the bones of the joint (Fig. 8). Calcification rarely occurs.

Ochronosis. This is a very rare disease which causes calcification of every disc

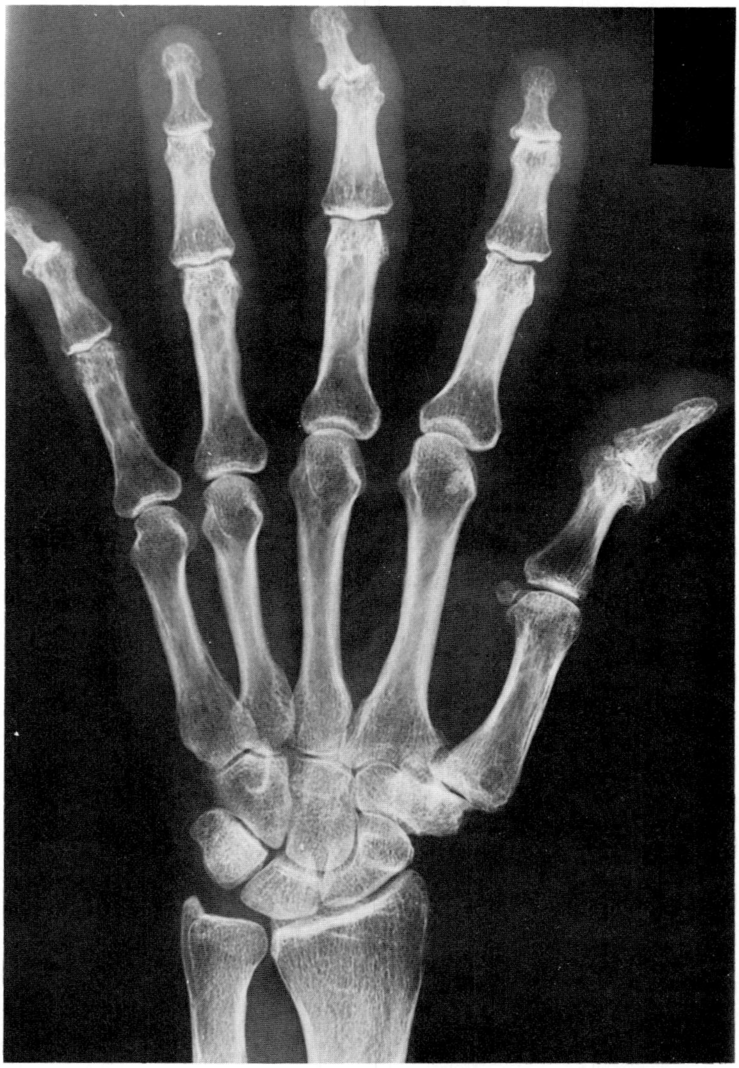

FIG. 7. Erosive osteoarthritis. There is narrowing of some of the distal interphalangeal joints with subchondral sclerosis. There is arthrosis of the first carpometacarpal joint. There is sparing of the ulnar styloid process.

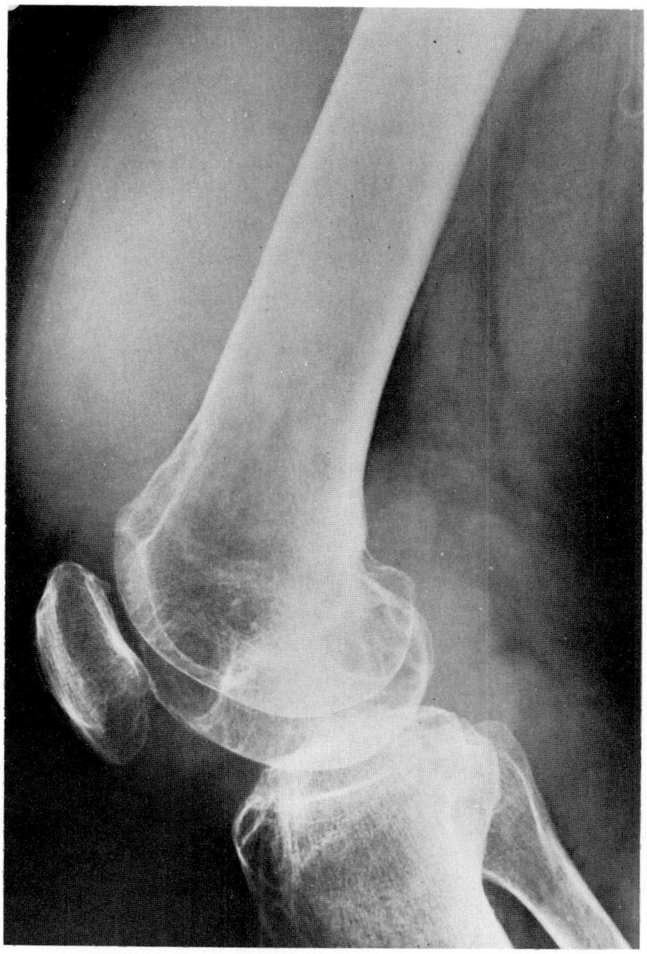

FIG. 8. Pigmented villonodular synovitis. There is a large soft tissue mass in the suprapatella region and erosions of the distal end of the femur and patella and proximal portion of the tibia anteriorly. There are also erosive changes of the posterior aspect of the femur.

of the spine late in the course of the disease (Fig. 9). Hypertrophi : arthritis may be found in the peripheral joints. Usually the disease has been known in infancy, but has been forgotten, and the arthritic changes that occur in early or late middle age are the dramatic findings.

Early rheumatoid arthritis. Arthritis may occur before the rheumatoid factor is positive and within 1 month or so after the onset of the disease. There are two findings that may be helpful. (1) A resorption of the articular cortex may occur on the radial aspect of the metacarpals, usually the second and third. This is almost pathognomonic of rheumatoid arthritis (Fig. 10). (2) There may be a slight radioulnar dislocation in the wrist and a small erosion or irregularity of the ulnar styloid process. Ulnar styloid involvement in rheumatoid arthritis is almost a constant feature, although it may be seen in other arthritides.

Reiter's disease. This disease has been discussed as one of the clinical arthritides, but very often a patient is referred to the radiologist without the diagnosis being made. It should be suspected in all young men who have foot pain, and when this occurs, the classical history usually may be elicited.

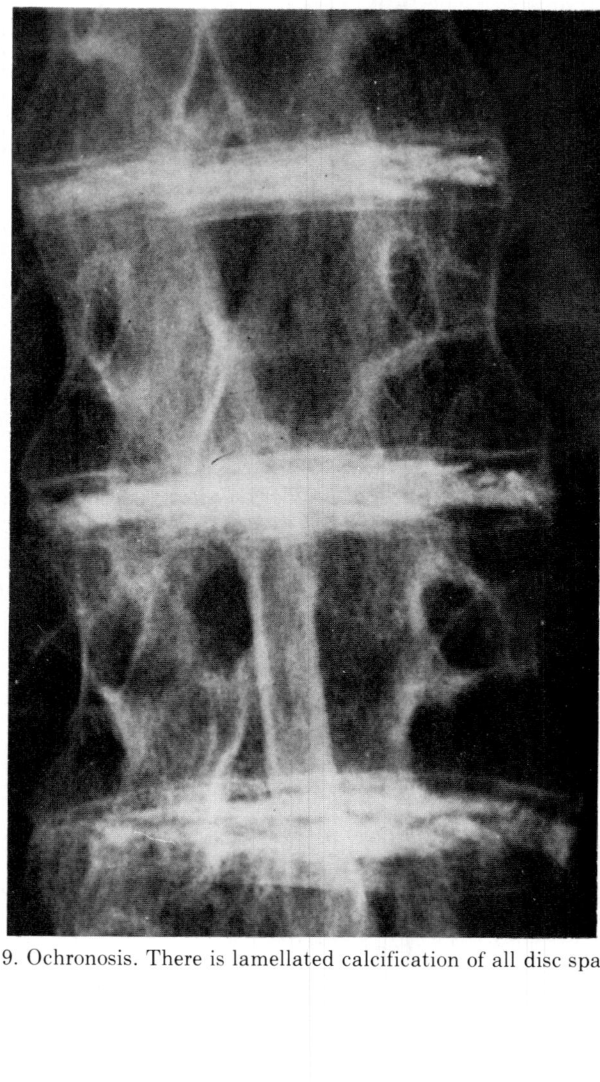

FIG. 9. Ochronosis. There is lamellated calcification of all disc spaces.

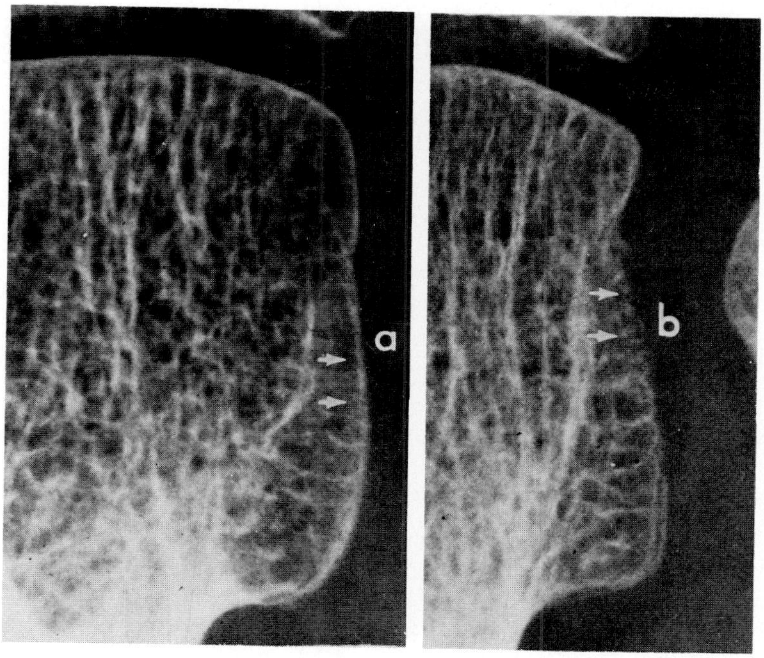

FIG. 10. Early rheumatoid arthritis. The roentgenograms of the distal portions of the second and third metatarsals are presented. *a*, normal articular cortex (*arrows*). *b*, erosion of the articular cortex (*arrows*). This sign is almost pathognomonic of rheumatoid arthritis.

SUMMARY

If the patient with arthritis is approached as a consultation and not as an x-ray, it is simple to make the diagnosis. The clinical arthritides are usually well known by the referring physician, or the diagnosis may be elicited from the patient. On the other hand, the radiologic arthritides occur in patients where the diagnosis is not made, but the roentgen features are so characteristic that the diagnosis is assured.

Chapter 8

Osteoarthritis

LEON SOKOLOFF

Osteoarthritis (degenerative joint disease) is the principal cause of rheumatic disability among the elderly, but it also has a great economic impact on the gainfully employed population. In the United States, people who are unable to work for more than 6 months because of illness become eligible for Social Security benefits. The National Health Survey (1957 to 1959) disclosed that of all persons so certified because of arthritis, 56% had osteoarthritis and only 27% had rheumatoid arthritis.[11] The general pathologist has long been familiar with the ubiquitous minor degenerative changes in the peripheral joints and spine in the autopsy population. The lesions have come to the attention of the surgical pathologist more recently because of the advent of the joint replacement procedures. Total hip arthroplasty has been a major medical triumph of the last decade and already more than 100,000 patients have been treated in this way. About 56% of these operations have been carried out for osteoarthritis.[14]

Although the lesions are complex and vary among different joints,[46] the endstage deformities have two components: disintegration and detachment of articular cartilage, and proliferation of new articular tissue at the margins and base of the joint surface (Fig. 1). The sequence of these events and their mechanisms are not clearly established.[70] Although overly simplistic, it is useful to recognize two broad but distinct mechanisms that may be involved. One postulates that osteoarthritis begins in an intrinsic senescent or other degeneration of articular cartilage; the other, that osteoarthritis is caused by abnormal mechanical stresses acting on joints. In reality both are involved.

AGING OF JOINTS

The concept that the earliest changes in osteoarthritis are a systemic senescence of cartilage was derived from autopsy studies. Even during the 3rd decade of life, fibrillation may occur on the surface of the patella. The frequency and severity increase almost linearly thereafter until by the 6th decade it is virtually universal.[26] Degenerative changes, furthermore, are widely distributed throughout the body. These findings and the occurrence of deteriorative changes in other cartilages, such as those of the ribs, suggested that some age-dependent change is the substrate on which the fibrillation and osteoarthritis develop.[3]

The problem with this is to define senescence. A recent workshop among experienced orthopedic pathologists and systems analysts failed to devise a

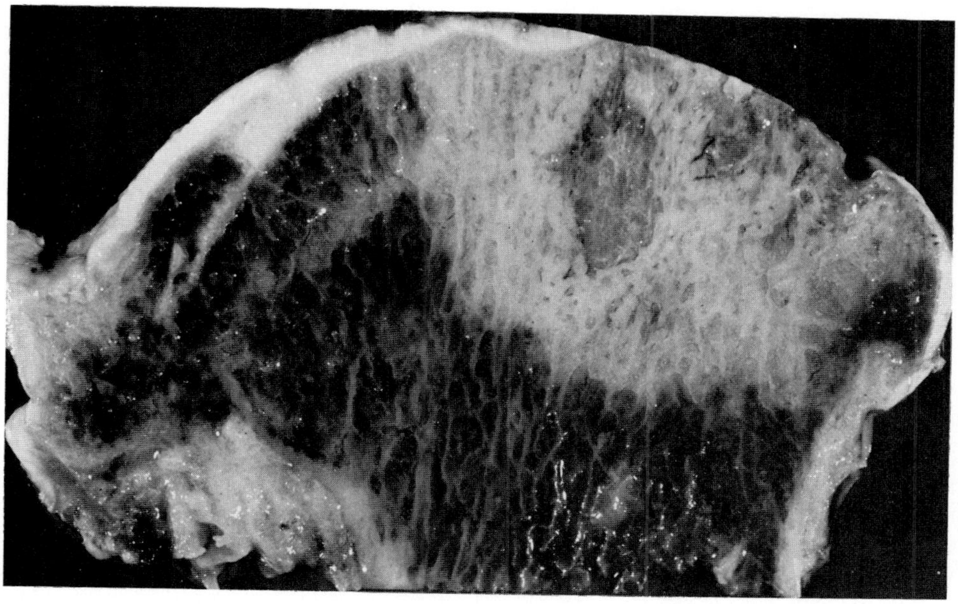

FIG. 1. Advanced osteoarthritis, head of femur. The contour is deformed both by loss of white articular cartilage and by the formation of marginal osteophytes. The spur at the left has grown not only to the side but superiorly onto the original joint surface. It is capped by newly formed cartilage. Subchondral pseudocysts approach the joint surface through slender crevices. The pallor of the eburnated tissue reflects the condensation of bony trabeculae and fibrous tissue in contrast to the darker hematopoietic marrow. (From Sokoloff, L., The pathology and pathogenesis of osteoarthritis. *In Arthritis and Allied Conditions*, edited by Hollander, J. L., and McCarty, D. J., Jr., Ed. 8. Philadelphia, Lea and Febiger, 1972. Used with permission.)

language for degenerative joint disease that would reconcile widely divergent concepts.[5] Some used the term aging of joints to indicate self-limited mild fibrillary changes or marginal osteophyte formation, while osteoarthritis was restricted to the severely deformed, symptom-producing lesions.[7] It seems more useful to this reviewer to regard senescence as the events in the articular cartilage that are associated with chronologic age exclusive of and distinct from osteoarthritis itself. For operational purposes, fibrillation may be considered the starting point of osteoarthritis. Even if one cannot identify age-dependent changes in the absence of fibrillation, the concept is worthwhile because it provides a handle for investigating the problem of biologic aging. At least one age-dependent change of this sort has been found: senescent pigmentation of the cartilage.[77] All other findings, chemical,[29, 42] physical,[33, 34] and morphologic[70] are associated more with fibrillation rather than age changes in intact portions of the joint cartilage.

Aging of joints in this sense may be resolved into two components: (1) a loss of self-replicating activity of the chondrocytes or (2) physico-chemical changes in the cartilage matrix taking place independently of cell functions.

Matrix changes

Articular cartilage, unlike most other tissues, is avascular and its cells are entirely dependent on a copious water-rich matrix for their metabolic exchanges.

This necessitates a low turnover of cells and is nature's way of maintaining a structural stability of the bearing surface of the joints. The matrix is a composite material in which the fibrous component is collagen, and the filler, the proteoglycan ground substance. The collagen is the source of the tissue's tensile strength; under conditions of health it turns over very little if at all. By contrast, the ground substance is quite labile. The half-life of chondroitin sulfate in rabbit cartilage is estimated as 8 to 40 days; in man, 250 or more days.[41] Because collagen persists throughout life, it is subject to slow molecular changes that may over the long run profoundly alter the physical properties of the tissue. There is an enormous literature on thermo-oxidation and cross-linking as mechanisms in the aging of connective tissues.[27]

In osteoarthritic fibrillation, the surface of the cartilage is disrupted, and there must necessarily be a disintegration of the preexisting collagen fibrils in the tangential layer. As the lesions become more advanced, tearing of the collagen extends more deeply into the radial zone until ultimately the cartilage is sheared off. Microscopically the fibrils in the vicinity of the tears appear discontinuous, disheveled, and unduly prominent ("unmasked"); these changes correspond to a diminution of the ground substance, which is readily confirmed histochemically and chemically.[43] It is not possible by morphologic means to distinguish which of these intimately associated events, fatigue and disruption of the fibers or depletion of the proteoglycans, comes first. Experimentally these components may be modified individually by physical and chemical means, but one is soon followed by the other.[82]

"Unmasking" of the collagen of older femoral head cartilage in the absence of overt fibrillation has been cited as an example of age changes in cartilage.[79] Unmasking and straightening of fibrils has often been referred to as amianthoid or asbestoid degeneration in this tissue by analogy to the fibrillary degeneration seen in rib and laryngeal cartilages. The argyrophilia and enormous diameter of the collagen fibrils of true amianthoid degeneration[31] are, in our experience, not characteristic of aging or osteoarthritic cartilage and have not been described in other accounts of the fine structure of this tissue.[83] The analysis of this phenomenon is complicated by the fact that reparative phenomena in osteoarthritic joints result in a largely fibrous rather than a hyaline cartilage. Thus reports of a Type I molecular species of collagen in osteoarthritic cartilage are difficult to interpret because the latter was obtained from surgically excised femoral heads.[54] Lesions so severe as to require joint replacement lack the original joint surface, and cartilage available for study in them must be obtained from the osteophyte. This phenomenon must also be reckoned with in many other chemical analyses of osteoarthritic tissues. This sort of sampling problem probably accounts for major disparities between the findings on proteoglycan synthesis and composition reported in this disorder.[29, 30]

Cellular aging

It has long been taught that articular chondrocytes, following cessation of skeletal growth, are incapable of mitotic division. The assumption that these cells are unable to replicate themselves has been one of the premises on which the wear and tear concept of osteoarthritis has been based. According to this view, articular cartilage degenerates with age because the cells cannot replenish structural components which are depleted by mechanical strains. That this is not strictly true is suggested by the fact that clusters of chondrocytes are seen regularly at the margins of the fibrillated fronds and, to a lesser extent, deeper in the cartilage. The clusters have the appearance of newly proliferated clones, an interpretation supported by autoradiographic demonstration of thymidine incorporation by the cells.[32, 62] Furthermore, radiosulfate is taken up by these cells and deposited into matrix proteoglycans.[45]

An additional argument in favor of a replicative capability of chondrocytes is the formation of thick layers of cartilage about joint mice detached in cases of osteochondritis dissecans. Similar structures are seen at times in osteoarthritis (Fig. 2). This evidence is not too secure, because the possibility that the detached nidus was at one time displaced into synovial tissue and so evoked a cartilaginous proliferation cannot be excluded.

The ultimate proof that articular chondrocytes can indeed divide has come from *in vitro* cell culture studies. These are accomplished by freeing the cells through mechanical and enzymatic disintegration of the tissue, phenomena structurally analogous to the finding of chondrocyte clusters close to the edges of matrix-depleted or fibrillated cartilage in osteoarthritis. The findings suggest that the failure of articular chondrocytes to divide in mature articular cartilage ordinarily is not an inherent deficiency in the cells' replicating mechanism but results from their sequestration in a matrix that denies them access of

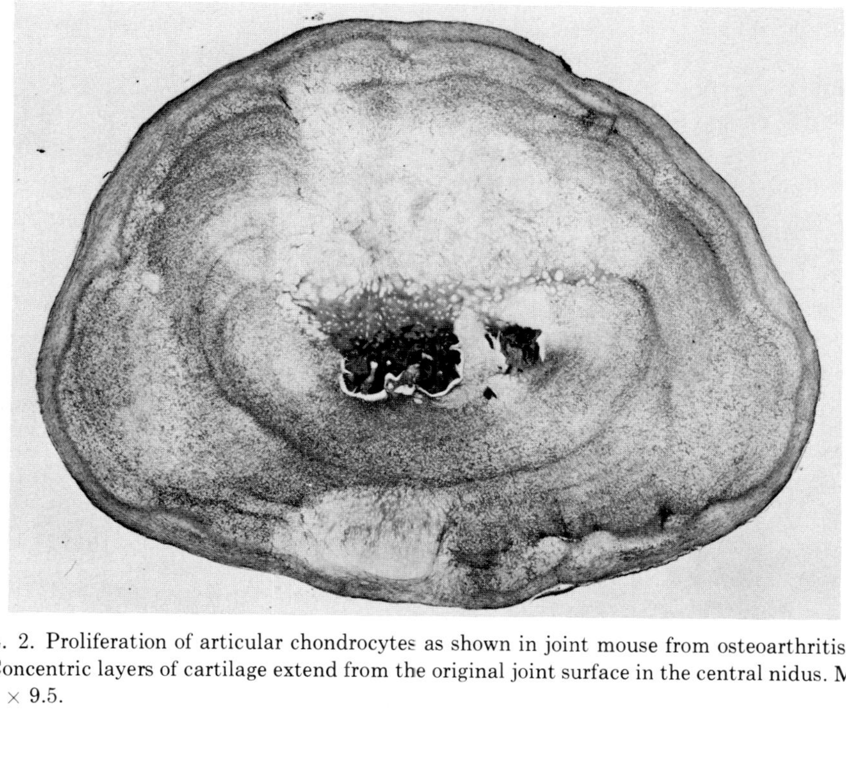

FIG. 2. Proliferation of articular chondrocytes as shown in joint mouse from osteoarthritis of the hip. Concentric layers of cartilage extend from the original joint surface in the central nidus. Masson stain; $\times$ 9.5.

macromolecular growth factors. Dissolution of the matrix seems to be the stimulus required for the cells to divide. Articular chondrocytes have been grown with varying degrees of success from several mammalian species.[81] Although human chondrocytes have failed to thrive under these conditions, there is no reason to believe that human osteoarthritis results from a species-specific failure of its chondrocytes to behave like other animal types. Depending on the conditions of culture, rabbit chondrocytes faithfully recapitulate *in vitro* both the proteoglycan profile[72] and collagen species (unpublished studies by D. Norby) that are produced *in vivo*. Furthermore, cells from 3-year-old rabbits divide and synthesize as much sulfated macromolecular material as do cells from young growing animals.

Articular chondrocytes contain proteases that can dissolve proteoglycans at neutral, naturally occurring *p*H[63] as well as cathepsins and other hydrolases[65] that have lower optimal acidity. The levels of catheptic activity are increased in osteoarthritic lesions.

Much of the cellular proliferation in osteoarthritis does not arise from articular chondrocytes but from a callus-like reaction both in the osteophytes and in the subchondral bone marrow of eroded areas. Side by side with islands of new hyaline cartilage there proliferate bone, fibrous scar and fibrocartilage. A large portion of the eroded joint surface is occupied by such tissue, and a palisaded synovial-like layer can be confused with a rheumatoid pannus.

PATHOLOGIC ANATOMY OF OSTEOARTHRITIS

Roentgenographic studies of slab sections are a necessary part of pathologic examination of osteoarthritic joints as well as other skeletal specimens.[47] A low kilovolt technique is desirable. The Faxitron (Hewlett-Packard) is a convenient and not too expensive equipment for this purpose; it has a sensor permitting automatic exposures and does not require a separate shielded room. For femoral heads, coronal slab sections approximately 0.8 mm thick are suitable (Fig. 3). The osteoarthritic lesions are so distorted that orientation may be difficult. A useful landmark in such cases is the calcar, the thick cortex on the posteromedial aspect of the femoral neck. The use of dilute India ink to stain minute breaks in the surface has been recommended to identify the earliest stages of fibrillation.[44]

Degeneration of the cartilage surface

The traditional description of the normal joint surface being very smooth has been reexamined by numerous investigators in recent years because of its importance in lubrication and wear in osteoarthritis. It had been the belief that minute breaks in the surface, arising from collapse of lacunae of necrobiotic ("effete") chondrocytes were the site of origin of the tears in fibrillation. Reflected light, transmission and scanning electron microscopy, and tallysurf measurements have been adduced to show that there normally is a degree of irregularity;[12, 21, 49, 80, 86] that the irregularity increases with age and imperceptibly goes over into fibrillation. There are significant technical limitations on the validity of these measurements, mostly stemming from unavoidable dehydration artefacts which result in collapse of the water-rich ground substance sols. The data reported often are contradictory. The so-called lamina splendens, a putative

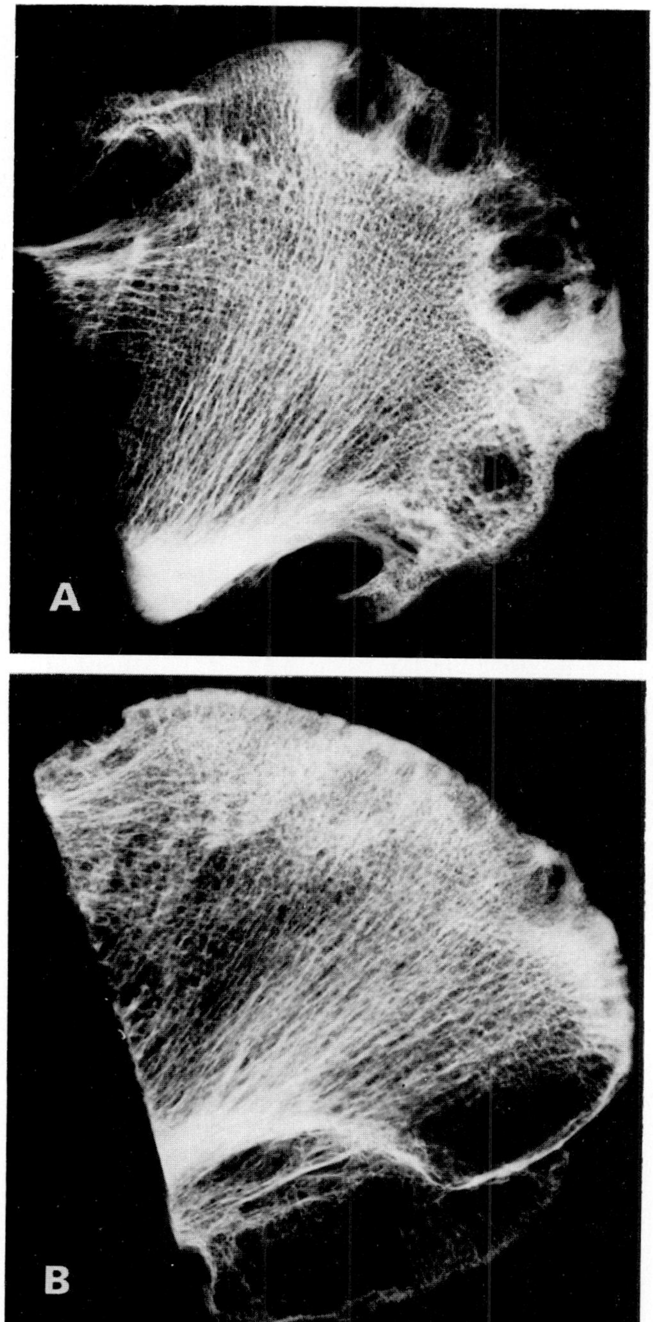

FIG. 3. Roentgenograms of coronal slabs of femoral heads showing different configurations of osteoarthritic deformity. The specimens are oriented as *in situ*. The superolateral surface is identified by the subjacent wedge-shaped spray of trabeculae. The latter converge onto the thick inferomedial edge of the femoral neck. *A*, numerous subchondral pseudocysts are present, particularly on the superolateral aspect. The osteophytes are small. *E*, buttress osteophytes are present on both aspects of the femoral neck. An enormous inferomedial osteophyte has merged with the adjacent buttress so that the entire femoral head has assumed an externally ovoid configuration. The surface is eburnated.

noncollagenous layer forming the surface of the cartilage, may or may not be a true structure. There presently are no techniques for distinguishing rigorously between such a layer and an absorbed film of synovial mucin. A recent scanning electron microscopy study has suggested that normal articular cartilage is relatively smooth, but when the elastic properties of the deep portion of the cartilage are reduced, the surface becomes unstable and rippled as the joint fluid flows over it under load.[51] Exaggeration of this process might then be instrumental in initiating the fibrillation.

It has often been postulated that the superficial tangential layer is not only structurally different from the deeper layers of the cartilage,[83] but serves as an "armor plate" in protecting the latter from mechanical injury.[51] The only empiric data for testing this hypothesis, actual measurement of resistance to an artificial abrader *in vitro*, have given no support to it.[68] Engineering analyses indicate that because friction is so low, articular cartilage is more likely to be damaged by impact than by abrasive forces.[58] Detachment of articular cartilage first takes place at the tidemark, the interface between the noncalcified and calcified layers of the cartilage rather than at the osteoarticular junction.[30]

There is one body of thinking that the initial degenerative changes or nonprogressive aging of joints occurs in relatively little stressed portions of the cartilage.[4] The bulk of the cartilage loss and exposure of underlying bone in osteoarthritis ultimately is found in the more central rather than the peripheral portions of the joint surface. In the femoral head, it is most marked in the superolateral region. This corresponds to the wedge-shaped spray of trabeculae seen in roentgenograms (Fig. 3) and usually is called the "weight-bearing" portion. Weight is, of course, supported in different parts of the joint surface depending on the position of the extremity. It has been argued that the superolateral surface is not the point of maximal weight bearing; there are two singular points of maximum contact and initial fibrillation on the anterior and posterior surfaces, respectively, instead.[4, 76]

The loss of joint surface is not confined to the cartilage. Subchondral bone also is eroded and polished. The latter, backed up by reactive new bone formation is responsible for the ivory-like (eburnated) appearance of the surface. Even in advanced eburnation, the exposed bony surface is perforated in many areas by nubbins of fibrous tissue and cartilage proliferating out of the subchondral marrow.

Necrosis of bone in osteoarthritis

Two major patterns of bone necrosis are commonly seen in osteoarthritis. One is a necrobiosis of osteocytes in the superficial layer of eburnated bone. It is conceivable that local frictional heat is responsible for killing the cells. The other is a more extensive segmental necrosis of subchondral bone. The latter most often results from minute fractures of the subchondral bone in areas of eburnation. These fractures are the rule rather than the exception in severe osteoarthritis and probably account for much of the deformity even if they are not at the heart of the process.[73, 74] In other cases, focal areas of aseptic necrosis occur in which microfractures cannot be identified. Occlusion of minute intramedullary arteries has been demonstrated by angiography in such cases by Trueta. Nevertheless, Streda's suggestion[75] that all osteoarthritis of the hip is secondary to aseptic necrosis of the femoral head goes beyond the anatomic evidence.

Other events also shape the subchondral bone. The sequence usually taught, that bony changes are secondary to initial degeneration of the cartilage, may not be valid. A reshaping of the articular ends of the bones with age has been described repeatedly.[4] It has been proposed by some that this remodeling, when it exceeds the rate at which cartilage can accommodate to the change in shape, is the basic process in osteoarthritic degeneration. Most of the published data on the subject have not come to grips with the problem of whether the surface of the cartilage has indeed remained intact while the bone changes its shape. Perhaps the best evidence for this comes from the temporomandibular joint, but the point remains moot. There can be no question that the changes in the osteochondral junction and reduplication of the tidemark do take place throughout adult life even in the absence of fibrillation.[25] The point is worth making because there is some engineering logic behind the thinking that articular cartilage is not a good shock absorber for impact loading, and that such impacts are the important events in causing osteoarthritis.[58] This places a greater importance on primary changes in the subchondral bone.

There is considerable variation in density of subchondral bone in osteoarthritis. Aside from the eburnation and pseudocysts described below, there also are regions of osteoporosis. Daracott and Vernon-Roberts have emphasized the rarefaction of the subchondral plate as the anatomic feature distinguishing chondromalacia of the patella from ordinary osteoarthritic fibrillation.[17] In areas of remodeling bone in osteoarthritic femoral heads, considerable osteoid material is found.[2] The new bone formation is the basis for increased uptake of bone-seeking isotopes in clinical scintigraphy of osteoarthritis.[15]

Comparison of osteoarthritis and aseptic necrosis

More than 5% of total hip replacements nowadays are performed for aseptic necrosis. The most frequent etiologic factor is corticosteroid therapy for rheumatoid arthritis or other rheumatic problems. Immunosuppressive agents used during organ transplantation or neoplastic disorders, late decompression syndrome, myeloproliferative disorders, gout, and alcoholism account for others, but there persists a good proportion for which no etiologic factor is found. Excluding obvious factors such as fractures of the femoral neck, our experience coincides with that of others[37] that vascular occlusion cannot be identified. There has been considerable speculation that fat emboli, initiated by the corticosteroids and other factors indicated above, may become impacted in medullary vessels and cause infarction. Formidable technical obstacles prevent satisfactory documentation of such emboli. Another mechanism, suggested by L. C. Johnson, deserves serious consideration although it too is difficult to prove. By analogy with myeloproliferative disorders, the hypothesis is that swelling of medullary components against the noncompliant, rigid bony cortex may compress the capillary-sinusoidal vessels and so cause ischemia. In the case of a Cushingoid response to corticosteroids, the yellow marrow of the bone might enlarge as do the subcutaneous adipose tissues of the buccal and dorsal region.

There are two distinct stages in the evolution of the necrotic lesion: (1) infarction of the subchondral bone and its marrow; and (2) subsequent fracture of the dead bone beneath the articular cartilage. Most of the dead bone prior to fracture remains inert indefinitely. Only at the interface of viable and dead tissue is there some minor osteoclastic resorption, as well as minute foci of calcification of necrotic adipose tissue and apposition of new bone on dead spicules. Because the overlying cartilage is avascular and derives its nourishment principally from the synovial fluid, it remains viable initially. Only when the fracture develops and the joint surface collapses does pain appear. The cartilage then is torn at one or more points, and a new false joint surface forms at the base of the callus tissue (Fig. 4). Secondary osteoarthritic changes, including subchondral pseudocysts and marginal osteophytes are a feature. The radiographs disclose, in addition to the fracture cleft, areas of radiolucency caused by focal new cartilage formation and the osteoelastic resorption already mentioned. Apparent areas of increased radiodensity mostly result from the contrast of unresorbed dead bone with the radiolucent regions, but there is also some focal reactive new bone formation at the callus.

In most cases it is not too difficult to distinguish cases of aseptic necrosis of the femoral head from ordinary osteoarthritis because of the extent of the infarction

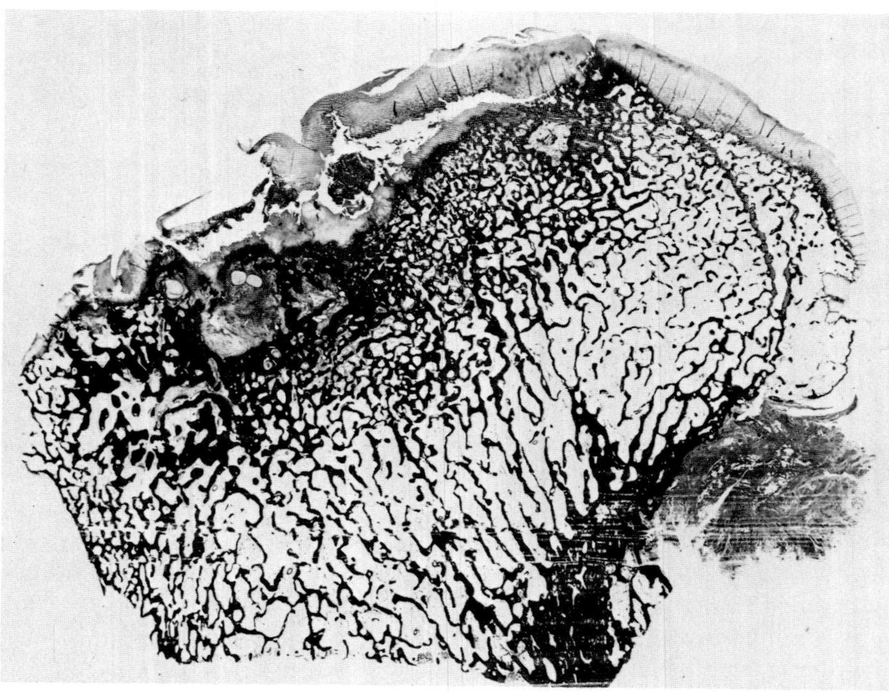

FIG. 4. Aseptic necrosis of femoral head in a 42-year-old alcoholic patient. The weight-bearing surface is jagged and depressed into a fracture cavity. An irregular cartilaginous surface has formed at the base of the fracture cleft, and pseudocysts are present beneath it.

and collapse of the joint surface. The contours differ as a result: the collapsed surface is more jagged, and the overall dimensions are reduced rather than enlarged. Aseptic necrosis, no matter what the cause, has a predilection for the femoral head. The basis for the localization is not evident. There has been some speculation that the nutrient vessels, traversing the synovial retinaculum before perforating the bone, may be particularly prone to intraarticular compression in this joint. Other joints are by no means immune to aseptic necrosis, and involvement of the knee, shoulder, and smaller joints is increasingly being recognized.

Subchondral pseudocysts (geodes)

Globoid or pyriform defects in subchondral bone are common in osteoarthritis of the hip and the base of the thumb but not in other joints.[22] The explanation offered for their occurrence is that the joint surface supports extremely high pressures during weight-bearing, and that when localized discontinuities in the subchondral plate develop, pressure intrudes into the subchondral marrow and disturbs the circulation.[70] Three sorts of processes are seen histologically to account for the loss of bony tissue in the center of these pseudocysts: (1) osteoclastic resorption associated with the formation of a fibromyxoid connective tissue (Fig. 5); (2) localized osteoporosis, probably the least common form; and (3) necrosis and microfractures of the bone and adjacent marrow. The centers of these areas contain fluid in only a relatively small percentage of cases. When present, the cysts form as puddles in the myxoid tissue and lack a synovial lining. They are morphologically similar to the periarticular cysts of Heberden's nodes and to ganglia. Rather similar pseudocysts are seen frequently about the knee of several laboratory rodents prone to osteoarthritis. They form by liquefaction of the periarticular fibroadipose tissue rather than protrusion and pinching off of synovial pouches from the joint (Fig. 5*B*).

The character of the cyst varies with the age of the lesion. Areas of hemorrhage are sometimes seen. The defect in the overlying bone plate is seen at the apex of the pseudocyst and often does not appear for this reason in random sections. The periphery of the geode is more cellular than the center, and may be replaced by compact fibrous tissue, sometimes mixed with cartilage. External to these, congested sinusoidal vessels are common and new bone is laid down to form a sclerotic rim. The pseudocysts in the hip are larger on the acetabular than the femoral side. They often are multiple and sometimes individually are more than 3 cm in diameter.

Structure of the osteophyte

Osteophytes form in different locations of individual joints but share common pathogenetic sequences. Among the earliest seen are those growing into the marginal no-mans-land of cartilage, synovium, capsule, periosteum, and subchondral bone plate. These often occur in regions where the immediately overlying cartilage is not eroded. At a later period, osteophytes may grow into ligamentous-capsular attachments to the joint, or protrude directly into the joint cavity. They are covered characteristically by a primarily fibrous cartilage and,

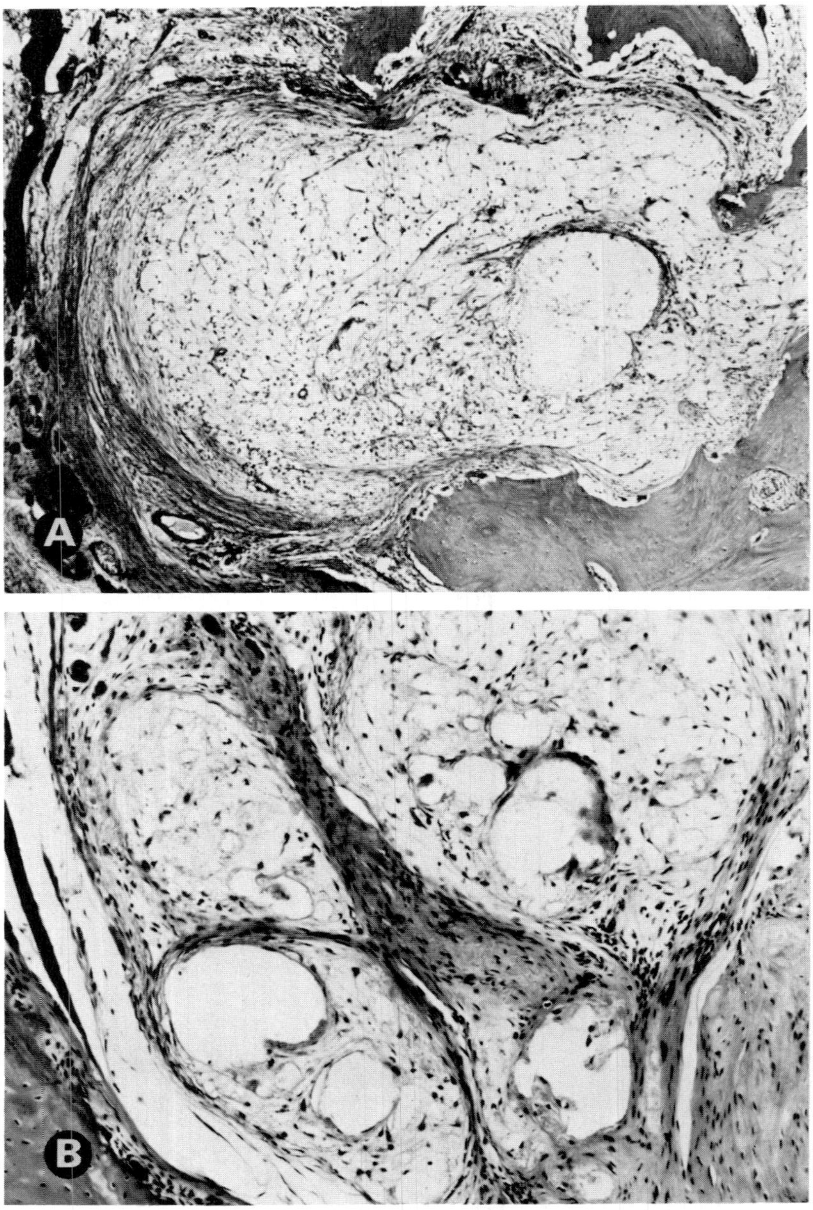

FIG. 5. Mucoid pseudocysts in osteoarthritis. *A*, subchondral pseudocyst in human femoral head. A fibrous rim is forming at the periphery, and osteoclastic activity is seen in the adjacent bone. Hematoxylin and eosin stain; × 60. *B*, early lesion in popliteal adipose tissue, 16-month-old STR/1N mouse. These mice have an inherited predisposition to severe degenerative joint disease. Hematoxylin and eosin stain; × 123.

peripherally, by synovial fibrous tissue. The subchondral bone of the osteophyte is fragile. The surface of the osteophyte itself commonly is caught up in the osteoarthritic process and becomes fibrillated and abraded. In the femoral head, the osteophyte extends along the retinaculum and may merge with the cortex of the femoral neck (so-called buttress osteophyte, Fig. 3). At times the entire osteophyte and femoral head become so remodeled that they form a single continuous ovoid structure. In the femoral head, osteophytes also form early about the fovea of the ligamentum teres but may become obliterated during progression of the eburnation.

Although the osteophyte may be regarded teleologically as an attempt to enlarge the bearing surface of the joint and thereby reduce pressure on it (pressure = force/area), it also is true that osteophytes interfere mechanically with excursions of the joint. Several prospective studies have demonstrated that small osteophytes often are present at the knee[16] and hip for long periods of time without apparent narrowing of the joint space or progressive deterioration. This is one of the reasons that have been offered for the belief held by some that aging changes should be distinguished from osteoarthritis. In evaluating this, it should be kept in mind that considerable anatomic destruction of joint cartilage may be present and not detected in conventional roentgenographic films. For this purpose, it is desirable to examine the osteoarthritic joint in a weight-bearing (erect) posture rather than while reclining.

Soft tissues in osteoarthritis

Although degenerative joint disease by definition is not inherently inflammatory, focal areas of chronic synovitis and fibrosis are the rule in advanced cases. Mostly this is characterized by small focal infiltrates of lymphocytes and mononuclear cells in the retinaculum; occasionally it is sufficiently severe to raise a question of rheumatoid arthritis. A foreign body giant cell reaction to joint detritus also occurs and must be responsible for pain and effusion in acute cases. Secondary synovial osteochondromatosis is usually of minor degree. Synovial hypertrophy and fibrosis are the rule rather than the exception, and the synovium may appear quite villous in surgical material. Fibrous contracture of the capsule and ligaments contributes to the loss of mobility of the hip, and this forms the basis for older surgical procedures in which the ligaments were simply cut across. Amyloid deposits have been described in the capsule by one group of observers.[71] The ligamentum teres usually has disintegrated and is absent in resected specimens. In the knee joint, cruciate ligaments and menisci also become frayed, and a degree of instability results.

Heberden's nodes sometimes present primarily as paraarticular mucoid cysts of the sort described above and come to the attention of the dermatologist. Recent experience has confirmed that these consistently arise in association with osteoarthritis of the fingers; and that simple surgical excision of the cysts without removing at the same time the associated marginal osteophytes will result in recurrence of the cysts.[13, 18, 35] The cysts characteristically lack a synovial lining even though they may have communicated at one time with a joint.

Degenerative spinal disease

The traditional distinction between spondylosis and spinal osteoarthritis, *i.e.*, degenerative disease of the intervertebral discs and the posterior facet joints, respectively, is more artificial than real. Although they do not usually occur on the same vertebral body, the lesions alternate with each other on adjacent ones.

A considerable emphasis has been placed on the fact that vertebral osteophytes may occur without apparent narrowing of the intervertebral disc and therefore be distinguished from intervertebral disc degeneration. The admonition noted above seems relevant here: disc narrowing may not be apparent in roentgenographic films unless the latter are made in an upright position. Vertebral osteophytes in the lumbar spine are so frequent that it is difficult to know whether their presence in any given individual with backache is satisfactory evidence for their contributing to the clinical discomfort.

Most vertebral osteophytosis occurs on the anterolateral aspects of the lumbar vertebrae. In the cervical spine, the osteophytes often occur more posteriorly. Where they impinge on the Luschka (neurocentral) joints, they are prone to cause brachial neuralgias. More posteriorly, they protrude into the neural canal proper, and particularly by interfering with the vertebral vascular circulation, result in cervical myelopathy. The danger of posterior cervical osteophytosis is increased in persons with congenitally narrow cervical canals and sudden death following whiplash injuries likely in the elderly.[84]

Hyperostotic ankylosing spondylosis is a special form of degenerative disease found with frequency in the lower dorsal spine during the 7th and 8th decades.[78] Local bony bridges unite individual vertebral bodies on the periosteal aspect of their anterolateral surfaces. Several investigators have emphasized in careful studies the infrequency with which narrowing of the disc occurs in these cases. I am impressed with the destructive changes in the bone cortex beneath these bridges, and the extension of the ossific reaction into the adjacent disc. Older views that there is an association between this lesion and diabetes mellitus do not receive support from recent studies.

MECHANICAL FACTORS IN PATHOGENESIS OF OSTEOARTHRITIS

Osteoarthritis is classified as being primary or secondary depending on whether some antecedant abnormality of the joint can be identified. In the case of the hip, the frequency of the two types varies according to the criteria employed, but the overall frequency is about equally distributed. Rheumatoid arthritis predisposes to secondary osteoarthritis, but the most frequent cause is congenital dysplasia or subluxation of the hip. This is one or another type of poor fit of the ball and socket, usually a shallow acetabulum.[85] As a result the full brunt of the force on the hip joint is supported only by a small area of the acetabulum, and the high pressure presumably is responsible for the damage to the structure. Overt dysplasia occurs sporadically or else in high prevalence in certain population isolates such as Navajo Indian reservations. The extent to which the endemic forms are genetically rather than culturally determined is a fascinating biologic and societal problem. Coxa vara, a configuration of the hip favoring osteoarthritic degeneration, is sometimes an inherited condition in man.[64]

There has been considerable extrapolation from the preceding to the role of unsuspected dysplasia being the cause of much idiopathic or primary osteoarthritis of the hip. Standard radiologic techniques which demonstrate that the calculated center of the femoral head is located outside of its expected position with respect to the acetabulum are adduced to show this.[28] It is doubtful that this is correct, since it is quite clear that large osteophytes forming on the medial aspect of the femoral head themselves can cause rather than result from the apparent displacement. Others have analyzed radiologic patterns of early changes in the hip to distinguish different etiologic factors. Narrowing of the medial side of the joint space is said to be more characteristic of idiopathic and superolateral involvement, of a long-leg origin. The latter postulates that in persons having one lower extremity more than 1.2 cm longer than the other, the increased leverage on the longer sides results in overloading the hip and thereby causing osteoarthritic degeneration.[23] This thesis has not gained universal acceptance because of technical uncertainties inherent in the measurements. In any event, this pattern should more often be unilateral than the dysplastic varieties. The surgical pathologist is unable to resolve this difference because the lesions in resected specimens are too far advanced and deformed for such an analysis. By and large, it has not been possible to distinguish primary and secondary types of osteoarthritis on anatomic grounds. The exception, other than obvious infarcts, fracture deformities, and so forth, is the osteoarthritis following Legg-Perthes disease and slipped capital epiphysis; in these, the disturbance in the growth of the epiphysis of a young child leaves its own calling card (Fig. 6).

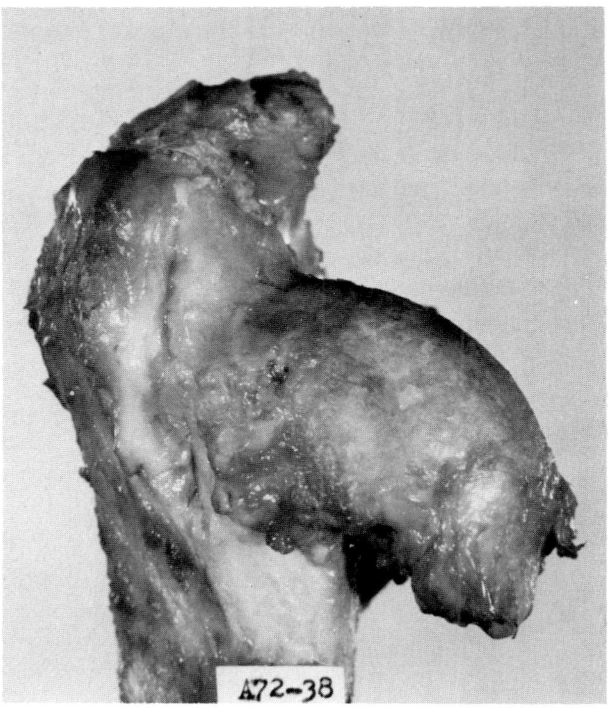

FIG. 6. Secondary osteoarthritis of the hip following Legg-Perthes disease. The patient was 59 years old. The shortening of the femoral neck reflects the damage to the growing epiphysis at an early age. Because of the massive osteophytes on the inferomedial margin, the femoral head was extracted from the acetabulum at necropsy only with great difficulty.

The role of recurrent or single instance of trauma in causing degenerative joint disease is difficult to determine. Probably the only clear examples of single traumatic insults causing osteoarthritis are those that follow overt fracture of the joint surface. Compensation courts wrestle every day with this problem, with respect to both peripheral and spinal joints. Occupational hazards[50] and athletic injuries[52] are all said to contribute to this. A deleterious mechanical contribution of obesity has also been cited frequently.[36] Although it would be unwise for a person with severe osteoarthritis not to control his weight, there is much evidence that obesity contributes relatively little to the severity of osteoarthritis of weight-bearing or non-weight-bearing joints.[70]

REPAIR OF OSTEOARTHRITIS

A limited potential for replication of chondrocytes in adult articular cartilage has already been noted, and so has the fact that new cartilage commonly is formed as part of the callus reaction in the subchondral marrow.[48] The question has therefore been asked with increasing frequency whether repair or reversal of osteoarthritis is possible. Numerous examples of an increase of roentgenologic joint space, suggesting formation of a new cartilage, have been reported clinically.[55] All recent experimental information[9, 59] is in agreement with older findings that surface wounds in articular cartilage do not fill in, but that defects extending into subchondral bone repair to varying degrees of perfection. Surprisingly little anatomic material from human subjects following osteotomies or shaving of articular cartilage (as is sometimes done for chondromalacia patellae) has been reported. What there is indicates only at best a fibrous and new fibrocartilaginous repair.[6] It is likely that much of the apparent increase in the joint space in roentgenographic films is the result of the angle of exposure rather than a measure of the cartilage regenerated. Subchondral pseudocysts and osteophytes, once formed, persist indefinitely.

It would be an error to conclude from these facts that there is no inherent potential for joints to repair themselves. Many clinical attempts are being made to influence the course of osteoarthritis by stimulating the chondrocytes to synthesize ground substance or to retard its degradation by medical means.[10] *A priori* there is no reason for believing that administering surrogate ground substance materials intraarticularly or systemically, or even stimulating the production of natural ground substance in itself, would offer an advantage to the osteoarthritic patient. The key to the repair of cartilage would seem to be that the chondrocytes can fulfill themselves only when there is a proper coupling of removal with synthesis of matrix, and necessarily too under conditions where the cartilage is not being subjected to mechanical insults as it is being formed.

SYSTEMIC INFLUENCES IN OSTEOARTHRITIS

Although local mechanical factors are major determinants of osteoarthritis in particular joints, there also are systemic factors. Aging and the widespread fibrillation of joints at routine necropsy attest to this. The literature on possible hormonal, biochemical (*e.g.*, ochronotic), and genetic factors through 1968 has been reviewed elsewhere,[70] and relevant data have been presented more recently.

Heberden's nodes are a case in point. Persons with osteoarthritis of the hip are more likely to have degenerative changes in the hands than age- and sex-matched individuals who do not have osteoarthritis of the hip.[61] This corresponds to what others have called primary generalized osteoarthritis. Although handedness has some influence on their development,[1] Heberden's nodes tend to form symmetrically. Possible mechanical explanations have been offered for their development: the area of the surfaces of the small joints is so small that high pressures can arise from even small compressive forces.[57] Despite this there is no documentation that applied forces account for the notable predilection of women in certain families to develop the nodes. The suggestion that a single dominant gene, fully penetrant in women although not in men, still seems attractive.

Senile osteoporosis, another degenerative disorder of the aging skeleton, typically does not favor and may actually militate against the development of osteoarthritis.[8, 20, 60] This pathologic finding should be remembered in the context of the previously mentioned uncertainties about the role of subchondral bone in the inception and pathogenesis of the cartilage degeneration in osteoarthritis.

Population studies have indicated that there are genetic contributions to degenerative joint disease in man as there also are in experimental animals and livestock. A recent study of one Zulu community disclosed severe generalized osteoarthritic changes in about half of the adult population.[38] It was considered likely that this represented an inherited epiphyseal dysplasia, but the possibility of an environmentally acquired etiology could not be ruled out.

Chondrocalcinosis is a disorder of pyrophosphate metabolism that, in long-standing cases, leads to degenerative joint disease. Increased levels of inorganic pyrophosphate in synovial fluid in ordinary osteoarthritis unassociated with chondrocalcinosis have been reported recently.[66, 67] Its significance has yet to be determined; perhaps it has to do with mineralizing aspects of the remodeling.

ANATOMIC BASIS FOR SYMPTOMS IN OSTEOARTHRITIS

Anatomic changes of degenerative joint disease may cause little clinical discomfort but there is a general correlation between complaints and the severity of the lesions. The principal complaints are pain and restriction of motion. Pain arises from several sources: (1) vascular engorgement of the bone;[53, 56] (2) collapse of subchondral bone; (3) detritic synovitis; (4) microtears in the capsular and ligamentous structures; and (5) particularly in the case of spinal roots, of impingements on nerves and nerve roots. Orthopedists have observed pain to disappear immediately following osteotomy and cite this as evidence that interruption of peripheral pain fibers rather than correction of mechanical or other disturbance is responsible for the relief. Limitation of movement results from (1) mechanical deformation and irregularity of the joint contours; and (2) the soft tissue fibrosis noted.

In the early stages of Heberden node formation, considerable reddening and swelling of periarticular soft tissues are common. Often this is associated with the periarticular mucoid cysts described. Considerable inflammation is present at times in the synovium in such cases,[24, 40] and there may be a difficulty in distinguishing this "erosive" osteoarthritis from rheumatoid arthritis.[19] The distribution of the lesions, predominantly in the distal rather than proximal parts of the fingers, and also at the base of the thumb is a useful clinical guide. Effusion into joints in osteoarthritis typically is associated with detritic synovitis. Ankylosis typically does not occur in degenerative joint disease except in hyperostotic spondylosis, but it is occasionally present in particularly severe osteoarthritis of the fingers.[69]

CONCLUDING REMARKS

The lesions of osteoarthritis have been reproduced with varying degrees of completeness by local mechanical and chemical abuses of joints, too many to be recounted here.[70] These findings do not indicate that naturally occurring degenerative joint disease arises always from some local peculiarity of an individual joint. Osteoarthritis is not a single disease but a pattern of biomechanical failure of joints. One or more components of the interacting mechanical and biologic feedback loops may lead to a malfunction of this complex system. Biologic modifiers have variable net effects depending on the particular target and timing of their actions.

REFERENCES

1. Acheson, R. M., Chan, Y. K., and Clemett, A. R. New Haven survey of joint diseases. XII. Distribution and symptoms of osteoarthrosis in the hands with reference to handedness. *Ann. Rheum. Dis. 29:* 275–286, 1970.
2. Batra, H. C., and Charnley, J. Existence and incidence of osteoid in osteoarthritic femoral heads. A preliminary report. *J. Bone Joint Surg. 51B:* 366–371, 1969.
3. Bennett, G. A., Waine, H., and Bauer, W. *Changes in the Knee Joint at Various Ages; with Particular Reference to the Nature and Development of Degenerative Joint Disease.* New York, Commonwealth Fund, 1942.
4. Bullough, P., Goodfellow, J., and O'Connor, J. The relationship between degenerative changes and load-bearing in the human hip. *J. Bone Joint Surg. 55B:* 746–758, 1973.
5. Byers, P. D. Conclusions of a working party of morbid anatomists. *Ann. Rheum. Dis.* (in press).
6. Byers, P. D. The effect of high femoral osteotomy on osteoarthritis of the hip. An anatomical study of six hip joints. *J Bone Joint Surg. 56B:* 279–290, 1974.
7. Byers, P. D., Contepomi, C. A., and Farkas, T. A. A *postmortem* study of the hip joint including the prevalence of the features of the right side. *Ann. Rheum. Dis. 29:* 15–31, 1970.
8. Byers, P. D., Hoaglund, F. T., Purewal, G. S., and Yau, A. C. M. C. Articular cartilage changes in Caucasian and Asian hip joints. *Ann. Rheum. Dis. 33:* 157–161, 1974.
9. Campbell, C. J. The healing of cartilage defects. *Clin. Orthop. 64:* 45–63, 1969.
10. Chrisman, O. D., Snook, G. A., and Wilson, T. C. The protective effect of aspirin against degeneration of human articular cartilage. *Clin. Orthop. 84:* 193–196, 1972.
11. Chronic conditions causing limitation of activities. U. S. National Health Survey. Health Statistics. United States, July 1959–June 1961 Ser. B. No. 36. U. S. Department of Health, Education and Welfare, Public Health Service. Washington, D. C.
12. Clarke, I. C. The microevaluation of articular surface contours. *Ann. Biomed. Eng. 1:* 31–43, 1972.
13. Constant, E., Royer, J. R., Pollard, R. J., Larsen, R. D., and Posch, J. L. Mucous cysts of the fingers. *Plast. Reconstr. Surg. 43:* 241–246, 1969.
14. Coventry, M. B., Beckenbaugh, R. D., Nolan, D. R., and Ilstrup, D. M. 2,012 total hip arthroplasties: a study of postoperative course and early complications. *J. Bone Joint Surg. 56A:* 273–284, 1974.
15. Crutchlow, W. P. Sr^{85} scintimetry of the hip in osteoarthritis and osteonecrosis. *Am. J. Roentgenol. Radium Ther. Nucl. Med. 109:* 803–812, 1970.

16. Danielsson, L., and Hernborg, J. Clinical and roentgenologic study of knee joints with osteophytes. *Clin. Orthop. 69:* 302–312, 1970.
17. Daracott, J., and Vernon-Roberts, B. The bony changes in "chondromalacia patellae." *Rheum. Phys. Med. 11:* 175–179, 1971.
18. Eaton, R. G., Dobranski, A. I., and Littler, J. W. Marginal osteophyte excision in treatment of mucous cysts. *J. Bone Joint Surg. 55A:* 570–574, 1973.
19. Ehrlich, G. E. Inflammatory osteoarthritis. I. The clinical syndrome. *J. Chron. Dis. 25:* 317–328, 1972.
20. Foss, M. V. L., and Byers, P. D. Bone density, osteoarthrosis of the hip and fracture of the upper end of the femur. *Ann. Rheum. Dis. 31:* 259–264, 1972.
21. Gardner, D. L., and Longmore, R. B. Age related studies of human and articular cartilage. In *Normal and Osteoarthrotic Articular Cartilage*, edited by Ali, S. Y., Elves, M. W., and Leaback, D. H., pp. 141–152. London, Institute of Orthopaedics, 1974.
22. Gerber, N. J., and Dixon, A. St. J. Synovial cysts and juxta-articular bone cysts (geodes). *Semin. Arthritis Rheum. 3:* 323–348, 1974.
23. Gofton, J. P. Studies in osteoarthritis of the hip. Parts 1–4. *Can. Med. Assoc. J. 104:* 679–683, 791–799, 911–915, 1007–1011, 1971.
24. Goldie, I. Erosive osteoarthritis of the distal finger joints. *Acta Orthop. Scand. 43:* 469–478, 1972.
25. Green, W. T., Jr., Martin, G. N., Eanes, E. D., and Sokoloff, L. Microradiographic study of the calcified layer of articular cartilage. *Arch. Path. 90:* 151–158, 1970.
25a. Harrison, M. H. M., Schajowicz, F., and Trueta, J. Osteoarthritis of the hip; a study of the evolution and nature of the disease. *J. Bone Joint Surg. 35B:* 598–626, 1963.
26. Heine, J. Ueber die Arthritis deformans. *Virchows Arch. 260:* 521–663, 1926.
27. Herbage, D., Huc, A., Chabrand, D., and Chapuy, M. C. Physicochemical study of articular cartilage from healthy and osteo-arthritic human hips. Orientation and thermal stability of collagen fibers. *Biochim. Biophys. Acta 271:* 339–346, 1972.
28. Hermodsson, I. Roentgen appearance of coxarthrosis. Relation between the anatomy, pathologic changes and roentgen appearance. *Acta Orthop. Scand. 41:* 169–187, 1970.
29. Hjertquist, S. O. and Lemperg, R. Identification and concentration of the glycosaminoglycans of human articular cartilage in relation to age and osteoarthritis. *Calcif. Tissue Res. 10:* 223–237, 1972.
30. Hough, A. J., Banfield, W. G., Mottram, F. C., and Sokoloff, L. The osteochondral junction of mammalian joints. An ultrastructural and microanalytic study. *Lab. Invest. 31:* 685–695, 1974.
31. Hough, A. J., Mottram, F. C., and Sokoloff, L. The collagenous nature of amianthoid degeneration of human costal cartilage. *Am. J. Pathol. 73:* 201–216, 1973.
32. Hulth, A., Lindberg, L., and Telhag, H. Mitosis in human osteoarthritic cartilage. *Clin. Orthop. 84:* 197–199, 1972.
33. Kempson, G. E., Muir, H., Swanson, S. A. V., and Freeman, M. A. R. Correlations between stiffness and the chemical constituents of cartilage on the human femoral head. *Biochim. Biophys. Acta 215:* 70–77, 1970.
34. Kempson, G. E., Spivey, C. J., Swanson, S. A. V., and Freeman, M. A. R. Patterns of cartilage stiffness on normal and degenerative human femoral heads. *J. Biomechan. 4:* 597–609, 1971.
35. Kleinert, H. E., Kutz, J. E., Fishman, J. H., and McCraw, L. H. Etiology and treatment of the so-called mucous cyst of the finger. *J. Bone Joint Surg. 54A:* 1455–1458, 1972.
36. Leach, R. E., Baumgard, S., and Broom, J. Obesity: its relationship to osteoarthritis of the knee. *Clin. Orthop. 93:* 271–273, 1973.
37. Leventhal, G. H., and Dorfman, H. D. Aseptic necrosis of bone in systemic lupus erythematosus. *Semin. Arthritis Rheum. 4:* 73–93, 1974.
38. Lockitch, G., Fellingham, S. A., Wittmann, W., De Villiers, P. D., De Wet, I. S., and Du Toit, G. T. Mseleni joint disease: The pilot clinical survey. *South Afr. M. J. 47:* 2283–2293, 1973.
39. Mankin, H. J. Biochemical abnormalities in articular cartilage in osteoarthritis. In *Normal and Osteoarthrotic Articular Cartilage*, edited by Ali, S. Y., Elves, M. W., and Leaback, D. H., pp. 153–172. London, Institute of Orthopaedics, 1974.
40. Marmor, L., and Peter, J. B. Osteoarthritis of the hand. *Clin. Orthop. 64:* 164–174, 1969.
41. Maroudas, A. Transport through articular cartilage and some physiological implications. In

Normal and Osteoarthrotic Cartilage, edited by Ali, S. Y., Elves, M. W., and Leaback, D. H., pp. 33–40. London, Institute of Orthopaedics, 1974.

42. Maroudas, A., Evans, H., and Almeida, L. Cartilage of the hip joint. Topographical variation of glycosaminoglycan content in normal and fibrillated tissue. *Ann. Rheum. Dis. 32:* 1–9, 1973.
43. McDevitt, C. A., Biochemistry of articular cartilage. Nature of proteoglycans and collagen of articular cartilage and their role in ageing and in osteoarthrosis. *Ann. Rheum. Dis. 32:* 364–378, 1973.
44. Meachim, G. Light microscopy of Indian ink preparations of fibrillated cartilage. *Ann. Rheum. Dis. 31:* 457–464, 1972.
45. Meachim, G., and Collins, D. H. Cell counts of normal and osteo-arthritic articular cartilage in relation to the uptake of sulphate ($^{35}SO_4$) *in vitro. Ann. Rheum. Dis. 21:* 45–50, 1962.
46. Meachim, G., and Emery, I. H. Cartilage fibrillation in shoulder and hip joints in Liverpool necropsies. *J. Anat. 116:* 161–179, 1973.
47. Meachim, G., Hardinge, K., and Williams, D. R. Methods for correlating pathological and radiological findings in osteoarthrosis of the hip. *Brit. J. Radiol. 45:* 670–676, 1972.
48. Meachim, G., and Osborne, G. V. Repair at the femoral articular surface in osteo-arthritis of the hip. *J. Pathol. 102:* 1–8, 1970.
49. Meachim, G., and Roy, S. Surface ultrastructure of mature adult human articular cartilage. *J. Bone Joint Surg. 51B:* 529–539, 1969.
50. Mintz, G., and Fraga, A. Severe osteoarthritis of the elbow in foundry workers. An occupational hazard. *Arch. Environ. Health 27:* 78–80, 1973.
51. Mow, V. C., Lai, W. M., Eisenfeld, J., and Redler, I. Some surface characteristics of articular cartilage. II. On the stability of articular surface and a possible biomechanical factor in etiology of chondrodegeneration. *J. Biomech. 7:* 457–468, 1974.
52. Murray, R. O., and Duncan, C. Athletic activity in adolescence as an etiological factor in degenerative hip disease. *J. Bone Joint Surg. 53B:* 406–419, 1971.
53. Müssbichler, H. Arteriographic findings in patients with degenerative osteoarthritis of the hip. *Radiology 107:* 21–27, 1973.
54. Nimni, M., and Deshmukh, K. Differences in collagen metabolism between normal and osteoarthritic human articular cartilage. *Science 181:* 751–752, 1973.
55. Perry, G. H., Smith, M. J. G., and Whiteside, C. G. spontaneous recovery of the joint space in degenerative hip disease. *Ann. Rheum. Dis. 31:* 440–448, 1972.
56. Phillips, R. S. Venous pathology in osteoarthritis of the knee. *J. R. Coll. Surg. Edinb. 17:* 195–199, 1972.
57. Radin, E. L., Parker, H. G., and Paul, I. L. Pattern of degenerative arthritis; preferential involvement of the distal finger joints. *Lancet 1:* 377–379, 1971.
58. Radin, E. L., Parker, H. G., Pugh, J. W., Steinberg, R. S., Paul, I. L., and Rose, R. M. Response of joints to impact loading. III. Relationship between trabecular microfractures and cartilage degeneration. *J. Biomechan. 6:* 51–57, 1973.
59. Riddle, W. E., Jr. Healing of articular cartilage in the horse. *J. Am. Vet. Med. Assoc. 157:* 1471–1479, 1970.
60. Roh, Y. S., Dequeker, J., and Mulier, J. C. Cortical bone remodeling and bone mass in primary osteoarthrosis of the hip. *Invest. Radiol. 8:* 351–354, 1973.
61. Roh, Y. S., Dequeker, J., and Mulier, J. C. Osteoarthrosis at the hand skeleton in primary osteoarthrosis of the hip and in normal controls. *Clin. Orthop. 90:* 90–94, 1973.
62. Rothwell, A. G., and Bentley, G. Chondrocyte multiplication in osteoarthritic articular cartilage. *J. Bone Joint Surg. 55B:* 588–594, 1973.
63. Sapolsky, A. I., Howell, D. S., and Woessner, J. F., Jr. Neutral proteases and cathepsin D in human articular cartilage. *J. Clin. Invest. 53:* 1044–1053, 1974.
64. Say, B., Tunçbilek, E., Pirnar, T., and Tokgözoglu, N. Hereditary congenital coxa vara with dominant inheritance? *Humangenetik 11:* 266–268, 1971.
65. Shoji, H., and Granda, J. L. Acid hydrolases in the articular cartilage of the patella. Normal, Chondromalacia patellae and osteoarthritis. *Clin. Orthop. 99:* 293–297, 1974.
66. Silcox, D. C., and McCarty, D. J., Jr. Elevated inorganic pyrophosphate concentrations in synovial fluids in osteoarthritis and pseudogout. *J. Lab. Clin. Med. 83:* 518–531, 1974.
67. Silcox, D. C., and McCarty, D. J., Jr. Measurement of inorganic pyrophosphate in biological

fluids. Elevated levels in some patients with osteoarthritis, pseudogout, acromegaly, and uremia. *J. Clin. Invest. 52:* 1863–1870, 1973.

68. Simon, W. H. Wear properties of articular cartilage *in vitro*. *J. Biomechan. 4:* 379–389, 1971.
69. Smukler, N. M., Edeiken, J., and Giuliano, V. J. Ankylosis in osteoarthritis of the finger joints. *Radiology 100:* 525–530, 1971.
70. Sokoloff, L. *The Biology of Degenerative Joint Disease*. Chicago, University of Chicago Press, 1969.
71. Sorenson, K. H., and Christensen, H. E. Local amyloid formation in the hip joint capsule in osteoarthritis. *Acta Orthop. Scand. 44:* 460–466, 1973.
72. Srivastava, V. M. L., Malemud, C. J., and Sokoloff, L. Chondroid expression by lapine articular chondrocytes in spinner culture following monolayer growth. *Connect. Tissue Res. 2:* 127–136, 1974.
73. Storey, G. O. Bone necrosis in joint disease. *Proc. R. Soc. Med. 61:* 961–969, 1968.
74. Storey, G. O., and Landells, J. W. Restoration of the femoral head after collapse in osteoarthrosis. *Ann. Rheum. Dis. 30:* 406–412, 1971.
75. Streda, A. Participation of osteonecrosis in the development of severe coxarthrosis. *Acta Univ Carol. (Med. Monogr.) (Praha) 46:* 1–164, 1971.
76. Tillman, B. Zur Lokalisation von degenerativen Veränderungen am Femurkopf bei der Coxarthrose. *Z. Orthop. 111:* 23–27, 1973.
77. van der Korst, J. K., Sokoloff, L., and Miller, E. J. Senescent pigmentation of cartilage and degenerative joint disease. *Arch. Pathol. 86:* 40–47, 1968.
78. Vernon-Roberts, B., Pirie, C. J., and Trenwith, V. Pathology of the dorsal spine in ankylosing hyperostosis. *Ann. Rheum. Dis. 33:* 281–288, 1974.
79. Vignon, E., Arlot, M., Meunier, P., and Vignon, G. Quantitative histological changes in osteoarthritic hip cartilage. Morphometric analysis of 29 osteoarthritic and 26 normal human femoral heads. *Clin. Orthop. 103:* 269–278, 1974.
80. Walker, P. S., Dowson, D., Longfield, M. D., and Wright, V. "Boosted lubrication" in synovial joints by fluid entrapment and enrichment. *Ann. Rheum. Dis. 27:* 512–520, 1968.
81. Webber, R. H., Malemud, C. J., and Sokoloff, L. Species differences in cell culture of mammalian articular chondrocytes. (Submitted for publication.)
82. Weightman, B. O., Freeman, M. A. R., and Swanson, S. A. V. Fatigue of articular cartilage. *Nature. 244:* 303–304, 1973.
83. Weiss, C. Ultrastructural characteristics of osteoarthritis. *Fed. Proc. 32:* 1459–1466, 1973.
84. Wilkinson, M. (ed.) *Cervical Spondylosis, Its Early Diagnosis and Treatment*. 2nd ed. Philadelphia, W. B. Saunders Co., 1971.
85. Woolf, C. M., Koehn, J. H., and Coleman, S. S. Congenital hip disease in Utah: the influence of genetic and nongenetic factors. *Am. J. Human Genet. 20:* 430–439, 1968.
86. Zimny, M. L., and Redler, I. Morphological variations within a given area of articular surface of cartilage. *Z. Zellforsch. Mikrosk. Anat. 147:* 163–167, 1974.

Chapter 9

Rheumatoid and Related Arthritides

HOWARD D. DORFMAN

Inflammatory arthritis, in contrast to degenerative joint disease, takes its origin in the synovial membrane of diarthrodial joints. Because this primary site of the disease is vascular and innervated, it can react to injurious stimuli with the full range of exudative and proliferative inflammatory changes. The ensuing damage to the articular cartilage is secondary to the synovial inflammatory process. If the synovitis is of limited duration and extent, there may be little or no cartilage damage or permanent impairment of joint function. Persistent and progressive synovitis or recurrent attacks will, on the other hand, result in joint damage either by cartilage lysis or by pannus erosion, depending upon the etiologic agent. Early extensive loss of cartilage by either mechanism leads to fibrous or bony adhesions between the ends of the bones. Associated thickening and contraction of the joint capsule and muscle spasm may lead to partial immobilization and contractures, while inflammatory weakening and rupture of involved ligaments and tendons contribute to subluxations and other deformities. Decreased density in the juxta-articular bone may extend for a considerable distance away from the inflamed joint. This atrophy of bone trabeculae is due in part to hyperemia and is partly dependent on neurotrophic or reflex mechanisms. It is a change which is most pronounced in rheumatoid arthritis and tuberculous arthritis. Should the inflammatory process subside short of total cartilage destruction, permitting articular function to continue, secondary degenerative joint disease with eburnation of exposed subchondral bone and marginal osteophyte formation can evolve in a joint initially the site of inflammatory arthritis.

The histologic details of synovial inflammation depend on the etiologic agent. Inflammatory arthritis due to known etiologic factors (infectious arthritis) can be classified as of bacterial suppurative, bacterial granulomatous, mycotic, and viral origin. In the inflammatory arthritides of undetermined etiology, principally rheumatoid arthritis and related conditions, the synovial changes lack histologic specificity. However, characteristic morphologic changes do occur. This discussion will deal with the clinical and morphologic interrelationships between adult rheumatoid and related arthritides—juvenile rheumatoid arthritis (juvenile chronic polyarthritis), ankylosing spondylitis, psoriatic arthritis, Reiter's syndrome, enteric arthritides, and the joint involvement of systemic lupus erythematosus. The use of the term "rheumatoid variants" in no way implies that these entities are simply atypical forms of rheumatoid arthritis. The enormous literature on rheumatoid and related arthritides with regard to their pathologic aspects can only be superficially alluded to here. Recent extensive reviews have been published by Gardner[15] and by Jaffe.[19]

RHEUMATOID ARTHRITIS

Rheumatoid arthritis (RA) is a chronic systemic disease in which a nonsuppurative inflammatory process affects diarthrodial joints and in which various nonarticular tissues are also involved. The course of the disease is extremely variable, and some patients manifest only a mild degree of synovitis involving few joints and clearing without severe impairment of joint function. While the disease shows a marked tendency toward spontaneous remissions and exacerbations, a chronic progressive course results in disability and characteristic deformities of joints. In the more classic adult form of the disease, there is almost always symmetrical involvement of the peripheral small joints of the hands and feet, but the knees, wrists, ankles, and elbow joints are also commonly involved. The hip joint is the least often involved of the large joints. The early changes of intra-articular synovial membrane inflammation and the periarticular soft tissue swelling are responsible for the stiffness which is so characteristic of the intitial stage. Later, the joint involvement is characterized by juxta-articular bone erosions, muscle spasm, flexion deformities, subluxations, and ankylosis.

The fact that rheumatoid arthritis is a systemic process (rheumatoid disease) is borne out by the early appearance of constitutional symptoms such as fever and weakness. A mild to moderate anemia usually appears, and this is similar to the anemia associated with chronic infections.

Because the etiology of rheumatoid arthritis is unknown, the synovial changes lack specificity, and even the subcutaneous nodule and rheumatoid factor in the serum are seen in other conditions; the early diagnosis is based on clinical criteria. The American Rheumatism Association's diagnostic criteria for classical, definite, probable, and possible rheumatoid arthritis and the even more restrictive New York criteria are based upon a combination of clinical features (stiffness, tenderness, swelling), number and distribution of the joints involved, erosive roentgenographic changes, and serologic positivity (rheumatoid factor).[5, 31] The diagnosis cannot be made unequivocally by biopsy, and in the early stages the characteristic laboratory findings are often absent.[20, 33]

Etiology and pathogenesis. Attention has been directed toward three main areas in attempts to identify the cause and pathogenetic factors in this disease, namely infectious agents, immune mechanisms, and the role of lysosomal enzymes.

Bland and Phillips[4] have reviewed the evidence for an infectious etiology. In the search for microorganisms, *Mycoplasma* or pleuropneumonia organisms have been investigated because of reports of their isolation from human synovium and joint fluid and because they are associated with arthritis in swine and other animals. Most investigators have failed to isolate Mycoplasma organisms from human rheumatoid arthritis tissue.[9, 32] Viruses have not been isolated from joint tissues of rheumatoid patients or observed with the electron microscope. Early reports that cultured rheumatoid synovial cells were more resistant to infection with rubella and Newcastle disease viruses than normal synovial cell lines have not been confirmed by recent investigations.[32, 41]

The finding of lymphoid cell infiltration of rheumatoid synovium, follicle formation, prominence of plasma cells synthesizing IgG and rheumatoid factor, decreased complement in serum and synovial fluid, and the demonstration of antigen-antibody complexes with rheumatoid factor in rheumatoid granulation tissue, synovial fluid, and free synovial leukocytes have all tended to implicate immune mechanisms in the rheumatoid process.

Yu and Peter[42] have recently reviewed the cellular immunologic aspects of rheumatoid arthritis with particular reference to the possibility of cell-mediated immunity factors.

The recent growth of basic knowledge of the role of T and B lymphocytes in the normal immune response has provided new approaches to our understanding of rheumatoid disease. These cells can now be differentiated in the laboratory. It has been proposed that the autoantibodies in such disorders as rheumatoid arthritis and systemic lupus erythematosus (SLE) are the result of interruptions of the normal T cell–B cell cooperation in the recognition of antigens. For example this might be caused by a virus which attaches to and alters a self-component. It this self component is itself an antibody, the B cells could produce an antibody to an antibody *i.e.*, rheumatoid factor.[25]

Evidence that T cell abnormalities do occur in RA and SLE is accumulating, and the therapeutic effectiveness of reducing the number of lymphocytes in rheumatic disorders lends support to the hypothesis. Thus the beneficial effect of cytostatic drugs and antilymphocytic sera suggests a direct action on T and B lymphocytes. Preliminary studies of the percentage of T and B lymphocytes in the peripheral blood and synovial fluid in rheumatoid arthritis have yielded inconsistent results, but there is some evidence that the number of T cells in the blood may be decreased during periods of activity.

The evidence to date suggests that IgG is produced by some unknown initiating factor in rheumatoid synovium. This immune globulin in turn provokes the production of anti-IgG or rheumatoid factor by the synovial cells and regional lymph nodes. Rheumatoid factor which is itself either IgG or IgM forms aggregates with the synovial IgG and the complement sequence is activated. There follows a local reduction in complement and the attraction of polymorphonuclear leukocytes into the joint to ingest the IgG-rheumatoid factor-complement aggregates. The so-called RA cells are thus produced and can be recognized by microscopic examination of joint fluid. Phagocytosis of the immune complexes is followed by the discharge of lysosomal hydrolases from the leukocytes in the synovial fluid and rheumatoid granulation tissue. It is likely that these acid hydrolases, the level of which is increased in rheumatoid joint fluids, play a direct role in chondromucoprotein breakdown.[40] The depletion of acid mucopolysaccharide seen in articular cartilage in advance of pannus replacement may be initiated by the action of these lysosomal enzymes acting in concert with certain nonlysosomal collagenases.[20] Waxman and Sledge[39] using operative specimens demonstrated a significant correlation between acid phosphatase content of rheumatoid synovium, histologic severity of inflammation, and clinical activity.

Genetic factors in rheumatoid "variants". It has been shown recently that a high proportion of patients with ankylosing spondylitis and their relatives have the histocompatibility antigen HL-A W27.[35] This relationship also extends to Reiter's syndrome and other seronegative rheumatic diseases associated with sacroiliitis and spondylitis such as juvenile chronic polyarthritis, inflammatory bowel disease, and psoriatic arthritis,[26] but the antigen is not related to rheumatoid arthritis itself.

Acute reactive arthritis is one which is associated with infection elsewhere, but the organism is not present in the joint. Reactive arthritis has followed or coexisted with streptococcal infection as in rheumatic fever, intestinal infections with *Shigella*, *Salmonella*, and *Yersinia*, and genitourinary infections due to the gonococcus. Recent studies have shown that, except for rheumatic fever, only a small proportion of the patients with these infections develop reactive arthritis. Those who do, show a very high incidence of the histocompatibility antigen HL-A W27. Thus, in patients with yersinia-reactive arthritis, 90% have HL-A W27, and this is also true of patients with post-*Shigella* arthritis.

The HL-A data for patients with rheumatic diseases indicate that host genetic factors play a role in determining susceptibility to certain diseases and may determine the common clinical and pathologic manifestations of multiple etiologic factors.

Pathologic changes. Early in the course of RA, when joint symptoms have been present for up to several months, the synovium shows hyperplasia of the lining cells, hyperemia and edema of the sublining layer, and perivascular inflammatory cell infiltrates (Fig. 1). In a study of biopsy material from 9 patients with adult and juvenile rheumatoid arthritis of less than 1 month's duration, Schumacher and Kitridou[36] found that plasma cells were uncommon in the initial stages and that polymorphonuclear leukocytes were present. The inflammatory infiltrate was not nodular in distribution but was predominantly around veins. An interesting observation was a lack of synovial fluid findings in some cases of established synovial membrane inflammation. The diagnosis of rheumatoid arthritis was substantiated in the cases in this study by their subsequent course in from 1 to 3 years. No specific ultrastructural changes have been found.[27] Later in the course of the disease, a chronic hypertrophic villous synovitis develops in which prominent synovial villi are infiltrated by large numbers of lymphocytes, sometimes arranged in follicles with reactive centers (Fig. 2, *A* and *B*). Plasma cells may be numerous. These changes are characteristic but not diagnostic, and they are properly reported as chronic nonspecific synovitis.[38] The biopsy findings are useful in excluding gouty and mycobacterial synovitis as well as pigmented villonodular synovitis. However, the identical histologic features can be observed in psoriatic arthritis, Reiter's syndrome, ankylosing spondylitis, juvenile rheumatoid arthritis, and in some cases of systemic lupus erythematosus.[10, 36, 37] In the active stages of synovial inflammation, fibrin exudation is also a prominent feature appearing in patches overlying thickened synovial villi and in their interstices. Later the fibrin may become organized or may form inspissated masses designated as rice bodies. In addition to lymphocytes, plasma cells, and polymorphonuclear leukocytes, the inflammatory infiltrates contain collections of mononuclear phagocytic cells with ingested hemosiderin pigment or lipid.

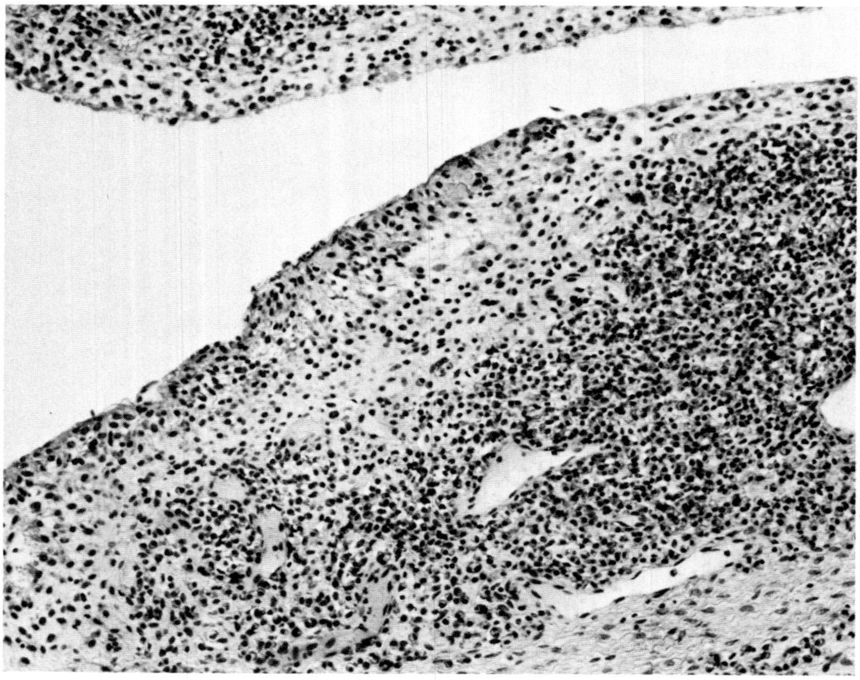

FIG. 1. Knee joint synovium in a 33-year-old woman with rheumatoid arthritis of 4 months duration. Note hyperplasia of synovial lining cells and intense mononuclear inflammatory cell infiltration of the sublining layer, predominantly perivascular. Hematoxylin and eosin stain, × 120.

The presence of synovial multinucleated giant cells was first noted by Collins[15] and later extensively studied by Grimley and Sokoloff[17] and others.[3, 12, 30] They are a characteristic, though not specific, finding, and the cells appear to arise through abnormal division of synovial lining cells from which they can be traced (Fig. 3). Fragments of cartilage and necrotic bone may also be found embedded in rheumatoid synovium.[30]

Chronicity of the synovial inflammation is always associated with damage to the articular cartilage. This results from the release of lysosomal hydrolases and other enzymes related to the synovial inflammation and by the outgrowth of inflammatory pannus which extends from the marginal synovial attachment over the surface of the articular cartilage (Fig. 4, *A* and *B*). This inflammatory mantle also burrows beneath the articular surface into the subchondral bone. Its proliferation in these sites produces the lytic defects known to the radiologist as marginal bone erosions. Pannus extends to involve other intra-articular structures such as menisci and ligaments. With repeated exacerbations of the inflammatory process further and further extension of the pannus and the cartilage erosion leads ultimately to total loss of cartilage. The bone ends are now covered by rheumatoid granulation tissue, which becomes organized into a fibrous ankylosis. Bony bridging sometimes follows but is less common in rheumatoid arthritis than in some variants.[10] Subsidence of the inflammatory process before total loss of articular cartilage and while continued function of the joint is possible, results in the development of secondary osteoarthritis.[19]

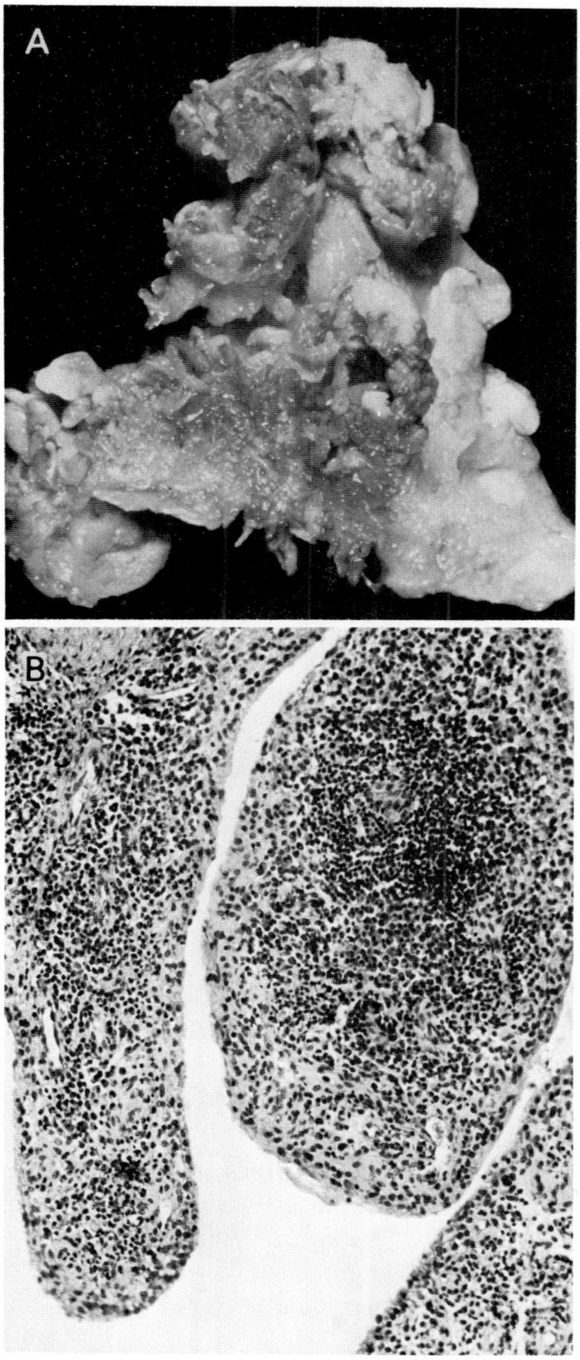

FIG. 2. *A*, inflamed knee joint synovium of a 42-year-old woman with multiple small and large joint involvement of 4 years' duration. The thickened and inflamed synovial membrane shows villous proliferation, and it appears edematous. *B*, the inflamed synovium in *A* showing the features of chronic hypertrophic villous synovitis. The thickened synovial villi are intensely infiltrated by mononuclear cells with a tendency to form lymphoid follicles. Hematoxylin and eosin stain, × 120.

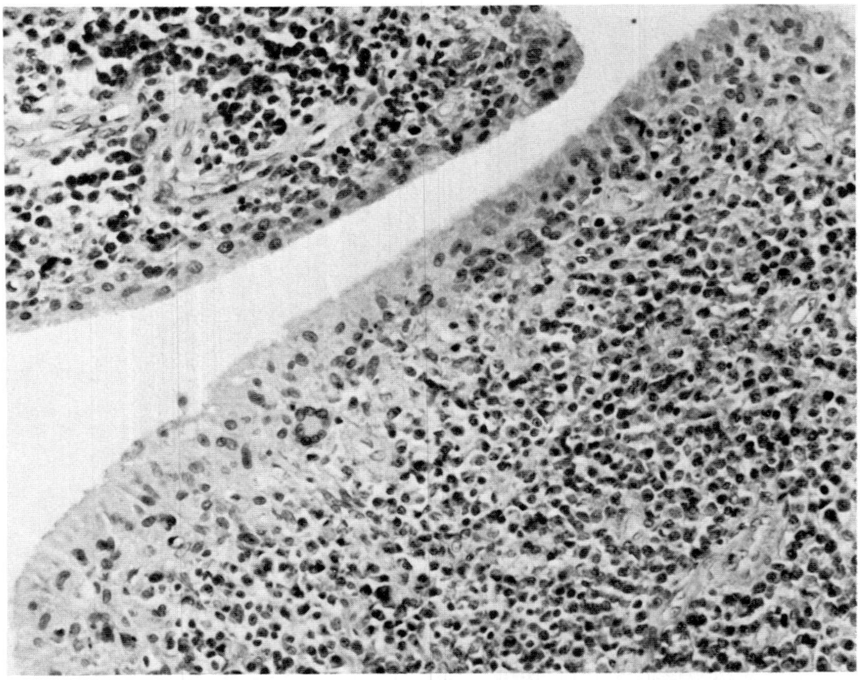

FIG. 3. Synovium in rheumatoid arthritis showing the formation of characteristic multinucleated giant cells which appear to arise in the deep layers of the hyperplastic synovial lining cells. Several stages in the development of these cells can be traced. The sub-lining layer is heavily infiltrated by plasma cells and lymphocytes. Hematoxylin and eosin stain, × 200.

Subcutaneous nodules are perhaps the most characteristic pathologic finding in rheumatoid arthritis. They are seen in 20 to 25% of cases, usually relatively late in the disease and almost invariably in patients with rheumatoid factor in their sera. Their presence indicates active disease and a poorer prognosis. Histologically similar nodules may be found in asymptomatic children who are seronegative, and these have been designated as "pseudorheumatoid" nodules. A recent study in which 10 of these children developed rheumatoid factor 2 to 16 years later suggests that the pseudorheumatoid nodule of childhood should be included in the spectrum of rheumatoid disease.[2] The rheumatoid nodule most often develops in the periarticular tissues such as joint capsule, tendon sheath, and bursa. They may also be found in periosteum causing bony erosion,[13] in other sites subjected to friction (occiput, pretibial region, Achilles tendon area), and in the pleura, dura mater, pulmonary parenchyma, and the heart. The nodules are firm, nontender, measure from 0.5 to 3.0 cm in diameter, and tend to persist for many months or years. They may be difficult to distinguish clinically from gouty tophi.

Microscopically, the center of a rheumatoid subcutaneous nodule is composed of fibrinoid material surrounded by a richly cellular palisade of histiocytes and fibroblasts (Fig. 5). Some lymphocytic infiltration may be present at the periphery, and in the fibrinoid centers, polymorphonuclear leukocytes may be

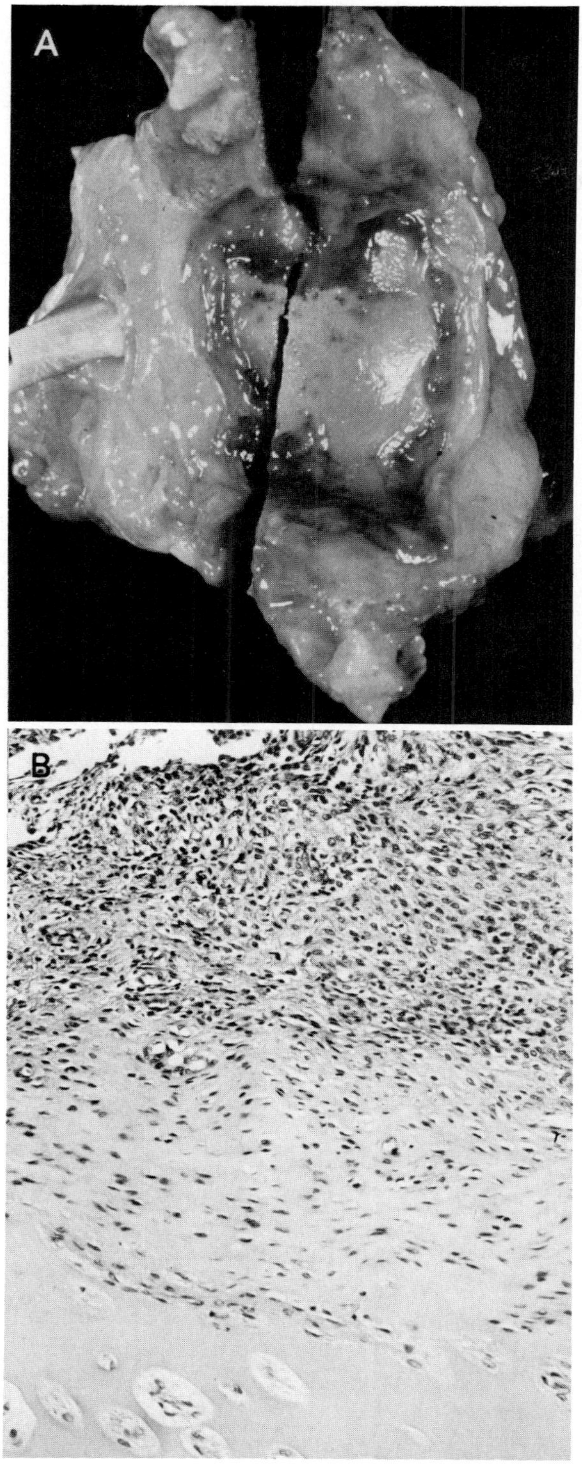

FIG. 4. *A*, superior aspect of talus of a 58-year-old woman with rheumatoid arthritis of 8 years' duration. Note the edematous thickened synovium with granulation tissue extensions encroaching upon the periphery of the articular cartilage. This inflammatory pannus replaces the cartilage by centripetal growth and will form the basis for eventual fibrous ankylosis of the joint. *B*, Rheumatoid pannus (granulation tissue) extending over articular cartilage (below) at periphery of joint. Hematoxylin and eosin stain, × 200.

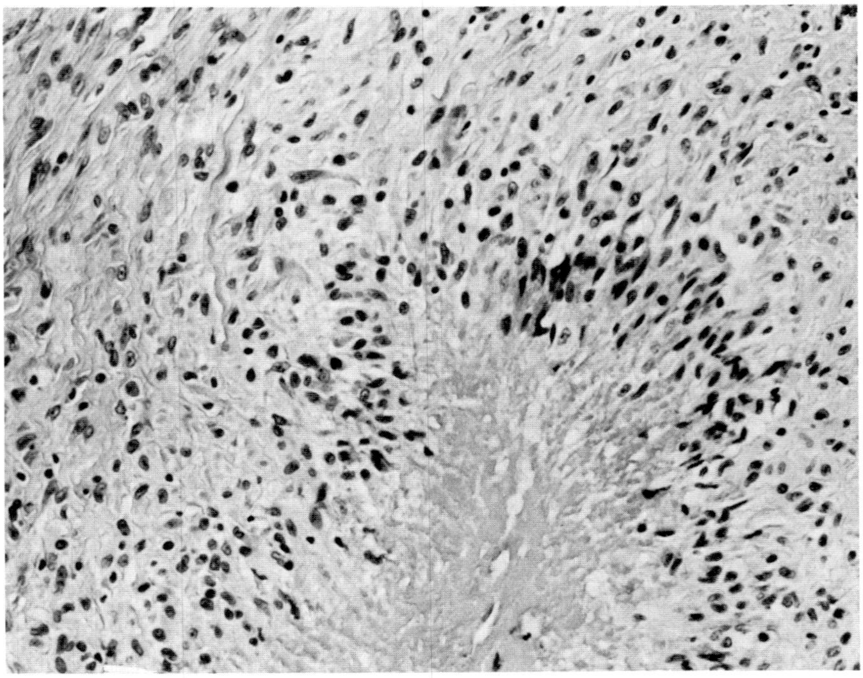

FIG. 5. Margin of a rheumatoid subcutaneous nodule or granuloma. Central amorphous eosinophilic zone containing fibrin is bordered by palisaded histiocytes and fibroblasts. Some lymphocytes are present external to the border of radially arranged cells. Hematoxylin and eosin stain, × 200.

numerous. Occasionally, multinucleated histiocytic giant cells of the foreign body type may be seen in the palisade and may give rise to confusion with a tophus. Sokoloff[10] has proposed that the rheumatoid nodule results from fibrinoid necrosis of blood vessels with ischemic breakdown of collagen.

Involvement of any diarthodial joint by the rheumatoid inflammatory process may lead to weakening of the joint capsule and herniation of the synovium when the effect of increased intraarticular pressure is superimposed. This results in the characteristic para-articular synovial cyst such as a Baker's cyst of the popliteal space which may dissect its way into the calf. These cysts may also rupture to form pseudocysts.[19]

The extra-articular manifestations also include a systemic vasculitis which may be characterized by simple intimal thickening, by subacute inflammation, or by necrotizing panarteritis. The latter form may be associated with so-called "malignant rheumatoid disease," which is characterized by neurologic complications, intestinal and digital infarcts and renal and coronary arteritis.[29] Anyloidosis occurs in 5 to 10% of cases and may lead to renal insufficiency.[19]

JUVENILE RHEUMATOID ARTHRITIS

Rheumatoid arthritis having an onset before 16 years of age is considered to be the juvenile form. In addition to the early appearance it differs from the adult disease in that it affects fewer joints initially or even presents as a mono-articular arthritis.[6, 34] There is also a high incidence of systemic manifestations such as spiking fever, dermatitis, hepatosplenomegaly, lymphadenopathy, and pericarditis which may antedate the joint localization. The term Still's disease has usually been applied to this systemic form of involvement, but it is also used to denote juvenile rheumatoid arthritis in general. Another term in common use is juvenile chronic polyarthritis. Although the symptoms and signs may begin as early as 6 weeks of age there is a biphasic peak of onset between 1½ and 8 years and 11 and 14 years.[19] Iridocyclitis is a serious complication, and it may precede the onset of arthritis. Band keratopathy may be noted clinically. Cervical spine involvement in juvenile rheumatoid arthritis often results in fusion of the apophyseal joints. Premature closure of the epiphyses may lead to growth disturbances such as micrognathia and generalized skeletal stunting.

The incidence of rheumatoid factor is low (10 to 15%), as is the occurrence of subcutaneous nodules. Histologically, the synovial findings are those of hyperplasia of the lining cells, focal lymphocyte, and plasma cell infiltrates and hyperemia (Fig. 6). These changes do not differ from those seen in the adult disease.

ANKYLOSING SPONDYLITIS

This chronic progressive form of arthritis is principally a disease of young males, in a male to female ratio of about 10:1. It begins in the sacroiliac joints and

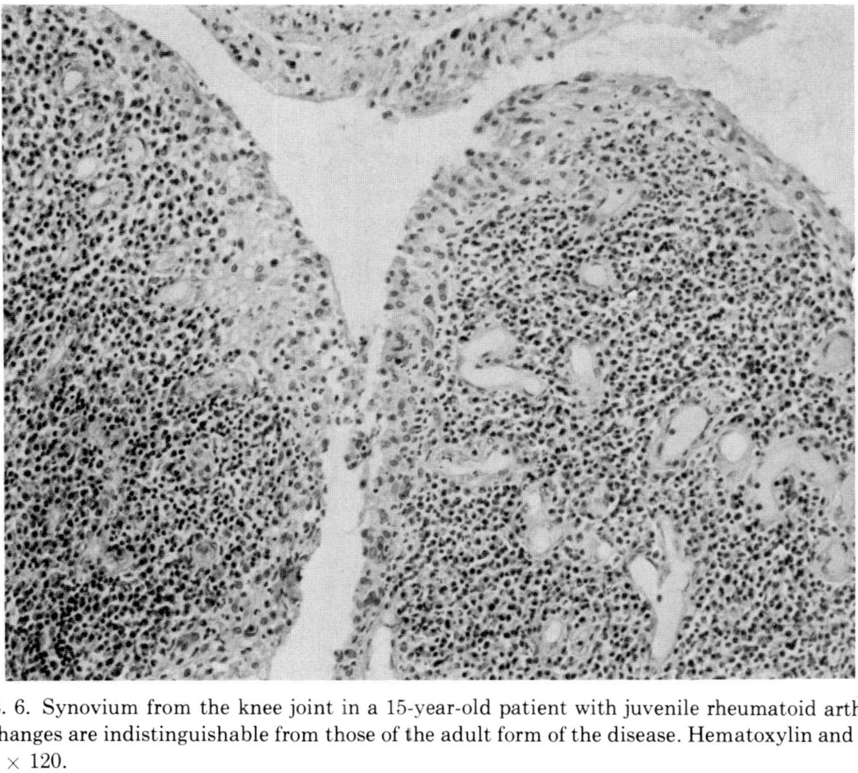

FIG. 6. Synovium from the knee joint in a 15-year-old patient with juvenile rheumatoid arthritis. The changes are indistinguishable from those of the adult form of the disease. Hematoxylin and eosin stain, × 120.

spreads progressively upward to involve the synovial and fibrocartilaginous joints of the spine and the vertebral ligaments.[11] The peripheral joints may be involved, but this is much less common than in rheumatoid arthritis. This type of arthritis has in the past been classified as a manifestation of rheumatoid arthritis. Because of the difference in age and sex incidence, the distribution of joint involvement, the lower frequency of rheumatoid factor and subcutaneous nodules, and the differing visceral lesions, the American Rheumatism Association has since 1963 separated this condition from rheumatoid spondylitis and adopted the term ankylosing spondylitis.[5] A recent finding by Schlosstein and co-workers[35] of a high association of a histocompatibility antigen, HL-A W27, in ankylosing spondylitis provides an important diagnostic adjunct in the work-up of patients suspected of having ankylosing spondylitis. Histologically, the synovial changes in a diarthrodial joint are identical with those of rheumatoid arthritis in that synovial lining cell hyperplasia, lymphocyte, and plasma cell infiltrates are present. The surfaces of the articular cartilages tend to become covered with inflammatory granulation tissue, and early fibrosis is seen. The adhesions which develop in diarthrodial joints have a much greater tendency to progress through fibrous to bony ankylosis than in rheumatoid arthritis. In the fibrocartilaginous joints of the spine, inflammatory changes are seen in the adjacent bone, which later extend to the intervertebral disc and to the adjacent anterior spinal ligaments. The discs are eventually ossified as are the spinal ligaments. Bony fusion is principally within the anatomic outlines of the adjacent vertebral bodies. The bony bridges or syndesmophytes result in bony fusion of the column, and the posterior facet and sacroiliac joints also show bony ankylosis eventually. Involvement of the other amphiarthroses, symphysis pubis and manubriosternal joints, is quite common in contrast to rheumatoid arthritis. The spinal syndesmophytes in ankylosing spondylitis are quite similar to those seen in the spondylitis associated with ulcerative colitis and regional enteritis, in that they are marginal in location.[24] The syndesmophytes in psoriatic arthritis and Reiter's syndrome are not limited to marginal locations. Aortitis and aortic insufficiency is a rare extra-articular manifestation and is characterized by nongranulomatous inflammation and medial necrosis at the aortic root. Amyloidosis develops in about 5% of cases and may be a cause of death through renal impairment.[19]

PSORIATIC ARTHRITIS AND RHEUMATOID ARTHRITIS

Approximately 7% of patients with psoriasis have associated inflammatory joint disease,[28] and it is now accepted as a distinct entity, psoriatic arthritis. The polyarthritis has a predilection for the distal interphalangeal joints and metatarsophalangeal joints in an asymmetric distribution. Serologic tests for rheumatoid factor are almost always negative, and subcutaneous nodules are absent, though some cases of combined seropositive rheumatoid arthritis and psoriasis have been seen. The prognosis for the articular involvement in psoriasis is generally better than that of rheumatoid arthritis, but occasional cases show a particularly deforming type of mutilating arthritis, with whittling deformities of the ends of the phalanges and telescoping of the digits (Fig. 7). The synovial changes are

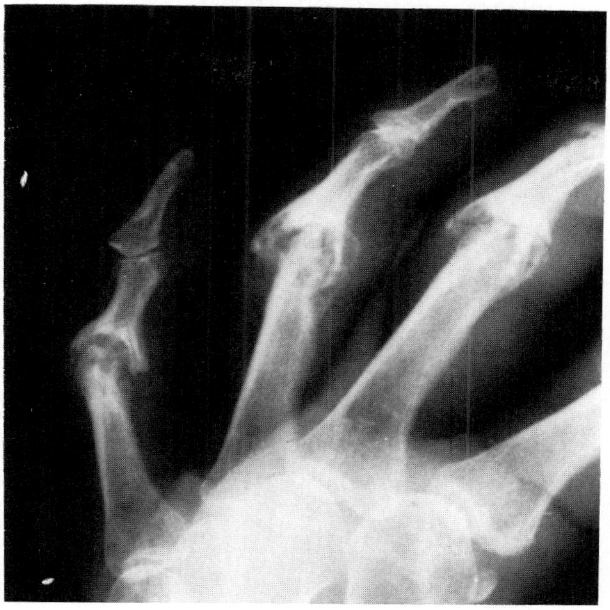

FIG. 7. Psoriatic arthritis whittling deformity of phalangeal distal bone ends and cupping of proximal ends producing "pencil in cup" deformity. These changes, distributed asymmetrically, are characteristic findings but are relatively uncommon. Note the relative sparing of the metacarpophalangeal joints.

indistinguishable from those of rheumatoid arthritis, and there is no similarity to the inflammatory changes in the skin.[15] The sequence of appearance of the skin and joint lesions varies, but the skin lesions usually precede the joint manifestations. Spondylitis in psoriasis differs from that seen in ankylosing spondylitis in the asymmetry of sacroiliac involvement and the nonmarginal syndesmophytes which arise from the surfaces of vertebral bodies.[24]

Studies of HL-A W27 frequency in psoriatic arthritis show an increase (35%) in those with psoriatic spondylitis.[26]

REITER'S SYNDROME

This clinical entity in its classic form principally affects young males and is characterized by arthritis, urethritis, and conjunctivitis. Ulcerations of the buccal mucosa, particularly the palate, circinate balanitis, hyperkeratotic dermatitis known as keratodermia blennorrhagicum, iritis, and uveitis are sometimes present. Joint involvement, usually asymmetrically distributed, is seen in the knees, ankles, and small joints of the hands and feet.[14, 16, 19] Fluffy deposits of new bone are also found in sites of tendon insertion, particularly in the calcaneal region. Sacroiliac joint involvement, often asymmetrical, and a form of spondylitis with syndesmophytes occurring outside of the margins of the vertebral bodies resemble the changes seen roentgenologically in psoriatic arthritis.[24] The predilection of small joint involvement for the distal interphalangeal joints and its asymmetry are further points of similarity.

The etiology of Reiter's syndrome is still uncertain. Among the proposed infectious causes are *Mycoplasma*, a pleuropneumonia-like organism, the *Bedsonia* group of viruses (psittacosis-lymphogranuloma venereum-trachoma organisms) and an abnormal response to gonococcal or *Shigella* organisms.[19] The laboratory findings are nonspecific, and these patients do not show rheumatoid factor or subcutaneous nodules. The synovial inflammatory changes in long-standing cases are indistinguishable from chronic hypertrophic villous synovitis in rheumatoid arthritis,[14] but early stages may show large numbers of polymorphonuclear leukocytes. A small number of patients develop pericarditis, myocarditis, and even aortic insufficiency due to aortitis. Most cases of Reiter's syndrome undergo complete resolution in several months without permanent joint sequelae.

The histocompatibility antigen studies show a definite relationship between the frequent finding of HL-A W27 in Reiter's patients (96%) and the tendency to develop this postinfective syndrome.

SYSTEMIC LUPUS ERYTHEMATOSUS AND RHEUMATOID ARTHRITIS

Joint manifestations are common in systemic lupus erythematosus, and there are clinical and pathologic features which overlap with rheumatoid arthritis. Positive serologic tests for rheumatoid factor occur in one-fourth to one-third of patients with SLE, usually in low titre. Conversely, between 3 and 27% of patients with rheumatoid arthritis give a positive test for LE cells.[15] Rheumatoid-like subcutaneous nodules have been found in otherwise typical cases of SLE.[18] The synovial findings are quite similar to those of rheumatoid arthritis (Fig. 8), with the exception that the fibrin on the synovial surface appears to lie directly on the subsynovial connective tissue in the arthritis of SLE.[15] Pannus formation is distinctly less common than in rheumatoid arthritis, and the finding of hematoxylin bodies in the synovium helps in the differentiation.

Clinical and serologic overlap between SLE and RA is further complicated by the finding of antinuclear factors in many patients with RA, most often with low titres. RA patients with positive LE cell tests and antinuclear factors tend to have greater serologic reactivity to rheumatoid factor, subcutaneous nodules, and extra-articular manifestations. They should not, however, be classified as having SLE without the appropriate clinical findings.

ENTERIC ARTHRITIDES

An acute migratory polyarthritis is found in about 5 to 10% of patients with regional enteritis and about one-fifth of patients with ulcerative colitis.[23] The onset is usually coincident with the appearance of the intestinal disorder. Involvement of the large joints of the extremities with resolution over a few months is the usual pattern. Some cases show only arthralgias without roentgenographic changes, while others have definite roentgenologic evidence of disease without symptoms.[8] Spondylitis similar to ankylosing spondylitis is seen in some, and the sacroiliitis is also similar. The frequency of this spondyliitis is

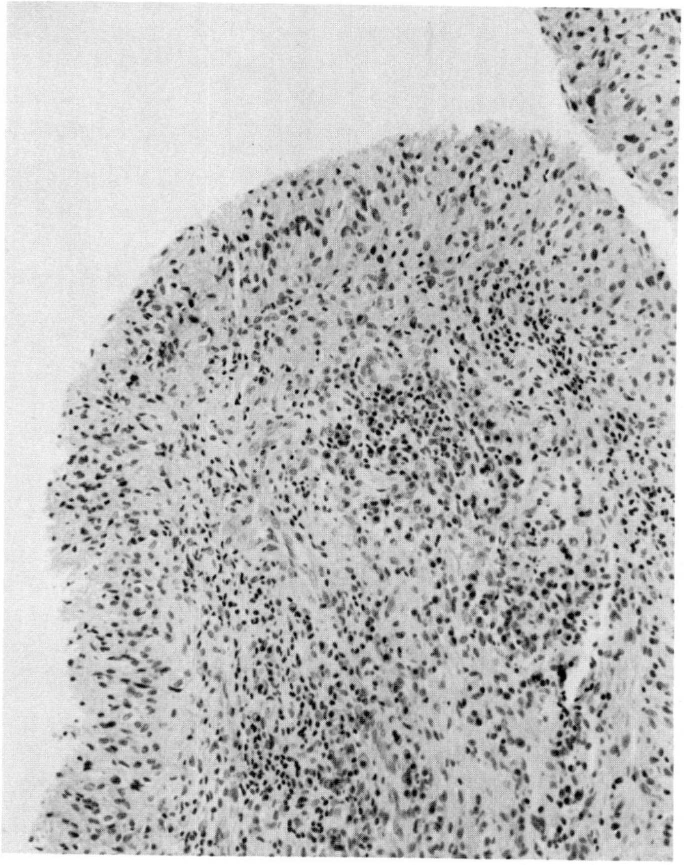

FIG. 8. Synovitis in systemic lupus erythematosus is characterized by nonspecific chronic inflammatory cell infiltrate like that seen in rheumatoid arthritis. In the absence of hematoxylin bodies, the distinction cannot be made on histological grounds. Hematoxylin and eosin stain, × 120.

much higher in ulcerative colitis than in regional ileitis.[24] Flare-ups of the intestinal inflammation sometimes correspond to exacerbations in joint symptoms. No rheumatoid factor or subcutaneous nodules can be demonstrated in these patients, and permanent joint damage is rare.[23]

In Whipple's disease, intermittent migratory arthritis may be present. The onset may precede the intestinal and systemic features by years.[7] The joint involvement leads to little or no permanent damage. The synovial tissue shows nonspecific chronic inflammation similar to the early stages of rheumatoid arthritis.[21, 22] The sickle-shaped particles described in histiocytes in the intestinal mucosa, lymph nodes, and other sites have not as yet been reported in the synovium.

Accuracy in diagnosis of this interesting group of interrelated diseases depends to a large extent on a full awareness of the range of overlapping clinical manifestations and laboratory findings. The nonspecificity of the histologic changes should stimulate further application of the techniques of electron microscopy, immunofluorescence, and enzyme histochemistry to the clarification of their differential features. The newly acquired data on the genetic factors as reflected in the distribution of histocompatibility antigens points toward a gene-controlled common mechanism, namely that of postinfective chronic immune response, to link together the so-called rheumatoid variants.

REFERENCES

1. Aho, K., Ahvonen, P., Lassus, A., Sievers, K., and Tiilikainen, A.: HL-A 27 in reactive arthritis; a study of Yersinia arthritis and Reiter's disease. *Arthritis Rheum. 17:* 521–526, 1974.
2. Berardinelli, J. L., Hyman, C. J., Campbell, E. E., and Fireman, P.: Presence of rheumatoid factor in ten children with isolated rheumatoid-like nodules. *J. Pediatr. 81:* 751–757, 1972.
3. Bhan, A. K., and Roy, S.: Synovial giant cells in rheumatoid arthritis and other joint diseases. *Ann. Rheum. Dis. 30:* 294–298, 1971.
4. Bland, J. H., and Phillips, C. A.: Etiology and pathogenesis of rheumatoid arthritis and related multisystem diseases. *Semin Arthritis Rheum. 1:* 339–359, 1972.
5. Blumberg, B. S., Bunim, J. J., Calkins, E., Pirani, C. L., and Zvaifler, N. J.: ARA nomenclature and classification of arthritis and rheumatism (tentative) *Arthritis Rheum. 7:* 93–97, 1964.
6. Bywaters, E. G. L.: Diagnostic criteria for Still's disease (Juvenile RA). Proc of the Third International Symposium. Population Studies of the Rheumatic Diseases. Edited by Bennett, P. H., and Wood, P. H. N., pp. 235–240. New York, Excerpta Medica Foundation, 1968.
7. Caughey, D. E., and Bywaters, E. G. L.: The arthritis of Whipple's syndrome. *Ann. Rheum. Dis. 22:* 327–335, 1963.
8. Clark, R. L., Muhletaler, A., and Margulies, S. I.: Colitic arthritis; clinical and radiographic manifestations. *Radiology 101:* 585–594, 1971.
9. Cole, B. C., Ward, J. R., Smith, C. B.: Studies on the infectious etiology of rheumatoid arthritis. *Arthritis Rheum. 16:* 191–198, 1973.
10. Cooper, N. S.: Pathology of rheumatoid arthritis. *Med Clin. North Am. 52:* 607–621, 1968.
11. Cruickshank, B.: Pathology of ankylosing spondylitis. *Clin Orthop. 74:* 43–58, 1971.
12. Donald, K. J., and Kerr, J. F. R.: Giant cells in the synovium in rheumatoid arthritis. *Med. J. Aust. 1:* 761–765, 1968.
13. Dorfman, H. D., Norman, A., and Smith, R. J.: Bone erosion in relation to subcutaneous rheumatoid nodules. *Arth. Rhem. 13:* 69–74, 1970.
14. Ford, D. K.: Reiter's syndrome. *Bull Rheum. Dis. 20:* 588–591, 1970.
15. Gardner, D. L.: *The Pathology of Rheumatoid Arthritis*, pp. 168–176. Baltimore, Williams & Wilkins Co., 1972.
16. Good, A.: Reiter's disease; a review with special attention to cardiovascular and neurologic sequellae. *Semin. Arthritis Rheum. 3:* 253–286, 1974.
17. Grimley, P. M., and Sokoloff, L.: Synovial giant cells in rheumatoid arthritis. *Am J. Pathol. 49:* 931–954, 1966.
18. Hahn, B. H., Yardley, J. H., and Stevens, M. B.: "Rheumatoid" nodules in systemic lupus erythematosus. *Ann. Intern. Med. 72:* 49–58, 1970.
19. Jaffe, H. L.: Inflammatory arthritis of undetermined origin. In *Metabolic Degenerative and Inflammatory Diseases of Bones and Joints*, pp. 779–846. Philadelphia, Lea and Febiger, 1972.
20. Johnson, J. S., Vaughan, J. H., Hench, P. K., and Blomgren, S. E.: Rheumatoid arthritis, 1970–1972. *Ann. Intern. Med. 78:* 937–953, 1973.
21. Kelly, J. J., III, and Weisiger, B. B.: The arthritis of Whipple's disease. *Arthritis Rheum. 6:* 615–632, 1963.
22. LeVine, M. E., and Dobbins, W. O.: Joint changes in Whipple's disease. *Semin. Arthritis Rheum. 3:* 79–93, 1973.
23. McEwen, C.: Arthritis accompanying ulcerative colitis. *Clin. Orthop. 57:* 9–17, 1968.
24. McEwen, C., Di Tata, D., Lingg, C., Porini, A., Good, A., and Rankin, T.: Ankylosing spondylitis and spondylitis accompanying ulcerative colitis, regional enteritis, psoriasis and Reiter's Disease; a comparative study. *Arthritis Rheum. 14:* 291–318, 1971.
25. Messner, R. P.: Clinical aspects of T- and B- lymphocytes in rheumatic disease. *Arthritis Rheum. 17:* 339–346, 1974.

26. Metzger, A. L., Morris, R. I., Bluestone, R., and Terasaki, P. I.: HL-A W27 in psoriatic arthropathy. *Arthritis Rheum. 18:* 111–115, 1975.
27. Mitchell, N., and Shepard, N.: The ultrastructure of articular cartilage in rheumatoid arthritis; a preliminary report. *J. Bone Joint Surg. 52A:* 1405–1423, 1970.
28. Moll, J. M. H., and Wright, V.: Psoriatic arthritis. *Semin. Arthritis Rheum. 3:* 55–78, 1973.
29. Mongan, E. S., Cass, R. M., Jacox, R. F., and Vaughan, J. H.: A study of the relation of seronegative and seropositive rheumatoid arthritis to each other and to necrotizing vasculitis. *Am. J. Med. 47:* 23–35, 1969.
30. Muirden, K. D.: Giant cells, cartilage and bone fragments with rheumatoid synovial membrane; clinico-pathological correlations. *Australas. Ann. Med. 19:* 105–110, 1970.
31. O'Sullivan J. B., and Cathcart, E. S.: The prevalence of rheumatoid arthritis; followup evaluation of the effect of criteria on rates in Sudbury, Massachusetts. *Ann. Intern. Med. 76:* 573–577, 1970.
32. Person, D. A., Sharp, J. T., and Rawls, W. E.: A search for viruses and mycoplasmas in connective tissue diseases. *Arthritis Rheum. 16:* 677–687, 1973.
33. Ropes, M. W., Bennett, G. A., Cobb, S., Jacox, R., and Jessar, R. A.: Revision of diagnositc criteria for rheumatoid arthritis. *Bull. Rheum. Dis. 9:* 175–176, 1958.
34. Schaller, J., and Wedgwood, R. J.: Juvenile rheumatoid arthritis; a review. *Pediatrics 50:* 940–953, 1972.
35. Schlosstein, L., Terasaki, P. I., Bluestone, R., and Pearson, C. M.: High association of an HL-A antigen, W27 with ankylosing spondylitis. *N. Engl. J. Med. 288:* 704–706, 1973.
36. Schumacher, H. R., and Kitridou, R. C.: Synovitis of recent onset; a clinicopathologic study during the first month of disease. *Arthritis Rheum. 15:* 465–485, 1972.
37. Schumacher, H. R., and Kulka, J. P.: Needle biopsy of the synovial membrane; Experience with the Parker-Pearson technic. *New Engl. J. Med. 286:* 416–485, 1972.
38. Sherman, M. S.: The non-specificity of synovial reactions. *Bull. Hosp. Joint Dis. 12:* 110–125, 1951.
39. Waxman, B. A., and Sledge, C. B.: Correlation of histochemical, histologic and biochemical evaluations of human synovium with clinical activity. *Arthritis Rheum. 16:* 376–382, 1973.
40. Weissmann, G.: Lysosomal mechanisms of tissue injury in arthritis. *N. Engl. J. Med 286:* 141–147, 1972.
41. Wilkes, R. M., Simsarian, J. P., Hopps, H. E., Rothe, H., Decker, J. L., Aptekar, R. G., and Meyer, H. M., Jr.: Virologic studies on rheumatoid arthritis. *Arthritis Rheum. 16:* 446–454, 1973.
42. Yu, D. T. Y., and Peter, J. B.: Cellular and immunological aspects of rheumatoid arthritis. *Semin. Arthritis Rheum. 4:* 25–52, 1974.

Chapter 10

Paget's Disease of Bone

H. A. SISSONS

Since its description by Paget in 1877,[11] this condition, then termed "osteitis deformans," has come to be recognized as a fairly common skeletal abnormality of obscure etiology and an important precursor of primary malignant bone tumors in older people. While it is quite rare in its fully developed form, as described by Paget, subsequent work has shown that lesser degrees of skeletal involvement, often without clinical manifestations, are more frequent. The pathologic studies of Schmorl[14] drew attention to certain histologic features of the abnormal bones which have become accepted as pathognomonic.

The characteristic histologic abnormality takes the form of mosaic areas, outlined by markedly crenated cement lines (Figs. 1–3 and 7), and results from disordered and active bone remodeling. Although osteoclastic resorption and osteoblastic bone formation are active during the early stage of the development of a lesion (Fig. 7, *left*), such a lesion, or an area of a lesion, may lack the pattern of cement lines: these are more readily apparent in the relatively dense bone of a more established lesion (Fig. 7, *right*).

INCIDENCE OF PAGET'S DISEASE

Paget's disease is rarely seen in patients under 40 years of age and usually becomes apparent after the age of 50 years. Juvenile cases with somewhat similar features have occasionally been reported.[18, 21] They are sometimes known as "hyperphosphatasia" and are probably unrelated to adult Paget's disease.

The incidence of Paget's disease varies considerably in different parts of the world. Relatively few cases have been reported in African or Asian populations, while many have been found in Britain and some other European countries.[16]

The most detailed and informative study of the incidence of Paget's disease is still that of Schmorl.[14] In Dresden, Germany, during the period 1926 to 1930, Schmorl found 138 cases of Paget's disease in a series of 4614 autopsies on patients over 40 years of age. The skeleton, particularly the vertebral column and pelvis, was examined with special care. No cases of Paget's disease were found during the period of study in autopsies on patients of less than 40 years of age. Schmorl's results, summarized in Table 1, show an increase in frequency of Paget's disease with increasing age in both males and females. Approximately 10% of individuals in the oldest age groups were affected, and the overall incidence was 3.0% (males, 3.5%; females, 2.5%).

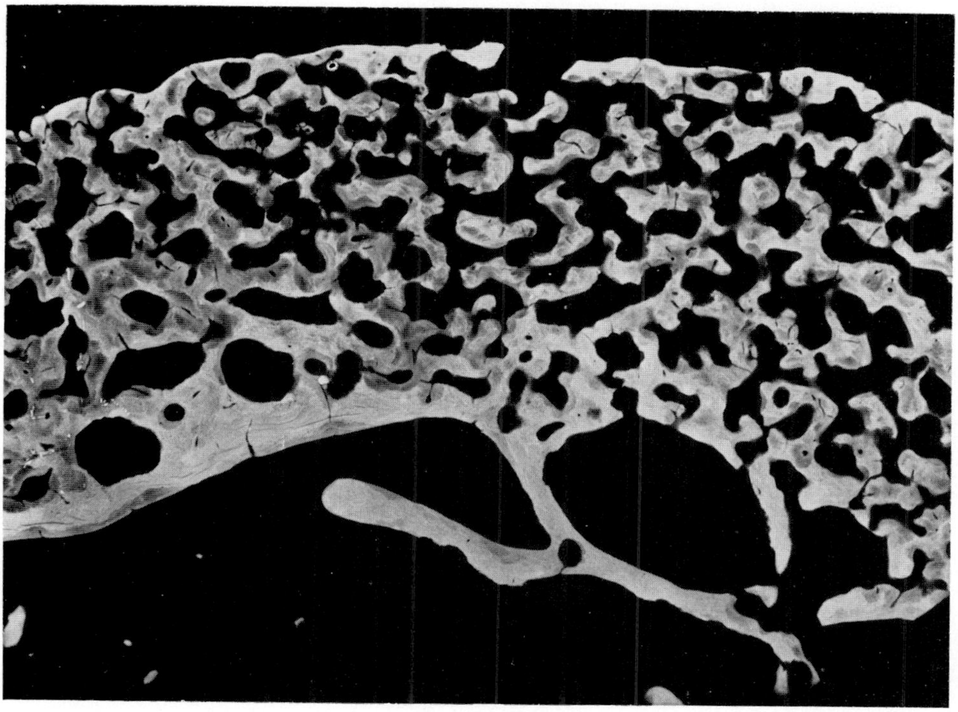

FIG. 1. Microradiograph through cortex of femur in typical (advanced) lesion of Paget's disease. The compact cortical bone is replaced by a network of thick trabeculae (×8).

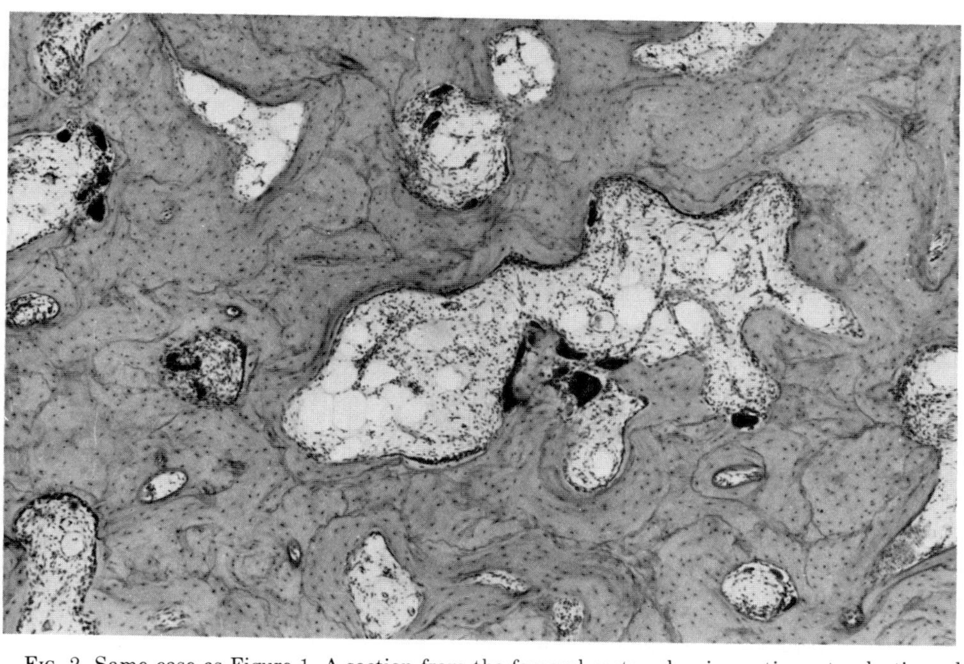

FIG. 2. Same case as Figure 1. A section from the femoral cortex showing active osteoclastic and osteoblastic activity. The enlarged spaces are occupied by vascular tissue. The thick trabeculae show a network of cement lines with a mosaic pattern. Hematoxylin and eosin stain; × 50.

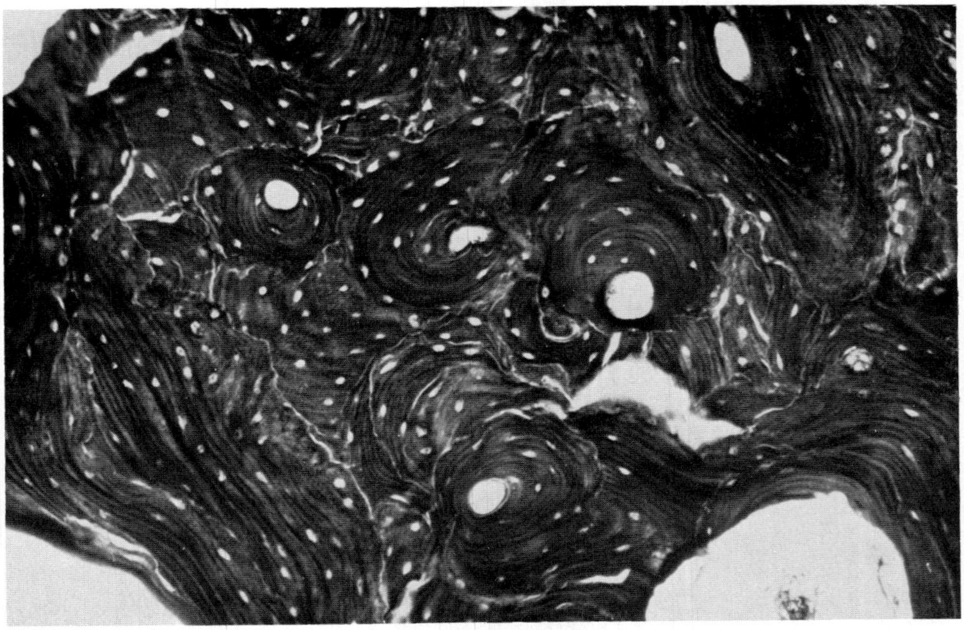

FIG. 3. Same case as Figure 1. A more magnified view, in which the cement lines show up because of their negative staining. Reticulin stain; × 130.

A similar autopsy study was carried out in Leeds and Sheffield, England, by Collins.[3] Twenty-four cases of Paget's disease were found in 650 autopsies on patients over 40 years of age, an overall incidence of 3.7% (males 3.5%; females 4.0%). When allowance is made for the smaller group of cases, the results, summarised in Table 2, are very similar to those of Schmorl's study, both with regard to total incidence and to age and sex distribution.

DISTRIBUTION OF LESIONS

The anatomic distribution of lesions in Schmorl's material is shown in Table 3, and has been broadly confirmed by subsequent pathologic and radiologic studies. The vertebral column, including the sacrum, is the part of the skeleton most frequently affected: other common sites include the skull, sternum, pelvis, and femur. The tibia is less frequently involved, although its bowing is one of the characteristic features of the disease. In some cases only a single bone is affected; in others many bones are involved. Whether solitary or multiple, the lesions are focal, being clearly demarcated from the adjacent uninvolved bone tissue.

PATHOLOGIC FEATURES

The gross appearance of the bone lesions varies. At an early stage in the development of a lesion the involved area of bone may be porotic. Later, both cortical and cancellous bone come to be replaced by a characteristic network of coarse trabecular structures, and this, together with an increase in the thickness of cortical bone, can result in a radiologic appearance of increased density (Fig. 4). Long bones commonly become bowed as well as thickened. Skull involvement usually takes the form of thickening of the vault with loss of distinction between the inner and outer tables; less often, areas of focal rarefaction are encountered and are sometimes termed "osteoporosis circumscripta."[4, 15] Involvement of the base of the skull may occur, and is occasionally accompanied by deafness or other evidence of cranial nerve compression, or by platybasia.[23]

The mosaic pattern of cement lines resulting from disordered and active bone remodeling has already been noted as the characteristic feature of Paget's

TABLE 1. INCIDENCE OF CASES OF PAGET'S DISEASE IN A SERIES OF 4614 AUTOPSIES[a]

Age	Number of Autopsies	Number of Cases	% of Autopsies in Age Groups	% of All Paget Cases
Males				
40 to 49	340	4	1	5
50 to 59	570	16	3	20
60 to 69	725	26	4	33
70 to 79	442	17	4	21
80 to 89	192	15	8	19
90 to 100	9	1	11	1
>100	1	1	100	1
Total	2279	80	3.5	100
Females				
40 to 49	249	2	1	3
50 to 59	406	10	3	17
60 to 69	524	16	3	28
70 to 79	805	14	2	24
80 to 89	332	14	4	24
90 to 100	20	2	10	3
>100				
Total	2335	58	2.5	100

[a] From Schmorl.[14]

TABLE 2. INCIDENCE OF CASES OF PAGET'S DISEASE IN A SERIES OF 650 AUTOPSIES[a]
Males and females.

Age	Number of Autopsies	Number of Cases	% of Autopsies in Age Group	% of All Paget Cases
40 to 49	88	1	1	4
50 to 59	160	8	5	33
60 to 69	190	4	2	17
70 to 79	174	7	4	29
80 to 89	35	4	1	17
>90	3			
Total	650	24	3.7	100

[a] From Collins.[3]

TABLE 3. DISTRIBUTION OF LESIONS OF PAGET'S DISEASE IN A SERIES OF 4614 AUTOPSIES[a]

Location	Number of Cases	% of Paget Cases
Sacrum	78	56.52
Spine	69	50.00
Lumbar	36	
Thoracic	23	
Cervical	10	
Right femur	43	31.15
Skull	39	28.26
Sternum	32	23.18
Pelvis	30	21.73
Left femur	21	15.21
Clavicle	18	13.24
Tibia	11	7.97
Ribs	10	7.24
Humerus	6	6.34

Total number of cases of Paget's disease: 138.

[a] From Schmorl.[14]

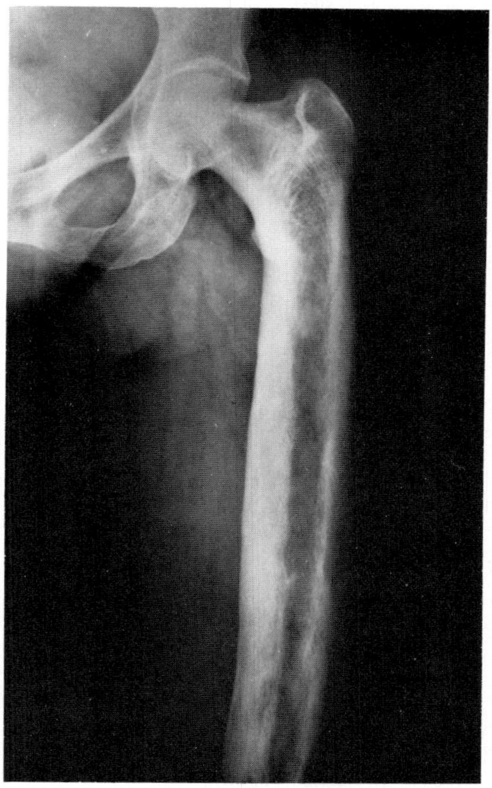

FIG. 4. *Case 1*. Radiograph of femur, showing thickening and coarse trabeculation of cortical bone.

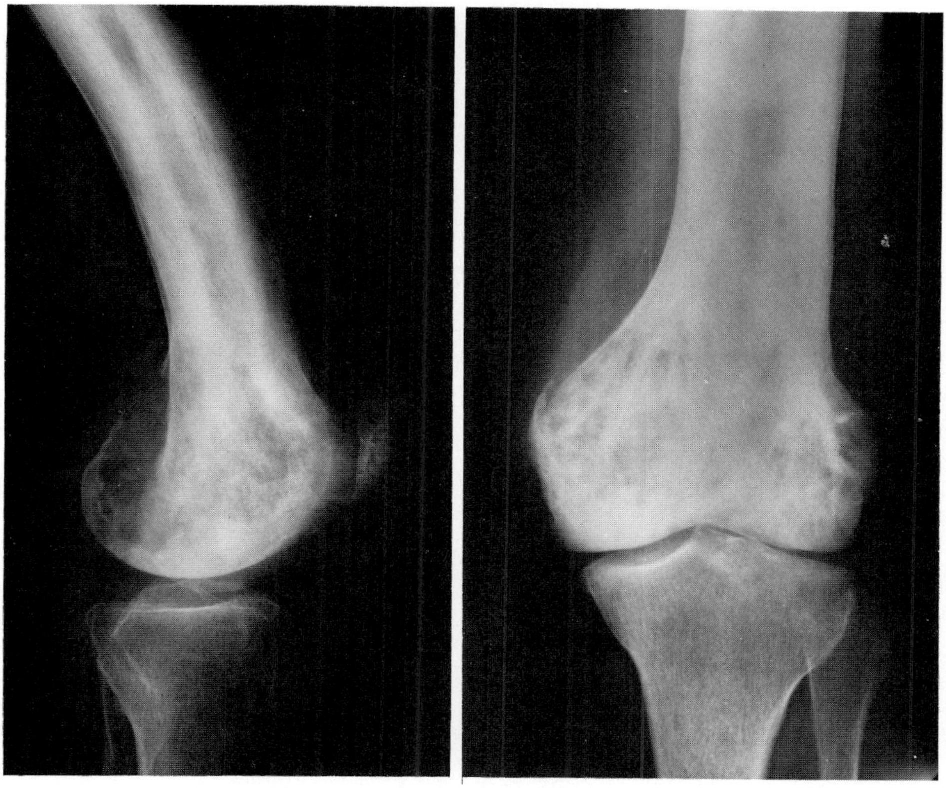

FIG. 5. *Case 1. Left*, lateral radiograph of lower end of femur, showing osteolytic lesion of medial condyle. *Right*, anteroposterior radiograph of same.

disease. Each cement line indicates a surface where bone resorption has been followed by bone deposition, and their complicated pattern indicates an alternation of these two processes at any point.

The lesions of Paget's disease are sometimes extremely vascular, and there can be a great increase in blood flow through the affected bone.[6, 7, 19] In effect, the bone lesions behave as arteriovenous shunts, and in extreme cases the consequent increase in cardiac output can result in cardiac failure.[6, 17]

Bones involved by Paget's disease are more liable to fracture than normal: after fracture, repair proceeds normally.

The use of isotopes for the study of mineral exchange in Paget's disease has shown high rates for skeletal accretion and turnover of calcium, with an increase in the size of the exchangeable pool.[1, 5, 9] The serum calcium and phosphate levels are usually normal in Paget's disease, but active lesions are associated with high values for serum alkaline phosphatase.

Calcitonin, the calcium-lowering hormone of the thyroid, finds a clinical application in the treatment of Paget's disease, particularly in the presence of bone pain or hypercalcemia.[21]

PAGET'S DISEASE AND BONE TUMORS

Paget's disease is a precancerous condition, and is an important precursor of bone tumors: indeed the association was noted by Paget in his original account of the condition. In more recent years many studies, such as those of Coley & Sharp[2] Gerstel and Janker,[8] Thomson and Turner-Warwick,[20] Mackenzie, Court Brown, Doll, and Sissons,[10] and Price,[12] have established that a disproportionate number of primary malignant bone tumors developing after the age of 40 years occur in individuals with Paget's disease. Information from Britain indicates that approximately 30% of primary malignant bone tumors developing after the age of 40 years occur in individuals with Paget's disease, although these individuals constitute only 3% of the population.[16] Any part of the skeleton may be involved, but tumors have been observed most frequently in the major long bones and in the pelvis and skull.[13] The majority of the tumors are pleomorphic osteosarcomas, but chondrosarcomas and fibrosarcomas are also found. The bone tumors in Paget's disease are highly malignant: most patients die rapidly with pulmonary metastases.

ILLUSTRATIVE CASES

The following 2 cases illustrate some points of interest in connection with Paget's disease.

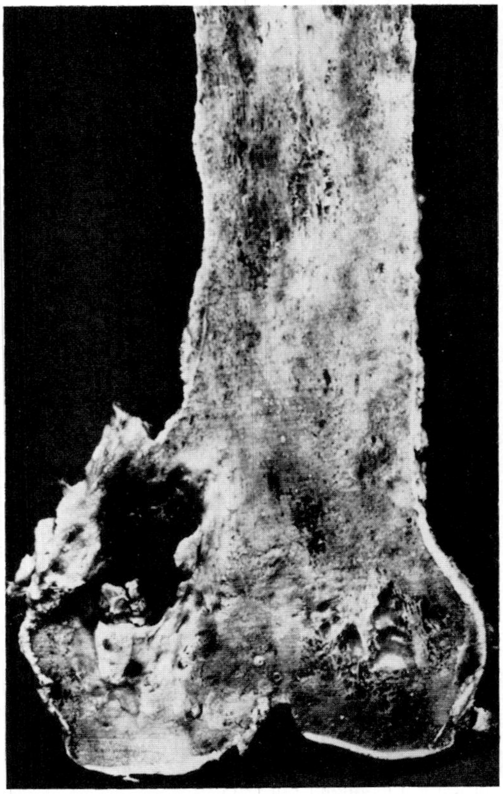

FIG. 6. *Case 1.* Tumor of lower end of femur.

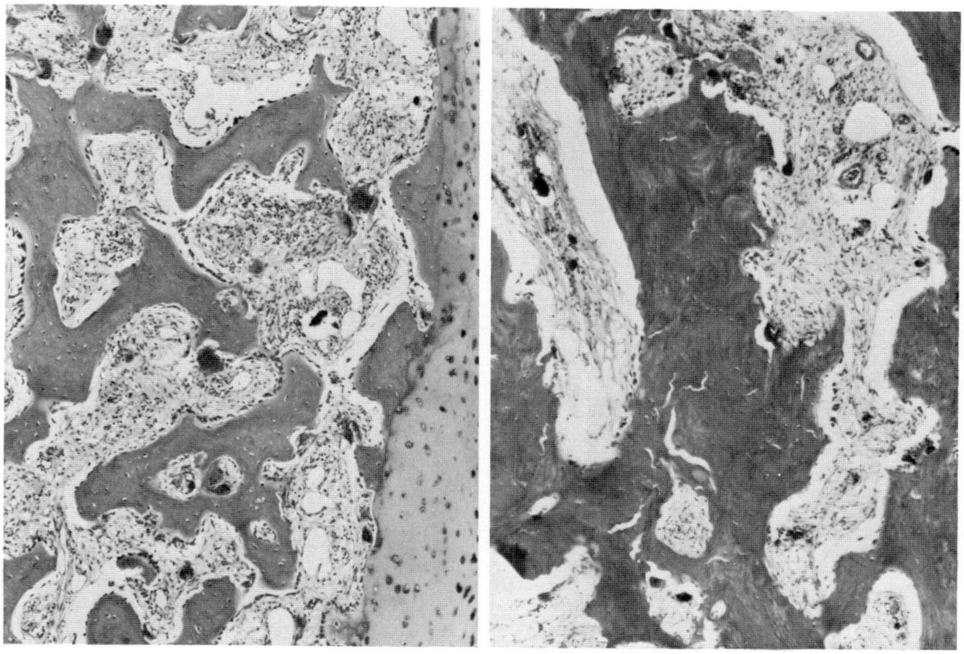

FIG. 7. *Case 1, Left,* histologic section from cancellous bone of lower femur, showing changes of "early" Paget's disease. There is active osteoclastic and osteoblastic activity, but the slender trabeculae do not yet show the mosaic pattern of cement lines. *Right,* Histologic section from area where changes are more advanced. Numerous irregular cement lines are present in the thick trabeculae, and the bone shows artefactual fragmentation along these lines. Hematoxylin and eosin stain; ×50.

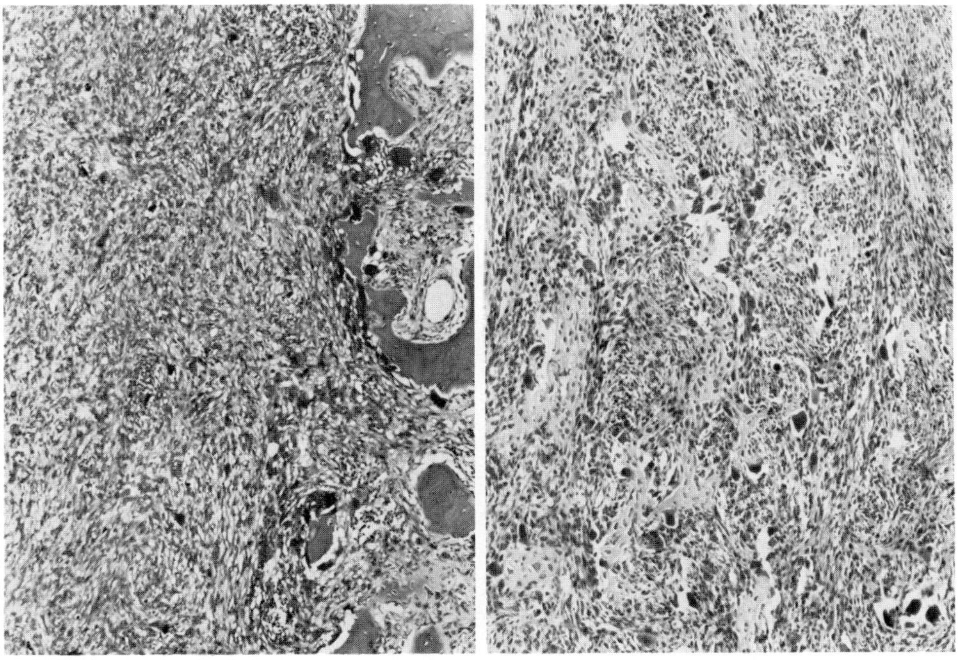

FIG. 8. *Case 1. Left,* histologic section from margin of tumor of lower femur. The histologic structure is that of an undifferentiated sarcoma, and the tumor is causing destruction of bone trabeculae. *Right,* another part of the tumor where the presence of a network of tumor bone establishes a diagnosis of osteosarcoma. Hematoxylin and eosin stain; × 50.

Case 1. A female 65 years of age complained of pain and bowing of the left femur for many years, recently becoming more severe. X-ray examination showed evidence of Paget's disease in the form of increased thickness and coarse trabeculation of the femoral cortex (Fig. 4). An irregular area of bone destruction was present in the medial condyle of the femur (Fig. 5) and was suspected of being a malignant tumor. Laboratory investigations gave the following values: serum calcium, 2.5 mmol/liter (10.0 mg per 100 ml); serum phosphorus, 0.85 mmol/liter (2.5 mg per 100 ml), and serum alkaline phosphatase 108 IU/liter (15 King-Armstrong (K. A.) units/100 ml). A biopsy of the medial condyle of the femur was carried out, and the diagnosis of sarcoma confirmed; this was followed by a disarticulation through the hip joint.

The gross pathology of the tumor is shown in Fig. 6, and its histologic structure in Fig. 8. Most of the tumor showed the structure of an undifferentiated sarcoma, but in some areas the presence of a network of tumor bone established a diagnosis of osteosarcoma. The rest of the bone showed characteristic changes of Paget's disease (Fig. 7).

Despite the unfavorable prognosis usually associated with malignant bone tumors in Paget's disease, the patient is alive and well 7 years after amputation.

Case 2. A male 32 years of age complained of pain in the back, radiating to the

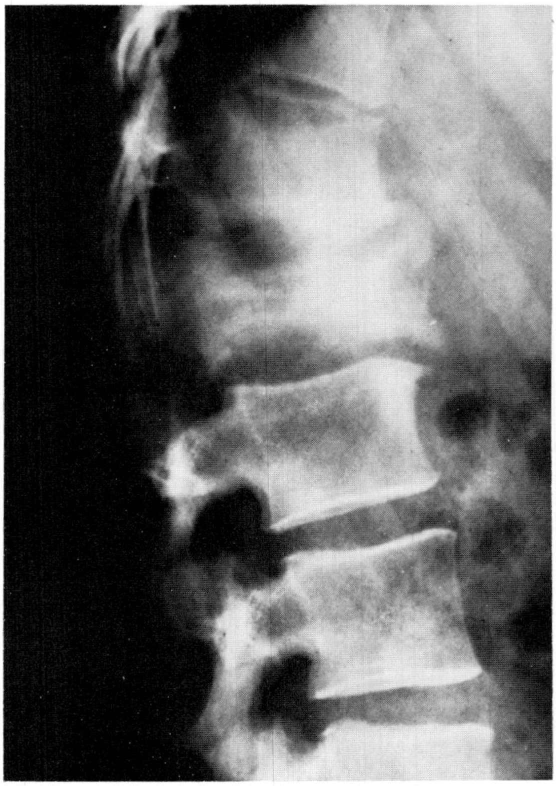

FIG. 9. *Case 2.* Radiograph of spine, showing increased anteroposterior diameter of the body of the 1st lumbar vertebra, with vertical compression.

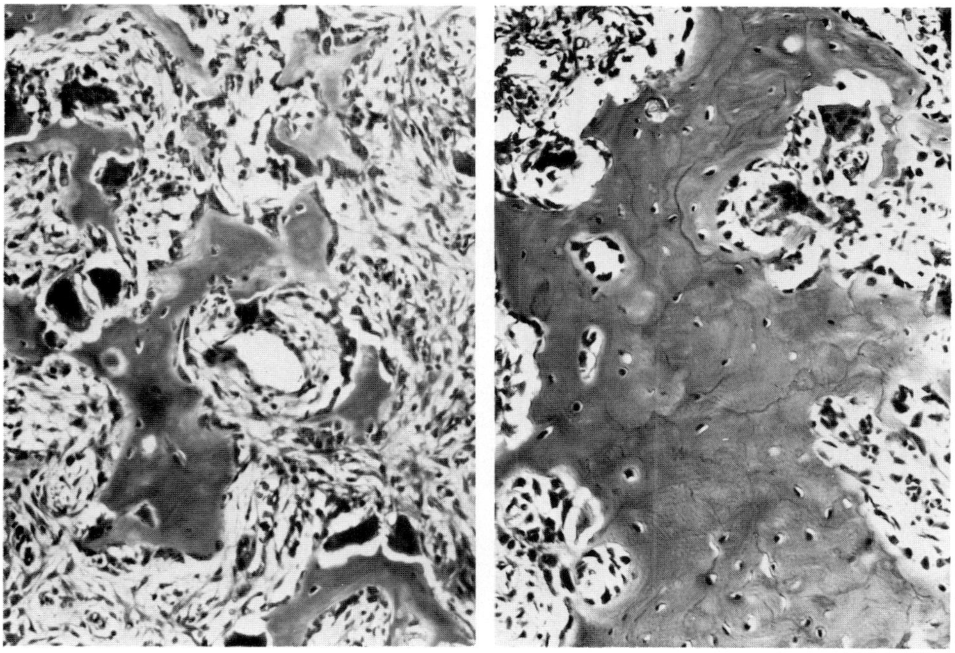

FIG. 10. *Case 2. Left*, histologic section of lesion, showing newly formed bone trabeculae without mosaic pattern of cement lines. *Right*, an area where the characteristic pattern of cement lines is present. Hematoxylin and eosin stain; × 130.

legs, for 4 years. There was no history of injury. Clinical examination showed evidence of incipient spinal cord involvement in the form of an abnormal plantar response. X-ray examination showed an abnormal appearance of the body of the 1st lumbar vertebra, which was compressed vertically and had an increased anteroposterior diameter (Fig. 9). Laboratory investigations gave the following values: serum calcium, 2.5 mmol/liter (10.0 mg per 100 ml); serum phosphorus, 1.0 mmol/liter (3.1 mg per 100 ml); and serum alkaline phosphatase, 400 IU/liter (56 K. A. units/100 ml).

The lesion was explored using a dorsal approach, and a laminectomy was performed to decompress the spinal cord. The bone was observed to be soft and spongy and to bleed easily. Histologic sections showed typical changes of Paget's disease (Fig. 10). After operation, the abnormal plantar response disappeared, but 3 years later further symptoms of spinal cord compression reappeared. These again disappeared, however, following treatment with calcitonin.

Despite the age of the patient, the presence of a characteristic mosaic pattern of cement lines establishes a diagnosis of Paget's disease. The clinical presentation with developing paraplegia is unusual (it not uncommonly indicates the presence of a malignant tumor), and the response to calcitonin treatment is of interest.

REFERENCES

1. Bauer, G. C. H., and Wendeberg, B.: External counting of Ca^{47} and Sr^{85} in studies of localised skeletal lesions in man. *J. Bone Joint Surg. 41B:* 558–580, 1959.

2. Coley, B. L., and Sharp, G. S.: Paget's disease. A predisposing factor to osteogenic sarcoma. *Arch. Surg. 23:* 918–936, 1931.
3. Collins, D. H.: Paget's disease of bone; incidence and subclinical forms. *Lancet 2:* 51–57, 1956.
4. Collins, D. H., and Winn, J. M.: Focal Paget's disease of the skull (osteoporosis circumscripta). *J. Pathol. 69:* 1–9, 1955.
5. Deuxchaisnes, C. N. de, and Krane, S. M.: Paget's disease of bone; clinical and metabolic observations. *Medicine 43:* 233–266, 1964.
6. Edholm, O. G., and Howart, S.: Studies on the peripheral circulation in osteitis deformans. *Clin. Sci. 12:* 277–285, 1953.
7. Edholm, O. G., Howarth, S., and McMichael, J.: Heart failure and bone blood flow in osteitis deformans. *Clin. Sci. 5:* 249–260, 1945.
8. Gerstel, G., and Janker, R.: Über die Entwicklung eines Spindelzellsarkoms auf dem Boden einer monostotischen Ostitis deformans Paget. *Dtsch. Z. Chir. 238:* 577–603, 1933.
9. Heaney, R. P., and Whedon, G. D.: Radiocalcium studies of bone formation rate in human metabolic bone disease. *J. Clin. Endocrinol. Metab. 18:* 1246–1267, 1958.
10. Mackenzie, A., Court Brown, W. M., Doll, R., and Sissons, H. A. Mortality from primary tumours of bone in England and Wales. *Br. Med. J.* 1782–1790, 1961.
11. Paget, J.: On a form of chronic inflammation of bones (Osteitis Deformans). *Med. Chir. Trans. Lond. 60:* 37–63, 1877.
12. Price, C. H. G. The incidence of osteogenic sarcoma in South-West England and its relationship to Paget's disease of bone. *J. Bone Joint Surg. 44B:* 366–376, 1962.
13. Price, C. H. G., and Goldie, W. Paget's sarcoma of bone. A study of eighty cases from the Bristol and the Leeds Bone Tumour Registries. *J. Bone Joint Surg. 51B:* 205–224, 1969.
14. Schmorl, G.: Über Ostitis deformans Paget. *Virchows Arch. Pathol. Anat. 283:* 694–751, 1932.
15. Schüller, A.: Dysostosis hypophysaria. *Br. J. Radiol. 31:* 156–158, 1926.
16. Sissons, H. A.: Epidemiology of Paget's disease. *Clin. Orthop. 45:* 73–79, 1966.
17. Sornberger, C. F., and Smedal, M. I.: Mechanisms and incidence of cardiovascular changes in Paget's disease (osteitis deformans); a critical review of the literature with case studies. *Circulation 6:* 711–726, 1952.
18. Stemmermann, G. N.: An histologic and histochemical study of familial osteoectasia (chronic idiopathic hyperphosphatasia). *Am. J. Pathol. 48:* 641–651, 1966.
19. Storsteen, K. A., and Janes, J. M.: Arteriography and vascular studies in Paget's disease of bone. *J. A. M. A. 154:* 472–474, 1954.
20. Thomson, A. D., and Turner-Warwick, R. T.: Skeletal sarcoma and gaint-cell tumour. *J. Bone Joint Surg. 37B:* 266–303, 1955.
21. Woodhouse, N. J. Y.: Paget's disease of bone. *Clin. Endocrinol. Metabol. 1:* 125–141, 1972.
22. Woodhouse, N. J. Y., Fisher, M. T., Sigurdsson, G., Joplin, G. F., and MacIntyre, I.: Paget's disease in a 5-year-old; acute response to human calcitonin. *Br. Med. J. 4:* 267–269, 1972.
23. Wycis, H. T.: Basilar impression (platybasia); a case secondary to advanced Paget's disease with severe neurological manifestations. Successful surgical result. *J. Neurosurg. 1:* 299–305, 1944.

Chapter 11

Neoplasms and Neoplasm-like Lesions of the Synovium

ROBERT E. FECHNER

The synovium is the source of histologically diverse neoplasms and neoplasm-like proliferations, virtually none of which bears the least resemblance to normal synovium. In fact, if it were not for the anatomic location, most would completely belie their synovial origin. For example, the histologic patterns of synovial sarcoma, clear cell sarcoma, synovial chondromatosis, and synovial chondrosarcoma simply have no normal histologic counterpart. To appreciate this divergence fully, it is appropriate to outline briefly the components and functions of the normal synovium before dealing with its tumors.

NORMAL SYNOVIUM

The synovial membrane of joints, tendon sheaths, and bursae is a highly specialized mesodermal derivative facilitating mobility between a variety of cartilaginous or connective tissue surfaces. The cells in the synovium are capable of numerous functions including phagocytosis, mucin production, and the physiologic maintenance of the synovial fluid which nourishes the avascular articular cartilage. In addition to lubrication, the synovium also provides mechanical flexibility during the physical rearrangements of joint or soft tissue spaces in motion.

The embryonic development of the joint includes two major morphologic phases: the formation of an interzone and the subsequent appearance of a cleft within it. The interzone forms in the mesenchyme remaining between the ends of the cartilaginous skeletal precursors, which also have arisen from mesenchyme. The periphery of the interzone becomes vascularized and is the site of formation for the joint capsule and ligaments. After the articular outline is established, minute clefts appear in the interzone mesenchyme, and the joint space becomes recognizable by the end of 6 to 8 weeks of embryonic life.[1] The mechanism certainly is more than a mere dissolution of cells, because the cleft from its inception is lined with intact cells.[2] One necessary factor in some species is the ability to move the embryonic limb, since complete cavitation of the joint fails to occur in experimentally paralyzed limbs in the chick embryo[3] and in mice with dysgenesis of the skeleton muscle with its concomittant lack of limb movement.[4]

The mature synovium (synovial membrane) consists of an inner layer of synovial lining cells (synovial intima) and a subsynovial layer (subintima) of connective tissue with varying quantities of collagen, elastic fibers, adipose tissue, and blood vessels. This layer merges imperceptibly into the denser, fibrous outer joint capsule. The gross and microscopic appearance of the synovium is variable even within the same joint depending on the character of the subsynovial layer. For example, the synovium over intraarticular ligaments and the more rigid areas of the joint capsule will be grossly smooth and microscopically covered with attenuated synovial cells forming a layer one cell thick. In some areas, the synovial cells may not be visible,[5] and this apparent absence has been verified by electron microscopy.[6, 7] When overlying adipose tissue, synovial cells form a layer up to five cells in thickness, and these areas correspond to the folds and villi seen grossly. Synovial villi are present in all joints occurring as a delicate fringe around the margin of the articular cartilage where the synovium inserts into the intraarticular periosteum.[8, 9] The number and size of villi increase with age,[10] although no qualitative microscopic alterations are detectable in synovia of patients ranging from 14 to 68 years of age.[5]

Cytologically, the synovial lining cells vary considerably in size and shape, which is most easily seen in the areolar and adipose synovium. The commonest cells are polyhedral (type A cells) with a more elongated cell (type B) intermixed. Ultrastructurally, the type A cell has filopodia, microvilli, many vacuoles and pinocytic vesicles, abundant Golgi, numerous mitochondria, and sparse ergastoplasmic reticulin. By contrast, the type B cell is elongated, has a fairly smooth border, few vacuoles and pinocytic vesicles, scant Golgi, and abundant rough ergastoplasmic reticulin. There are no specialized attachments between the cells, although some adherence is provided by cell invaginations.[11] Many cells have a configuration and complement of organelles which are neither clearly type A or B and are considered to be intermediate cells. Most authors believe that the A, B, and intermediate cells are not separate species of cells, but are morphologic variants reflecting different functional activities of the same basic cell.[6]

The matrix between the synovial cells consists mainly of aperiodic fibers and finely granular material with only a rare collagen fiber in the deepest portion of the layer. There is no basement membrane between the synovial intima and the subsynovial layer,[6, 12] although an inconstant thin amorphous layer of greater density than the matrix has been seen adjacent to small sectors of a few synovial cells.[6]

The synovial fluid is in part a selective dialysate of plasma, but in addition contains hyaluronic acid, a lubricating substance contributed by the synovial cells.[13] The site of production has long been a matter of debate, but recent studies by electron microscopic radioautography on cultures of human synovial cells indicate localization of precursors of hyaluronate in the Golgi apparatus of synovial lining cells.[14] Colloidal iron, a traditional stain for connective tissue mucins has also been localized in the Golgi vesicles in rabbit synovium.[15] Presumably, these are type A cells because of their abundance of Golgi.

Besides the production and reabsorption of fluid, the synovial cells remove particulate matter. They are capable of engulfing material as large as whole erythrocytes.[16] The subsynovial layer is rich in lymphatic vessels as well as blood vessels, and soluble material injected into the joint space will appear in lymph or blood within a few minutes. The pinocytic vesicles and filopodia of the type A cells are visible evidence of this clearing process, resulting in cells with phagocytized debris which are morphologically indistinguishable from the macrophages in the subsynovial connective tissue. The latter probably represents synovial cells that have migrated downward after removing material from the joint fluid or synovial matrix.[6]

BENIGN NEOPLASMS AND NEOPLASM-LIKE LESIONS

The nonspecialized soft tissues of the subsynovium can give rise to tumors such as hemangiomas and lipomas with conventional histologic patterns and natural histories identical to those occurring in other soft tissue sites. On the other hand, the synovial cells themselves or primitive cells within the synovium give rise to tumors which are peculiar to synovium, *e.g.*, synovial chondromatosis and the various types of nodular synovitis. These lesions are considered by some as neoplasms and by others as reactive lesions; a distinction of neither clinical nor pathologic importance.

Synovial Chondromatosis

The term synovial chondromatosis is preferred to osteochondromatosis since ossification is not always present. The disease has been defined in different ways with a few older reports accepting the presence of four or more loose bodies within a joint as adequate evidence for the diagnosis in the absence of degenerative joint disease, osteochondral fracture, or osteochondritis dissecans.[17] Jaffe's[18] more stringent definition demands a chondromatous component in the synovial membrane (Fig. 1) in addition to the loose bodies, and the number of free bodies is not crucial. The author adheres to this definition.

The process begins with the formation of cartilage in the subintimal connective tissue of the synovial membrane. The nodules eventually project above the surface, and some are shed into the joint space. It is possible that there is continued growth of cartilage once the nodule drops into the joint space. This

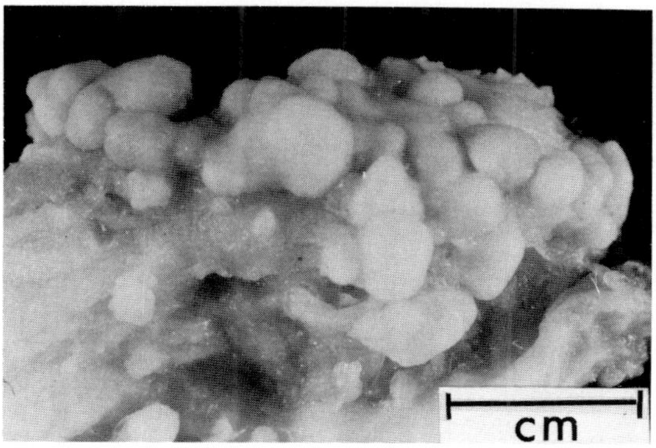

FIG. 1. The presence of intrasynovial cartilaginous nodules is the prime criterion for the diagnosis of synovial chondromatosis. (Baylor Neg. 47194.)

cannot be directly verified in chondromatosis, but data from cases of osteochondritis dissecans may be pertinent in that the size of the original exfoliated fragment can be determined by the radiologic defect and compared with the size of the surgically removed specimen. In some instances, the loose body has been larger than the defect,[18] and by analogy, it is reasonable to assume that some loose bodies in chondromatosis may also enlarge as they float in the joint space.

Tendon sheaths occasionally contain free cartilaginous bodies,[19] and some have free bodies plus a synovial component.[20]Bursae also may be the site of morphologically typical synovial chondromatosis.[21] Some patients have had pedunculated osseous and cartilaginous masses attached to the lining of tendon sheaths as solitary or multiple nodules but lacking large numbers of intrasynovial nodules, thereby differing from chondromatosis.[22] Such lesions have been designated as tenosynovial osteochondroma,[23] but probably are only less florid examples of chondromatosis.

Clinical features. As with practically every orthopedic disease involving an extremity, a definite history of trauma will be elicited in a minority of patients but denied by most. The growing population of heavily traumatized knees of amateur and professional athletes has not been associated thus far with an epidemic of synovial chondromatosis, and the etiologic role of trauma is doubtful.[24]

The knee is the site of involvement in about two-thirds of patients, with the hip or elbow about equally divided as the next most frequent site.[25] Lesions of the shoulder, ankle, carpus, tarsus, temporomandibular joint,[26] and finger have been reported on isolated occasions.[27] About 10% of the knee, hip, elbow, and shoulder lesions are bilateral.[25] One case of triple joint involvement (shoulder, hand, and foot) has been described.[28] Males are afflicted twice as often as females, and ages have ranged from 14 to 67 years with a peak in the 5th decade.[29]

The clinical findings are not distinctive, and the patients complain of various combinations of pain, swelling, and limited motion for durations of 1 month to 5 decades. On the average, patients are symptomatic for about 5 years.[29] The radiologic findings may be strongly suggestive of the diagnosis if numerous calcified bodies are visualized; however, not all loose bodies are calcified, and in about 10% of patients none whatsoever will be seen radiologically.[29] One joint contained 395 loose bodies, none of which was detected radiologically:[30] arthrography may be of value in this situation.[25] Another radiologic clue in hip lesions is a distinctive conical deformity of the femoral neck resulting from bone erosion, a process which is reversible after the loose bodies are removed.[25] Certainly the most extraordinary clinical presentation of synovial chondromatosis in the hip was the mass encountered on a routine pelvic examination.[31]

Gross and operative findings. The synovium may be diffusely studded with hundreds of nodules, or less commonly, only a few square centimeters may be affected. The area near the synovial cartilaginous junction tends to be more heavily involved. The synovial surface is irregular with flat bumps, polypoid nodules of various shapes, and pedunculated masses, some on long delicate stalks. The individual nodules, whether free or attached, vary in size from less than a millimeter to 3 cm. The loose bodies, which can number over 400,[32] may have a smooth surface or be granular, suggesting fusion of smaller nodules.

Microscopic findings. The earliest stage of synovial chondromatosis is the formation of round, cellular islands of cartilage in the synovial connective tissue beneath but not involving the synovial lining cells. Concentric layers of collagen may form a distinct cuff around the chondroid islands. Occasionally the smallest microscopic foci consist exclusively of round nodules of loosely arranged trabeculae of bone. Their small size and lack of cartilage suggest that they are osseous from their inception rather than ossified cartilage. In addition to well organized foci of cartilage or bone, the synovial membrane may contain minute jagged fragments of calcified material identical to those found in the synovium from patients with degenerative joint disease. This is not unexpected since degenerative changes are present in at least half the joints involved by chondromatosis with the degenerative joint disease considered as either a coincidental aging process or in younger patients a secondary manifestation of mechanical derangement and trauma due to the loose bodies.

Larger nodules, including those protruding above the synovial membrane and lying free in the joint, may have a mixture of cartilage and bone with fatty marrow. The free-floating nodules are sometimes still covered with a layer of synovium, and the surface cartilage is usually intact even when there is necrosis of the inner bone or cartilage.[19]

The cytologic atypia of the chondrocytes is often worrisome (Fig. 2). Enlarged nuclei, pleomorphism, and binucleated cells can be found in about two-thirds of cases.[29] One must follow the same philosophy in evaluating synovial chondromatosis as in evaluating cartilaginous neoplasms of bone. In the latter

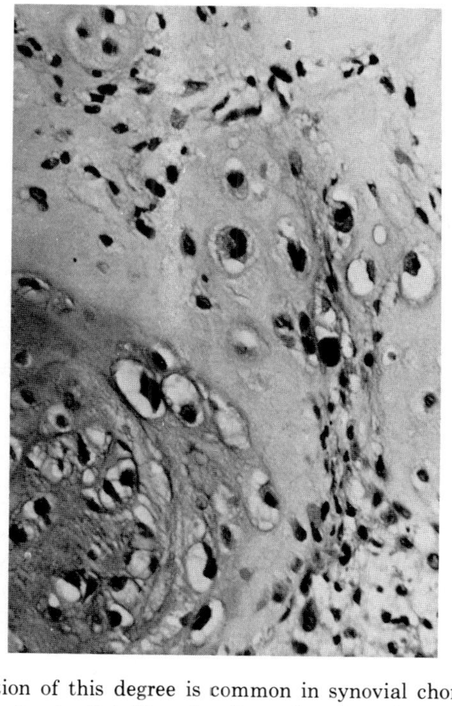

FIG. 2. Cytologic variation of this degree is common in synovial chondromatosis and does not constitute proof of malignant potential. Hematoxylin and eosin stain, × 200.

situations, one is required to take into account the entire clinical setting before deciding the significance of cytologic atypia in the chondrocytes. Similarly, when the clinical and gross findings of chondromatosis show the disease confined to the synovium and joint space, the microscopic atypia can be discounted for all practical purposes since these lesions rarely behave differently from those without atypia. The presence of orderly ossification in juxtaposition to the cartilage further favors a benign process. The extremely rare exceptions to these statements are detailed in the discussion of synovial chondrosarcoma.

Prognosis. Therapy usually consists of the removal of loose bodies and the involved synovial membrane. Radiotherapy is not beneficial.[29] Many authors have pointed out that the disease appears to be self-limited since even in the absence of total synovectomy, recurrence is virtually nonexistent.[29, 32, 33] On the basis of long range observations, it would appear that most patients have reached a quiescent stage of loose body formation by the time they decide to have a surgical procedure. An alternative explanation is that the enlargement of chondromatosis bodies is so slow that there simply is not enough remaining life to regrow nodules to a symptomatic size or number.

A few instances of alleged spontaneous regression have been described. In one case, the arthrogram was the basis of the initial diagnosis, and 7 months later the joint was explored and no bodies were found.[34] The author is not convinced that the arthrogram can be considered unequivocal proof of the diagnosis in this particular instance. In another case, sequential films showed progressively fewer bodies.[30] This may only reflect demineralization rather than total dissolution of the cartilage or bone, since the joint was not explored and there was no objective proof of a decreased number.

A few cases have had extraarticular masses of cartilage.[33, 35] These masses, one to three in number, are easily shelled out, and the patients have not followed a course different from ordinary chondromatosis, although such cases must be closely studied to exclude their being synovial chondrosarcoma. Extraarticular extensions have been left in a few patients without evidence of further growth.[36]

Pigmented Villonodular Synovitis

Proliferation of the synovium includes two lesions, pigmented villonodular synovitis and localized nodular synovitis, which have caused considerable confusion in the literature. Both are characterized microscopically by a variable mixture of synovial cells, foam cells, hemosiderin-laden cells, and multinucleated giant cells. The separation of pigmented villonodular synovitis (PVNS) and localized nodular synovitis (LNS) can be determined by the gross appearance (Fig. 3). PVNS is predominately villous and almost invariably involves most or all of the synovium. By contrast, localized nodular synovitis is a circumscribed tumor with a predominantly smooth surface arising from a small area of synovium. The localized tumors may be contained completely within a joint space or may be present in an extraarticular location even though originating from joint synovium, whereas PVNS is almost exclusively a disease of articular synovium.

It is possible that the diffuse villous lesions and at least some of the solitary

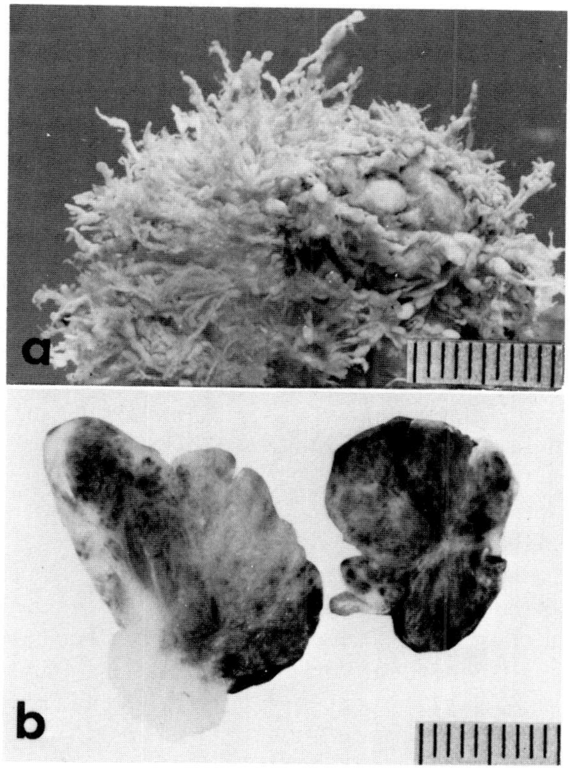

FIG. 3. Both photographs are of synovial lesions from the knee joint. *a*, pigmented villonodular synovitis from a 16-year-old girl (see text). *b*, bisected solitary lesion with the smooth outer surface and mottled cut surface typical of localized intraarticular nodular synovitis (millimeter ruler). (Baylor Neg. 32817; Methodist Neg. 7139897.) (*b*, from Fraire, A. E., and Fechner, R.E. [62]Used with permission.)

intraarticular circumscribed lesions are related. For example, one can see multiple smooth nodules in otherwise diffuse villous lesions, and some solitary lesions are spongy, appearing to be formed by the coalescence of closely packed villi.[37] Even more persuasive is Wright's demonstration that a single lesion may be villous when growing into a joint space or tendon sheath space, whereas the opposite side of the same mass growing into the soft tissues results in a solid, smooth-surfaced nodule.[38] Despite this possible relationship between villous and nodular synovitis, it is important to separate PVNS and LNS sharply when dealing with intraarticular tumors because of fundamental differences in natural history and therapeutic response. For these reasons, PVNS and LNS will be discussed separately.

Pigmented villonodular synovitis is defined by a combination of gross and microscopic features. Grossly, most or all of the synovium is covered with tan to brown papillary projections ranging from slender villi to globoid nodules. Microscopically a polymorphic population of synovial cells, foam cells, and hemosiderin-laden histiocytes is intermixed with fibrous tissue. By adhering to these gross and microscopic criteria, one will eliminate several lesions having some, but not all, of the above features.[39] In examining a grossly villous synovium, one must remember that the normal synovium has delicate villi near the chondrosynovial junction, and a wide variety of diseases and stimuli such as rheumatoid arthritis, degenerative joint disease, and hemorrhage will result in villous enlargement. For example, PVNS has been said to occur in hemophiliacs because the synovium of hemophilic arthropathy may contain great amounts of hemosiderin and have villi. Nonetheless, the villi lack large numbers of foam cells and multinucleated giant cells and thereby fail to qualify as PVNS.[40] The synovium in the joint with degenerative arthritis is occasionally quite villous, but usually lacks heavy hemosiderin deposits and never has the polymorphic infiltrate.[41]

The etiology of PVNS is unknown. The abundance of hemosiderin and the presence of sanguineous joint fluid has raised the possibility that hemorrhage, perhaps on a traumatic basis, might be causative, but a history of trauma can be elicited in less than a quarter of patients.[42] There is no evidence that repeated hemorrhages will result in changes such as are seen in PVNS. Cases of hemophilia or synovial hemangiomas can have huge accumulations of hemosiderin both in the synovium and subsynovial tissues which may or may not be associated with prominent villi, but as stated before, they lack further microscopic features of PVNS.[43, 44] Patients with hemochromatosis who have long-standing deposits of iron in type B synovial cells[45] and subsynovial stroma will have a grossly brown synovium and occasional villous formation without the other changes of PVNS.

Experimentally, multiple injections of fresh blood into the knee joints of dogs and rabbits will produce synovial changes resembling pigmented villonodular synovitis.[46, 47] However, similar changes have been produced by repeated injections of sterile normal saline, thereby suggesting that the trauma of the injection rather than blood *per se* may be the major cause for the alterations in this experimental model. Furthermore, in the latter experiment, the changes regressed 6 months after cessation of injections,[43] which is unlike the natural course of PVNS and throws considerable doubt on the relevance of these experiments to the etiology of the disease in humans.

Clinical features. There is a preponderance of females with the ratio reaching as high as 2:1 in one series.[37] Patients have been from 16 to 60 years old with a fairly even age distribution per decade including the 3rd and 4th decades. The duration of symptoms has ranged from 6 months to 25 years with an average of 6 years. Pain is a constant symptom, and most patients complain of swelling which is either intermittent or steadily progressive. Many patients have had the joint aspirated with recovery of a yellow to brown clear or turbid fluid. Limitation of motion is a frequent symptom, but "locking" is uncommon. On physical examination tenderness, limitation of motion, swelling, and occasionally palpable masses are found. Radiologic changes can be identified in about two-thirds of patients including soft tissue masses, unilocular or multilocular cystic changes in the subchondral region of adjacent bones, and alterations of degenerative joint disease.[48-50] Arthrography may demonstrate a diagnostic pattern.[51]

More than 80% of all cases of PVNS have been in the knee. The hip accounts for about 15%,[51, 52] with a few cases reported in the ankle,[42] foot or hand,[49] elbow,[51] and shoulder.[53] Over 200 cases of PVNS are reported in the literature, but only a few have involved more than one joint. The distribution of multiple joints involved and the ages of these patients are: knee-knee (56 years old),[54] knee-hip (60 years old),[54] knee-knee (24 years old),[55] and ankle-ankle (age unknown).[42] In addition. we have seen a girl with bilateral involvement by histologically typical PVNS of wrists, knees, and ankles. These six areas became symptomatic within a few months of each other at the age of 10 years, and all except one knee have been operated upon because of cosmetic deformity and limitation of motion. The surgical procedures were performed between 16 and 18 years of age with no progression of disease in the ensuing 3 years.

A few instances of PVNS arising in bursae have been described. An amazing clinical presentation of a bursal lesion was a large inguinal mass in a 28-year-old man thought to be a hernia, but turning out to be PVNS arising in the iliopectineal bursa.[56] Whether the bursa communicated with the hip joint was not determined. Popliteal bursae have been resected for PVNS in which the knee joint has apparently not been involved.[37] The case reported by Peterson, Johnson, and Woolner[57] is perhaps the most convincing for extraarticular PVNS. A large lesion was present in the soft tissues of the anterior-lateral aspect of the knee, and although attached to the outer capsule of the knee joint, the joint itself was uninvolved.

Gross and operative findings. The synovium is reddish brown with occasional yellow foci. Usually it is diffusely involved although small patches of normal synovium can remain. The villous projections are quite variable in size and shape. There may be hundreds of filamentous villi, and there may be smooth nodules, either projecting above the surface or forming flat pads. Either the filamentous or the multinodular gross pattern may dominate.

Uncommonly, only a small area of synovium is affected. In one group of 23 cases, 3 consisted of localized spongelike masses which suggested a fusion of villi.[37] Such cases can be considered as a localized villonodular synovitis and may be an early stage of the solid lesion which will be discussed under intraarticular localized nodular synovitis.

The bone lesions seen radiologically may contain only fibrous or myxomatous tissue such as that seen in conjunction with degenerative joint disease.[49] In other cases, there is direct extension of villonodular tissue into the osseous defect which is in continuity with the joint space.[50] The extension probably occurs by growth of synovium through the points of entry of nutrient vessels near the joint capsule. We have seen 1 case of extension into the femoral head through the insertion of the ligamentum teres (Fig. 4).

Microscopic findings. The villi are covered by a thickened layer of synovial cells containing hemosiderin. Mitotic figures are usually easy to find and in some cases are quite numerous.[37] The synovial layer merges imperceptibly into the cellular infiltrate occupying the central core of the villus, and many of the central cells are cytologically identical to the synovial cells. Others have a distinctly foamy appearance, and sheets of such cells correlate with the grossly yellow foci. Multinucleated cells are invariably present. The grossly solid nodules have a

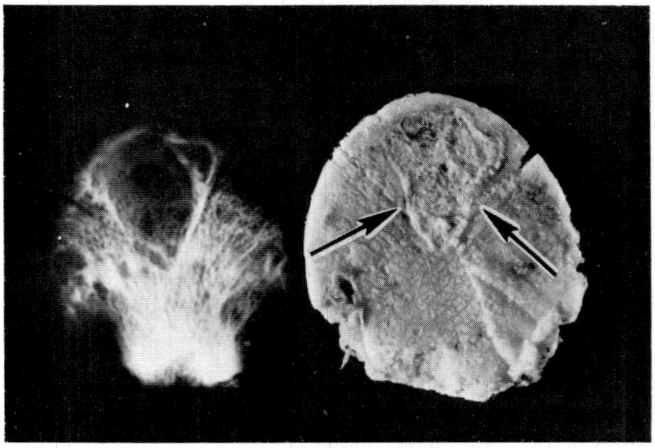

FIG. 4. Specimen radiograph of half of a femoral head shows defect due to osseous extension by pigmented villonodular synovitis at insertion of ligamentum teres. The area demarcated by *arrows* (which corresponds with lytic area on radiograph) contained polypmorphic mixture of foam cells, giant cells, and hemosiderin-filled cells similar to synovial lesion. (Methodist Neg. 7457159.)

variable appearance. Some contain clefts lined by synovial cells and apparently represent remnants of matted villi. Others are truly solid, lack clefts, and consist only of sheets of cells with an admixture of fibrous and hyalinized tissues. These areas are indistinguishable from the lesions of LNS. Occasional lymphocytes are present, but they rarely form large collections, and other inflammatory cells are notably absent. The degree of iron deposition was found to correlate somewhat with the duration of symptoms in one study with the more extensive deposits being found in patients with long-standing symptoms.[37]

Prognosis. The management of PVNS is difficult, except in the rare localized cases. In common with intraarticular LNS, nearly all patients with a localized mass of fused villi remain well after excision.[37] There is only one case reported which may represent a progression from a localized to a diffuse disease. A 2- by 2-cm localized area of distinctly multinodular and multivillous tumor was excised, but diffuse joint involvement was demonstrated at a subsequent operation. However, it is not clear as to how thoroughly the joint space was explored at the initial operation, and therefore it is uncertain whether this is indeed a case of "progression" from a localized villonodular synovitis to a diffuse disease.[38]

Unlike the localized disease, the diffuse form has a high long term morbidity despite therapy. Surgical excision and radiotherapy generally fail to yield satisfactory results. Extensive synovectomy removes most of the disease, but patients may end up with a less functional joint and greater pain than before the operation.[42] Irradiation has been used as an adjunct to surgery, but usually without resulting in significant benefit compared to surgical excision alone.[37] Byers et al.[42] state that both bone and soft tissue lesions regress with radiation therapy, but a completely satisfactory outcome occurred in only 2 of 8 patients. Many of these patients were treated with old techniques and variable dosages, and there remains a distinct possibility that newer radiotherapeutic techniques may yield better results. However, since so many patients are young or early middle-aged, the potential hazard of postradiation sarcoma must be kept in mind, although no such case has thus far been reported.

Intraarticular Localized Nodular Synovitis

Clinical features. All reported cases of intraarticular LNS have occurred in the knee except for one in the hip. Unlike PVNS, there is a 2:1 male predominance.[44, 58–60] The age distribution has been fairly uniform from the 2nd to the 7th decade with a slight peak between 30 and 40 years. Patients invariably have had pain varying from 12 hours to 11 years duration. About half of the patients have had signs or symptoms consistent with internal mechanical derangement such as locking or clicking. The patient with the hip lesion had findings consistent with degenerative joint disease, and a 1.5-cm lesion of the synovium was removed at the time of cup arthroplasty.[61] Some patients cite a specific episode of trauma, but two-thirds recall no such incident.[58]

Gross and operative findings. The mass may be sessile, but more often there is a pedicle, and rarely it floats as a loose body.[37] Most are 2 to 4 cm in greatest diameter with the size ranging from 0.9 to 8.2 cm. The mass is often irregular and may be flat. The colors cover a spectrum from bright yellow to dark brown.

Microscopic findings. The histologic features are the same as extraarticular LNS and are described under that heading. In addition, there is a distinct synovial lining which in contrast to PVNS does not have hemosiderin in the lining cells.[58]

Prognosis. Simple excision has resulted in cure in every instance in which full clinical information is available.[58, 62] Byers et al.[42] refer to 2 patients with recurrences, but no details are given, and the adequacy of the initial surgical procedure cannot be evaluated. Brashear[60] says that solitary lesions "may recur" but does not document the statement, and none of his cases developed recurrence. Thus, in contrast to both PVNS and extraarticular LNS, there appears to be no documented case of recurrence of intraarticular LNS.

Extraarticular Localized Nodular Synovitis

For the purposes of this discussion the term localized nodular synovitis is used simply because it seems to enjoy the widest usage. Other terms such as giant cell tumor of tendon sheath, fibrous histiocytoma, xanthofibroma, and benign synovioma have their devoted adherents and cannot be faulted either semantically or conceptually since the basic nature of localized nodular synovitis is debatable. Some authors have viewed the lesion as a reactive process based on the polymorphic infiltrate, which includes cells with obvious phagocytic properties and multinucleated giant cells identical to those seen in other well recognized inflammatory conditions. However, it should be noted that aside from histiocyte-like cells, other inflammatory cells are sparse, and in this sense the suffix "itis" is inaccurate. Ackerman and Rosai[63] have commented on the similarity of LNS to the currently fashionable diagnostic category of fibrous histiocytoma, which is considered neoplastic. Wright[38] also has preferred to view LNS as a true neoplasm, but of synovial cell origin (benign synovioma). He considered the benign synovioma to be at one end of a spectrum with transitional forms leading on up to malignant metastasizing synovioma, but this line of reasoning was questioned sharply by Lichtenstein[64] after his review of Wright's "malignant" cases. Ultrastructural studies cannot be expected to resolve the problem. Eisenstein[65] studied two tumors of LNS by electron microscopy and demonstrated cells compatible with both type A and type B synovial cells. He believed that the foam cells, histiocyte-like cells, and giant cells seen by light microscopy could have arisen from the synovial cells since transitions between all of these cell types was evident. However, synovial cells have no distinctive ultrastructural features, and since they are capable of phagocytosis, they become indistinguishable from histiocytes. It is useless to try to decide whether the histiocyte-like cells deep in the tissue are of synovial origin or of nonsynovial histiocytic origin, and certainly there is no clue as to whether they are reactive or neoplastic.[66] Whatever the exact cell of origin, the lesion seems clearly to arise in synovium and, therefore, warrants inclusion in a discussion of neoplasm or neoplasm-like lesions of the synovium.

Clinical features. Over 90% of extraarticular LNS occurs in the fingers with a few cases in the hands, toes, feet, wrists, ankles, or knees. There is a distinct female predominance. In the three largest series, almost exactly two-thirds of the 263 cases were women.[38, 58, 61] Patients have ranged from 8 to 80 years of age with most between 40 and 60 years. A history of trauma can be obtained in about half of the patients, but the other half will specifically deny it. A few have suffered trauma at the geographically precise site of the subsequent tumor, including cuts from saws, glass, hooks, and a stab by a knitting needle.[38] Even in these instances, however, one wonders if the trauma is more than coincidence. Symptoms are limited almost exclusively to a painless mass which may have been noted for a week to 15 years, but most are present between 3 months and 3 years. Pain and tenderness occur rarely and only in association with arduous manual labor.[58] Radiographic findings include a soft tissue mass and approximately 10 to 20% will show erosion of the cortex of the phalanges and occasional cortical perforation.[58, 61, 67]

Except for a slightly lower frequency in the ring finger and a slight preponderance in the index and middle fingers, the distribution of lesions is fairly uniform.[38, 61, 68] About one-third are located adjacent to the distal interphalangeal joint with the remainder near the proximal interphalangeal joint or interarticular segments. They are about equally divided between the volar and dorsal surfaces with an occasional tumor confined to the medial or lateral soft tissues. Larger lesions may encircle the finger. About half of the cases have radiographic evidence of degenerative joint disease in the adjacent joint.[61] Rarely, the lesions are multiple either in the same digit, in two different digits of the hand, or both hands.[58, 69] A few instances of metachronous lesions in different digits have been reported.

Gross and operative findings. The typical specimen is a smooth solitary mass which may be lobulated. The size varies from a few millimeters to 7 cm,[70] but most lesions in the fingers are 1 to 2 cm.[58] The color varies from yellow to brown, depending on the proportions of lipid, hemosiderin, and fibrous tissue. Occasionally the specimen is resected piecemeal as it is dissected from around digital nerves or vessels. In fact, the prevalent concept that these lesions are only single spherical masses pushing structures aside is misleading. By failing to appreciate the infiltrative capacity with small extensions radiating from the main mass, portions of tumors are sometimes left behind and continue to grow. Invasion and fixation to the skin occur rarely.[38] Another gross feature which should be fully appreciated is the involvement of the inner surface of either a tendon sheath or a joint lining despite the main mass lying in subcutaneous tissues. The intraarticular or intrasheath component may consist only of small villous structures, and these may even extend for a considerable distance away from the point where the main mass is in continuity with the inner synovial lining. Therefore, the surgeon should not only remove the tumor down to the joint capsule, but should open the joint space and excise any articular synovial lining which is abnormal. LNS can also invade through the cortex into the medullary portion of phalangeal bone, and in one instance, invasion of the ends of long bones by a massive extraarticular lesion raised the possibility of a primary bone tumor.[69] Nonetheless, the subsequent course in these cases indicates that one is dealing only with a locally invasive process.

The exact site of origin may be difficult to identify with confidence. Certainly, some flexor lesions have been clearly shown to arise in the flexor tendon sheath. But Wright[38] has pointed out that extensor lesions are almost invariably associated with an involved interphalangeal joint space. He states that there is a long proximal dorsal prolongation of the synovial joint sac beneath the extensor tendon, and although the tendon is certainly involved or surrounded by the ensuing growth, it is not the precise site of origin.

Microscopic findings. There is enormous variation of patterns between different tumors or even from one area to another within the same tumor. Giant cells or foam cells may be found in only a few isolated foci. In this situation, the marked cellularity, pleomorphism, and mitotic activity commonly seen in the fibrous stroma may tempt the unwary to consider a malignant tumor (Fig. 5, *left*). On the other hand, some lesions are almost entirely hyalinized fibrous tissue. Phalen, McCormack, and Gazale[58] were unable to correlate the degree of fibrosis with the age of the tumor as determined by the duration of clinical symptoms. Foci of necrosis may be seen in both small and large masses. Hemosiderin is always present as are multinucleated giant cells which may contain hemosiderin or lipid and rarely have asteroid bodies.[71] Cholesterol deposits may be abundant, and intracytoplasmic deposits in the foam cells have been verified.[46] About one-third to a half of the lesions will have clefts[37, 58] lined either by attenuated cells or by plump cells, including multinucleated forms (Fig. 5, *right*). The presence of clefts may cause confusion with synovial sarcoma, but the epithelium-like cells resulting in the glandular structures of synovial sarcoma are not present.

One other process which might be confused with LNS is the giant cell reaction of phalangeal or metacarpal bones.[72, 73] However, these lesions are predominantly fibrous, produce osteoid, and have minimal hemosiderin. Most importantly, the radiograph shows the lesion to be arising from within the bone rather than eroding into it from the outside.

Prognosis. The local recurrence rate has been high reflecting the difficulties of

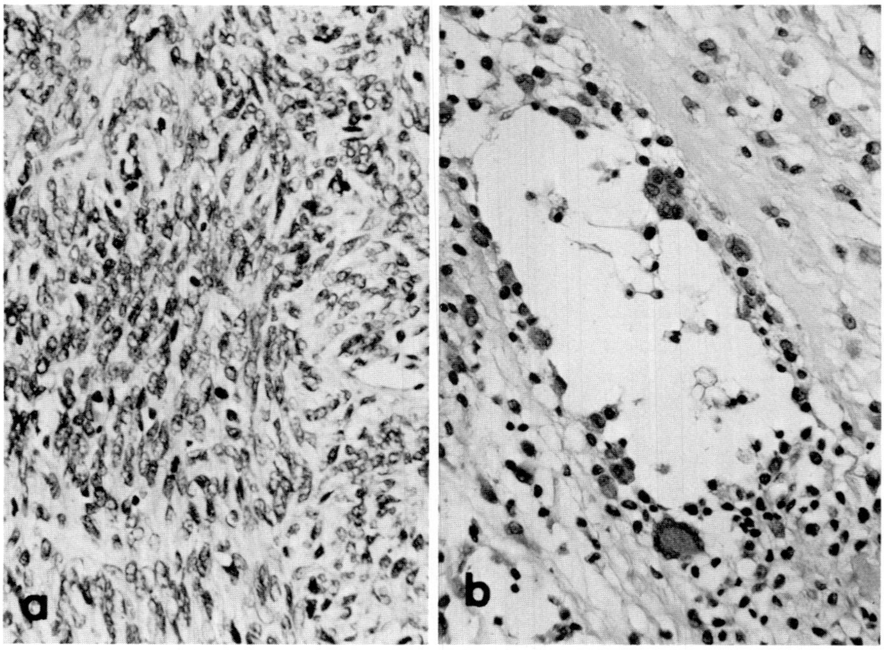

FIG. 5. *Left*, densely cellular foci with mitotic figures are common in extraarticular localized nodular synovitis and are not indicative of malignancy. Hematoxylin and eosin stain, × 200. (Methodist Neg. 7457247.) *Right*, intraarticular nodular synovitis may contain spaces lined by synovial-like cells with similar cells scattered in the stroma. This contrasts with the more cuboidal epithelium-like cells of synovial sarcoma. Hematoxylin and eosin stain, × 200. (Methodist Neg. 7138982.) (*Left*, from Fraire, A. E., and Fechner, R. E.[62] Used with permission.)

total excision. From 10 to 20% of lesions recur one or more times with most recurrences appearing within 5 years and about half of these within 2 years.[61] Recurrences usually do not seem to act any more aggressively than the initial lesion, and, in one instance, a recurrence was left in place and grew slowly for 34 years.[74] The degree of cellularity and the proportions of different elements does not seem to correlate with recurrences.[75] However, one case with as many as 5 mitotic figures per high power field recurred within 2 weeks and was treated with amputation of the finger.[76] The patient was well 14 months later.

The metastatic potential of LNS may be nil. Only 2 cases of what have been considered malignant LNS have followed a course culminating in metastases. Decker and Owen[77] published a case of LNS which was apparently of 14 years duration, recurred twice after surgical excision, and invaded tarsal bones. The patient eventually had clinical evidence of vertebral and pulmonary metastases, but these were not histologically verified. Kobak and Perlow[78] described a lesion arising adjacent to the triceps insertion near the elbow which recurred, involved axillary nodes, and within a year had widespread visceral metastases. A definite origin from tendon sheath cannot be verified because of the size and the extensive local invasion. It must be recognized that these lesions had cytologic atypia and were not garden variety nodular synovitis. They may have been examples of malignant giant cell tumors of soft parts, neoplasms which metastasize frequently. Malignant giant cell tumor as defined by Guccion and Enzinger[79] has considerable cytologic atypia and should not be confused with LNS. Certainly it can be said that a lesion clearly arising from tendon or synovium and having the typical histologic pattern of LNS has never been reported to metastasize.

Ganglion Cyst and Synovial Cyst

Conflicting viewpoints on the pathogenesis of the soft tissue ganglion enliven the study of this commonplace lesion. Discussion centers around the gross or microscopic relation of the ganglion to the joint space and whether the gelatinous fluid is altered synovial fluid or the result of connective tissue degeneration. The situation is aggravated semantically by the interchangeable use of the terms ganglion and synovial cyst, especially in certain juxtaarticular bone defects. The author believes that the term synovial cyst should be reserved for a lesion lined unequivocally by synovium, whereas a cyst filled with gelatinous material devoid of a distinct lining should be designated as a ganglion.[80]

At the present time, the preponderance of evidence fails to support a relationship of ganglion to synovial origin even though there is almost a constant attachment of a ganglion of the wrist to the underlying joint capsule. Ultrastructural studies of the wall and contents of ganglia have failed to demonstrate synovial cells.[81] One study purporting to show continuity of ganglia to the joint space is difficult to interpret,[82] and it is not clear from the illustrations whether the small clefts represent joint spaces or are the small intracapsular cysts so clearly demonstrated by McEvedy[83] His meticulous operative dissections of ganglia with special attention to their relation to intracapsular cysts failed to show any communication with the joint space. The tiny cysts within the joint capsule are lined by an intact layer of attenuated cells which superficially resembles synovium. However, even if these are synovial cells, they seem to be arising in this site as an adventitial bursa rather than a herniation from the joint space.

A lesion morphologically indistinguishable from the soft tissue ganglion occurs within bone and has been variously labeled subchondral cyst, synovial cyst, ganglionic cyst, or ganglion. Regardless of the diagnostic label, none of these has shown continuity with synovium or a synovial lining. Instead, the mass consists of gelatinous material surrounded by a fibrous rim devoid of a specific cell lining. The subjacent bone forms a sclerotic rim, and there is fibrosis in the bone marrow. It is of interest that 7 of the 15 patients reported by Kambolis, Bullough, and Jaffe[84] had a mass of degenerated connective tissue characteristic of ganglion covering the bone defect, and in 4 of these there was communication between the intraosseous and extraosseous components.

The commonest true synovial cyst is the popliteal cyst arising either as a herniation of the joint space of the knee or from the gastrocnemiosemimembranosus bursa.[85] Patients with a primary synovial cyst complain of a mass, dull aching pain, and stiffness. The excised specimen shows a cyst wall varying from 0.1 to 0.8 cm in thickness lined by inflammatory cells, attenuated unidentifiable cells, and definite synovium. The lesion is cured by excision. Synovial cysts have also been seen adjacent to joints afflicted with rheumatoid arthritis where they apparently serve as a safety valve to relieve increased intraarticular pressure.[86]

Hemangioma

Clinical features. Hemangiomas may be localized either to the tendon sheath or the intraarticular synovium as well as paraarticular soft tissues. The lesions in the tendon sheaths have been located almost exclusively in the hand or wrist forming localized masses which can be completely resected and do not recur.[87]

About 135 cases of intraarticular hemangiomas have been reported, and with the exception of one in the elbow joint and one in the ankle, all have been in the knee. In one series, half of the patients had hemangiomas elsewhere.[88] Most patients are teenagers who have a long history of dull pain, limitation of motion, and an intermittently palpable mass, although an occasional adult gives only a short history of symptoms.[89] Muscle atrophy in the quadriceps group is present in the majority of patients and seems out of all proportion to the amount expected from disuse alone. The atrophy coupled with a long but intermittent history of swelling and pain in the presence of a mass which decreases in size when the extremity is elevated are a constellation of features allowing a correct preoperative diagnosis.[90] Radiographs may show phleboliths, degenerative joint changes, a periosteal reaction in the bone immediately adjacent to the joint, or lucent areas in the end of the bone. Arteriography has been recommended in suspected cases in order to detect the location of arteriovenous shunts,[88] and to define the extent of the lesion.[91]

Gross and operative findings. Some hemangiomas form a sessile nodule within the synovium or a polypoid mass which may be pedunculated and amenable to total removal. Unfortunately, most are diffuse, penetrate the joint capsule, and spread without sharp demarcation into the surrounding soft tissues.

Microscopic findings. The lesions are usually characterized as cavernous hemangiomas and occasionally as capillary angiomas[88] or venous hemangiomas.[90] There is no correlation of these various patterns with the localized or diffuse gross configurations.

Prognosis. The localized lesions are totally resectable and do not recur.[89] The diffuse lesions defy complete resection and may recur even after complete synovectomy.[92] Radiotherapy has been used with relief of symptoms,[88] although persistence after radiotherapy may necessitate additional surgery.[90]

Lipoma

Lipoma occurring as a circumscribed mass of the articular synovium is a very rare lesion. The tumor consisting of mature adipose tissue without histologic peculiarity may be pedunculated and produce signs of mechanical derangement.[17] It is easily excised.

A more common tumor of synovial adipose tissue is the arborescent lipoma involving the synovium diffusely with papillary fatty excrescenses which may be of sufficient volume to be seen by arthrogram.[93] In effect it looks like a diffuse yellow villonodular synovitis. Obese individuals may have prominent projections of fat into the joint space, but some cases of arborescent lipoma have been seen in thin persons so it is more than an accentuation of synovial folds of adipose tissue.[94] Microscopically, well vascularized fat is covered with a uniform synovial layer. Plasma cells and lymphocytes may be prominent leading to the consideration of a reactive inflammatory lesion.[17, 95] Occasionally there is bilateral involvement such as the girl with onset in one knee at age 9 and the other knee at age 16 producing grotesque deformities cured by bilateral synovectomy.[96]

Lipomas within the tendon sheath have been reported more commonly than articular lipomas. Patients have ranged from 6 to 70 years of age with most being younger than 40 years. They complain of dull aching and a mass of several weeks to 20 years duration. The tendon sheaths of the hands and the wrists are the usual sites with about a third presenting as bilateral and symmetrical lesions. Rarely there are multiple tumors in various tendons of a single extremity.[97] Lipomas of tendon sheath are about equally divided between discrete lesions and the arborescent configuration. The latter is occasionally extensive with small erosions into cortical bone and involvement of adjacent joint spaces.[98] As a rule, however, total excision of the sheath is readily accomplished and there is no recurrence.

MALIGNANT NEOPLASMS OF SYNOVIUM

Four histologically distinctive types of primary malignant tumors are considered to arise from synovium: synovial sarcoma, clear cell sarcoma of tendon sheaths, synovial chondrosarcoma, and epithelioid sarcoma. Another category occasionally appearing in the literature is "malignant giant cell tumor of tendon sheath." The cases in those reports are probably better viewed as variants of the above groups rather than a specific lesion. One other malignant tumor consists of secondary synovial involvement by direct extension of primary bone tumors or by metastatic carcinoma.

Synovial Sarcoma

Whether synovial lining cells have malignant potential has never been substantiated despite the use of the deeply entrenched term of synovial sarcoma for a neoplasm with a highly distinctive pattern which by definition must include an "epithelioid" element plus a malignant spindle cell stroma.[80] Cadman, Soule, and Kelly[99] rather accurately characterized synovial sarcoma as "at best a crude caricature of synovial tissue," and one detailed ultrastructural study of a synovial sarcoma has demonstrated features not found in normal human synovium.[100] Nevertheless, the anatomic relationships of a few synovial sarcomas indicate origin from synovium whether or not the precise cell of origin is the synovial lining cell *per se*.

Clinical features. Synovial sarcoma makes up about 10% of all soft tissue sarcomas.[99] About half of the cases occur between 15 and 30 years of age, and an additional quarter by 50 years of age. A few cases in children have recently been reported.[101] Males are more often affected by a slight margin (3:2). About two-thirds of lesions are in the lower extremity with knee, thigh, lower leg, and foot involved in descending order. Conversely, the upper extremity lesions are more common in the hand and progressively less frequent in the forearm, elbow region, and upper arm. An origin in the finger or toe is exceedingly rare. The tumor may arise in areas which one does not ordinarily associate with synovium such as retroperitoneum,[102] neck,[103] and anterior abdominal wall.[104]

There are enormous variations in the clinical presentation, both as to types of symptoms and their duration, before the diagnosis is established. Patients rarely present with symptoms referable to metastatic disease although metastases may become clinically apparent a few months after the primary lesion is diagnosed.[105] The primary complaint may be a painless mass, a painful mass, or pain in the absence of a mass. The latter group is at special risk for prolonged misdiagnosis as arthritis or internal derangement of the knee, because the pain can be aggravated by weight bearing.[102] Bone destruction and calcification of a neoplasm may be demonstrable without a palpable tumor.[106] In most patients, the duration of symptoms is from 6 to 12 months, but about 15% will give a history of more than 5 years.[107] The pain may precede a palpable mass by up to 18 years as it did in one case in which the patient was a physician.[99] In several instances, a painless mass has been present, seemingly unchanged in size for many years (7 to 30), before beginning to enlarge conspicuously and becoming painful.[99, 102] Despite histories of this type, there is no convincing morphologic evidence that a benign lesion (specifically nodular synovitis) is a precursor of the sarcoma. One must simply concede that in some patients the neoplasm grows exceedingly slowly and may be symptomatic for a long time.

Destruction of adjacent bone is seen in about 1 of 6 cases. A similar proportion have large amorphous calcifications, which is far more frequent than other soft tissue sarcomas, and the presence of calcium in a soft tissue mass is suggestive of synovial sarcoma.[99] Nodular synovitis, by contrast, almost never is calcified.[38]

Gross and operative findings. The lesions tend to be sharply circumscribed but can extend along fascial planes, incorporate tendon and nerves into the substance of the tumor, and invade bone. Only a small minority have a demonstrable anatomic association with synovium at the time that they are excised. Even when they are in continuity with the capsule of a large joint, the joint space is rarely invaded, although it may contain a secondary effusion. Cytologic examination of synovial fluid was postive in one reported instance where there was a far advanced lesion.[108] Regional lymph node metastases have been present in as many as 25% of cases.[105]

Microscopic findings. The proportions of the epithelioid and spindle components and the patterns of the epithelioid component vary enormously from tumor to tumor and even within the same lesion. The spindle cell component usually predominates, and less often the epithelioid element is dominant. The least common variant is a fairly even distribution of both elements.[109] Pulmonary metastases show both elements.[109, 110] The epithelioid element varies from slits lined by small cuboidal cells to round glandular structures lined by tall columnar epithelium to irregular spaces lined by complex papillary configurations. Occasionally the epithelioid cells are in solid sheets. Mucin production is considered characteristic, but in fact is demonstrable in only about 15%.[99] The periodic acid-Schiff and Alcian blue positivity are shared by both hyaluronic acid and other connective tissue mucins.

The stroma may be indistinguishable from fibrosarcoma, but more often consists of plumper cells in broad sheets. The cells may be almost rounded, and this particular cytologic and histologic appearance has led to the concept of a monophasic synovial sarcoma when there is no demonstrable epithelioid component. However, the diagnosis of monophasic synovial sarcoma is unprovable and has generally fallen into disfavor.[80]

The biphasic character required for the diagnosis of synovial sarcoma by light microscopy has been confirmed by ultrastructural studies.[100, 111] The spindle cells seem to be different from normal fibroblasts by lacking well developed ergastoplasm. They differ further by being equipped with specialized cell junctions and filopodia. The epithelial cells also have attachment sites (both maculae adherentes and desmosomes) just below the luminal surface. Such attachment sites are not a feature of normal synovial cells, but may be found in non-neoplastic reactions of synovium, *e.g.*, rheumatoid or osteoarthritis.[6] A distinct, but discontinuous, basal lamina separates the epithelium-like cells from the spindle cells. In short, the neoplastic cell and stroma (the basal lamina) of synovial sarcoma possess features not seen in normal synovium, but one can reconcile these discrepancies by stating that the differences are consistant with changes which synovial cells are capable of undergoing, at least in reactive lesions.

Prognosis. Therapeutic approaches have included numerous combinations of various types of surgery and radiotherapy with inconstant results. Patients have been subjected to enucleation, wide local excision, or amputation, with and without preoperative or postoperative radiation. Most reported series have been so variably treated and contain so few cases in the different groups from various anatomic locations that it is impossible to compare different therapeutic modalities. Nonetheless, two statements do appear justified. First of all, local excision is followed by a high rate of recurrence (50 to 70%) and second, amputation does not seem to alter the rate of distant metastases. The local recurrence may be anywhere from a few months to 11 years later, yet some of these patients have become long term survivors following further multiple local excisions[109] or amputation.[99] There appears to be no correlation of histologic pattern (number and degree of differentiation of glandular elements) with prognosis.[109]

Until recently, the effect of radiotherapy on synovial sarcomas has been considered unpredictable, although a few cases of local tumor "sterilization" have occurred as has objective regression of pulmonary metastases.[112] A more consistent result has been recently reported using current techniques in 14 cases treated by simple local excision followed by radical radiotherapy. There was only one recurrence at the margin of the irradiated field and not within the field itself.[113] Naturally, it is not possible to know how many might have been controlled by local excision alone, but knowing the natural history of this sarcoma there should have been many more than one recurrence. Two patients subsequently required amputation for radiation damage. Nonetheless, the preservation of a useful extremity and complete control in 11 of 14 cases is strong preliminary evidence to support this as the preferred method of therapy for local control. Four patients have gone 44 months or longer without evidence of disease, and such a trend would indicate that this modality of therapy will produce a survival at least equal to amputation and certainly with less morbidity. Nevertheless, 5 patients are dead with distant metastases, and that facet of the disease appears unaltered by radiotherapy. The technique of isolation perfusion is another form of therapy that was followed by a 10-year survival for 4 of 7 patients.[114]

Epithelioid Sarcoma

Epithelioid sarcoma is the term employed for a morphologically distinctive tumor occurring at different depths within the soft tissues including superficial fascia, deep fascia, tendon sheaths, and periosteum.[115] The pertinence to a discussion of synovial neoplasms is seen both in the gross relation to tendon sheath and one ultrastructural study interpreted as demonstrating a similarity of epithelioid sarcoma to synovial sarcoma. In retrospect, epithelioid sarcomas have been included in reports of synovial sarcoma and often were specifically separated as atypical variants.[116, 117] The four cases of large cell sarcoma of tendon sheath described by Bliss and Reed[118] also seem to be identical to epithelioid sarcoma.

Clinical features. About three-fourths of patients are between the ages of 10 and 34 years, and there is a male predominance even after correcting for the military bias of an AFIP series[115] The commonest sign is a painless mass located on the fingers, hand, wrist, forearm, or lower leg in descending order of frequency. In one large series, epithelioid sarcoma was the commonest soft tissue sarcoma of the hand.[119] The superficial lesions commonly ulcerate even when less than a centimeter in size.[120] The tumors are closely associated with fascia or tendon sheaths. A nodular pattern is conspicuous with central necrosis in the larger nodules.

Microscopic findings. There is a wide spectrum of cytologic and histologic features which contribute to the difficulty of making the diagnosis. Epithelioid sarcoma is unique among sarcomas in that it may be readily interpreted as an inflammatory granulomatous process at one extreme or a metastatic carcinoma at the other.[115, 121] The characteristic nodular pattern contributes to this confusion (Fig. 6, *left*). The neoplastic cells range from fusiform to large polygonal cells (Fig. 6, *right*). This cytologic variation is on a continuous spectrum and does not result in a sharply biphasic pattern as seen in synovial sarcoma. There may be active fibrous tissue proliferation around the nodules, hyalinization of collagen, and aggregates of lymphocytes in the stroma.

Several cases of epithelioid sarcoma have been examined by electron microscopy. Fisher and Horvat[122] favored a fibrocytic derivation. However, Frable et al.[123] thought that their sarcoma was related to both synovial sarcoma and fibrohistiocytic sarcomas with the fibroblast as the interlinking cell capable of differentiating both toward a synovium-like cell and a histiocyte-like cell. Gabbiani et al.[124] specifically denied any relation between epithelioid sarcoma and histiocytes. They thought the neoplastic cells resembled the stromal areas of classical synovial sarcoma. The features common to epithelioid and synovial

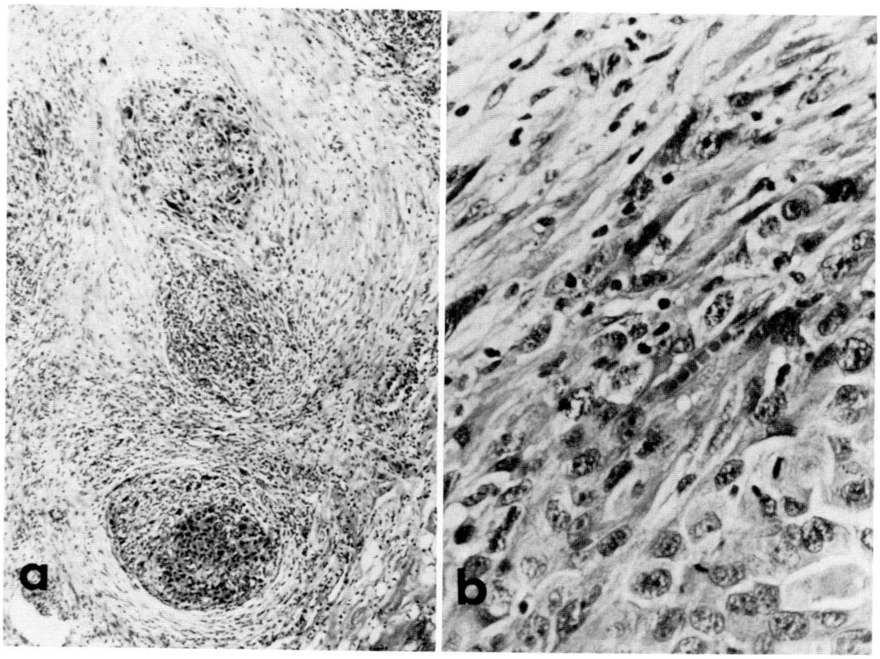

FIG. 6. *a*, epithelioid sarcoma has a nodular pattern at low power which may be confused with granuloma. Hematoxylin and eosin stain, × 32. *b*, polyhedral and spindle cells are intermixed without the sharp separation seen in synovial sarcoma. Hematoxylin and eosin stain, × 200. (Baylor Neg. 47233.)

sarcoma were cells with distorted nuclei, few lysosomes, large lipid droplets, scanty ergastoplasm, few mitochondria, and numerous cytoplasmic microfilaments around the nucleus. However, there were conspicuous differences, including the absence of true glands and the lack of basal lamina.

Prognosis. When treated by local resection, recurrence is the rule—usually within 6 months. Only 2 of 30 patients followed by Enzinger for 5 years were free of recurrences or metastases.[115] The lungs have been the commonest site of detectable metastases. Lymph nodes and, oddly, the scalp have been the next most frequent sites of metastases. The neoplasm is slowly progressive with a median of 5 years between the initial diagnosis and the detection of metastases. Even after the metastases were identified, one patient lived 8 years. This strikingly variable course of disease in different patients is similar to synovial sarcoma and clear cell sarcoma, thereby forming a common bond of clinical capriciousness in contrast to most other soft tissue sarcomas.

CLEAR CELL SARCOMA

Enzinger[125] has given the name clear cell sarcoma to a neoplasm arising in tendons or aponeuroses.

Clinical features. The mass is usually painless, often of long duration (average of 3½ years), and about half have been located in the area of the ankle, heel, or plantar region. Four specifically involved the Achilles tendon. At operation the lesions are inseparably attached to the tendon, range from 2 to 6 cm in size, and may have mucoid foci or cystic degeneration.

Microscopic findings. Cytologically, the tumor cells are pale, may be finely vacuolated, and are polyhedral or more fusiform, but without a biphasic pattern (Fig. 7). Glycogen is demonstrable in most tumors. The 3 cases reported by Dutra[126] had a predominating fusiform shape to the cells, and he also emphasized the lack of a true biphasic pattern. About two-thirds of the cases have multinucleated giant cells containing 10 to 15 bland nuclei. Mitoses are scarce and occasionally absent altogether. The cells are arranged in solid nests or fascicles set off by fibrous septa which are continuous with the preformed tendon or aponeurosis. Recurrences or metastases generally have the same appearance, although in some instances there is a less orderly arrangement of cells, greater pleomorphism, more necrosis, and more frequent mitotic figures. However, a few metastases may bear virtually no resemblance to the primary and could easily be diagnosed as undifferentiated carcinoma.[125]

Clear cell sarcoma was studied ultrastructurally by Kubo,[127] who identified two types of tumor cells, acinar structures, and a basement membrane. The two types of cells included a large cell with fairly clear cytoplasm and oval nucleus and a small cell with indented nucleus and scant cytoplasm. The lesion differed from synovial sarcoma by lacking special attachments and having abundant glycogen. Nonetheless, it was considered as a possible variant of synovial sarcoma because of the two cell types and the presence of acini. Hoffman and Carter[128] studied an

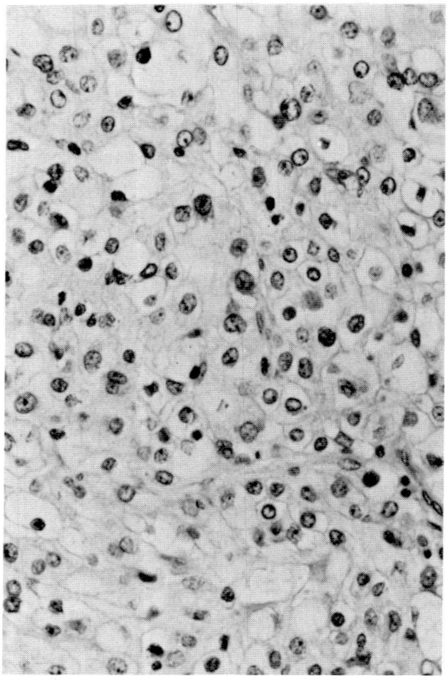

FIG. 7. Clear cell sarcoma resembles an epithelial neoplasm. Only the clinical location within a tendon sheath raises the possibility of primary sarcoma. Hematoxylin and eosin stain, × 200. (Baylor Neg. 47233A.)

otherwise typical clear cell sarcoma which was ultimately found to have melanosomes. The histogenetic significance of this case is baffling.

Prognosis. Local excision is almost always followed by recurrence with the persisting lesions being less well circumscribed and extending along tendinous structures. The time between initial diagnosis and the appearance of metastases varies from a few months to 30 years with an average of 6 years. The mortality rate is at least 70% and probably higher as survivors are followed for longer periods.

Enzinger[125] could not demonstrate any difference in survival between those patients treated radically at an early stage and those treated with multiple local excisions. There does not appear to be a correlation between duration of symptoms and length of survival.

Malignant Giant Cell Tumor of Tendon Sheaths and Soft Tissue

Upper extremity lesions from 5 patients have been viewed as malignant giant cell tumor of tendon sheath and all died of distant metastases. This diagnosis stemmed from the presence of polymorphic populations of foam cells, multinucleated giant cells, and spindle cells, thereby imparting a similarity to nodular synovitis (benign giant cell tumor of tendon sheath). Four of the cases were reported by Bliss and Reed[118] prior to the coining of the term epithelioid sarcoma and seem to fall into that category. It should be noted that they actually preferred the term large cell sarcoma of tendon with the designation of malignant giant cell tumor as a parenthetic appellation.[118] Kahn's[129] case of malignant giant cell tumor of tendon sheath contains areas indistinguishable from clear cell sarcomas as he points out, and perhaps his case is better considered a variant of that sarcoma. In short, malignant giant cell tumor of tendon sheath has not been convincingly proven as a specific histologic category.

Guccion and Enzinger[79] have reviewed 32 cases which they call malignant giant cell tumor of soft parts. The deep seated tumors often involved tendons, but in no case were they localized to a tendon or tendon sheath. In addition, the anatomic distribution of the malignant giant cell tumors was different from nodular synovitis, further weakening any consideration that they represent the malignant counterpart of nodular synovitis.

Synovial Chondrosarcoma

Eight cases of synovial chondrosarcoma have been reported as compared to about 250 cases of synovial chondromatosis.[33] Synovial chondrosarcoma is characterized by multiple nodules of cytologically malignant cartilage invading through the joint capsule into the surrounding soft tissues. The one possible exception to this gross appearance was a solitary intraarticular cartilage mass interpreted as synovial chondrosarcoma and treated by local excision.[130] The presence of cartilage in the fibrous portion of the joint capsule does not automatically mean invasion. On rare occasions, a solitary chondroma or osteochondroma has been found within the fibrous capsule, and in the absence of cytologic atypia a diagnosis of chondrosarcoma should not be made.[131]

There are 2 cases of chondrosarcoma which raise the possibility of origin in preexisting synovial chondromatosis. One case had a 14-year history of a very slowly enlarging knee followed by the abrupt onset of rapid growth.[132] Even in this case, there was moderate cellular pleomorphism in the synovectomy specimen 2 years before the onset of the rapid growth. Similarly, another case contained atypia in a synovectomy specimen 4 years before invasive chondrosarcoma was found. Although initially thought to be within the limits of atypia of chondromatosis, the lesion was interpreted in retrospect as being chondrosarcoma from its inception.[133] In addition to these cases, 1 patient had a mass palpable in the knee for 25 years before rapid enlargement began. This is interpreted as evidence of antecedent synovial chondromatosis.[134]

Clinical features. Seven of the lesions were in the knee and one in the hip. One patient was a 43-year-old woman, and the others were males ranging from 34 to 71 years of age with 5 between the ages of 34 and 43 years. Except for the 3 cases mentioned above, the duration of symptoms was less than 2 years. Five patients had partial synovectomy with the clinical and pathologic diagnosis of synovial chondromatosis. All had recurrence of symptoms (usually in a few months), reexploration, the identification of extraarticular invasion, and subsequent amputation. The two exceptions to this sequence were the man with a solitary pedunculated mass treated successfully by local excision,[130] and 1 patient with an initial biopsy diagnosed as chondrosarcoma and immediately treated by amputation.[135]

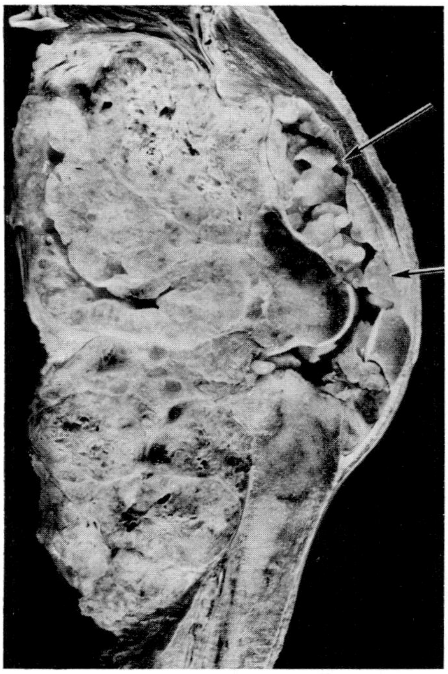

FIG. 8. Synovial chondrosarcoma fills extracapsular soft tissues (*left*). Intrasynovial cartilaginous component is marked by *arrows*. (From Dunn, E. J., McGavran, M. H., Nelson, P., and Greer, R. B.,[134] courtesy of Malcolm H. McGavran, M.D. Used with permission.)

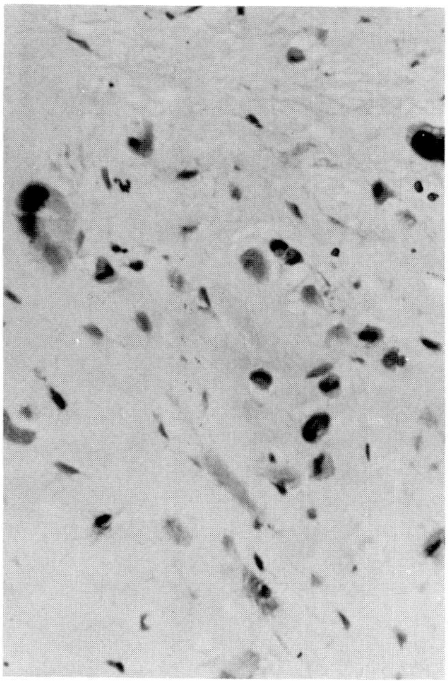

FIG. 9. Pleomorphism of chondrocytes of synovial chrondrosarcoma. Hematoxylin and eosin, × 200. (Baylor Neg. 19655.) (From King, J. W., Spjut, H. J., Fechner, R. E., and Vanderpool, D. W.[133] Used with permission.)

Gross and operative findings. The intraarticular space contains various numbers of loose bodies, and the synovium has the same variegated nodular appearance described under synovial chondromatosis. The diagnostic feature is the extension of lobulated cartilaginous masses out through the joint capsule into the surrounding soft tissues (Fig. 8). In one case, vein invasion was grossly evident.[132]

Microscopic findings. The cartilage has the features of malignant cartilage such as that seen in chondrosarcoma of any site, *i.e.*, enlarged, atypical nuclei, binucleated cells, and rarely mitotic figures (Fig. 9).

Prognosis. Three patients have developed metastases 9, 20, and 30 months after diagnosis.[132, 134, 135] The man with the solitary nodule was well 3 years later, and the outcome in the other patients is not known.[136]

METASTATIC NEOPLASMS

Synovial involvement by metastatic carcinoma has been reported rarely, and thus far has always been secondary to an osseous metastasis with extension secondarily into the joint.[137, 138] The resulting effusion may contain malignant cells on cytologic examination.[108]

REFERENCES

1. Gardner, E., and O'Rahilly, R.: The early development of the knee joint in staged human embryos. *J. Anat. 102:* 289–299, 1968.

2. Henrikson, R. C., and Cohen, A. S.: Light and electron microscopic observations of the developing chick interphalangeal joint. *J. Ultrastruct. Res. 13:* 129–162, 1965.
3. Drachman, D. B., and Sokoloff, L.: The role of movement in embryonic joint development. *Dev. Biol. 14:* 401–420, 1966.
4. Pai, A. C.: Developmental genetics of a lethal mutation, muscular dysgenesis (mdg) in the mouse. II. Developmental analysis. *Dev. Biol. 11:* 93–109, 1965.
5. Castor, C. W.: The microscopic structure of normal human synovial tissue. *Arthritis Rheum. 3:* 140–151, 1960.
6. Ghadially, F. N., and Roy, S.: *Ultrastructure of Synovial Joints in Health and Disease.* New York, Appleton-Century-Crofts, 1969.
7. Wysocki, G. P., and Brinkhous, K. M.: Scanning electron microscopy of synovial membranes. *Arch. Pathol. 93:* 172–177, 1972.
8. Collins, D. H.: *The Pathology of Articular and Spinal Diseases.* Baltimore, Williams & Wilkins Co., 1950.
9. Lever, J. D., and Ford, E. H. R.: Histological, histochemical and electron microscopic observations on synovial membrane. *Anat. Rec. 132:* 525–539, 1958.
10. Barnett, C. H., Davies, D. V., and MacConaill, M. A.: *Synovial Joints: Their Structure and Mechanics.* London, Longmans, 1961.
11. Barland, P., Novikoff, A. B., and Hamerman, D.: Electron microscopy of the human synovial membrane. *J. Cell Biol. 14:* 207–220, 1962.
12. Coulter, W. H.: The characteristics of human synovial tissue as seen with the electron microscope. *Arthritis Rheum. 5:* 70–80, 1962.
13. Hamerman, D., Rosenberg, L. C., and Schubert, M.: Diarthrodial joints revisited. *J. Bone Joint Surg. 52A:* 725–774, 1970.
14. Barland, P., Smith, C., and Hamerman, D.: Localization of hyaluronic acid in synovial cells by radioautography. *J. Cell Biol. 37:* 13–26, 1968.
15. Roy, S., and Ghadially, F. N.: Synthesis of hyaluronic acid by synovial cells. *J. Pathol. 93:* 555–557, 1967.
16. Ghadially, F. N. and Roy, S.: Phagocytosis by synovial cells. *Nature 213:* 1041, 1967.
17. Mussey, R. D., Jr., and Henderson, M. S.: Osteochondromatosis. *J. Bone Joint Surg. 31A:* 619–627, 1949.
18. Jaffe, H. L.: *Tumors and Tumorous Conditions of the Bones and Joints.* Philadelphia, Lea and Febiger, 1958.
19. Jones, H. T.: Loose body formation in synovial osteochondromatosis with special reference to the etiology and pathology. *J. Bone Joint Surg. 6:* 407–458, 1924.
20. Curr, J. F.: Synovial osteochondromatosis; two uncommon examples. *Br. Med. J. 2:* 1020–1022, 1949.
21. Symeonides, P.: Bursal chondromatosis. *J. Bone Joint Surg. 48B:* 371–373, 1966.
22. Shepherd, J. A.: Osteochondromata of tendon-sheaths; a case arising from the flexor sheath of the index finger. *Br. J. Surg. 30:* 179–181, 1942.
23. Murphy, A. F., and Wilson, J. N.: Tenosynovial osteochondroma in the hand. *J. Bone Joint Surg. 40A:* 1236–1240, 1958.
24. Fain, R. H.: Personal communication, 1974.
25. Bloom, R., and Pattinson, J. N.: Osteochondromatosis of the hip joint. *J. Bone Joint Surg. 33B:* 80–84, 1951.
26. Ballard, R., and Weiland, L. H.: Synovial chondromatosis of the temporomandibular joint. *Cancer 30:* 791–795, 1972.
27. Lewis, M. M., Marshall, J. L., and Mirra, J. M.: Synovial chrondromatosis of the thumb; a case report and review of the literature. *J. Bone Joint Surg. 56A:* 180–183, 1974.
28. Paul, G. R., and Leach, R. E.: Synovial chondromatosis of the shoulder. *Clin. Orthop. 68:* 130–135, 1970.
29. Murphy, F. P., Dahlin, D. C., and Sullivan, C. R.: Articular synovial chrondromatosis. *J. Bone Joint Surg. 44A:* 77–86, 1962.
30. Freund, E.: Chondromatosis of the joints. *Arch. Surg. 34:* 670–686, 1937.
31. Eisenberg, K. S., and Johnston, J. O.: Synovial chondromatosis of the hip joint presenting as an intrapelvic mass; a case report. *J. Bone Joint Surg. 54A:* 176–178, 1972.

32. McIvor, R. R., and King, D.: Osteochondromatosis of the hip joint. *J. Bone Joint Surg. 44A:* 87-97, 1962.
33. Jeffreys, T. E.: Synovial chondromatosis. *J. Bone Joint Surg. 49B:* 530–534, 1967.
34. Swan, E. F., and Owens, W. F., Jr.: Synovial chondrometaplasia; a case report with spontaneous regression and a review of the literature. *South. Med. J. 65:* 1496–1500, 1972.
35. Dunn, A. W., and Whisler, J. H.: Synovial chrondromatosis of the knee with associated extracapsular chondromas. *J. Bone Joint Surg. 55A:* 1747–1748, 1973.
36. Wilmoth, C. L.: Osteochondromatosis. *J. Bone Joint Surg. 23:* 367–374, 1971.
37. Atmore, W. G., Dahlin, D. C., and Ghormley, R. K.: Pigmented villonodular synovitis; a clinical and pathologic study. *Minn. Med. 39:* 196–202, 1956.
38. Wright, C. J. E.: Benign giant-cell synovioma; an investigation of 85 cases. *Br. J. Surg. 38:* 257–271, 1951.
39. Jaffe, H. L., Lichtenstein, L., and Sutro, C. J.: Pigmented villonodular synovitis, bursitis and tenosynovitis. *Arch. Pathol. 31:* 731–765, 1941.
40. Rodnan, G. P., Brower, T. D., Hellstrom, H. R., Didisheim, P., and Lewis, J. H.: Postmortem examination of an elderly severe hemophiliac, with observations on the pathologic findings in hemophiliac joint disease. *Arthritis Rheum. 2:* 152–161, 1959.
41. Lloyd-Roberts, G. C.: The role of capsular changes in osteoarthritis of the hip joint. *J. Bone Joint Surg. 35B:* 627–642, 1953.
42. Byers, P. D., Cotton, R. E., Deacon, O. W., Lowy, M., Newman, P. H., Sissons, H. A., and Thomson, A. D.: The diagnosis and treatment of pigmented villonodular synovitis. *J. Bone Joint Surg. 50B:* 290–305, 1968.
43. Collins, D. H.: Haemosiderosis and haemochromatosis of synovial tissues. *J. Bone Joint Surg. 33B:* 436–441, 1951.
44. McCollum, D. E., Musser, A. W., and Rhangos, W. C.: Experimental villonodular synovitis. *South. Med. J. 59:* 966–970, 1966.
45. Schumacher, H. R., Jr.: Ultrastructural characteristics of the synovial membrane in idiopathic haemochromatosis. *Ann. Rheum. Dis. 31:* 465–473, 1972.
46. Young, J. M., and Hudacek, A. G.: Experimental production of pigmented villonodular synovitis in dogs. *Am. J. Pathol. 30:* 799–811, 1954.
47. Roy, S., and Ghadially, F. N.: Synovial membrane in experimentally produced chronic haemarthrosis. *Ann. Rheum. Dis. 28:* 402–414, 1969.
48. Breimer, C. W., and Freiberger, R. H.: Bone lesions associated with villonodular synovitis. *Am. J. Roentgenol. Radium Ther. Nucl. Med. 79:* 618–629, 1958.
49. Smith, J. H., and Pugh, D. G.: Roentgenographic aspects of articular pigmented villonodular synovitis. *Am. J. Roentgenol. Radium Ther. Nucl. Med. 87:* 1146–1156, 1962.
50. Scott, P. M.: Bone lesions in pigmented villonodular synovitis. *J. Bone Joint Surg. 50B:* 306–311, 1968.
51. Nilsonne, U., and Moberger, G.: Pigmented villonodular synovitis of joints. Histological and clinical problems in diagnosis. *Acta Orthop. Scand. 40:* 448–460, 1969.
52. Chung, S. M. K., and Janes, J. M.: Diffuse pigmented villonodular synovitis of the hip joint; review of the literature and report of four cases. *J. Bone Joint Surg. 47A:* 293–303, 1965.
53. Levin, E. J., and Gannon, W.: Diffuse villonodular synovitis of the shoulder. *Am. J. Roentgenol. Radium Ther. Nucl. Med. 89:* 1302–1304, 1963.
54. Gehweiler, J. A., and Wilson, J. W.: Diffuse biarticular pigmented villonodular synovitis. *Radiology 93:* 845-851, 1969.
55. Greenfield, M. M., and Wallace, K. M.: Pigmented villonodular synovitis. *Radiology 54:* 350–356, 1950.
56. Weisser, J. R., and Robinson, D. W.: Pigmented villonodular synovitis of the iliopectineal bursa; a case report. *J. Bone Joint Surg. 33A:* 988-992, 1951.
57. Peterson, L. F. A., Johnson, E. W., Jr., and Woolner, L. B.: Extra-articular pigmented villonodular synovitis of the knee. *Am. J. Clin. Pathol. 30:* 158–162, 1958.
58. Phalen, G. S., McCormack, L. J., and Gazale, W. J.: Giant-cell tumor of tendon sheath (benign synovioma) in the hand; evaluation of 56 cases. *Clin. Orthop. 15:* 140–151, 1959.
59. Granowitz, S. P., and Mankin, H. J.: Localized pigmented villonodular synovitis of the knee; report of five cases. *J. Bone Joint Surg. 49A:* 122–128, 1967.

60. Brashear, H. R.: Pigmented villonodular synovitis. *South. Med. J. 49:* 679–684, 1956.
61. Jones, F. E., Soule, E. H., and Coventry, M. B.: Fibrous xanthoma of synovium (Giant-cell tumor of tendon sheath, pigmented nodular synovitis); a study of one hundred and eighteen cases. *J. Bone Joint Surg. 51A:* 76–86, 1969.
62. Fraire, A. E., and Fechner, R. E.: Intra-articular localized nodular synovitis of the knee. *Arch. Pathol. 93:* 473–476, 1972.
63. Ackerman, L. V., and Rosai, J.: *Surgical Pathology*, 5th ed., p. 1084. St. Louis, C. C. Mosby Co., 1974.
64. Lichtenstein, L.: Tumors of synovial joints, bursae, and tendon sheaths. *Cancer 8:* 816–830, 1955.
65. Eisenstein, R.: Giant-cell tumor of tendon sheath; its histogenesis as studied in the electron microscope. *J. Bone Joint Surg. 50A:* 476–486, 1968.
66. Wyllie, J. C.: The stromal cell reaction of pigmented villonodular synovitis; an electron microscopic study. *Arthritis Rheum. 12:* 205–214, 1969.
67. Fletcher, A. G., Jr., and Horn, R. C., Jr.: Giant cell tumors of tendon sheath origin; a consideration of bone involvement and report of two cases with extensive bone destruction. *Ann. Surg. 133:* 374–385, 1951.
68. Sherry, J. B., and Anderson, W.: The natural history of pigmented villonodular synovitis of tendon sheaths. *J. Bone Joint Surg. 37A:* 1005–1011, 1955.
69. Shafer, S. J., and Larmon, W. A.: Pigmented villonodular synovitis; a report of seven cases. *Surg. Gynecol. Obstet. 92:* 574–580, 1951.
70. Schajowicz, F., and Blumenfeld, I.: Pigmented villonodular synovitis of the wrist with penetration into bone. *J. Bone Joint Surg. 50B:* 312–317, 1968.
71. Arthaud, J. B.: Pigmented nodular synovitis; report of 11 lesions in non-articular locations. *Am. J. Clin. Pathol. 58:* 511–517, 1972.
72. Jernstrom, P., and Stark, H. H.: Giant cell reaction of a metacarpal. *Am. J. Clin. Pathol. 55:* 77–81, 1971.
73. D'Alonzo, R. T., Pitcock, J. A., and Milford, L. W.: Giant-cell reaction of bone; report of two cases. *J. Bone Joint Surg. 54A:* 1267–1271, 1972.
74. Stewart, M. J., and Wright, C. J. E.: A recurrent benign giant cell synovioma of tendon-sheath of 34 years' duration. *Br. J. Surg. 37:* 370, 1950.
75. Galloway, J. D. B., Broders, A. C., and Ghormley, R. K.: Xanthoma of tendon sheaths and synovial membranes: A clinical and pathologic study. *Arch. Surg. 40:* 485–538, 1940.
76. Wright, C. J. E.: Rapid recurrence of a giant-cell synovioma of tendon sheath. *J. Pathol. Bact. 61:* 271–274, 1949.
77. Decker, J. P., and Owen, B. J.: An invasive giant cell tumor of tendon sheath in the foot. *Bull. of the Ayer. Clin. Lab. of Penn. Hosp. 4:* 43–53, 1954.
78. Kobak, M. W., and Perlow, S.: Xanthomatous giant cell tumors arising in soft tissue; report of an instance of malignant growth. *Arch. Surg. 59:* 909–916, 1949.
79. Guccion, J. G. and Enzinger, F. M.: Malignant giant cell tumor of soft parts; an analysis of 32 cases. *Cancer 29:* 1518–1529, 1972.
80. Stout, A. P. and Lattes, R.: *Tumors of the Soft Tissues. Atlas of Tumor Pathology*, 2nd series, fascicle 1. Armed Forces Institute of Pathology, Washington, D. C., 1967.
81. Ghadially, F. N., and Mehta, P. N.: Multifunctional mesenchymal cells resembling smooth muscle cells in ganglia of the wrist. *Ann. Rheum. Dis. 30:* 31–42, 1971.
82. Tophøj, K., and Henriques, U.: Ganglion of the wrist—a structure developed from the joint; a histological study with serial sections. *Acta Orthop. Scand. 42:* 244–250, 1971.
83. McEvedy, B. V.: Simple ganglia. *Br. J. Surg. 49:* 585–594, 1962.
84. Kambolis, C., Bullough, P. G., and Jaffe, H. L.: Ganglionic cystic defects of bone. *J. Bone Joint Surg. 55A:* 496–505, 1973.
85. Burleson, R. J., Bickel, W. H., and Dahlin, D. C.: Popliteal cyst; a clinicopathological survey. *J. Bone Joint Surg. 38A:* 1265–1274, 1956.
86. Genovese, G. R., Jayson, M. I. V., and Dixon, A. St. J.: Protective value of synovial cysts in rheumatoid knees. *Ann. Rheum. Dis. 31:* 179–182, 1972.

87. Bate, T. H.: Hemangiomata of the tendon sheath. *J. Bone Joint Surg. 36A:* 104–109, 1954.
88. Halborg, A., Hansen, H., and Sneppen, H. O.: Haemangioma of the knee joint. *Acta Orthop. Scand. 39:* 209–216, 1968.
89. Karlholm, S., and Stjernsward, J.: Hemangioma of the knee joint. *Acta Orthop. Scand. 33:* 306–311, 1963.
90. Lewis, R. C., Jr., Coventry, M. B., and Soule, E. H.: Hemangioma of the synovial membrane. *J. Bone Joint Surg. 41A:* 264–271, 1959.
91. Forrest, J., and Staple, T. W.: Synovial hemangioma of the knee; demonstration by arthrography and arteriography. *Am. J. Roentgenol. Radium Ther. Nucl. Med. 112:* 512–516, 1971.
92. Moon, N. F.: Synovial hemangioma of the knee joint; a review of previously reported cases and inclusion of two new cases. *Clin. Orthop. 90:* 183–190, 1973.
93. Burgan, D. W.: Lipoma arborescens of the knee; another cause of filling defects on a knee arthrogram. *Radiology 101:* 583–584, 1971.
94. Gardner, D. L.: *Pathology of the Connective Tissue Diseases* p. 407. Baltimore, Williams & Wilkins Co., 1965.
95. Weitzman, G.: Lipoma arborescens of the knee; report of a case. *J. Bone Joint Surg. 47A:* 1030–1033, 1965.
96. Arzimanoglu, A.: Bilateral arborescent lipoma of the knee; a case report. *J. Bone Joint Surg. 39A:* 976–979, 1957.
97. Sullivan, C. R., Dahlin, D. C., and Bryan, R. S.: Lipoma of the tendon sheath. *J. Bone Joint Surg. 38A:* 1275–1280, 1956.
98. White, J. R.: Arborescent lipomata of tendon sheaths; a report of two cases. *Surg. Obstet. Gynecol. 38:* 489–490, 1924.
99. Cadman, N. L., Soule, E. H., and Kelly, P. J.: Synovial sarcoma. An analysis of 134 tumors. *Cancer 18:* 613–627, 1965.
100. Gabbiani, G., Kay, G. I., Lattes, R., and Majno, G.: Synovial sarcoma; electron microscopic study of a typical case. *Cancer 28:* 1031–1039, 1971.
101. Lee, S. M., Hajdu, S. I., and Exelby, P. R.: Synovial sarcoma in children. *Surg. Gynecol. Obstet. 138:* 701–704, 1974.
102. Ariel, I. M., and Pack, G. T.: Synovial sarcoma; review of 25 cases. *N. Engl. J. Med. 268:* 1272–1275, 1963.
103. Attie, J. N., Steckler, R. M., and Platt, N.: Cervical synovial sarcoma. *Cancer 25:* 758–761, 1970.
104. Lord, G. A., and Goodale, F.: Synovial sarcoma arising in the anterior abdominal wall. *Arch. Surg. 81:* 1020–1022, 1960.
105. Vincent, R. G.: Malignant synovioma. *Ann. Surg. 152:* 777–788, 1960.
106. Craig, R. M., Pugh, D. G., and Soule, E. H.: The roentgenologic manifestations of synovial sarcoma. *Radiology 65:* 837–846, 1955.
107. Tillotson, J. F., McDonald, J. R., and Janes, J. M.: Synovial sarcomata. *J. Bone Joint Surg. 33A:* 459–473, 1951.
108. Naib, Z. M.: Cytology of synovial fluids. *Acta Cytol. 17:* 299–309, 1973.
109. Mackenzie, D. H.: Synovial sarcoma; a review of 58 cases. *Cancer 19:* 169–180, 1966.
110. Bennett, G. A.: Malignant neoplasms originating in synovial tissues (synoviomata); a study of thirty-two specimens registered at the Army Institute of Pathology during the war-time period 1941–1945. *J. Bone Joint Surg. 29:* 259–291, 1947.
111. Kubo, T.: A note on fine structure of synovial sarcoma. *Acta Pathol. Jap. 24:* 163–168, 1974.
112. Raben, M., Calabrese, A., Higinbotham, N. L., and Phillips, R.: Malignant synovioma. *Am. J. Roentgenol. Radium Ther. Nucl. Med. 93:* 145–153, 1965.
113. Suit, H. D., Russell, W. O., and Martin R. G.: Management of patients with sarcoma of soft tissue in an extremity. *Cancer 31:* 1247–1255, 1973.
114. McBride, C. M.: Sarcomas of the limbs; results in adjuvant chemotherapy using isolation perfusion. *Arch. Surg. 109:* 304–308, 1974.
115. Enzinger, F. M.: Epithelioid sarcoma; a sarcoma simulating a granuloma or a carcinoma. *Cancer 26:* 1029–1041, 1970.

116. DeSanto, D. A., Tennant, R., and Rosahn, P. D.: Synovial sarcomas in joints, bursae, and tendon sheaths; a clincial and pathological study of sixteen cases. *Surg. Gynecol. Obstet. 72:* 951–981, 1941.
117. Berger, L.: Synovial sarcomas in serous bursae and tendon sheaths. *Am. J. Can. 34:* 501–539, 1938.
118. Bliss, B. O., and Reed, R. J.: Large cell sarcomas of tendon sheath. Malignant giant cell tumors of tendon sheath. *Am. J. Clin. Pathol. 49:* 776–781, 1968.
119. Bryan, R. S., Soule, E. H., Dobyns, J. H., Pritchard, D. J., and Linscheid, R. L.: Primary epithelioid sarcoma of the hand and forearm; a review of thirteen cases. *J. Bone Joint Surg. 56A:* 458–465, 1974.
120. Santiago, H., Feinerman, L. K., and Lattes, R.: Epithelioid sarcoma; a clinical and pathologic study of nine cases. *Hum. Pathol. 3:* 133–147, 1972.
121. Soule, E. H., and Enriquez, P.: Atypical fibrous histiocytoma, malignant fibrous histiocytoma, malignant histiocytoma, and epithelioid sarcoma; a comparative study of 65 tumors. *Cancer 30:* 128–143, 1972.
122. Fisher, E. R., and Horvat, B.: The fibrocytic derivation of the so-called epithelioid sarcoma. *Cancer 30:* 1074–1081, 1972.
123. Frable, W. J., Kay, S., Lawrence, W., and Schatzki, P. F.: Epithelioid sarcoma; an electron microscopic study. *Arch. Pathol. 95:* 8–12, 1973.
124. Gabbiani, G., Fu, Y. S., Kaye, G. I., Lattes, R., and Majno, G.: Epithelioid sarcoma; a light and electron microscopic study suggesting a synovial origin. *Cancer, 30:* 486–499, 1972.
125. Enzinger, F. M.: Clear-cell sarcoma of tendons and aponeuroses; an analysis of 21 cases. *Cancer 18:* 1163–1174, 1965.
126. Dutra, F. R.: Clear-cell sarcoma of tendons and aponeuroses; three additional cases. *Cancer 25:* 942–946, 1970.
127. Kubo, T.: Clear-cell sarcoma of patellar tendon studied by electron microscopy. *Cancer 24:* 948–953, 1969.
128. Hoffman, G. J., and Carter, D.: Clear cell sarcoma of tendons and aponeuroses with melanin. *Arch. Pathol. 95:* 22–25, 1973.
129. Kahn, L. B.: Malignant giant cell tumor of the tendon sheath. Ultrastructural study and review of the literature. *Arch. Pathol. 95:* 203–208, 1973.
130. Goldman, R. L., and Lichtenstein, L.: Synovial chondrosarcoma. *Cancer 17:* 1233–1240, 1964.
131. Kautz, F. G.: Capsular osteoma of the knee joint; report of four cases. *Radiol. 45:* 162–167, 1945.
132. Mullins, F., Berard, C. W., and Eisenberg, S. H.: Chondrosarcoma following synovial chondromatosis; a case study. *Cancer 18:* 1180–1188, 1965.
133. King, J. W., Spjut, H. J., Fechner, R. E., and Vanderpool, D. W.: Synovial chondrosarcoma of the knee joint. *J. Bone Joint Surg. 49A:* 1389–1396, 1967.
134. Dunn, E. J., McGavran, M. H., Nelson, P., and Greer, R. B.: Synovial chondrosarcoma; report of a case. *J. Bone Joint Surg. 56A:* 811–813, 1974.
135. Scully, R. E.: In case 23-1962; case records of the Massachusetts General Hospital; weekly clinicopathological exercises. *N. Engl. J. Med. 266:* 725–729, 1962.
136. Brannon, E. W., and Tracey, J. F.,: Hindquarter amputation for hip chondrosarcoma. *U. S. Armed Forces Med. J. 8:* 1517–1526, 1957.
137. Benedek, T. G.: Lysis of the patella due to metastatic carcinoma. *Arthritis Rheum. 8:* 560–567, 1965.
138. Gall, E. P., Didizian, N. A., and Park, Y.: Acute monarticular arthritis following patellar metastasis; a manifestation of carcinoma of the lung. *JAMA 229:* 188–189, 1974.

Chapter 12

Etiology of Human Skeletal and Soft Tissue Sarcomas: A Summary of Immunologic and Virologic Studies*

FREDERICK R. EILBER AND DONALD L. MORTON

In recent years there has been renewed interest in a possible viral etiology for human neoplasms. Studies of Burkitt's lymphoma,[11, 22, 26, 43] human leukemia,[1, 7] and carcinoma of the cervix[31] suggested circumstantial evidence for infectious agents associated with these tumors. Ever since Dr. Peyton Rous discovered a virus (RSV) as the cause for malignant soft tissue tumors in chickens in 1912,[46] the search for a virus etiologic agent has been undertaken in other laboratory animals. In 1966, Finkel, Biskis, and Jinkins[14] described a virus associated with soft tissue tumors in mice. Moloney[37] described a virus that caused malignant sarcoma in rodents (MSV), and a virus was described recently that caused fibrosarcomas in cats (FSV)[16, 50] and in woolly monkeys (SSV-1).[65] Therefore, it would appear that viruses have been isolated as the cause for skeletal and soft tissue sarcomas in a variety of animal species that include the nonhuman primates.

The renewed interest in a possible viral etiology of human sarcomas comes from several sources. A familial clustering of sarcomas was first reported by Roberts and Roberts.[45] The authors described 3 cases of concurrent osteogenic sarcoma in a brother and two sisters, an instance suggestive of a common genetic origin or adjuvant extraneous factors, including infection. Although these cases were reported in 1935, the investigators expressed surprisingly up-to-date speculation and discussion: "Unless the concurrence of the cases can be assigned to chance, the incidence offers the possibility of a specific infectious agent at the outset." This familial tendency in osteosarcoma has been observed repeatedly since then.[18, 19, 30, 39, 48, 53] However, the etiology of human skeletal and soft tissue sarcomas still remains unresolved.

Laboratory investigations to determine the origin of an immunologic response to human tumors present problems not encountered in the study of animal tumors. The original experiments by Prehn and Main,[42] that conclusively demonstrated the tumor-specific transplantation antigens of methylcholan-

* These investigations are supported by United States Public Health Service Grants CA 12582, CA 05252, CA 12285, and grants from California Institute for Cancer Research and Surgical Services, Sepulveda Veterans Administration Hospital.

threne-induced tumors, were performed in genetically identical (syngeneic) mice. In this way, it was possible to distinguish the tumor-specific antigens from the human leukocyte antigens (HLA) that also cause graft rejections. However, humans lack this genetic homogeneity, and it is not possible to use this valuable tool to provide the *sine qua non* of an immunologic reaction, *i.e.*, to prevent tumor growth by immunization. Thus, the study of human tumors on an immunologic basis has been confined to *in vitro* inspection of antibody activity directed against the tumor antigens.

Experimentation in animal systems has shown that tumors caused by chemical carcinogens contain tumor-specific transplantation antigens that are unique and distinct for each tumor. There is no antigenic cross-reactivity between carcinogen-induced tumors even if caused by the same chemical in the same animal. Protection against subsequent tumor challenge is afforded only by identical tumor antigens. However, immunologic studies of the virus-induced tumors revealed that protection from tumor growth can be achieved through a common cross-reacting antigen regardless of the histologic type of tumor caused by the virus.[25] Immunity can be accomplished by an injection of the virus itself, a subcellular fraction, or by whole tumor cells derived from the tumor. In some cases immune protection has been achieved between species in this manner.

Many of the animal tumor viruses have been identified and purified by injection into neonatal or chronically immunosuppressed animals.[16] This procedure allows a full expression of the viral genome and the actual creation of a particular virus thus making it possible to isolate, immunologically characterize, quantitate, and fulfill Koch's original postulates by reinjecting the viruses to produce tumor growth. Obviously such techniques are not possible in the study of human tumors.

The purpose of this chapter is to report the present status of virologic and immunologic studies of human skeletal and soft tissue sarcomas. All of the reports are from *in vitro* assays, using virologic and immunologic techniques in an effort to characterize and identify neoantigens associated with skeletal and soft tissue sarcomas.

COMMON TUMOR-ASSOCIATED ANTIGENS OF HUMAN SARCOMA

Biopsy specimens of human sarcomas and tissue culture cells from human sarcomas contain common tumor-associated antigens. This fact was initially described by Morton and Malmgren in 1968.[35] They found that human osteosarcomas contained a common tumor-associated antigen by the indirect immunofluorescence technique. The antigens were not present on normal cells derived from the same patients although these studies were performed with serum of patients from whom the tumors were derived. Therefore, the immunologic reaction was not due to histocompatibility, or HLA antigens, but was specific for tumor and was found to be cross-reactive. Because the antigens were common in different patients with sarcomas, it was postulated that these neoantigens could be due to an associated infectious agent. Subsequently these immunofluorescence studies have been expanded and confirmed by several investigators.[32, 33, 38, 40, 41, 44]

Three distinct types of immunofluorescent reactions have been noted. The first was that of a diffuse cytoplasmic fluorescence of the type described by Morton and Malmgren.[35] The second type was a particulate, cytoplasmic fluorescence described by Giraldo and co-workers.[17] It was apparent that the cytoplasmic immunofluorescence was not tumor-specific because it has been found in non-sarcoma-bearing patients. A third type of immunofluorescence noted by various investigators was on the cell surface. This type was described by Drewinko, Montgomery, and Trujillo in 1973,[8] and may also be tumor-specific as immunologic reactivity was seen only in sera from tumor-bearing patients.

The presence of tumor-associated antigens in human skeletal and soft tissue sarcomas has been detected by several other immunologic techniques. These include complement fixation,[9, 10] humoral cytotoxicity,[58] immunodiffusion,[59] lymphocyte blastogenesis,[57] and lymphocyte cytotoxicity.[5, 21] All of these studies have shown that human sarcomas contain a cross-reacting tumor-associated antigen(s).

The immunologic reactions described in the aforementioned studies that have demonstrated sarcoma-associated antigens were performed with lymphocytes or antibody derived from sera of human patients and, therefore, indicate that the antigens are immunogenic in patients. However, all of these studies were *in vitro* immunologic assays, and none were performed by the transplantation techniques used in animal systems to identify tumor-specific "transplantation" antigens.

Antibody distribution to sarcoma-associated antigens. The association of an infectious agent with human sarcomas is suggested by the observation that a higher incidence of antibodies to sarcoma-associated antigens is found in sarcoma patients, their family members, and close friends than is found in normal donors or in patients with other malignant diseases. This fact was originally described by Morton and Malmgren in 1968,[35] and was expanded by Eilber and Morton in 1970 and 1971,[9, 10] and by Priori, Wilber, and Dmochowski in 1971.[41] These studies showed an incidence of sarcoma antibody between 80 and 90% in tumor-bearing patients and an approximate incidence of 50 to 60% in close associates and family members. Antisarcoma antibody was found in only 20% of normal donors. However, none of the close friends or family members who had antisarcoma antibodies had evidence of tumor. These results implied that infection by, and immunologic reaction against, a possible etiologic agent was common, whereas induction of tumor was a relatively rare occurrence. In animal systems this antibody distribution is a common finding.[2] *In vitro* immunologic reactivity against viruses can be very high whereas the actual infection rate or tumor induction is relatively low.

Identification of virus-like particles of human tumors. Several reports have described electron microscopic examinations of biopsy specimens and tissue cultures derived from human sarcomas that have shown virus-like particles similar to those found in animal sarcoma.[12, 34, 41, 52] We have examined over 100 sarcoma specimens, and such particles were identified in only five. Morton and Malmgren[35] characterized the particles as morphologically similar to the "C" type particles known to cause animal sarcomas. Their occurrence in biopsy or tissue culture specimens is obviously very low, and their identification by electron microscopy is extremely difficult, because of the limited concentration of intact virus particles. It must be emphasized that the presence of these particles does not necessarily imply etiology. It is possible that they are merely a passenger or contaminants and not the causative agents.

Extracts from human sarcomas contain a filterable agent that can cause morphologic alterations in normal tissue culture cells. It was hypothesized that since the virus-like particles were in such low concentration in human tumors that amplification of their numbers as well as evidence for infectivity might be achieved by the application of filtered tumor extracts to tissue cultures of nonmalignant human cells. Morton, Malmgren, and Hall reported such an experiment in 1969.[36] Filtered extracts of human sarcomas were overlaid on normal human embryo fibroblasts, and morphologic transformation was observed approximately 21 days later. This transformation was manifest by loss of contact inhibition, a rounding up of the cells, and the formation of a tumor *in vitro*. This observation was confirmed by Giraldo, *et al.*[17] However, when the foci of morphologically transformed cells were examined by electron microscopy, no virus particles were seen. The incidence of this morphologic transformation again was extremely low, occurring in only 2% of the experiments. Additionally, horizontal infectivity could not be achieved, as it was not possible to infect normal cells with extracts from these transformed foci.

Human sarcomas contain a filterable substance which can induce antigenic transformation. Since morphologic transformation occurred sporadically, it was reasoned that it was very probable that antigenic transformation might be occurring more readily than the actual tumor formation.[51] Therefore, Morton, Malmgren, Hall, and Schidlovsky,[36] Eilber and Morton,[9] and Giraldo, *et al.*[17] described immunologic assays of normal cells that had been infected with filtered extract derived from human sarcomas. Antigenic transformation was described in approximately 60% of the cultures analyzed. The antigenic transformation occurred in approximately 14 to 21 days after the filtered extracts were overlayed on the normal cells, and two of these cell lines continue to express the sarcoma antigen 5 years after the original experiment. However, electron microscopic examinations of the transformed cultures failed to disclose intact virus particles.

It is apparent, therefore, that there is a filterable substance in sarcoma that is capable of inducing a neoantigen on previously normal cells. It is possible that this neoantigen is not a virus-induced antigen but is instead due to immune RNA or transfer factor. However, regardless of its exact nature, a neoantigen has been produced from extracts of human sarcomas.

Human sarcomas contain RNA related to murine leukemia virus. The discovery of a "reverse transcriptase" enzyme was certainly an important one for future study of animal and potential human viruses.[47, 49] Prior to this discovery it was not thought possible for RNA to synthesize DNA but only in the opposite direction, *i.e.*, DNA to RNA. This discovery made it understandable how a C-type RNA virus could, in fact, cause a permanent DNA change.[54] Kufe, Hehlmann, and Spiegelman, and Kufe, Peters, and Spiegelman[27, 28] described experiments using RNA from the polysome fraction of human sarcomas. They discovered that 68% of these fractions hybridized with labeled DNA complimentary to the RNA leukemia virus. This complimentary hybridization is a very significant finding and has been the technique utilized in animal systems by several investigators. Examination of the cells by electronmicroscopy did not show intact virus and thus these macromolecular techniques disclosed the "foot prints" of viral infection. Additionally, Gallo, Miller, Saxinger, and Gillespie[15] have utilized the same technique in human leukemia to suggest a viral etiology.

Characteristics of sarcoma antigens and modifications in tissue culture. When one appreciates the limitations of the experiments with human skeletal and soft tissue sarcomas, it becomes apparent that there are fascinating immunologic and virologic leads suggesting the association of an infectious agent in these tumors. However, to date the identification, purification, and characterization of such an agent have not been successful. There are several difficult and unresolved problems associated with any immunologic and virologic studies of these tumors. Since the work must be performed *in vitro*, it is desirable that tissue-cultured sarcoma cell lines be established in order to provide a constant source of materials for long term study.

It is apparent from several studies that human sarcomas contain several associated neoantigens rather than a single sarcoma-specific antigen. From the initial studies of Giraldo, *et al.*, in 1971,[17] it is clear that the particulate cytoplasmic fluorescence is a neoantigen found in human sarcoma and that it may not be specific for sarcomatous tumors. An epidemiologic study of the distribution of antibody to this antigen showed an equal distribution throughout the population. This information suggests that a "common cross-reactivity" to this antigen may not necessarily be an implication of viral etiology.[23] Irie and Irie[24] recently reported that tumor cells in culture acquire a new antigen from the culture medium. This heterologous membrane antigen was found on human cells supplemented with bovine serum. Since most tissue culture preparations contain fetal calf serum this antigen certainly must be recognized and not confused with a tumor-associated antigen.

From the work of Bloom,[4] it is evident that cultured cells can acquire other neoantigens related to blood group A that possibly may be responsible for some of the previously reported cytoxic reactions to sarcoma cells. Investigations must be carefully controlled to exclude the presence of fetal antigens,[38] which also may be expressed in tissue culture. Finally, it is apparent from several studies that contaminating microorganisms such as mycoplasma and bacteria also create new antigens in tissue cultures that were not present initially and also may be responsible for some of the immunologic reactions reported.

Interspecies transmission of oncogenic virus. It is interesting to note that many of the problems of viral identification and neoantigenic expression in human sarcomas have been encountered in studies of interspecies viral oncogenesis. Deinhardt and co-workers[6] have summarized recent experiments in primates that have been injected with SSV, RSV, and FSV viruses. When these viruses were injected into the marmoset, malignant fibrosarcomas developed within 7 to 10 days in almost 100% of the animals. By electron microscopy, intact virus particles were found in only the SSV-induced sarcomas even though known viruses induced the tumors in all animals. Horizontal transmission of infection by the injection of animals with filtered extracts of the tumor was only possible in the SSV system. Immunologic evidence for the viral etiology of the induced tumors was established by the demonstration of neoantigens, related to viral group specific (GS) antigens, in both the SSV and FSV systems. Although no GS antigens were observed in the RSV tumors, antibody to the RSV GS antigen was detected in the sera of the animals in whom the tumors were induced.

The results of these studies on primates are very interesting and have many similarities to the results of studies of human neoplasms. They also appear pertinent in view of recent studies that have identified macromolecular structures, homologous to the nucleic acids of animal viruses, in leukemia[3, 15, 20] and sarcomas.[27, 28] Whether an analogy of interspecies transmission of oncogenic virus can be made to man remains speculative. However, it is probable that future immunologic and viral studies in primates will result in a better understanding of the mode of viral transmission, provide additional techniques of viral particle identification, and possibly clarify the relationship of the viral GS antigen to the sarcoma neoantigen. This information would be very useful in helping to decipher the results obtained from the study of human sarcomas.

SUMMARY

There are numerous pieces of information that when taken collectively are highly suggestive for an association of an infectious agent with human skeletal and soft tissue sarcomas. Virus-like particles have been identified in biopsy specimens as well as in tissue cultures of human tumors. Filtered extracts from these tumors have caused morphologic and antigenic transformation of normal human cells. Neoantigen(s) have been detected on sarcoma cells, and antibody to these antigen(s) have been detected in sera of tumor-bearing patients. Whether the associated infectious agents are responsible for tumor induction and for the sarcoma antigens are important questions that remain unanswered. Hopefully, by continued studies of viral oncogenesis in primates and with the application of macromolecular techniques and newer tumor antigen purification procedures to the study of human sarcomas, these questions can be resolved.

REFERENCES

1. Ames, R. P., Sobota, J. T., Reagan, R. L., and Karon, M.: Virus-like particles and cytopathic activity in urine of patients with leukemia. *Blood 28:* 465–478, 1966.
2. Aoki, T., Boyse, E. A., and Old, L. J.: Occurrence of natural antibody to the G (Gross) leukemia antigen in mice. *Cancer Res. 26:* 1415–1419, 1966.
3. Baxt, W., Hehlmann, R., and Spiegelman, S.: Human leukaemic cells contain reverse transcriptase associated with a high molecular weight virus related RNA. *Nature* (*New Biol.*) *240:* 72–75, 1972.
4. Bloom, E. T.: Further definition by cytotoxicity tests of cell surface antigens of human sarcomas in culture. *Cancer Res. 32:* 960–967, 1972.
5. Cohen, A. M., Ketcham, A. S., and Morton, D. L.: Cellular immunity to a common human sarcoma antigen and its specific inhibition by sera from patients with growing sarcomas. *Surgery 72:* 560–567, 1972.
6. Deinhardt, F., Wolfe, L., Northrop, R., Marzynska, B., Ogden, J. McDonald, R., Falk, L., Shramek, G., Smith, R., and Deinhardt, J.: Induction of neoplasms by viruses in Marmoset Monkeys. *J. Med. Primatol. 1:* 29–50, 1972.
7. Dmochowski, L., Yumoto, T., Grey, C. E., Hales, R. L., Langford, P. L., Taylor, H. G., Freireich,

E. J., Shullenberger, C. C., Shively, J. A., and Howe, C. D.: Electron microscopic studies of human leukemia and lymphoma. *Cancer 20:* 760–777, 1967.

8. Drewinko, B., Montgomery, C. T., Trujillo, J. M.: Demonstration of common sarcoma-associated antigen(s) in an established human neurogenic sarcoma cell line. *Cancer Res. 33:* 601–605, 1973.
9. Eilber, F. R. and Morton, D. L.: Immunologic studies of human sarcomas; additional evidence suggesting an associated sarcoma virus. *Cancer 26:* 588–596, 1970.
10. Eilber, F. R., and Morton, D. L.: Immunologic response to human sarcomas; relation of antitumor antibody to the clinical course. *Progress in Immunology. First International Congress of Immunology*, edited by Amos, B., pp. 951–957. New York and London, Academic Press, Inc., 1971.
11. Epstein, M. A., Achong, B. G., and Barr, Y. M.: Virus particles in cultured lymphoblasts from Burkitt's lymphoma. *Lancet, 1:* 702–703, 1964.
12. Finkel, M. P., Biskis, B. O., and Farrell, C.: Osteosarcomas appearing in syrian hamsters after treatment with extracts of human osteosarcomas. *Proc. Natl. Acad. Sci. U. S. A. 60:* 1223–1230, 1968.
13. Finkel, M. P., Biskis, B. O., and Farrell, C.: Nonmalignant and malignant changes in hamsters inoculated with extracts of human osteosarcomas. *Radiology 92:* 1546–1552, 1969.
14. Finkel, M. P., Biskis, B. O., and Jinkins, P. B.: Virus induction of osteosarcomas in mice. *Science 151:* 698–700, 1966.
15. Gallo, R. C., Miller, N. R., Saxinger, W. C., and Gillespie, D.: Primate RNA tumor virus-like DNA synthesized endogenously by RNA-dependent DNA Polymerase in virus-like particles from fresh human acute leukemic blood cells. *Proc. Natl. Acad. Sci. U. S. A. 70:* 3219–3224, 1973.
16. Gardner, M. B., Rongey, R. W., Arnstein, P., Estes, J. D., Sarma, P., Huebner, R. J., and Rickard, C. G.: Experimental transmission of feline fibrosarcoma to cats and dogs. *Nature 226:* 807–809, 1970.
17. Giraldo, G., Beth, E., Hirshaut, Y., Aoki, T., Old, L. J., Boyse, E. A., and Chopra, H. C.: Human sarcomas in culture; foci of altered cells and a common antigen; induction of foci and antigen in human fibroblast cultures by filtrates. *J. Exp. Med. 133:* 454–478, 1971.
18. Goldenberg, G. J., Spurll, G. M., and Hogg, G. R.: Simultaneous occurrence of sarcomas in a husband and wife. *Can. Med. Assoc. J. 110:* 49–50, 1974.
19. Harmon, T. P., and Morton, K. S.: Osteogenic sarcoma in four siblings. *J. Bone Joint Surg. 48B:* 493–498, 1966.
20. Hehlmann, R., Kufe, D., and Spiegelman, S.: RNA in human leukemic cells related to the RNA of a mouse leukemia virus. *Proc. Natl. Acad. Sci. U. S. A. 69:* 435–439, 1972.
21. Hellström, I., Hellström, K. E., Pierce, G. E., Yang, J. P. S.: Cellular and humoral immunity to different types of human neoplasms. *Nature 220:* 1352–1354, 1968.
22. Henle, W., Henle, G., Gunven, P., Klein, G., Clifford, P., and Singh, S.: Patterns of antibodies to Epstein-Barr virus-induced early antigens in Burkitt's lymphoma; comparison of dying patients with long-term survivors. *J. Natl. Cancer Inst. 50:* 1163–1173, 1973.
23. Hirshaut, Y., Dawn, T. P., Marcove, R. C., Mukherji, B., Spielvogel, A. R., and Essner, E.: Seroepidemiology of human sarcoma antigen (S_1). *N. Engl. J. Med. 291:* 1103–1107, 1974.
24. Irie, K., and Irie, R. F.: Surface antigens of cultured human sarcomas detected by immune-adherence (abstract). *Proc. Am. Assoc. Cancer Res. 14:* 119, 1973.
25. Klein, G.: Tumor Antigens. *Annu. Rev. Microbiol. 20:* 223–252, 1966.
26. Klein, G., Clifford, P., Henle, G., Henle, W., Geering, G., and Old, L. J.: EBV-associated serological patterns in a Burkitt lymphoma patient during regression and recurrence. *Int. J. Cancer 4:* 416–421, 1969.
27. Kufe, D., Hehlmann, R., and Spiegelman, S.: Human sarcomas contain RNA related to the RNA of a mouse leukemia virus. *Science 175:* 182–185, 1972.
28. Kufe, D. W., Peters, W. P. and Spiegelman, S.: Unique nuclear DNA sequences in the involved tissue of Hodgkins and Burkitt's lymphomas. *Proc. Natl. Acad. Sci. U. S. A. 70:* 3810–3814, 1973.
29. Levy, J. A., and Henle, G.: Indirect immunofluorescence tests with sera from African children and cultured Burkitt lymphoma cells. *J. Bacteriol. 92:* 275–276, 1966.

30. Li, F. P., and Fraumeni, J. F., Jr.: Rhabdomyosarcoma in children; epidemiologic study and identification of a familial cancer syndrome. *J. Natl. Cancer Inst. 43:* 1365–1373, 1969.

31. Melnick, J. L., Adam, E., and Rawls, W. E.: The causative role of herpesvirus type 2 in cervical cancer. *Cancer 34:* 1375–1385, 1974.

32. Moore, M., and Hughes, L A.: Circulating antibodies in human connective tissue malignancy. *Br. J. Cancer (suppl. 1) 28:* 175–184, 1973.

33. Moore, M., Witherow, P. J., Price, C. H. G., and Clough, S. A.: Detection by immunofluorescence of intracytoplasmic antigens in cell lines derived from human sarcomas. *Int. J. Cancer 12:* 428–437, 1973.

34. Morton, D. L., Hall, W. T., and Malmgren, R. A.: Human liposarcomas; tissue cultures containing foci of transformed cells with viral particles. *Science 165:* 813–816, 1969.

35. Morton, D. L., and Malmgren, R. A.: Human osteosarcomas: Immunologic evidence suggesting an associated infectious agent. *Science 162:* 1279–1281, 1968.

36. Morton, D. L., Malmgren, R. A., Hall, W. T., and Schidlovsky, G.: Immunologic and virus studies with human sarcomas. *Surgery 66:* 152–161, 1969.

37. Moloney, J. B.: Biological studies on a lymphoid-leukemia virus extracted from sarcoma 37. I. Origin and introductory investigations. *J. Natl. Cancer Inst. 24:* 933–951, 1960.

38. Mukherji, B., Hirshaut, Y.: Evidence for fetal antigen in human sarcoma. *Science 181:* 440–442, 1973.

39. Pohle, E. A., Stovall, W. D., and Boyer, H. N.: Concurrence of osteogenic sarcoma in two sisters. *Radiology 27:* 545–548, 1936.

40. Priori, E. S., Wilbur, J. R., and Dmochowski, L.: Studies of sera from patients with osteosarcoma by immunofluorescence test (Abstract). *Proc. Am. Assoc. Can. Res. 11:* 64, 1970.

41. Priori, E. S., Wilbur, J. R., and Dmochowski, L.: Immunofluorescence tests of sera of patients with osteogenic sarcoma. *J. Natl. Cancer Inst. 46:* 1299–1308, 1971.

42. Prehn, R. T., Main, J. M.: Immunity to methylcholanthrene-induced sarcomas. *J. Natl. Cancer Inst. 18:* 769–778, 1957.

43. Reedman, B. M., Klein, G.: Cellular localization of an Epstein-Barr virus (EBV) associated complement-fixing antigen in producer and non-producer lymphoblastoid cell lines. *Int. J. Cancer 11:* 499–520, 1973.

44. Reilly, C. A., Pritchard, D. J., Biskis, B. O., and Finkel, M. P.: Immunologic evidence suggesting a viral etiology of human osteosarcoma. *Cancer, 30:* 603–609, 1972.

45. Roberts, C. W., and Roberts, C. P.: Concurrent osteogenic sarcoma in brother and sisters. *J. Am. Med. Assoc. 105:* 181–185, 1935.

46. Rous, P., Murphy, J. B., and Tytler, W. H.: A filterable agent the cause of a second chicken tumor, an osteochondrosarcoma. *J. Am. Med. Assoc. 59:* 1793–1794, 1912.

47. Sarngadharan, M. G., Sarin, P. S., Reitz, M. S., and Gallo, R. C.: Reverse transcriptase activity of human leukaemic cells; purification of the enzyme, response to AMV 70S RNA and characterization of the DNA product. *Nature (New Biol.) 240:* 67–72, 1972.

48. Schajowicz, F., and Bessone, J. E.: Chondrosarcoma in three brothers; a pathological and genetic study. *J. Bone Joint Surg. 49A:* 129–141, 1967.

49. Schlom, S., and Spiegelman, S.: Simultaneous detection of reverse transcriptase and high molecular weight RNA unique to oncogenic RNA viruses. *Science 174:* 840–843, 1972.

50. Snyder, S. P., Theilen, G. H.: Transmissible feline fibrosarcoma. *Nature 221:* 1074–1075, 1969.

51. Stanton, M. F., Law, L. W., Ting, R. C.: Some biologic immunogenic, and morphologic effects in mice after infection with a murine sarcoma virus. II. Morphologic studies. *J. Natl. Cancer Inst. 40:* 1113–1129, 1968.

52. Stewart, S. E., Kasnic, G., Jr., Draycott, C., Feller, W., Golden, A., Mitchell, E., and Ben, T.: Activation *in vitro* by 5-iododeoxyuridine, of a latent virus resembling C-Type virus in a human sarcoma cell line. *J. Natl. Cancer Inst. 48:* 273–277, 1972.

53. Swaney, J. J.: Familial osteogenic sarcoma. *Clin. Orthop. 97:* 64–68, 1973.

54. Temin, H. M.: Introduction to virus-caused cancers. *Cancer 34:* 1347–1352, 1974.

55. Theilen, G. H., Gould, D., Fowler, M., and Dungworth, D. L.: C-Type virus tumor tissue of a woolly monkey (lagothrix spp.) with fibrosarcoma. *J. Natl. Cancer Inst. 47:* 881–889, 1971.

56. Todaro, G. J., and Gallo, R. C.: Immunological relationship of DNA polymerase from human

acute leukemia cells and primate and mouse leukemia virus reverse transcriptase. Nature (London) *244:* 206–209, 1973.

57. Vansky, F., Stjernswärd, J., Klein, G., Steiner, L., and Lindberg, L.: Tumor-associated specificity of serum mediated inhibition of lymphocyte stimulation by autochthonous human tumors. *J. Natl. Cancer Inst. 51:* 25–32, 1973.
58. Wood, W. C., and Morton, D. L.: Host immune response to a common cell-surface antigen in human sarcomas. *New Engl. J. Med. 284:* 569–572, 1971.
59. Winters, W. D., and Morton, D. L.: Detection of human antisarcoma antibodies by immunodiffusion (abstract). *Proc. Amer. Assoc. Cancer Res. 14:* 55, 1973.

Chapter 13

The Radiologic Approach to Bone Tumors

ALEX NORMAN

The intuitive approach to a bone tumor is an effective means of diagnosis. However, this experience is difficult to impart to others. To the uninitiated, a disciplined review of radiographic features and a logical evaluation of these characteristics measured against a list of diagnostic possibilities is a more effective exercise in learning.

If the clinician, radiologist, and pathologist share information, an accurate diagnosis is possible in at least 95% of cases,[4] and through such cooperative efforts, the radiologist may often venture the correct histologic diagnosis. Whereas the clinical story is frequently nonspecific and of little help in diagnosis, it is important to know certain clinical features of the tumor such as (1) the preferred location in the skeleton and (2) the predilection for certain age groups (Chart 1).[8]

The radiograph is an accurate reflection of the gross pathology. It shows (1) the location of the lesion, (2) the extent of the tumor, (3) the perilesional reaction, and (4) the calcification or ossification of the matrix.[3] In essence, the radiograph is a measure of bone destruction caused by the enlarging tumor and the degree of reactive new bone formation.

If the radiographic pattern and clinical setting are reviewed, one of several categories of bone disease will be suggested by the roentgenographic appearance (table 1). Occasionally, the appearance of the lesion may suggest more than one of these categories. Indeed, tumors can be mistaken for other conditions such as infection, metabolic disorder, or traumatic lesion. Selecting a single category is not always a simple matter. However, once the lesion is considered a tumor, the next phase of the analysis is to compare the roentgenographic characteristics of a known list of tumors (classification) against the features of the lesion under discussion, gradually narrowing the field to the one most likely diagnosis.

THE ANALYTIC APPROACH

Clinical Features

Age. Benign tumors and tumor-like lesions occur in young patients, generally between the ages of 10 and 30 years (Chart 1). Exceptions to this are the non-ossifying fibroma and simple bone cysts, which are infrequent after the 2nd decade, and the solitary enchondroma, which may be seen from the 2nd to the 6th decades of life. In certain instances, as in giant cell tumor, the age

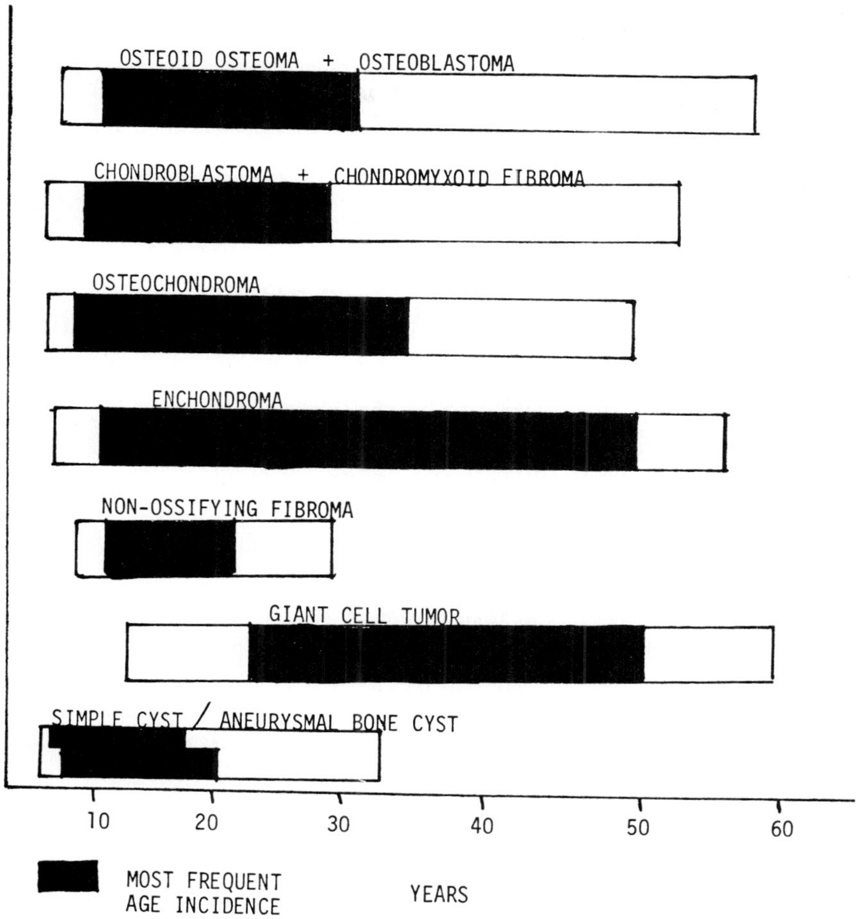

CHART 1. AGE RANGE OF BENIGN BONE TUMORS

TABLE 1. RADIOLOGIC CATEGORIES OF BONE DISEASE

1. Developmental disorder
2. Traumatic lesion
3. Ischemic necrosis
4. Infection
5. Tumor
6. Metabolic or endocrine disorder
7. Hematologic condition
8. Arthritis

significantly influences the diagnosis. Conventional giant cell tumors of bone occur between the ages of 20 and 50 years. In the adolescent, when the growth plates are still active, the diagnosis of giant cell tumor should be guarded, even if the histologic pattern is suggestive of this lesion.

Sarcomas of bone on the other hand, occur throughout a wide range of ages, from childhood to late adult life. Ewing's tumor is a lesion of the young, usually between 5 and 20 years of age. This tumor is extremely rare under 3 years of age and is seldom seen after the age of 20 years.

The predilection for specific decades of life is further emphasized by the age dependence of osteosarcoma. Conventional osteosarcomas occur in the adolescent and young adult. Only infrequently is it seen past the age of 40 years, unless it complicates a preexisting lesion or follows irradiation to bone. Differing from the classic osteosarcoma, the parosteal osteogenic sarcoma arises in a somewhat older age group and is rare in adolescence. With increasing age, chondrosarcomas and fibrosarcomas become more prevalent; usually the patients are between the ages of 30 and 60 years. Although chondrosarcoma is seen in the young, it seldom occurs before the age of 20 years. In fact, the diagnosis should be questioned if the patient is a child or a young adolescent. More often, the lesion is osteosarcoma and incorrectly called chondrosarcoma because of incomplete sampling of the tumor. In persons beyond 50 years of age, malignant bone tumors are statistically more likely to be metastatic than primary.

Location. The knowledge that bone tumors have a predilection for parts of the skeleton and particularly certain sites within bone is an additional aid to diagnosis. Some tumor sites are so specific, that a diagnosis can be suggested on the basis of location alone. Chondroblastoma, for one, singles out the epiphyses of long bones, particularly about the knee and proximal end of the humerus. Giant cell tumor has a decided predilection for the articular ends of long bones. Fifty percent are located in the distal end of the femur, proximal tibia, and distal end of the radius.

Further indications of the specific localization of bone lesions in the skeleton is the site of origin of the solitary bone cyst and nonossifying fibroma. Approximately half of simple bone cysts present in the proximal end of the humerus and an additional 15 to 20% in the proximal end of the femur; they arise centrally in the metaphysis and rarely extend into the epiphysis or articular end of the bone. Nonossifying fibroma arises eccentrically in the shaft of long bones, and predominantly in the lower extremity and near the cartilaginous growth plates about the knee. Other tumors with favored skeletal sites are the osteocartilaginous exostoses, which are common about the knee and also closely oriented to the cartilaginous growth plate. Indeed, they are the most common benign lesion of long bones.

Generalizations may be made for the sarcoma group as well. The epiphyses, with the exception of multifocal osteosarcoma, are rarely the sites of origin of a primary malignant bone tumor. Prior to epiphyseal plate closure, osteosarcoma is usually confined to the shaft and only occasionally erodes through the growth plate. However, once the cartilaginous growth plate is obliterated, the lesion may infiltrate the articular cortex. Few lesions have the specificity of location of the parosteal osteosarcoma. In approximately 70% of cases, the lesion arises at the posterior cortex of the distal end of the femur.[1]

Ewing's tumor is often limited to the metaphyseal and diaphyseal regions of long bones. Only in exceptional cases will it infiltrate the epiphysis.

Tumors affecting the spine also have preferred sites of origin. For example, osteoid osteoma, osteoblastoma, and aneurysmal bone cyst characteristically occur in the vertebral arch. If the vertebral body is affected, the lesion will usually involve the posterior half of the vertebra adjacent to the articulation with the pedicle. On the other hand, myeloma, lymphoma, and metastatic disease have a decided predilection for the vertebral body. It is of interest that the body of the sacrum is not an uncommon site for giant cell tumor, chordoma, and osteoblastoma.

Bone Destruction and Repair

Bone destruction is a consequence of tumor growth. The exact mechanism for destruction is not clearly understood, but several hypotheses have been proposed: (1) pressure erosion from encroachment of tumor cells on bone, (2) physical and chemical alterations on the surface of bone favoring resorption, and (3) destruction mediated through osteoclastic resorption.[6]

The extent of bone destruction is not related to the histologic characteristics of the neoplasm, but rather to its rate of growth. Three basic patterns of bone resorption are seen: geographic, moth-eaten, and permeative, and these reflect the aggressiveness of the lesion.[5]

The permeative lesion is the most aggressive of the three, and the geographic form of destruction, the least. A moth-eaten pattern is intermediate between the two. On occasion, so little bone destruction occurs with a permeative lesion that the tumor is not detected on the initial radiograph. When the tumor spreads through the marrow spaces and permeates the cortex, it will ultimately result in cortical resorption, sometimes saucerizing the surface[2] and eventually leading to trabecular destruction of lentil-shaped holes which fade imperceptibly into the surrounding bone. As the tumor penetrates the cortex and elevates the periosteum, it stimulates a new bone reaction. The Codman triangle is the periosteal reaction at the margin of the lesion (Fig. 1). Permeative and mottled destructive bone changes suggest a round cell tumor, Ewing's sarcoma, or malignant lymphoma of bone (Fig. 2). However, osteosarcoma, desmoplastic fibroma, and metastatic cancer may also present a similar picture.

The confluence of the lentil-shaped holes in a moth-eaten pattern may give the impression of multifocal tumor destruction.[5] The margins of the lesions are ill-defined, and the zone of transition is poorly demarcated. Such changes are indicative of rapid tumor growth and aggressiveness (Fig. 3). Although malignant bone tumors are suspected when these changes are seen, non-neoplastic lesions such as eosinophilic granuloma, Gaucher's disease, and osteomyelitis should be considered.

Gross or geographic bone destruction is more indicative of slow growth, and the radiographic appearance is dependent on the extent of cortical bone destruction.

New bone deposited within the lesional tissue or at its margins is the reparative reaction to bone destruction. The more pronounced the marginal sclerosis, the more prominent is the healing process.[5] Aggressive tumors rarely have a fine sclerotic edge, whereas slowly growing tumors are more often demarcated by a dense zone of sclerosis (Fig. 4, *A* to *D*). Although the reparative response is most pronounced about the edge of the lesion, sclerosis may occur within the

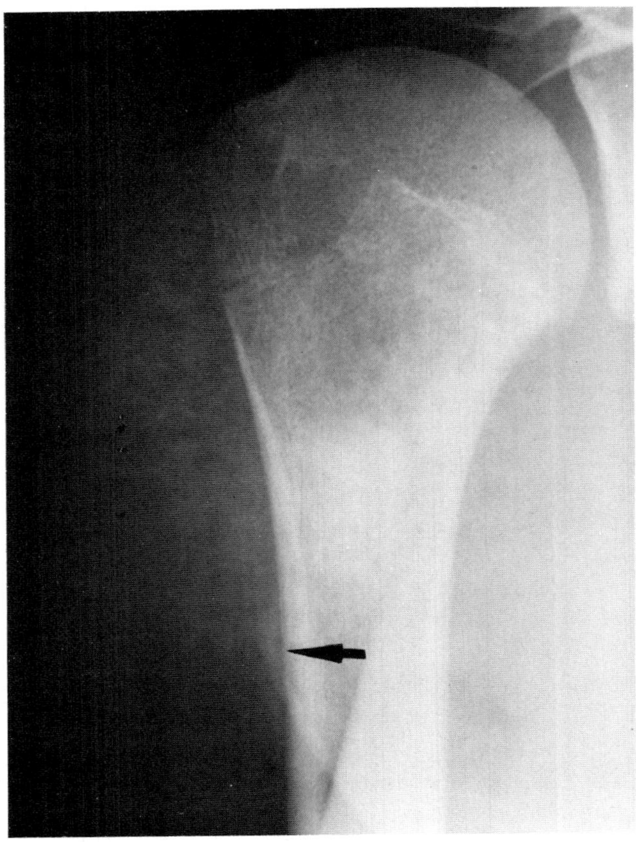

FIG. 1. The dense angle of periosteal new bone at the margin of an osteosarcoma (*arrow*) is the Codman triangle.

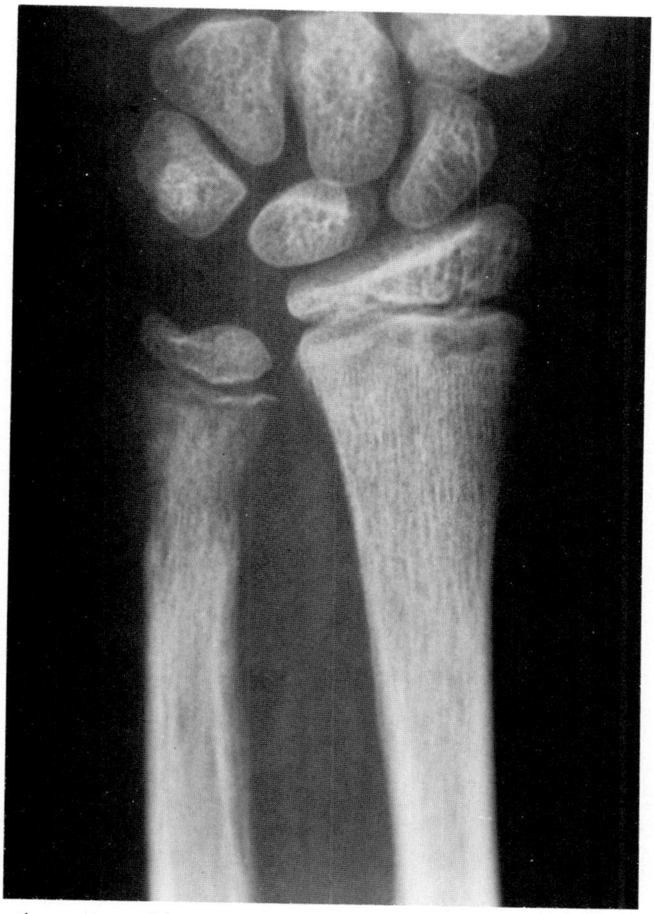

FIG. 2. Permeative pattern of bone resorption in the ulna of a child with lymphocytic leukemia. Note the whittled, saucerized surface of bone.

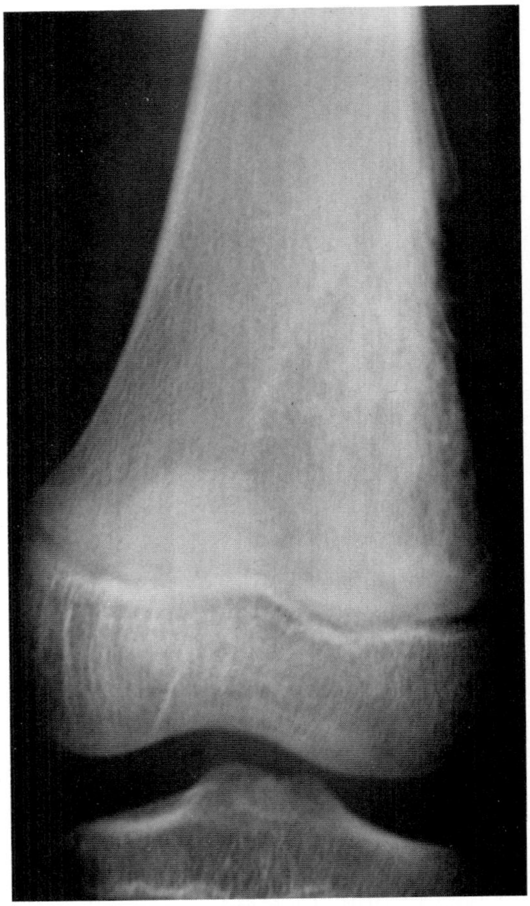

FIG. 3. Moth-eaten bone destruction in an 8-year-old child with osteosarcoma.

tumor, as for example, in round cell tumors and osteoblastic metastases (Fig. 5). Reparative reaction may also occur on the surface and thicken the cortex. The more intense the sclerosis, the more likelihood there is that the lesion is benign.

As the tumor enlarges, and erodes the cortex, it elevates and stimulates the periosteum to produce new bone. In slowly growing tumors, the lesion is usually contained by a shell of new-formed cortex and a buttress of dense lamellated or consolidated periosteal reactive bone at the edge of the neoplasm. The buttress response is generally associated with lesions that arise eccentrically or on the surface of bone (chondroblastoma and juxtacortical chondroma). Cyclic elevations of periosteum result in the lamellated or onion-skin appearance.

Although the type of periosteal reaction is nonspecific, a perpendicular or spiculated response is evidence of aggressive tumor behavior and malignant disease (Fig. 6). Reactive periosteal new bone is considered rare in metastatic disease, but this is not so.[7] In fact, Milch and Changus[6] observed that 80% of patients with osteoblastic metastasis had subperiosteal new bone formation,

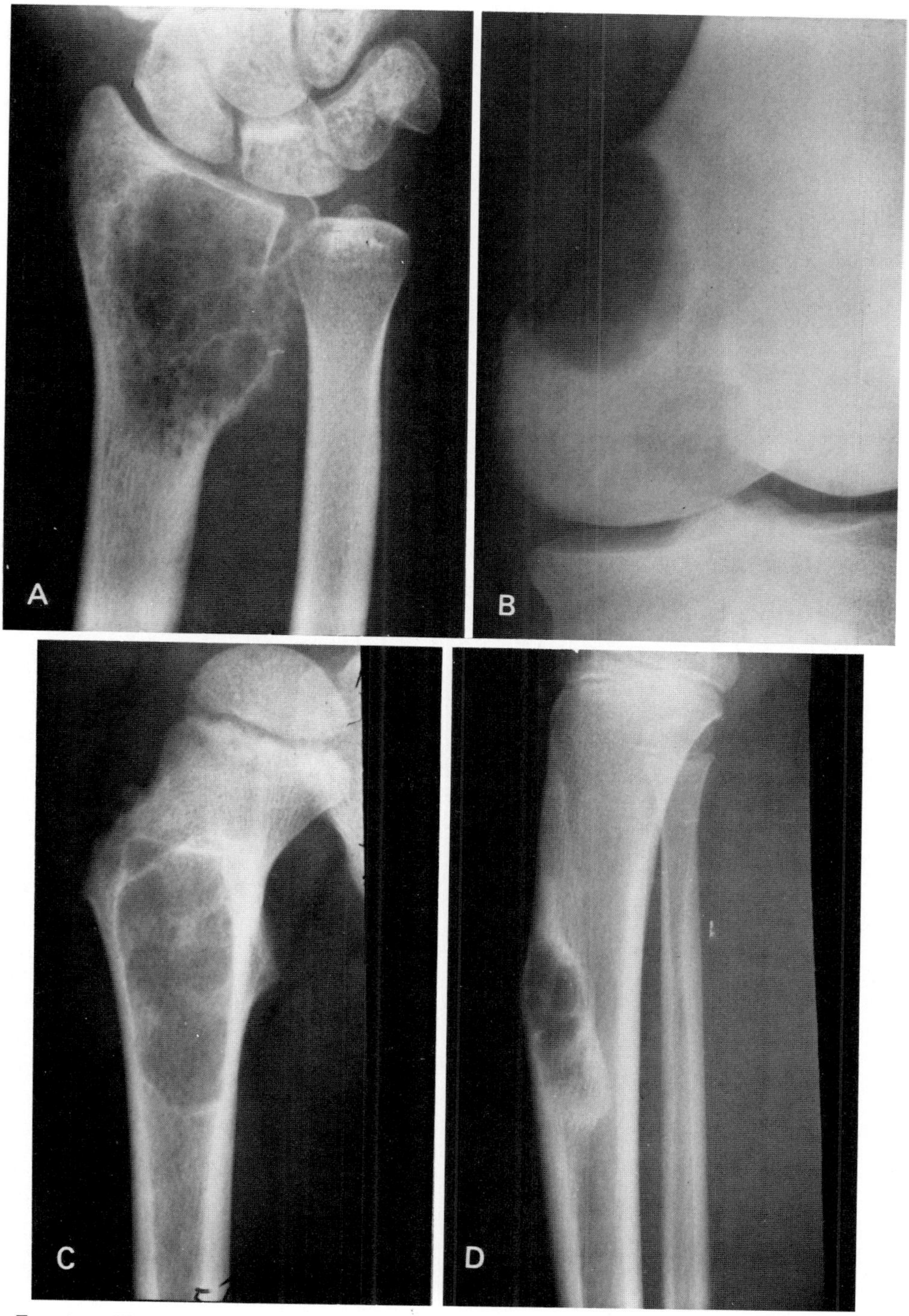

FIG. 4. *a*, The lack of sclerosis about the margin of this giant cell tumor indicates aggressive growth; *b*, chondromyxoid fibroma with a more sharply demarcated border, which indicates a less aggressive behavior; *c*, marginal sclerosis about a simple bone cyst suggesting slower growth; and *d*, a slowly growing ossifying fibroma in the tibia of a 7-year-old child. Note the dense margin of sclerosis.

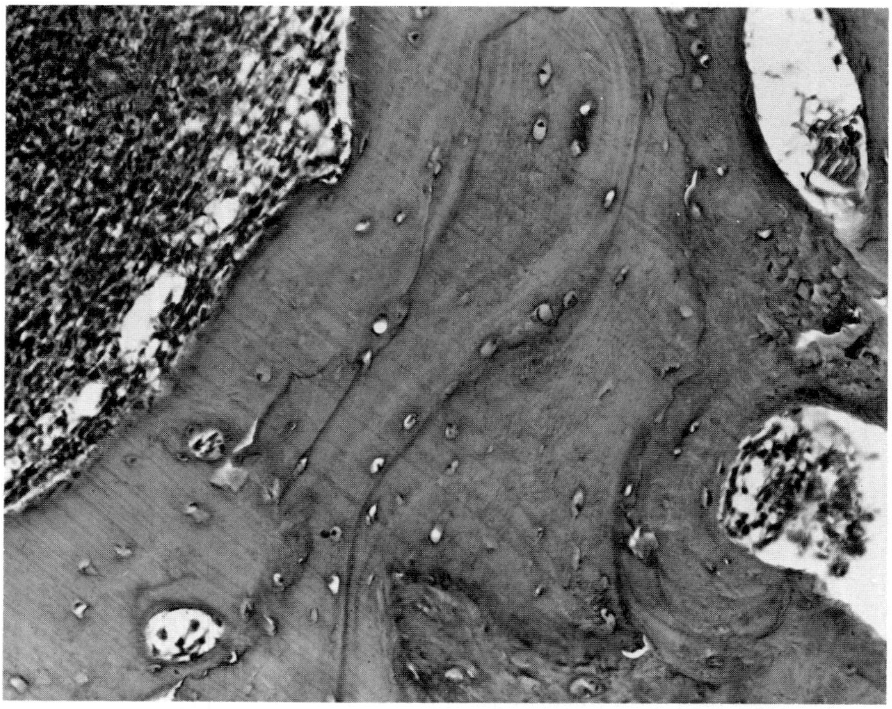

FIG. 5. Photomicrograph of an Ewing's sarcoma demonstrating reactive new bone on the right, in apposition to preexisting bone. Tumor is noted in the left upper quadrant. Hematoxylin and eosin stain; × 320.

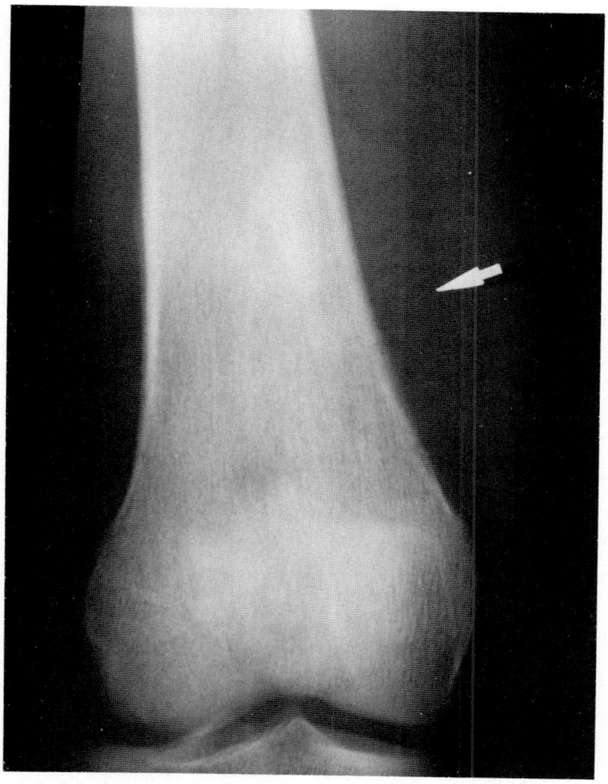

FIG. 6. Delicate spiculated periosteal reactive new bone (*arrow*) in a 16-year-old patient with osteosarcoma. A Codman triangle is seen at the upper margin of the lesion.

reemphasizing the frequency with which this response occurs in metastatic disease, and implying that the stimulus to periosteal new bone formation is multifactorial and that in addition to mechanical elevation of the periosteum there may also be a biochemical influence.

LESIONAL CALCIFICATION OR OSSIFICATION

The nature of the calcification or ossification in the matrix of tumors can be of help in their identification. Neoplasms may calcify or ossify, and the distinction between these two is not always easily indentifiable on the radiograph. Calcification in tumor cartilage is variable. The calcareous deposits may be granular, ringlike or fluffy. Some lesions, such as enchondroma or chondrosarcoma, may be lightly calcified, and the concretions may appear granular or punctate. In other instances, cartilage matrix may be heavily calcified. In such cases, the calcification is most pronounced about the periphery of the lobules creating a ringlike opacification on the radiograph (Fig. 7, *A* and *B*). At the same location, adjacent to vascular spaces, the matrix may even undergo ossification. Flocculent calcareous deposits are the nature of the calcification seen in chondroblastoma. In other cartilaginous tumors, such as chondromyxoid fibroma, the calcific deposits are of microscopic size and rarely visualized on the radiograph.

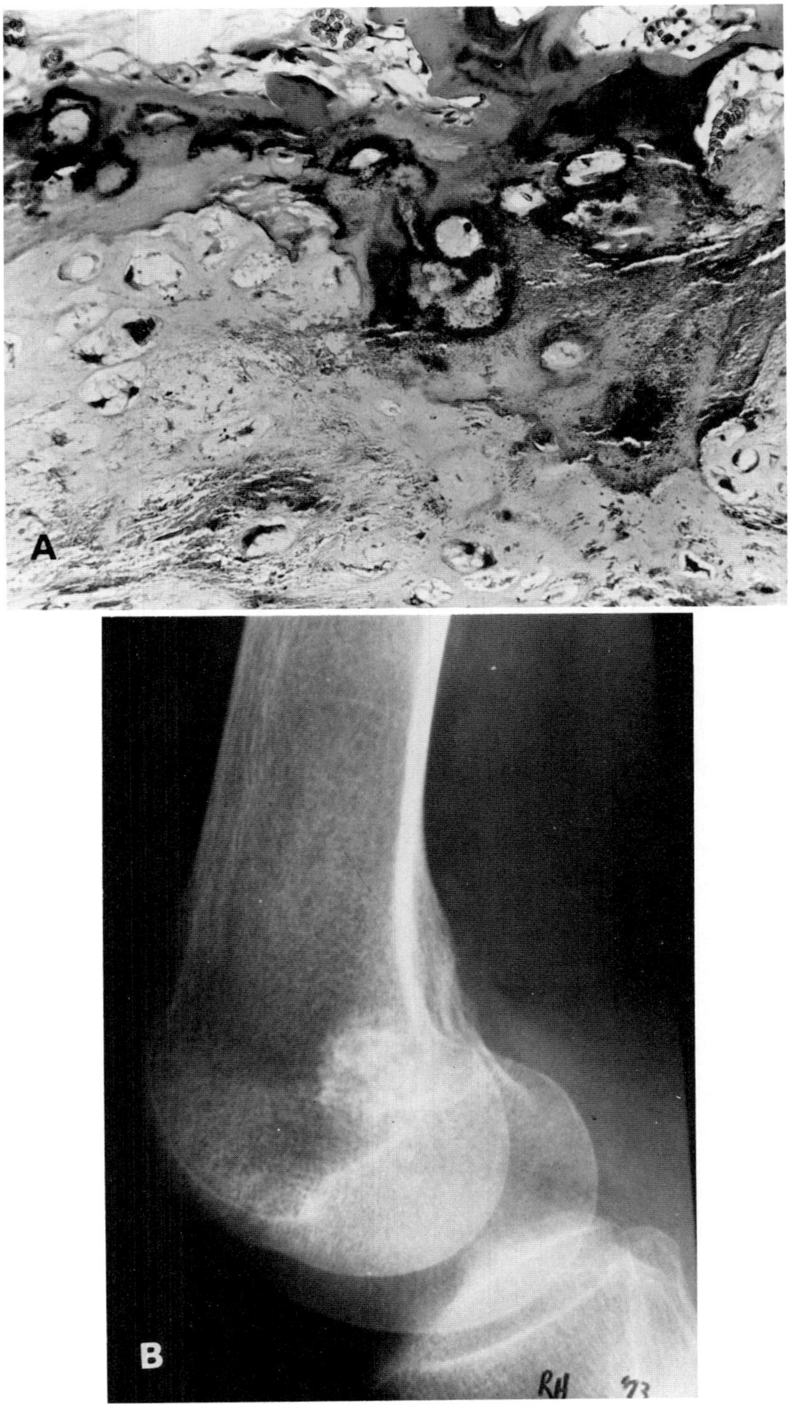

FIG. 7. *A*, Photomicrograph of an enchondroma showing the periphery of a lobule. There is granular calcification in the matrix in a ringlike fashion about the lobule. Hematoxylin and eosin stain, × 320. This corresponds to the densities on radiograph *B*.

Matrix ossification may occur in either benign or malignant tumors. The osteoid osteoma is representative of a benign osteoblastic lesion, and 25% of these will have an opacified nidus consisting of heavily ossified, broad or delicate bony trabeculae. Osteoblastoma, although possessing similar microscopic features, has a variable radiographic appearance. Poorly calcified masses of osteoid trabeculae may be present in one aspect of the lesion, and at other sites there are heavily calcified trabeculae of primitive bone. No distinct trabecular pattern can be discerned on the radiograph even when the tissue is converted to mature bone.[3] Osteoblastoma may vary from a destructive tumor surrounded by a delicate rim of periosteal new bone with little opacification within the lesion, to one that is heavily calcified or ossified.

Of the malignant neoplasms, osteosarcoma is the one tumor producing bone and osteoid from the sarcomatous stromal tissue. The wide range of radiographic appearances reflects the degree of tumor bone formed in the lesional tissue. Fifty percent of osteosarcomas are sclerosing in nature. Small scattered foci or large confluent areas of tumor bone are seen in the medullary cavity, filling the marrow spaces. The ossified tumor obliterates the last vestiges of preexisting normal trabeculation. In the soft tissue, the dense areas are an intermingling of tumor ossification and periosteal reactive new bone (Fig. 8).

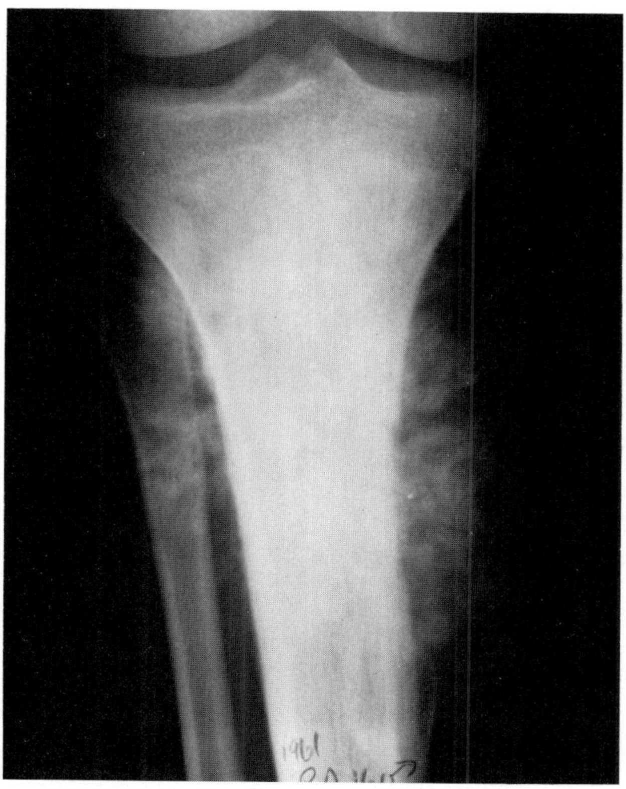

FIG. 8. Sclerotic foci of osteosarcoma obliterate normal trabecular pattern in the medullary cavity. Tumor bone in the soft tissue obscures the periosteal response.

SUMMARY

The age of the patient and the location of a lesion within bone are extremely helpful in deciding the diagnosis of a bone tumor. The aggressiveness of a lesion can be recognized from the pattern of destruction and repair on the radiograph, and frequently the appearance of the calcification or ossification of the matrix will suggest the histologic nature of the tumor. All of these factors must be considered in the radiologic analysis of a bone tumor.

REFERENCES

1. Dahlin, D. C.: *Bone Tumors: General Aspects and Data on 3,987 Cases*, p. 177. Springfield, Ill., Charles C. Thomas, 1967.
2. Edeiken, J.: Personal communication.
3. Jaffe, H. L.: *Tumors and Tumorous Conditions of the Bones and Joints*, p. 12. Philadelphia, Lea and Febiger, 1958.
4. Lodwick, G. S.: A systematic approach to the roentgen diagnosis of bone tumors. In *Tumors of Bone and Soft Tissue*, pp. 49–68. Chicago, Year Book Medical Publishers, Inc., 1965.
5. Lodwick, G. S.: *The Bones and Joints*, p. 42. Chicago, Year Book Medical Publishers, Inc., 1971.
6. Milch, R. A., and Changus, G. W.: Response of bone to tumor invasion. *Cancer 9:* 340–351, 1956.
7. Norman, A., and Ulin, R.: A comparative study of periosteal new-bone response in metastatic bone tumors (solitary) and primary sarcomas. *Radiology 92:* 705–708, 1969.
8. Spjut, H. J., Dorfman, H. D., Fechner, R. E., and Ackerman, L. V.: In *Atlas of Tumor Pathology*, fascicle 5, *Tumors of Bone and Cartilage*, pp. 20–21. Washington, D. C., Armed Forces Institute of Pathology, 1971.

Chapter 14

Fibro-osseous Lesions of Bone

LOUIS P. DEHNER

"Fibro-osseous lesions of bone" has evolved over the past 25 to 30 years as a clinicopathologic concept which has conventionally included the three histologic entities of fibrous dysplasia, ossifying fibroma, and cementifying fibroma. There has been no official sanctioning of the term "fibro-osseous lesions" by the World Health Organization in its *Histological Typing of Bone Tumours*[48] nor in the Armed Forces Institute of Pathology fascicle *Tumors of Bone and Cartilage.*[55] In the latter publication, ossifying fibroma and fibrous dysplasia are listed under the heading of "Tumor or tumor-like lesions of fibrous tissue origin." The issue is managed in a less definitive manner by the World Health Organization which categorized fibrous dysplasia as a "tumor-like lesion" but failed to mention ossifying fibroma.[48] It is obvious that the status of the fibro-osseous lesions as a fully defined concept still remains a controversial and elusive one in spite of the more or less conventional use of the term. It is, therefore, not surprising that many pathologists are confronted with a terminologic and sometimes diagnostic dilemma when they are presented with such a lesion from bone. There are also other tumors and tumor-like lesions, particularly in the jaws, which must be differentiated, if possible, from fibrous dysplasia, ossifying fibroma, and cementifying fibroma.

Fibrous dysplasia. Fibrous dysplasia was the first of the fibro-osseous lesions to be recognized and defined as a pathologic process. Albright and co-workers[2] and McCune and Bruch[39] independently described the syndrome of precocious puberty, multiple café-au-lait spots, and polyostotic fibrous dysplasia. In addition to these features, other abnormalities such as diffuse hyperplasia of the thyroid gland (Graves' disease) and myositis ossificans progressiva have been reported.[7, 20] Following the recognition of the polyostotic skeletal lesions, the monostotic variety of fibrous dysplasia was established as an entity by Lichtenstein and Jaffe[37] and later by Schlumberger[49] in his review of 67 bone lesions (rib, 29; femur, 9; tibia, 8; maxilla, 7; calvarium, 5; mandible, 2; humerus, 2; ulna, 2; vertebra, 1; pelvis, 1; and fibula, 1).

The etiology of fibrous dysplasia is unclear, as is the question of whether the lesion represents a true neoplasm or a developmental anomaly in the skeletal system. Its locally aggressive pattern of growth on occasion, the progressive involvement of multiple bones and the development of bone sarcomas such as osteosarcomas or fibrosarcomas without previous irradiation, have been advanced as arguments in favor of its neoplastic nature. The prevailing pathogenetic consideration, on the other hand, espouses the idea that fibrous dysplasia is a developmental process which is characterized by the active proliferation of connective tissue within the medullary cavity that gradually expands the cortex of the affected bone. The bone which forms within the dense fibrous tissue is immature and poorly organized and so is unable to provide the necessary structural support. In the case where multiple bones are involved, there are significant orthopedic abnormalities which are the direct and indirect results of this structural instability.[27] The proposed relationship between von Recklinghausen's neurofibromatosis and fibrous dysplasia is yet another line of argument advanced in favor of the latter disorder being a developmental abnormality.[46] There are some histologic similarities between the metaphyseal fibrous defect-like lesions of von Recklinghausen's neurofibromatosis and fibrous dysplasia. A third and quite obvious pathogenetic and etiologic consideration is that fibrous dysplasia is a manifestation of an incompletely defined endocrinopathy.[61] It has been estimated that 5 to 10% of patients with fibrous dysplasia have hyperparathyroidism, and the association with precocious puberty and hyperthyroidism is well documented when there are multiple bony lesions.[17]

Periodontal membrane. The periodontal membrane is that fibrous structure which surrounds and anchors the tooth within the alveolar bone. Hamner and associates[26] have proposed that the mesenchymal cells of this membrane have the ability to differentiate into cementum, osteoid, and fibrous tissue, and the membrane is, therefore, the site of origin for the ossifying and cementifying fibromas. These authors and Waldron and Giansanti[59] distinguish between the fibro-osseous lesions of periodontal membrane origin and other tumors in the jaws such as fibrous dysplasia, giant cell granuloma, osteoblastoma, desmoplastic fibroma, and aneurysmal bone cyst, which are primarily intramedullary in location. It is true, however, that a particular lesion may attain sufficient size that its relationship or lack of it to the periodontal membrane is not always established through roentgenographic examination.

One of the most important reasons cited in the literature for the differentiation of the periodontal fibro-osseous lesion (ossifying fibroma, cementifying fibroma) from fibrous dysplasia is that the former neoplasms may behave in an aggressive manner.[26] There still remains some question about the consistency and validity of this observation; however, a review of our experience with fibro-osseous lesions in the mandible and maxilla of children revealed a tendency for the cementifying fibromas to recur locally and in some cases require extensive surgery to control the spread of tumor.[15]

This discussion of the differential diagnosis of fibro-osseous lesions of bone is divided into two general headings based upon the anatomic site of the primary tumor, the head and neck including the jaws, and the long bones and other extragnathic locations. It is the spectrum of lesions in the former location which poses the greatest number of problems to the pathologist and to which simple morphologic solutions are the most difficult to apply.

FIBRO-OSSEOUS LESIONS OF THE HEAD AND NECK

Fibrous dysplasia. Fibrous dysplasia of the cranio-facial and jaw bones is generally a monostotic lesion; however, in polyostotic fibrous dysplasia, 40 to 50%

of patients have involvement of the base of the skull or other sites in the head and neck.[27] Approximately one-fourth of all monostotic lesions occur in the head and neck region with a predilection for the mandible and maxilla.[24, 28] Most individuals with solitary lesions are diagnosed before the age of 20 years, and there is a consistent female predilection (2:1)[15, 18] except in the series of 22 cases by Waldron and Giansanti.[58] A slight preference for the maxilla including the antrum and floor of the orbit is noted in a review of 140 lesions (table 1). The body of the mandible with extension posteriorly into the ramus or anteriorly into the symphysis when the lesion is quite large is the usual site and type of involvement in this location. Facial swelling, proptosis, and an intraoral mass are the presenting manifestations of the maxillary and mandibular tumors. Deformity of the skull, proptosis, and visual or auditory difficulties are the principal clinical features of cranial bone involvement.[34] Absence of circumscription and the lack of orientation to the periapical region of the tooth are characteristic roentgenographic findings of fibrous dysplasia in the jaws. The peripheral margins have a tendency to blend imperceptibly into the adjacent normal bone through a transitional zone which can measure 1 cm or more in thickness.[58] Including this zone, most lesions measure from 4 to 8 cm in greatest dimension. The internal pattern of the expansile mass in the mandible or maxilla varies from the homogeneous "ground glass" texture to a mixed radiolucent-radiodense mottled appearance (Fig. 1). Less frequently, the lesion is multilocular or densely sclerotic (Fig. 2). A diffusely sclerotic or hyperostotic type of process is a characteristic feature when the base of the skull or sphenoid ridges are involved (Fig. 3).[34] The frontal, sphenoid, and ethmoid bones are the usual sites of craniofacial fibrous dysplasia.

There is a paucity of macroscopic observations of fibrous dysplasia involving the bones of the head and neck, since in most cases, a limited surgical procedure is utilized in the procurement of tissue for microscopic examination. The exception to this statement occurs in those cases of fibrous dysplasia of the calvarium which is often removed *in toto* (Fig. 4). There is often symmetrical expansion of the medullary cavity by a firm, greyish tan gritty lesion which is poorly delimited from the surrounding normal bone (Fig. 5). On occasion, a solitary cyst or multiple small cysts are present within the mass. This latter feature is seemingly more common as judged by the radiographic changes within some mandibular or maxillary fibrous dysplasias. The cortical bone is invariably attenuated because of fibrous ingrowth and osteoclastic activity, but in the case

TABLE 1. FIBROUS DYSPLASIA OF MANDIBLE AND MAXILLA: DISTRIBUTION OF INVOLVEMENT

Authors	Total cases	Mandible	Maxilla	Both
Zimmerman *et al.*[62]	69	40	28	1
Houston[30]	8	5	3	
Henry[28]	12	6	6	
Dahlgren *et al.*[13]	20	4	16	
Gibson and Middlemiss[24]	9	4	5	
Waldron and Giansanti[58]	22	9	13	—
Total	140	68 (49%)	71 (51%)	1 (<1%)

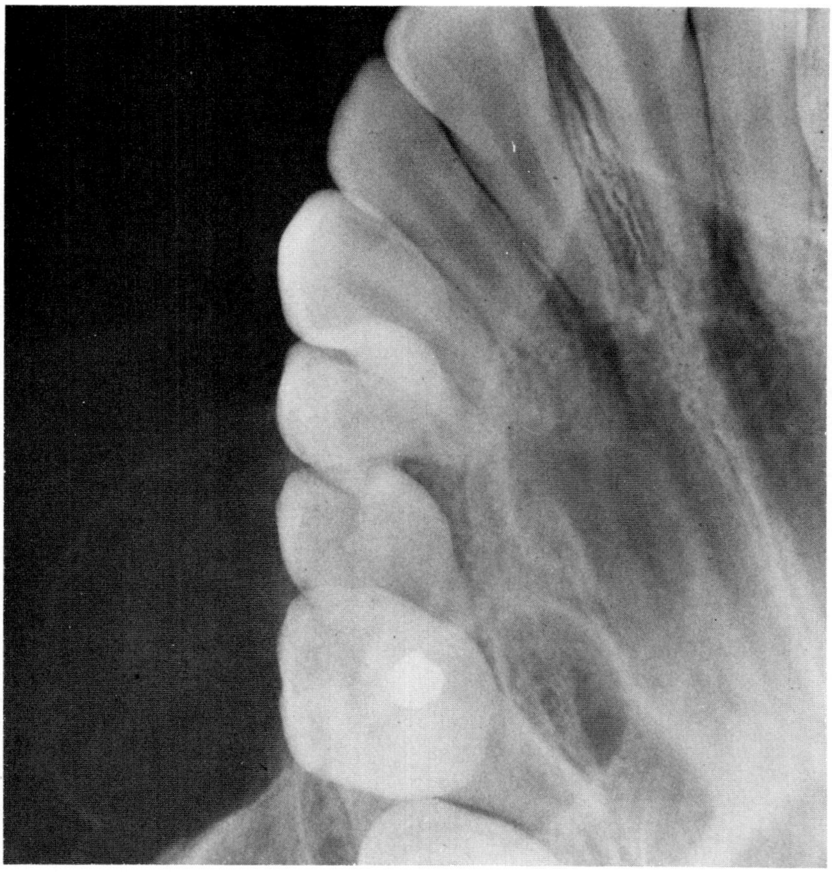

FIG. 1. Fibrous dysplasia of the maxilla in a 15-year-old boy occurring as an expansile, circumscribed radiolucent defect with a slight ground glass appearance.

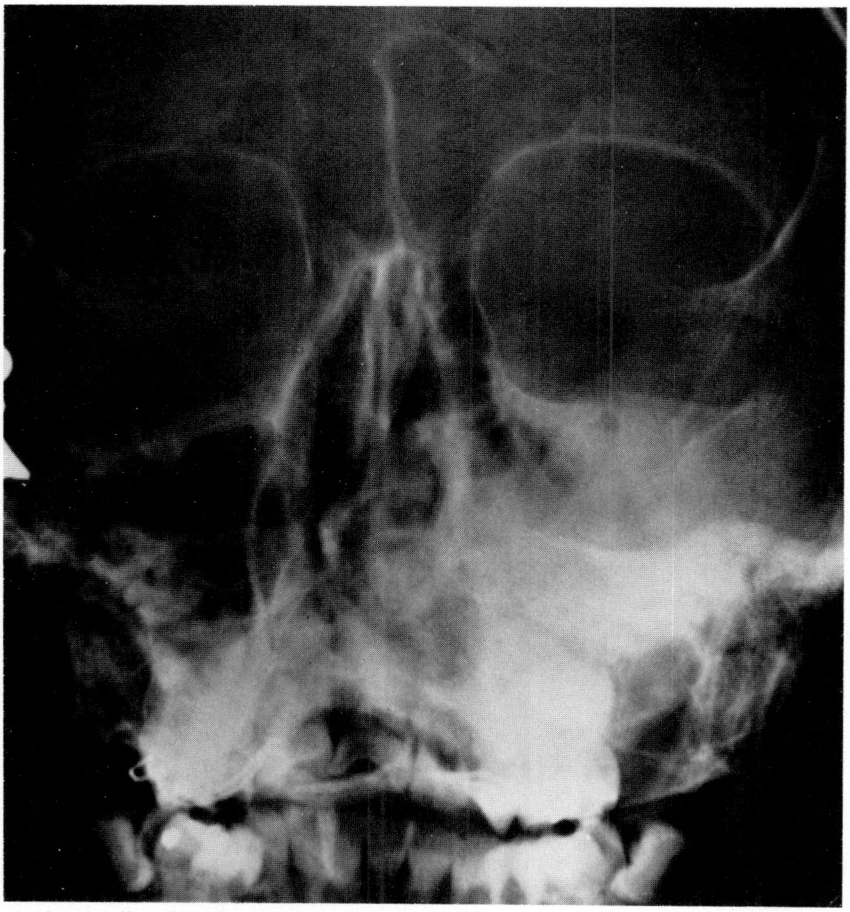

FIG. 2. A partially sclerotic, mottled density with obliteration of the maxillary antrum is another roentgenographic characterization of fibrous dysplasia in the facial bones.

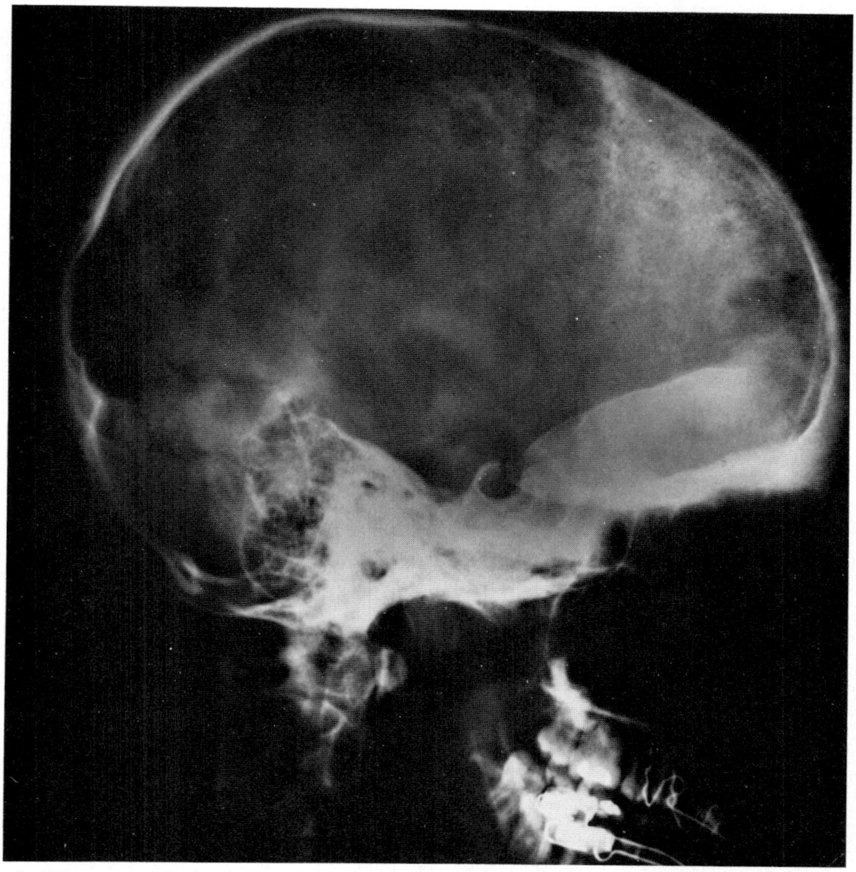

FIG. 3. Fibrous dysplasia of the sphenoid ridge with a densely sclerotic appearance, which must be differentiated from a meningioma in this region.

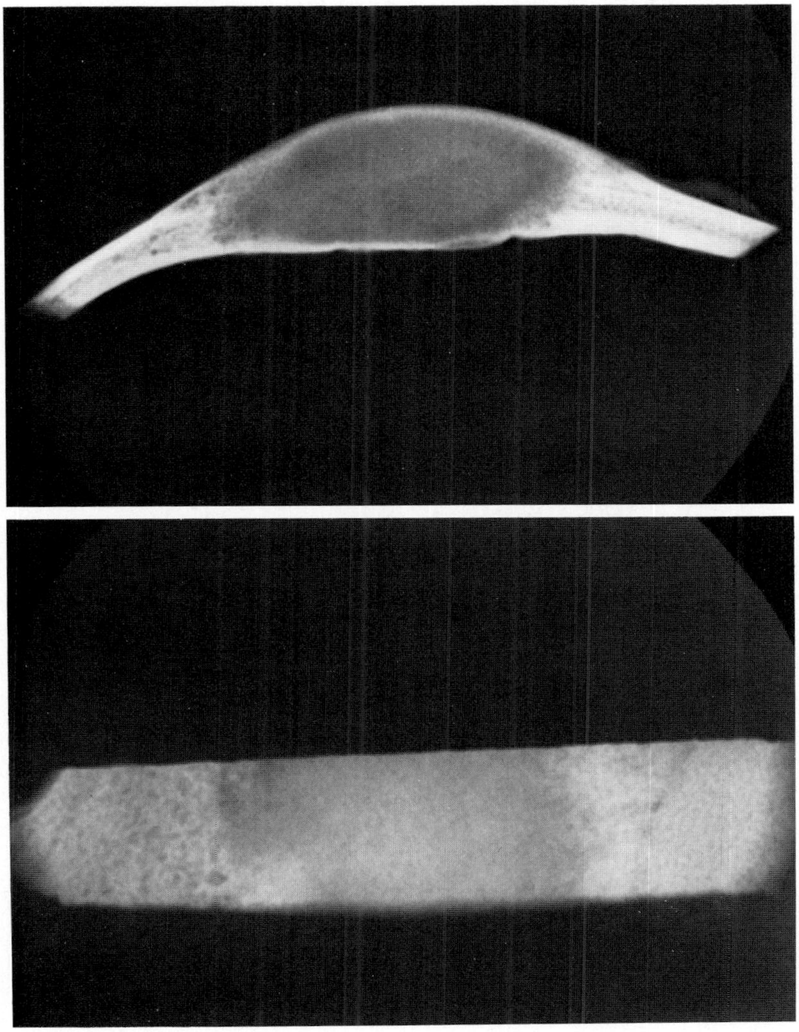

FIG. 4. Fibrous dysplasia of the calvarium as demonstrated in a specimen roentgenogram showing the characteristic ground glass pattern.

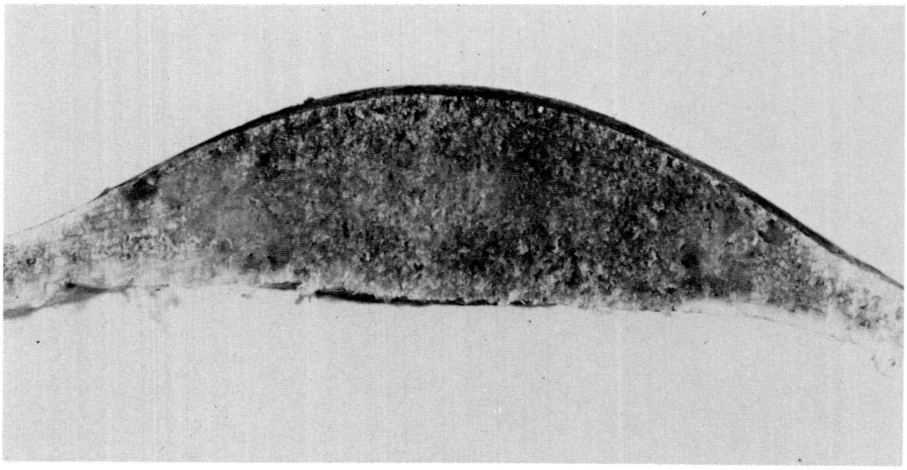

FIG. 5. Fibrous dysplasia of the calvarium showing the typical expansile growth of the lesion and the gradual zone of transition at the periphery.

of some calvarial and sphenoidal lesions, there is osseous thickening resulting from intense osteoblastic activity at the margins. MacMahon[38] has thoroughly documented the hyperostotic changes particularly in the skull at autopsy in a child with Albright-McCune-Sternberg syndrome.

The simplest histologic description of fibrous dysplasia is that of a lesion composed of irregular trabeculae of immature or woven bone set in a background of cellular fibrous stroma (Fig. 6, *A* and *B*). This classic pattern lends support to the hypothesis by Reed[43] that fibrous dysplasia represents an arrest in maturation at the woven bone stage. Unfortunately, especially in the head and neck region, many fibro-osseous lesions eventually designated as fibrous dysplasia do not have the uniform microscopic appearance which is repeatedly illustrated in various textbooks. Eversole and co-workers[18] and Waldron and Giansanti[58] have systematically analyzed the type of calcification and bone formation and noted as others before them that woven bone was the predominant mineralized element. Although many of these trabeculae lack a peripheral rim of osteoblasts, it is not uncommon in our experience to find moderately plump cells which are part of or merge with the adjacent fibrous stroma. In less than 5% of the fibrous dysplasias, multinucleated cells with features of osteoclasts may be quite conspicuous as isolated foci within the lesion. Osteocytes and a prominent internal mosaic pattern with an increase in the basophilic staining are other findings in the trabeculae of the woven bone.

Lamellar bone formation in fibrous dysplasia has been the source of some confusion in the past (Fig. 6*C*). It has been argued that its presence negates the diagnosis, but it has now been demonstrated that some lamellar bone does occur in fibrous dysplasia. In the review of 75 cases of monostotic fibrous dysplasia and 26 cases of craniofacial fibrous dysplasia, lamellar bone was identified in 39 and 27% of lesions, respectively.[18] When lamellar bone is identified, it should be differentiated from that which occurs at the periphery and is responsible, in part, for the marked hyperostosis noted roentgenographically in some lesions. A histologic correlation, although not absolute, has been documented between the

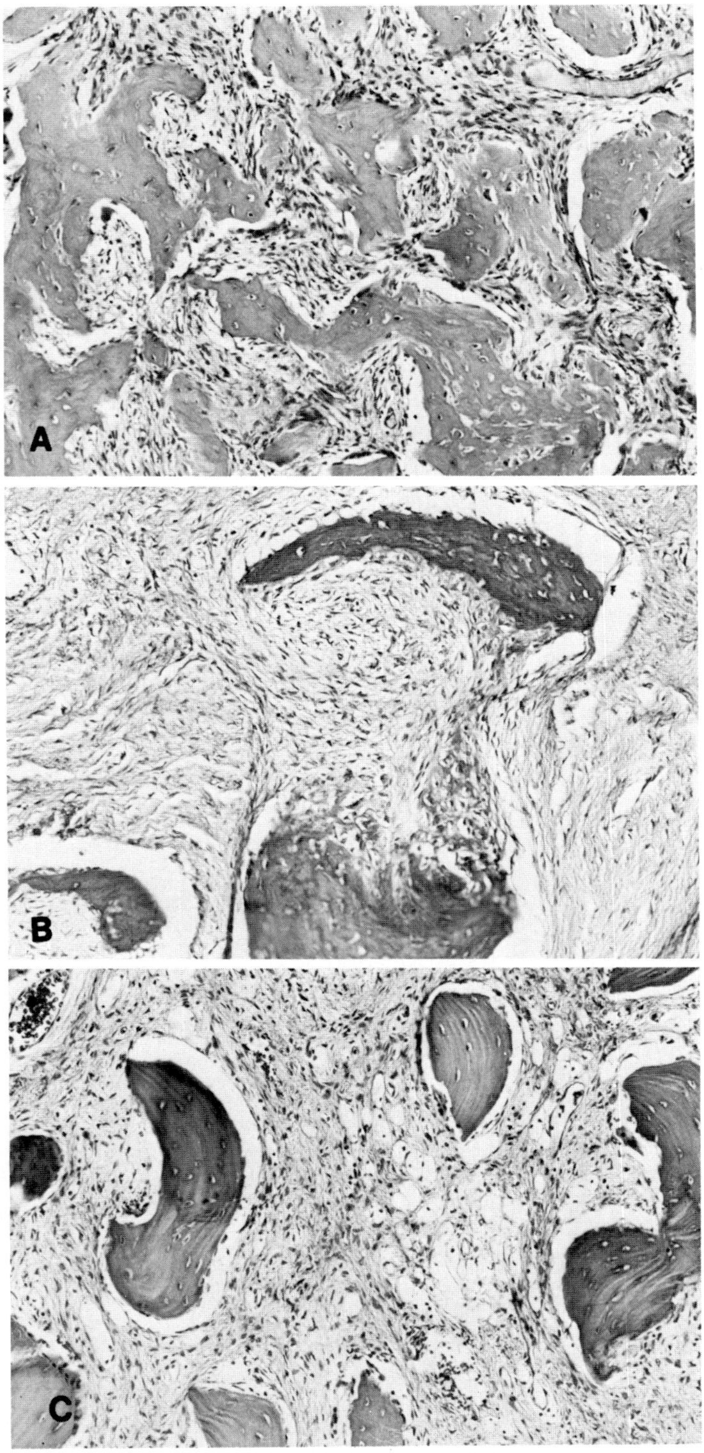

FIG. 6. Fibrous dysplasia of the maxilla with the characteristic pattern of woven bone formation (*A*); another area showing the intimate relationship between the stroma and the immature bone (*B*), and focal lamellar bone formation and foam cells in the stroma (*C*).

presence of thickened lamellar trabeculae and reduced fibrous stroma with the age of the patient.[13] Individuals over the age of 30 years tend to have the more sclerotic, inactive-appearing lesions. We have seen a few exceptions to this generalization.

Spherical islands or masses of mineralized material representing a part or the total pattern of a fibro-osseous lesion are difficult to evaluate in terms of their impact upon the diagnosis (Fig. 7).[62] In the past, such foci have been considered the characteristic appearance of cementum and therefore, they represented cementicles. Spheroid calcifications were identified in 15 to 20% of fibrous dysplasias examined by Eversole and co-workers.[18] A method for the differentiation of osteoid from cementum has been the subject of recent studies through the application of polarization microscopy by Giansanti.[22, 23] Microscopically, the spherical masses rarely dominate the histologic pattern but are noted focally in small clusters adjacent to areas of woven or lamellar bone. A spherical shape is not uniform with some slight variations in outline noted. At the periphery of these islands, a prominent eosinophilic band or immediate abutment of the cellular stroma is present, but rarely is there osteoblastic activity.

The fibrous stroma, especially in the lesions from younger individuals, has an extremely active appearance with plump basophilic nuclei and marked hypercellularity. It is generally difficult to identify mitotic figures. The pattern of spindle fibroblasts does not ordinarily attain a fascicular or storiform configuration. Some fibro-osseous lesions such as fibrous dysplasia may have a predominant fibroblastic appearance with only focal areas of woven bone present in the center of the lesion. In these circumstances when a biopsy of the periphery is taken, it is virtually impossible to distinguish the tumor from a fibromatosis, desmoplastic

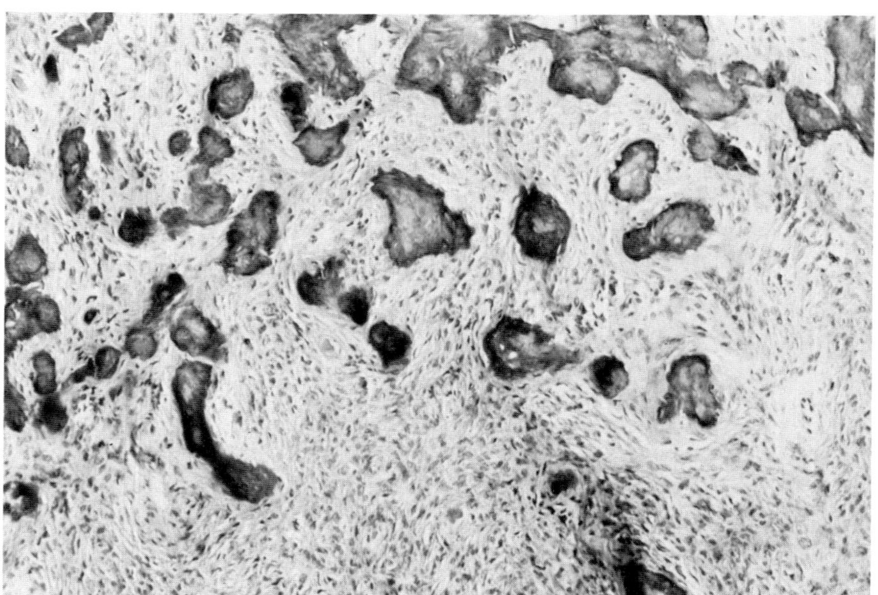

FIG. 7. Spherical islands of calcification resembling cementicles in a fibrous dysplasia of the mandible.

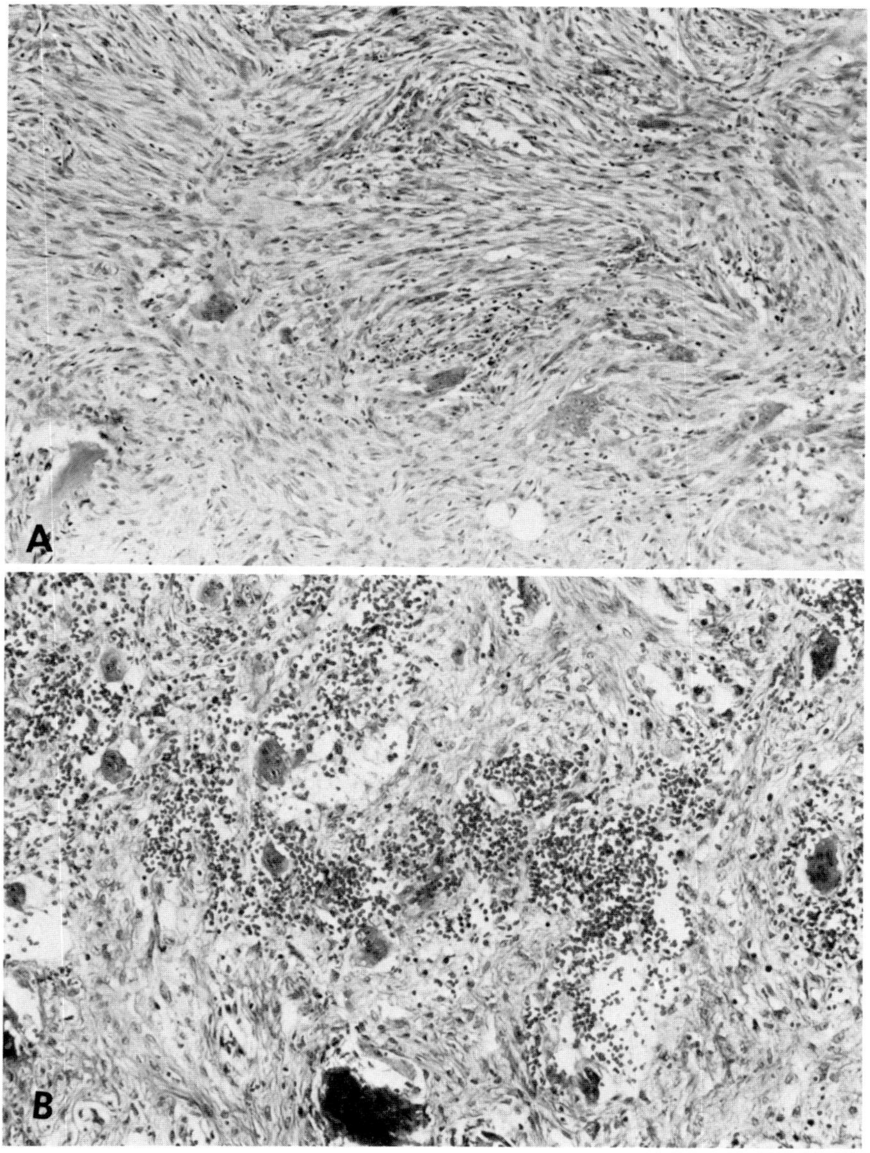

FIG. 8. Focal aggregates of giant cells in a background of fibrous stroma can simulate a giant cell granuloma in the jaws (*A*), particularly when some hemorrhage has occurred (*B*).

fibroma, reactive fibrosis, or a giant cell granuloma (Fig. 8, *A* and *B*). When the fibrous tissue is contained within a loose and edematous background, the differentiation from an odontogenic myxoma becomes necessary.

Dilated vascular spaces are noted sparingly in the stroma, and overall, fibrous dysplasia does not have many recognizable blood vessels. This feature is in marked contrast to the osteoid osteoma-osteoblastoma group of lesions. The focal occurrence of multinucleated giant cells and the cellular stroma in a small biopsy may pose the diagnostic possibility of a giant cell granuloma or fibrous histiocytoma. Aggregates of erythrocytes within luncunae in the stroma which are surrounded by giant cells are the characteristic features of the giant cell granuloma and are rarely observed in fibrous dysplasia or the other fibro-osseous lesions. Inflammatory cells and even foam cells are found in the giant cell granuloma but generally not in the fibro-osseous tumors.

Ossifying fibroma and cementifying fibroma. Ossifying fibroma and cementifying fibroma are considered by Hamner and colleagues[25] as histogenetically related lesions which originate in the periodontal membrane. It is obvious that this explanation is not completely satisfactory, since ossifying fibromas occur in the skull, paranasal sinuses, and even the long bones.[14, 33, 35] The difficulties in the separation of these lesions by clinical, radiographic, and histopathologic criteria has been appreciated in the dental literature through the use of the term "cemento-ossifying fibroma."[25, 54] In a combined review of 292 cases of fibro-osseous lesions of periodontal membrane origin, the patients ranged in age from 7 to 70 years with a female predilection which ranged from 60 to 80%.[26, 59] If symptoms are present, and they generally are not, a painless mass associated with some asymmetry is noted. Proptosis or loss of vision and/or smell are the clinical features when the mass is located in the paranasal sinuses. The mandible is the most common site and is involved in 70 to 80% of cases, particularly the posterior region adjacent to the premolars and molars (75 to 85% of mandibular sites). Midline lesions in the symphysis are infrequent. The remaining 20 to 30% of cementifying or ossifying fibromas, or both, occur in the maxilla with a preference for the posterior portion.[59] Multiple lesions in either the mandible or the maxilla, or both are encountered in less than 20% of patients. The highest reported incidence of multiplicity occurred among the cementoid lesions (18%) in the series from the Armed Forces Institute of Pathology.[26]

There is relatively little to differentiate the cementifying from ossifying fibroma on the basis of the roentgenographic examination in the mandible or maxilla. A well delineated radiolucent defect with minimal to moderate peripheral sclerosis is adjacent to the apex of the tooth. It is uncommon for the mass to measure in excess of 3 to 4 cm in diameter; however, we have seen large tumors fill and obliterate the maxillary antrum.[15] Focally opacified areas can alternate with radiolucent zones within the neoplasms and thus produce a mixed roentgenographic appearance. It is important to distinguish such an appearance in an edentulous area of the jaw as probable focal chronic osteomyelitis.[18] In the paranasal sinuses, the ossifying fibroma is identified as a circumscribed lobulated mass with a predominant lytic or mixed lytic-sclerotic appearance.

Numerous attempts have been made in the past to differentiate cementum and osteoid on the basis of tinctorial, histochemical, and optical variations, but none to date have been entirely satisfactory nor definitive. Hamner and co-workers[26] relied primarily upon the droplet or spheroid character of the cementum with a relatively acellular matrix (Fig. 9). Although plump cells or cementoblasts are recognized at the periphery, they are not as prominent nor as abundant as the osteoblasts in the classic type of ossifying fibroma. As an indication that the droplets or spheroid calcification is not uniformly accepted as characteristic of cementum, Eversole et al.[18] state that 55% of the ossifying fibromas which they examined contained these structures. Other features which have purportedly

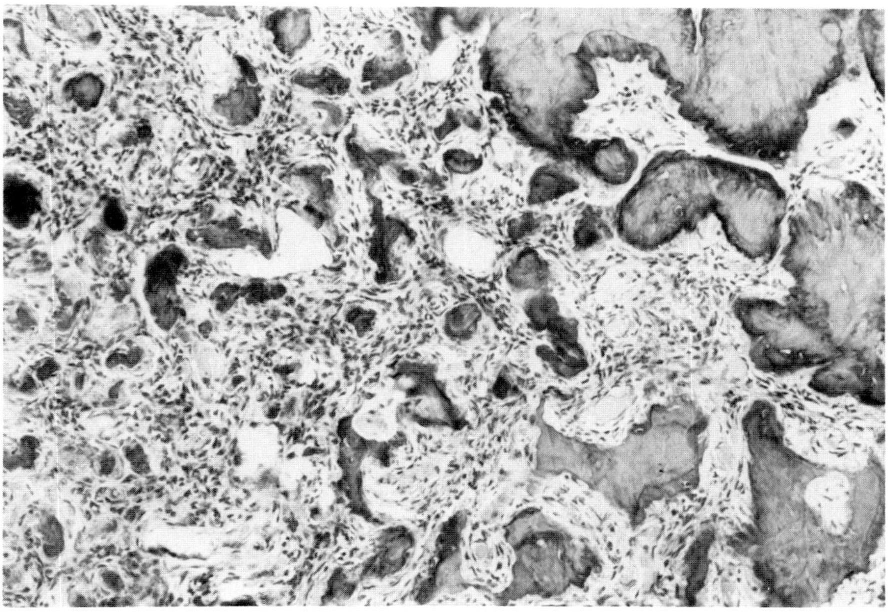

FIG. 9. Droplets of magenta staining material and larger acellular masses in a fibrous background are the features of a cementifying fibroma.

been successful in the identification of the cementum are the staining qualities, *i.e.*, the magenta or deep basophilia of cementum rather than the acidophilia of osteoid with the hematoxylin and eosin stain, and the unique pattern of the collagen bundles in cementum, which is demonstrated through polarization microscopy.[22, 23] The parallel lines of birefringence are delicate in cementum but are more coarse and broad in osteoid. Inconsistencies in these observations occur as evidenced by Eversole and co-workers' evaluation[18] of three periapical lesions which were designated as cementomas or "periapical cemental dysplasias." The curvilinear calcifications had histologic and polarization features of bone rather than cementum.

Once the calcified material within a jaw lesion has been successfully identified as cementum to the pathologist's satisfaction, the second problem is the type of cemental tumor. According to the World Health Organization[42] and in a later analysis of 15 lesions composed primarily of cementum,[59] four basic histologic types of tumors collectively designated as cementomas are recognized (table 2). The periapical cemental dysplasia and cementifying fibroma are the two lesions which are the most difficult to distinguish from fibrous dysplasia and ossifying fibroma, respectively. In some cases, the histologic differentiation is arbitrary and artificial. Cementoblastoma is a relatively uncommon tumor which occurs as a solitary, slowly expansile mass in the molar and premolar region of the mandible more frequently than in the maxilla.[1, 12] Most lesions are diagnosed in the 2nd and 3rd decades of life. Unlike the cementifying fibroma and periapical cemental dysplasia, which produces radiolucent defects, the cementoblastoma shows central sclerosis with a peripheral zone of radiolucency around the root of a normal tooth (Fig. 10, *A* and *B*). The size of the lesion usually does not exceed 2 to

TABLE 2. CHARACTERISTICS OF FOUR TYPES OF CEMENTOMA[a]

	Benign cementoblastoma	Cementifying fibroma	Periapical cemental dysplasia	Gigantiform cementoma
Location	Mandibular premolar or molar region. Attached to tooth	Mostly mandibular premolar or molar region	Mostly mandibular incisor region	Multiple; often symmetrical
Sex	Mostly male	No known sex predilection	Mostly female	Mostly Negro females
Age	Under 25 years	Middle age	Postmenopausal	Middle age
Radiographic features	Mottled or dense mass with radiolucent periphery; attached to roots; roots resorbed	Well demarcated radiolucent area containing varying amounts of dense material	Radiolucent in early stages, then central opacity; finally, may be dense throughout	Dense masses, often lobulated; no radiolucent border
Histological features	Hard tissue with very many reversal lines; sheets of uncalcified "cementoid," especially at periphery	Mainly rounded deeply-staining "cementicles," sometimes fusing	Mixture of rounded "cementicles," larger cementum-like masses, and woven bone	Large sheets of tissue closely resembling secondary cementum; many empty lacunae; few vascular channels

[a] From Pindborg, J. J., and Kramer, I. R. H.[42]

3 cm in diameter. Grossly, the curetted tissue has a gritty bonelike consistency as expected from the radiographic appearance. There is active proliferation of mineralized trabeculae with plump cells at the periphery and a hypervascular and hypercellular stroma (Fig. 10*C*). In general, the stroma lacks the compactness of the other fibro-osseous lesions such as the fibrous dysplasia and cemento-ossifying fibroma. The cementoblastoma in its roentgenographic and pathologic features most closely resembles osteoid osteoma and osteoblastoma.[10, 16] Both of these benign osteoblastic lesions, which are related morphologic variants, are uncommon in the head and neck region.[44] Still, the persistent problem remains for the pathologist to try to distinguish osteoid from cementum. Gigantiform cementoma can present as multiple, lobulated radiodense lesions in the jaws.[50] Large globular, acellular masses without a significant stromal background are the principal histologic findings associated with this tumor. There are some similarities with the osteoma of the paranasal sinuses.

Ossifying fibroma and fibrous osteoma are equivalent designations for the fibro-osseous lesion which in the mandible or maxilla is associated with identical roentgenographic findings as the cementifying fibroma. Among the 15 fibro-osseous lesions of the jaws in children which we reviewed, there were four (27%) ossifying fibromas, 2 each in the mandible and maxilla.[15] The well circumscribed nature of these tumors facilitates surgical enucleation. Microscopically, the bony trabeculae are composed entirely of lamellar bones which are lined by a more or less continuous rim of osteoblasts and occasionally multinucleated osteoclasts (Fig. 11, *A* and *B*). There are few, if any, cement lines producing a mosaic pattern in the ossifying fibroma in contrast to the fibrous dysplasia and occasionally the cementifying fibroma. Osteocytes are also evenly distributed within the osseous trabeculae, but the number of cells in the calcified islands of cementum is, for the most part, markedly reduced in quantity. The fibroblastic stroma of the ossifying fibroma, cementifying fibroma, and fibrous dysplasia is essentially identical. An important point in the differential diagnosis of the ossifying fibroma from osteoblastoma is the quality of the stroma which in the former lesion resembles

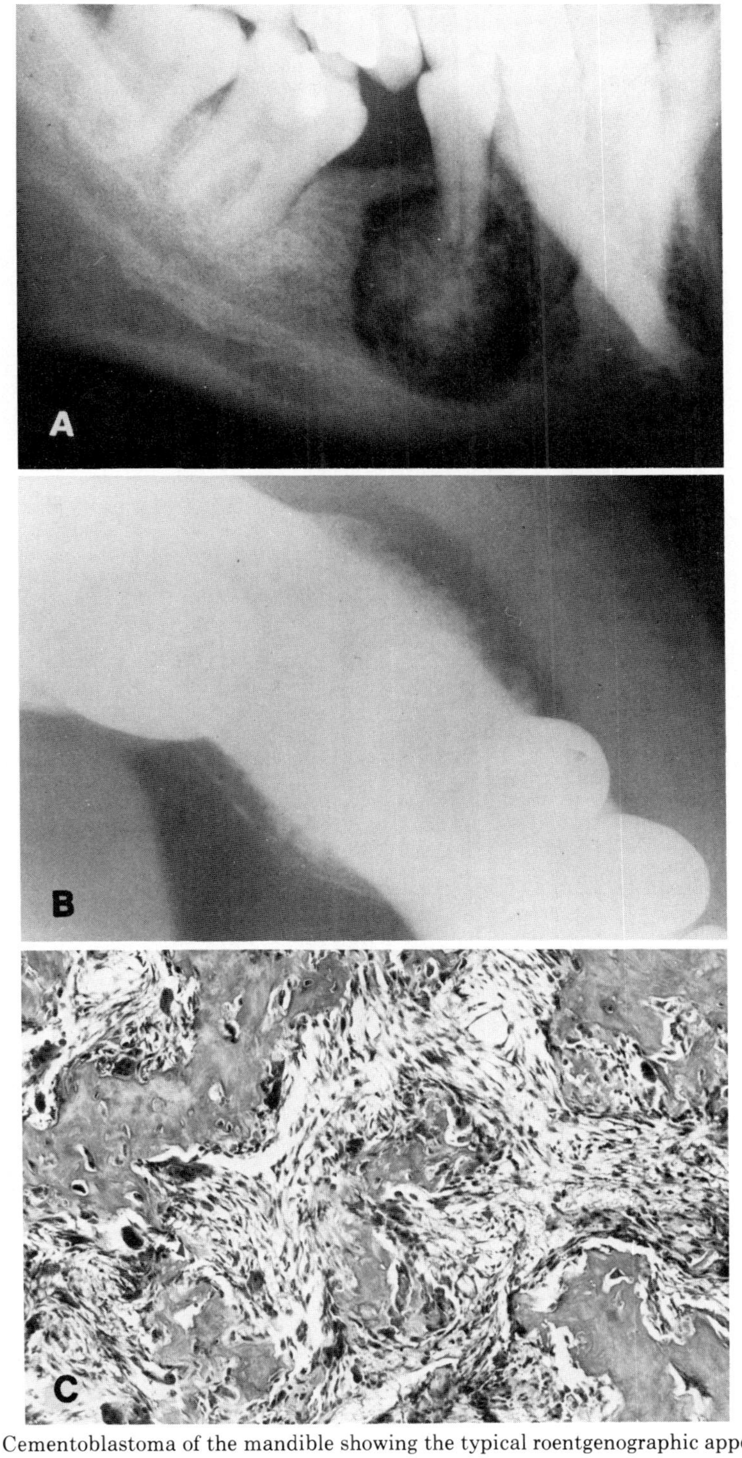

FIG. 10. Cementoblastoma of the mandible showing the typical roentgenographic appearance and orientation around the root of the tooth (*A*, *B*). The microscopic features are similar to those of an osteoblastoma (*C*). (*A* and *B* from Abrams, A. M., Kirby, J. W., and Melrose, R. J.[1] used with permission.)

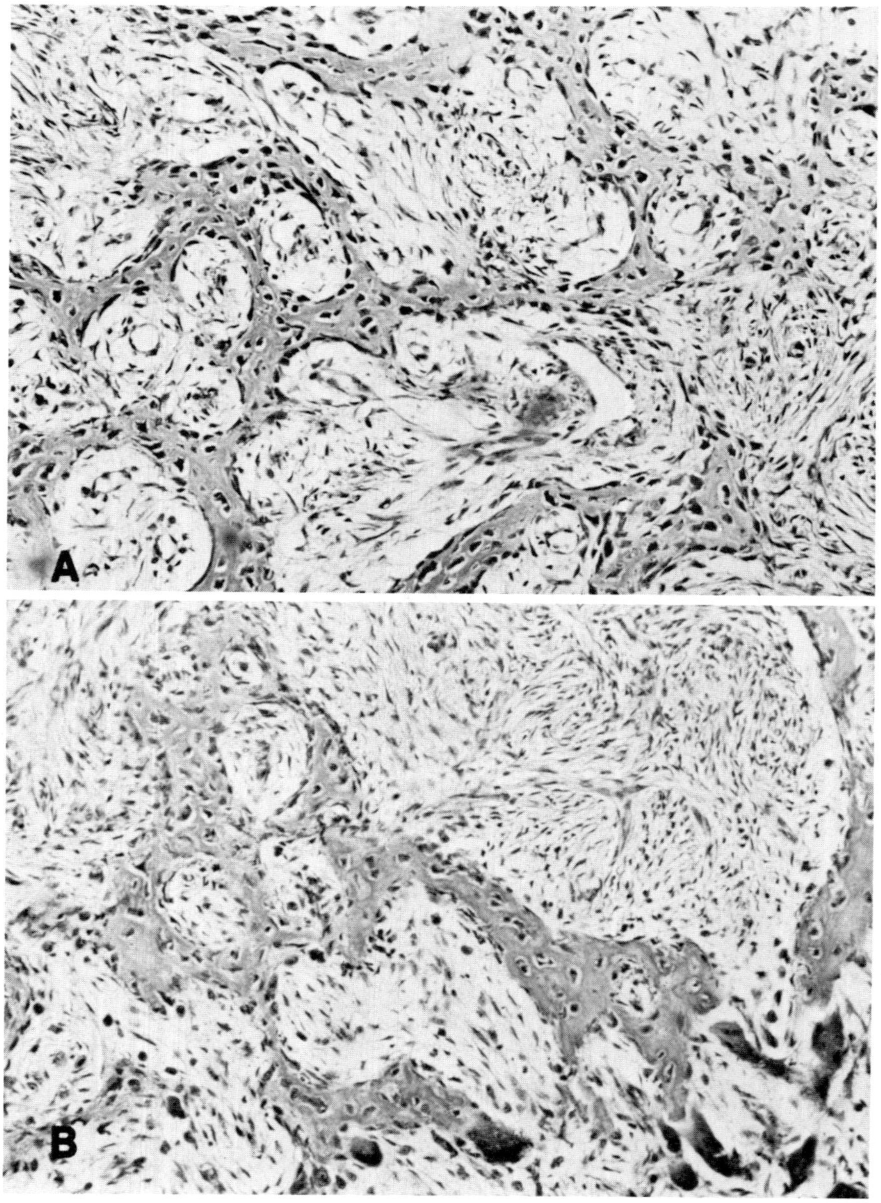

FIG. 11. Ossifying fibroma of the maxilla with osteoblasts lining the bony trabeculae (*A*) and foci showing some osteoclastic activity (*B*).

that of a fibromatosis. The stroma of the osteoblastoma is extremely vascular, and the individual cells are plump and loosely cohesive. Unlike the cellular mesenchyme of the osteosarcoma, there is little nuclear hyperchromatism and few bizarre gigantiform cells, or mitotic figures in either the ossifying fibroma or osteoblastoma.

Mixed fibro-osseous tumors. Mixed fibro-osseous tumors are those lesions with a combination of histopathologic features, usually cementoid and osteoid foci (cemento-ossifying fibroma).[26] The problems of an exact histologic designation are compounded further with the identification of areas of woven bone. Eversole and co-workers[18] have well illustrated and documented the morphologic variations associated with the fibro-osseous lesions. It has been our experience with the mixed fibro-osseous lesions that the roentgenographic appearance is that of a circumscribed radiolucent defect rather than the diffuse pattern of a fibrous dysplasia.

Central fibroma. Central fibroma is a tumor occurring in the periapical region of the tooth and according to Hamner and associates[26] originates from the periodontal membrane like the ossifying and cementifying fibromas. Its radiographic features are similar to the latter lesions, but its incidence is considerably lower. The histologic distinction between the central fibroma and the desmoplastic fibroma is subtle at best. A moderately cellular fibrous stroma characterizes both lesions; however, the degree of cellularity is more variable from one area of the tumor to another in the desmoplastic fibroma.[29] Osseous metaplasia and islands of odontogenic epithelium are absent in both tumors. The combination of fibrous stroma with foci of odontogenic epithelium are the histologic features of an ameloblastic fibroma.[56] Its multilocular character as demonstrated by roentgenography is significantly different from the fibro-osseous lesions. Intraosseous neurofibroma and odontogenic myxoma must also be included in the differential diagnosis of jaw masses resembling fibrous neoplasms.[5, 11, 52] Giant cell granuloma and cherubism are other tumor-like conditions of the jaws with a prominent fibrous component which in the periphery may be completely devoid of giant cells. There are also differences roentgenographically which allow for an accurate diagnosis.[3, 6, 60] Microscopically, the definitive areas are located toward the central zones where the multinucleated giant cells are aggregated around lacunae filled with erythrocytes and plasma. The "brown tumor" of hyperparathyroidism has histologic features which are virtually identical to the giant cell granuloma.

Chronic osteomyelitis. Chronic osteomyelitis associated with marked sclerosis particularly in the premolar and molar regions is confused, on occasion, with a fibro-osseous lesion.[18, 41] The admonition is given that the diagnosis of a fibro-osseous lesion in an edentulous area of the jaw should be made with extreme reluctance. There are many potential traps for the pathologist, since the reactive new bone formation and fibrosis of chronic osteomyelitis can simulate ossifying fibroma. If fragments of necrotic bone or plasma cells are identified in the biopsy, the potential error can be side-stepped. A certain reliance upon the radiographic findings is another method of avoiding a misdiagnosis.

CLINICOPATHOLOGIC CORRELATION AND PROGNOSIS

The confusion which tends to surround the histologic diagnosis of a fibro-osseous lesion of the head and neck, especially of the jaws, as one might expect, is transmitted to the clinicopathologic factors that affect the prognosis. There are contradictory statements regarding the malignant potential of fibrous dysplasia and the reduced rate of growth of this lesion with the onset of adolescence. Another point of variance is the constancy of locally aggressive behavior associated with the cementifying fibroma.[26, 59]

Fibrous dysplasia. Fibrous dysplasia as a recurrent process in the bone regardless of the anatomic location is a difficult problem to evaluate, for most lesions are not excised *in toto.* This particular point is emphasized by Zimmerman and associates,[62] who prefer to designate the lesion in such circumstances as a persistence. In the review of their experience at the Mayo Clinic, persistent fibrous dysplasia of the jaws occurred in 19% of patients who developed an increase in the size of the mass after initial surgery, usually within 2 or 3 years. The poor circumscription of the lesion contributes significantly to the relatively high frequency of persistence. We have been unable to correlate the degree of histologic activity, *i.e.*, the cellularity of the stroma and amount of woven bone formation, with the biologic behavior. It is generally correct that fibrous dysplasia from older individuals contains more lamellar bone and collagen, and there are fewer cells in the fibrous stroma.[32]

Primary sarcomas are reported in bones affected by fibrous dysplasia, and in a review of 33 cases of sarcomatous transformation, 13 involved the craniofacial bones.[53] The mandible (3 cases) was the only affected facial bone among the 12 patients with fibrous dysplasia and sarcoma of the bone studied by Huvos and co-workers.[31] A sarcoma developed 15 and 25 years after the original diagnosis of fibrous dysplasia in 2 patients, and a simultaneous diagnosis of fibrous dysplasia-sarcoma was established in the 3rd case. Prior irradiation therapy was not a historical consideration in the occurrence of the sarcoma in these 3 patients as it has been in some other patients. The question whether irradiation poses any greater hazard to the development of sarcoma in fibrous dysplasia above that reported in the literature with bones in general remains open at this time.[4] Osteosarcoma is the most common histologic type of neoplasm.

Although the author as well as others has studied examples of cementifying fibromas which behaved in an extremely aggressive manner with multiple local recurrences, the overall impression is that the majority of lesions is successfully controlled after the initial excision or curettage.[15] An analysis of the pathologic features in these two clinical groups (recurrent *versus* nonrecurrent tumors) fails to disclose any significant differences in terms of size and histopathologic characteristics. There is an impression, however, that cementifying fibromas of the maxilla are more prone to recur. Cementoblastoma responds well to local excision, and in spite of its disquieting microscopic features, the clinical behavior is rather indolent.[1]

Ossifying fibroma is usually a well circumscribed lesion, and for that reason, it is readily enucleated from the affected bone in most cases. It is uncommon for an ossifying fibroma to recur. Microscopically, the findings are rarely disturbing enough to consider the diagnosis of osteosarcoma, but we have seen cases where the differentiation from osteoblastoma was difficult.

FIBRO-OSSEOUS LESIONS OF THE LONG BONES AND EXTRAGNATHIC SITES

The interpretation of a fibro-osseous lesion in terms of the pathologic diagnosis is a far less complicated problem when sites outside of the head and neck region are affected. Fibrous dysplasia occurring as solitary (monostotic) or multiple (polyostotic) bony defects is, by far, the most common histologic type of fibro-osseous lesion in the extragnathic cranial skeletal system. There are individual case reports of cementomas and ossifying fibromas originating in the long bones.[21, 33]

Fibrous dysplasia. Fibrous dysplasia as a monostotic lesion occurs most frequently in the femur, tibia, and rib, but no bone is immune from involvement.[19, 24, 28, 32] Although most patients in the series from the Massachusetts General Hospital[27] had polyostotic lesions (74%), the general experience is that 75 to 80% of those with fibrous dysplasia have the solitary variety. There is a similar female predilection as noted in the head and neck area. The diagnosis is usually not established until late childhood or young adulthood when one bone is involved, but in the more severe types of polyostotic fibrous dysplasia, there are clinical manifestations present before 1 year of age. Bone pain unaccompanied by fracture, precocious puberty, and multiple fractures, many of which are pathologic in type, are some of the early symptoms and signs in patients with polyostotic lesions.[27] An incidental radiographic finding, a palpable mass, bone pain, or a pathologic fracture are the various means by which monostotic fibrous dysplasia comes to clinical attention. Most "silent" lesions are identified in a rib, whereas the pathologic fractures occur in long bones.[24]

A diaphyseal defect with cortical expansion and no sign of destruction is the characteristic radiographic appearance of a monostotic lesion. The central portion is generally radiolucent; however, a trabeculated or multicystic change may also occur. In some cases, these features are accompanied by a pathologic fracture. The differential diagnosis includes enchondroma, unicameral bone cyst, fibrous cortical defect (metaphyseal fibrous defect, nonossifying fibroma), aneurysmal bone cyst, and giant cell tumor. It is important to obtain a biopsy specimen of the solitary lesion because of the lack of roentgenographic specificity. Harris and co-workers[27] state that the diagnosis of monostotic fibrous dysplasia should not be accepted without histologic confirmation. The situation regarding the necessity for a biopsy is somewhat different when multiple bones are involved.[32] Among the bones which are affected in 50% or greater of cases of polyostotic fibrous dysplasia are the femur, tibia, fibula, ilium, metacarpals-metatarsals, ribs, and humerus.[24, 27] Expansion of the cortex with relatively little thinning by a diaphyseal-metaphyseal radiolucent process is the typical roentgenographic alteration (Fig. 12). A loculated or trabeculated appearance is another variation of the internal pattern which is less frequent than the translucent or ground glass change. The margins are either circumscribed with a sclerotic rim, or they blend into the adjacent bone. Marked bowing of the bones especially in the neck and proximal shaft of the femur produces the so-called "shepherd's crook" deformity (Fig. 13). Extension of previous lesions, formation of new lesions, and increasing deformities are the roentgenographic signs which are associated with the progression of polyostotic fibrous dysplasia.

An intact periosteum contains the symmetrically expansile, greyish tan granular lesion in the bone with a solitary fibrous dysplasia. The cortex is often completely eroded, which differs from the cortex in the polyostotic lesion, which may appear normal or even thickened as in the case of the skull or its base. One of the major histologic differences between fibrous dysplasia in bones outside of the head and neck region is the more uniform microscopic appearance. Trabeculae of

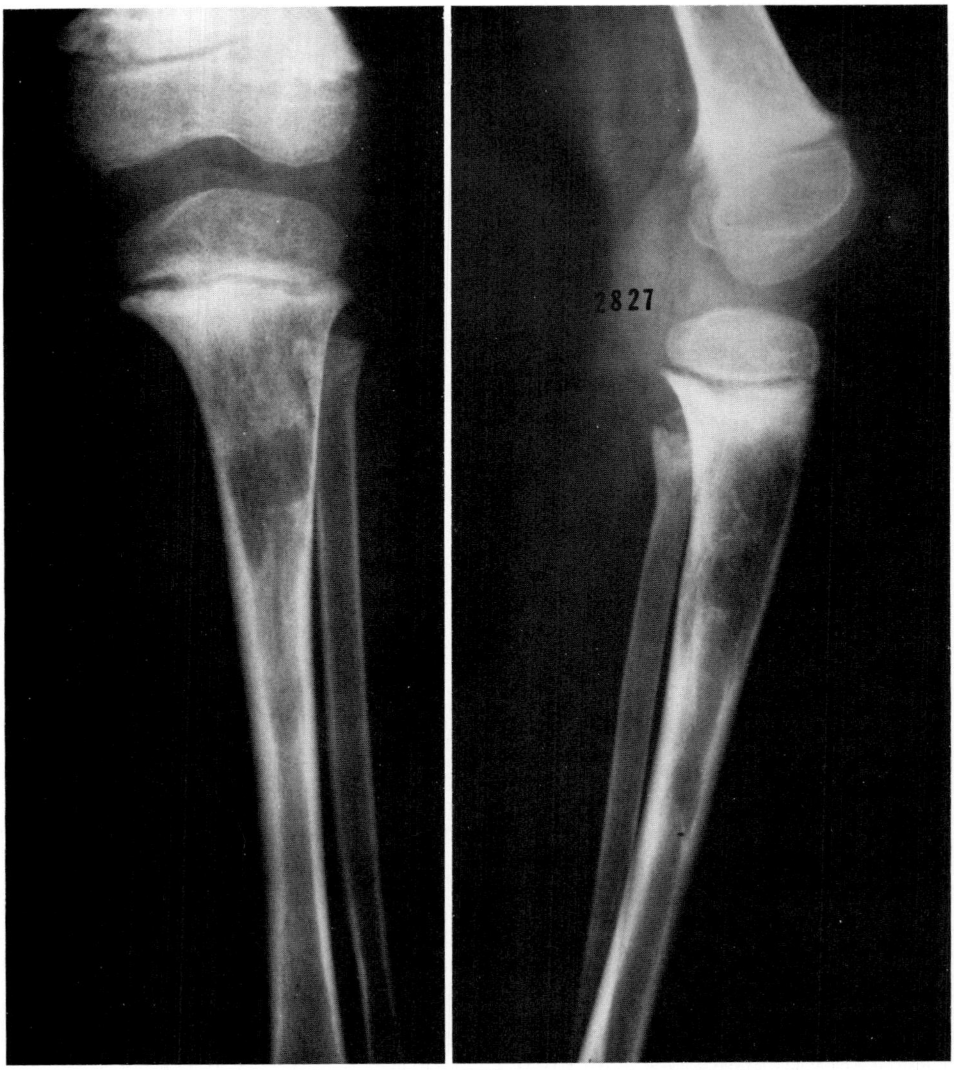

FIG. 12. Anteroposterior and lateral views of fibrous dysplasia of the tibia showing irregular expansion and trabeculation of the medullary canal.

woven bone are irregularly distributed within a connective tissue stroma. Occasional islands of bone outlined by osteoblasts and spherical masses are relatively uncommon when compared to their occurrence in the mandible and maxilla. There are some variations in the histology which can be the source of difficulties in the pathologic interpretation: (1) a fracture with the resulting hemorrhage, giant cells, foam cells, and new bone formation; (2) aneurysmal bone cyst with fibrous dysplasia; and (3) foci of hyaline cartilage occurring in a minority of cases (10 to 15%) of polyostotic fibrous dysplasia.[27, 38] The association between aneurysmal bone cyst and fibrous dysplasia has been thoroughly reviewed by Biesecker et al.,[8] Buraczewski and Dabska,[9] and Levy and co-workers.[36] A fibrous cortical defect or giant cell tumor is a consideration in the

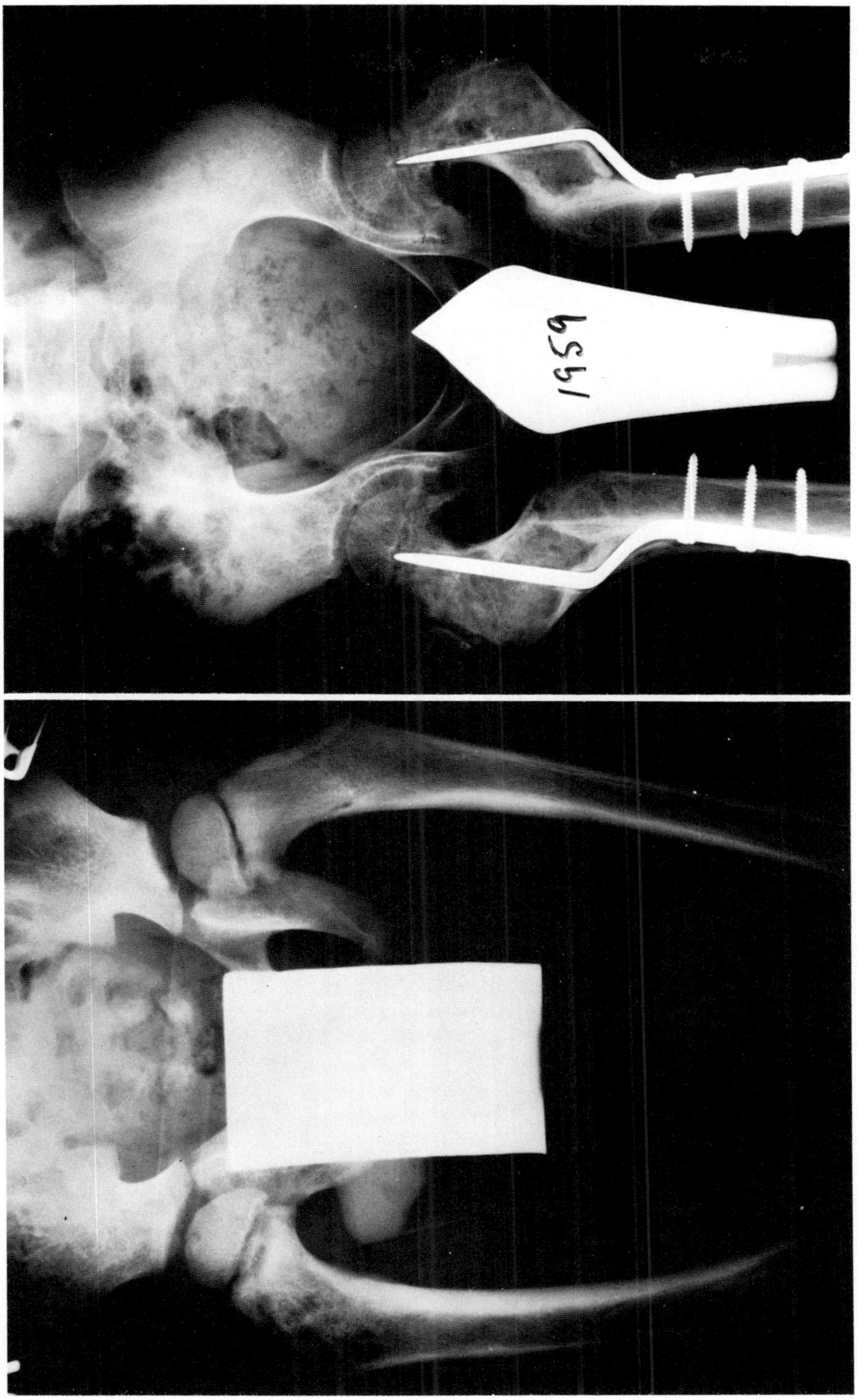

FIG. 13. Progression of the "shepherd's crook" deformities of the femora in a patient with polyostotic fibrous dysplasia.

histologic differential diagnosis when a limited biopsy fails to disclose the characteristic woven bone. If a biopsy is taken through a purely fibroblastic area, then desmoplastic fibroma and fibrosarcoma are other possible diagnoses. Osteosarcoma is simulated when a fracture occurs through fibrous dysplasia or in a lesion from a young child.[55]

Sarcomatous transformation of fibrous dysplasia. Sarcomatous transformation of fibrous dysplasia has been reported most often in the long bones particularly the femur and tibia.[45] This finding obviously corresponds to the frequency with which these bones are involved in fibrous dysplasia. Although the specific figures are not available, it must be assumed that the development of a sarcoma in fibrous dysplasia is a relatively rare event. The risk among patients with polyostotic lesions is seemingly greater, judging from the available reports.[31, 45] Osteosarcoma is the most common type of malignant tumor; however chondrosarcomas, fibrosarcomas, and anaplastic neoplasms without significant differentiation are also described (Fig. 14).[45] The prognosis, as one might anticipate, is rather poor.

Ossifying fibroma. Ossifying fibroma rarely occurs in sites other than the mandible, maxilla, or paranasal sinuses. Kempson[33] has thoroughly studied the features of the lesion in the tibias of two children, both 4 years of age. There was little to distinguish these tumors from fibrous dysplasia on the basis of the roentgenographic examination. Microscopically, the spicules of lamellar bone are surrounded by a continuous rim of osteoblasts and some osteoclasts. The number of cases of ossifying fibroma in the literature is insufficient to provide an adequate appraisal of the clinical behavior in extracranial and extragnathic location.

Cementoma. Cementoma has been reported in the femur and humerus of 2 children, ages 6 and 7 years, respectively.[21] In both cases, the roentgenographic appearance was that of a multicystic lesion located in the metaphysis associated with expansion of the cortex but with no evidence of destruction. Spheroid islands of calcification occurring in clusters and evenly distributed within a fibrous stroma are the principal histologic features (Fig. 15). One of these lesions was personally examined, and the findings including the polarization microscopy are essentially identical to those of the cementoid tumors of the jaws. An explanation for the occurrence of a cementoma in the long bones would obviously entail only hopeless speculation.

SUMMARY

In spite of all that has been written, including this review, the fibro-osseous lesions of bone continue as a problem to the pathologist in terms of histologic definition, nosology, and pathogenesis. A basic question regarding the developmental or neoplastic nature of fibrous dysplasia, ossifying fibroma, and cementifying fibroma remains unanswered, although the prevailing opinion exists that fibrous dysplasia, at least, represents some type of maturational defect in the bone. There are some generalizations about these lesions which are valid in the majority of cases. Fibrous dysplasia is the most common histologic variant of the fibro-osseous lesions, and in 75 to 80% of patients, it occurs as a solitary defect in one of the long bones, usually the femur and tibia. The remaining cases of fibrous

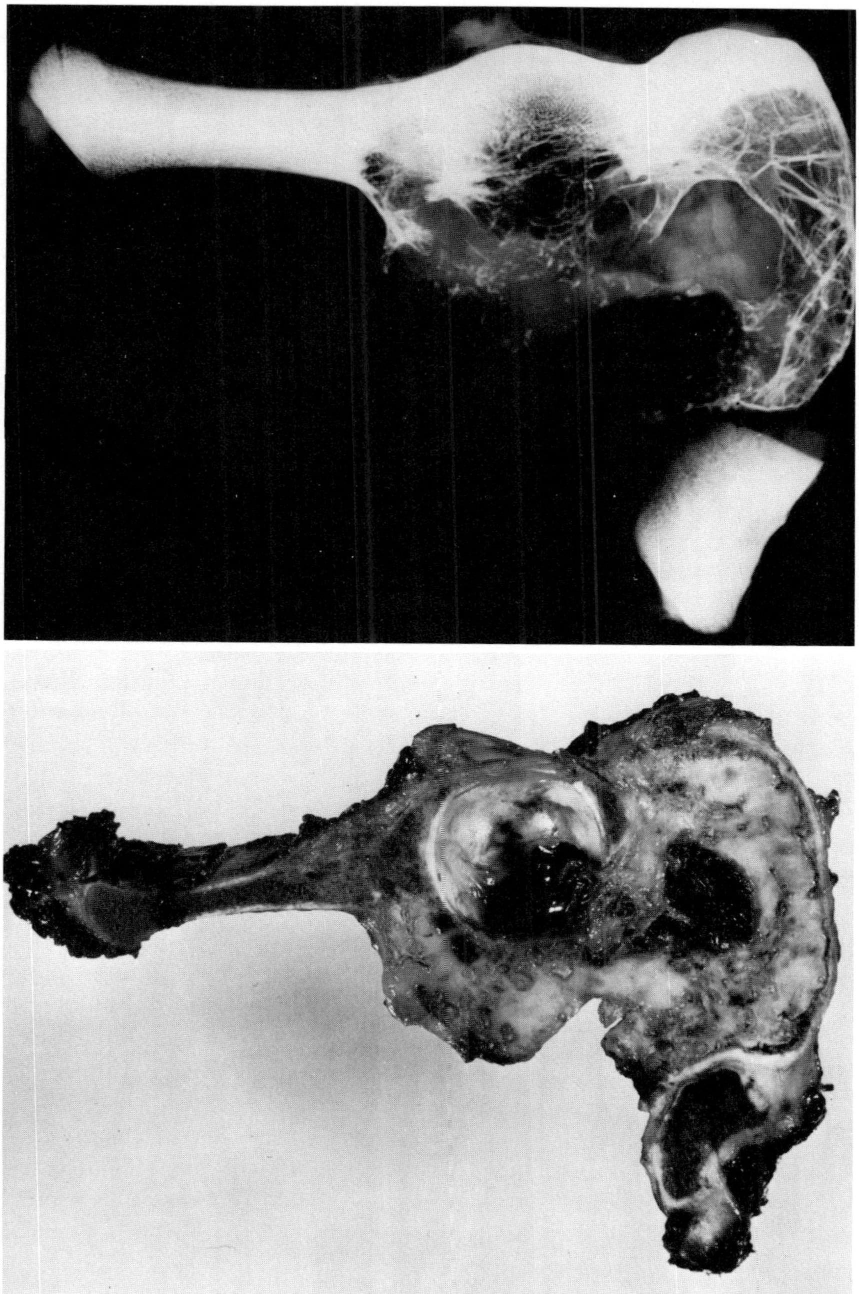

FIG. 14. Chondrosarcoma occurring in the ilium, ischium, and pubis of a 19-year-old female with proven fibrous dysplasia in these bones (From Huvos, A. G., Higinbotham, N. L., and Miller, T. R.[31] (Used with permission.)

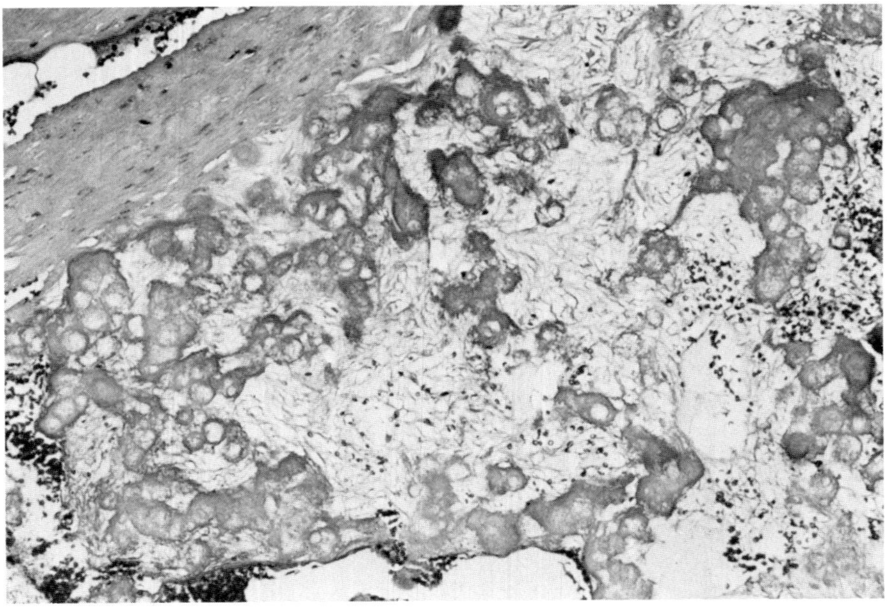

FIG. 15. Cementoma of the femur showing the characteristic spherical islands or droplets with the tinctorial and optical qualities of cementum. (Courtesy of Dr. N. B. Friedman, Los Angeles, California.)

dysplasia (20 to 25%) have multiple bone involvement. Craniofacial and jaw bones contain lesions in 40 to 50% of those individuals with polyostotic fibrous dysplasia, but only 20 to 25% of monostotic defects are located in the head and neck region. An earlier onset of symptoms and progression of the disease with severe orthopedic deformities are constant features of polyostotic fibrous dysplasia. The ill-defined roentgenographic appearance of fibrous dysplasia in the mandible and maxilla permits its differentiation from the other fibro-osseous lesions. In the long bones, the monostotic radiolucent defect requires a biopsy to establish its exact diagnosis. The uncomplicated histologic pattern of fibrous dysplasia is that of irregular trabeculae of immature or woven bone in a cellular fibrous stroma. With some exceptions, most monostotic lesions of long bones have this appearance. Difficulties in the histologic interpretation occur as a result of lamellar bone formation and spherical calcifications in fibrous dysplasia of the jaw bones.

Ossifying and cementifying fibromas are very similar lesions by any parameter which is examined. The cementifying fibroma like the other cemental tumors should, by definition, be related to the root of a tooth. An underlying problem in the differential diagnosis of ossifying and cementifying fibroma is the morphologic distinction between osteoid and cementum. Polarization microscopy among other techniques has been utilized to define this difference. It has been our experience that the results are often indeterminate. In some cases, a diagnosis of mixed fibro-osseous lesion or cemento-ossifying fibroma is the simplest and most honest interpretation. There is some evidence to show that the differentiation is important prognostically, since the cementifying fibroma can pursue a locally aggressive course which may require radical local surgery in order to control the disease.

REFERENCES

1. Abrams, A. M., Kirby, J. W., and Melrose, R. J.: Cementoblastoma; a clinical-pathologic study of seven new cases. *Oral Surg. 38:* 394–403, 1974.
2. Albright, F., Butler, A. M., Hampton, A. O., and Smith, P.: Syndrome characterized by osteitis fibrosa disseminata, areas of pigmentation and endocrine dysfunction, with precocious puberty in females. *N. Engl. J. Med. 216:* 727–746, 1937.
3. Andersen, L., Fejerskov, O., and Philipsen, H. P.: Oral giant cell granulomas; a clinical and histological study of 129 new cases. *Acta Pathol. Microbiol. Scand. A 81:* 606–616, 1973.
4. Arlen, M., Higinbotham, N. L., Huvos, A. G., Marcove, R. C., Miller, T., and Shah, I. C.: Radiation-induced sarcoma of bone. *Cancer 28:* 1087–1099, 1971.
5. Barros, R. E., Dominguez, F. V., and Cabrini, R. L.: Myxoma of the jaws. *Oral Surg. 27:* 225–236, 1969.
6. Batsakis, J. G., and Rice, D. H.: Diseases affecting the jaws. III. Giant cell lesions and fibrous dysplasia of the jaws. *Univ. Mich. Med. Cent. J. 35:* 162–169, 1969.
7. Benedict, P. H.: Endocrine features in Albright's syndrome (fibrous dysplasia of bone). *Metabolism 11:* 30–45, 1962.
8. Biesecker, J. L., Marcove, R. C., Huvos, A. G., and Miké, V.: Aneurysmal bone cysts, a clinicopathologic study of 66 cases. *Cancer 26:* 615–625, 1970.
9. Buraczewski, J., and Dabska, M.: Pathogenesis of aneurysmal bone cyst; a relationship between the aneurysmal bone cyst and fibrous dysplasia of bone. *Cancer 28:* 597–604, 1971.
10. Byers, P. D.: Solitary benign osteoblastic lesions of bone; osteoid osteoma and benign osteoblastoma. *Cancer 22:* 43–57, 1968.
11. Cassalia, P. T., and Miller, A. S.: Solitary central neurofibroma of the mandible. *Br. J. Oral Surg. 8:* 270–272, 1971.
12. Cherrick, H. M., King, O. H., Jr., Lucatorto, F. M., and Suggs, D. M.: Benign cementoblastoma; a clinicopathologic evaluation. *Oral Surg. 37:* 54–63, 1974.
13. Dahlgren, S. E., Lind, P. O., Lindbom, A., and Martensson, G.: Fibrous dysplasia of jaw bones; a clinical, roentgenographic and histopathologic study. *Acta Otolaryngol. 68:* 257–270, 1969.
14. Darsie, J. L., and Kenan, P. D.: Ossifying fibromas of the frontal-ethmoid sinuses. *South. Med. J. 64:* 1033–1038, 1971.
15. Dehner, L. P.: Tumors of the mandible and maxilla in children. I. Clinicopathologic study of 46 histologically benign lesions. *Cancer 31:* 364–384, 1973.
16. Dias, L. S., and Frost, H. M.: Osteoid osteoma-osteoblastoma. *Cancer 33:* 1075–1081, 1974.
17. Ehrig, U., and Wilson, D. R.: Fibrous dysplasia of bone and primary hyperparathyroidism. *Ann. Intern. Med. 77:* 234–238, 1972.
18. Eversole, L. R., Sabes, W. R., and Rovin, S.: Fibrous dysplasia; a nosologic problem in the diagnosis of fibro-osseous lesions of the jaws. *J. Oral Pathol. 1:* 189–220, 1972.
19. Fibrous dysplasia (unsigned editorial). *Br. Med. J. 1:* 685–686, 1971.
20. Frame, B., Azad, N., Reynolds, W. A., and Saeed, S. M.: Polyostotic fibrous dysplasia and myositis ossificans progressiva; a report of coexistence. *Am. J. Dis. Child. 124:* 120–122, 1972.
21. Friedman, N. B., and Goldman, R. L.: Cementoma of long bones. An extragnathic odontogenic tumor. *Clin. Orthop. 67:* 243–248, 1969.
22. Giansanti, J. S.: The pattern and width of the collagen bundles in bone and cementum. *Oral Surg. 30:* 508–514, 1970.
23. Giansanti, J. S.: The effects of acids upon the pathologic interpretation of the widths of the collagen bundles in bone. *Oral Surg. 30:* 151–157, 1970.
24. Gibson, M. J., and Middlemiss, J. H.: Fibrous dysplasia of bone. *Br. J. Radiol. 44:* 1–13, 1971.
25. Hamner, J. E., III, Lightbody, P. M., Ketcham, A. S., and Swerdlow, H.: Cemento-ossifying fibroma of the maxilla. *Oral Surg. 26:* 579–587, 1968.
26. Hamner, J. E., III, Scofield, H. H., and Cornyn, J.: Benign fibro-osseous jaw lesions of periodontal membrane origin; an analysis of 249 cases. *Cancer 22:* 861–878, 1968.
27. Harris, W. H., Dudley, H. R., Jr., and Barry, R. J.: The natural history of fibrous dysplasia. An

orthopaedic, pathological and roentgenographic study. *J. Bone Joint Surg. (Am.) 44A:* 207–233, 1962.

28. Henry, A.: Monostotic fibrous dysplasia. *J. Bone Joint Surg. (Br.) 51B:* 300–306, 1969.
29. Hinds, E. C., Kent, J. N., and Fechner, R. E.: Desmoplastic fibroma of the mandible; report of case. *J. Oral Surg. 27:* 271–274, 1969.
30. Houston, W. O., Jr.: Fibrous dysplasia of maxilla and mandible; clinicopathologic study and comparison of facial bone lesions with lesions affecting general skeleton. *J. Oral Surg. 23:* 17–39, 1965.
31. Huvos, A. G., Higinbotham, N. L., and Miller, T. R.: Bone sarcomas arising in fibrous dysplasia. *J. Bone Joint Surg. (Am.) 54A:* 1047–1056, 1972.
32. Jaffe, H. L.: Fibrous dysplasia. In *Tumors and tumorous conditions of the Bones and Joints*, pp. 117–142. Philadelphia, Lea and Febiger, 1958.
33. Kempson, R. L. Ossifying fibroma of the long bones; a light and electron microscopic study. *Arch. Pathol. 82:* 218–233, 1966.
34. Leeds, N., and Seaman, W. B.: Fibrous dysplasia of the skull and its differential diagnosis. A clinical and roentgenographic study of 46 cases. *Radiology 78:* 570–582, 1962.
35. Lehrer, H. Z.: Ossifying fibroma of the orbital roof; its distinction from "blistering" or "Intra-osseous" meningioma. *Arch. Neurol. 20:* 536–541, 1969.
36. Levy, W. M., Miller, A. S., Bonakdarpour, A., and Aegerter, E.: Aneurysmal bone cyst secondary to other osseous lesions. Report of 57 cases. *Am. J. Clin. Pathol. 63:* 1–8, 1975.
37. Lichtenstein, L., and Jaffe, H. L.: Fibrous dysplasia of bone; affecting one, several or many bones, the graver cases of which may present abnormal pigmentation of skin, premature sexual development, hyperthyroidism or still other extra-skeletal abnormalities. *Arch. Pathol. 33:* 777–816, 1942.
38. MacMahon, H. E.: Albright's syndrome—thirty years later (polyostotic fibrous dysplasia). *Pathol. Annul. 6:* 81–146, 1971.
39. McCune, D. J., and Bruch, H.: Osteodystrophia fibrosa; report of a case in which the condition was combined with precocious puberty, pathologic pigmentation of the skin and hyperthyroidism, with a review of the literature. *Am. J. Dis. Child. 54:* 806–848, 1937.
40. Meister, H. P., Lufft, W., and Schlegel, D.: Differential diagnosis of fibro-osseous jaw lesions (fibrous dysplasia vs. ossifying fibroma). *Beitr. Pathol. 148:* 221–229, 1973.
41. Meyer, I.: Infectious diseases of the jaws. *J. Oral Surg. 28:* 17–26, 1970.
42. Pindborg, J. J., and Kramer, I. R. H.: *Histological Typing of Odontogenic Tumours, Jaw Cysts, and Allied Lesions*, International Histological Classification of Tumours, No. 5. Geneva, World Health Organization, 1971.
43. Reed, R. J. Fibrous dysplasia of bone; a review of 25 cases. *Arch. Pathol. 75:* 480–495, 1963.
44. Remagen, W., and Prein, J.: Benign osteoblastoma. *Oral Surg. 39:* 279–283, 1975.
45. Riddell, D. M.: Malignant change in fibrous dysplasia; report of a case. *J. Bone Joint Surg. (Br.) 46B:* 251–255, 1964.
46. Rosenberg, R. N., Sassin, J., Zimmerman, E. A., and Carter, S.: The interrelationship of neurofibromatosis and fibrous dysplasia.: *Arch. Neurol. 17:* 174–179, 1967.
47. Royer, R. Q., and Neibling, H. E.: Osteomyelitis of the jaws. *Semin. Roentgenol. 6:* 391–396, 1971.
48. Schajowicz, F., Ackerman, L. V., and Sissons, H. A.: *Histological Typing of Bone Tumours*, International Histological Classification of Tumours, Geneva, World Health Organization, 1972.
49. Schlumberger, H. G.: Fibrous dysplasia of single bones (monostotic fibrous dysplasia). *Milit. Med. 99:* 504–527, 1946.
50. Schmaman, A., Smith, I., and Ackerman, L. V.: Benign fibro-osseous lesions of the mandible and maxilla; a review of 35 cases. *Cancer 26:* 303–312, 1970.
51. Scott, M., Peale, A. R., and Croissant, P. D.: Intracranial midline anterior fossae ossifying fibroma invading orbits, paranasal sinuses, and right maxillary antrum; case report. *J. Neurosurg. 34:* 827–831, 1971.
52. Shear, M., and Copelyn, M.: Myxofibroma of the jaws. In *Fourth Proceedings of the International Academy of Oral Pathology*, p. 195. New York, International Academy of Oral Pathology, 1969.
53. Slow, I. N., Stern, D., and Friedman, E. W.: Osteogenic sarcoma arising in a preexisting fibrous dysplasia; report of case. *J. Oral Surg. 29:* 126–129, 1971.

54. Small, I. A., and Goodman, P. A.: Giant cemento-ossifying fibroma of the maxilla; report of case and discussion. *J. Oral Surg. 31:* 113–119, 1973.
55. Spjut, H. J., Dorfman, H. D., Fechner, R. E., and Ackerman, L. V.: In *Atlas of Tumor Pathology*, 2nd series, fascicle 5, *Tumors of Bone and Cartilage.*
56. Trodahl, J. N.: Ameloblastic fibroma; a survey of cases from the Armed Forces Institute of Pathology. *Oral Surg. 33:* 547–558, 1972.
57. Waldron, C. A.: Fibro-osseous lesions of the jaws. *J. Oral Surg. 28:* 58–64, 1970.
58. Waldron, C. A., and Giansanti, J. S.: Benign fibro-osseous lesions of the jaws; a clinical-radiologic-histologic review of sixty-five cases. Part I. Fibrous dysplasia of the jaws. *Oral Surg. 35:* 190–201, 1973.
59. Waldron, C. A., and Giansanti, J. S. Benign fibro-osseous lesion of the jaws; a clinical-radiologic-histologic review of sixty-five cases. Part II. Benign fibro-osseous lesions of periodontal ligament origin. *Oral Surg. 35:* 340–350, 1973.
60. Waldron, C. A., and Shafer, W. G.: The central giant cell reparative granuloma of the jaws; an analysis of 38 cases. *Am. J. Clin. Pathol. 45:* 437–447, 1966.
61. Warrick, C. K.: Some aspects of polyostotic fibrous dysplasia. Possible hypothesis to account for the associated endocrinological changes. *Clin. Radiol. 24:* 125–138, 1973.
62. Zimmerman, D. C., Dahlin, D. C., and Stafne, E. C.: Fibrous dysplasia of the maxilla and mandible. *Oral Surg. 11:* 55–68, 1958.

Chapter 15

Differential Diagnosis of Giant Cell Lesions of Bone

C. P. SCHWINN

The differential diagnosis of giant cell lesions of bone (arbitrarily defined as lesions containing benign, multinucleated giant cells and occuring in bone) requires the surgical pathologist's consideration of a considerable number of possibilities. Some of the bone entities which contain benign multinucleated giant cells are described elsewhere in this monograph, *i.e.*, chronic granulomatous inflammation (Chapter 4), florid Paget's disease and Paget's sarcoma (Chapter 10), and fibro-osseous lesions of bone (Chapter 14). With a few exceptions, these lesions will be omitted from this presentation.

Jaffe[7] has emphasized "the necessity of bringing to [bear upon] the [differential] diagnosis of bone tumors [and related lesions] the light which can be shed jointly by the disciplines of radiology, surgery and pathology." In other words, the surgical pathologist when considering the differential diagnosis of a bone lesion containing benign multinucleated giant cells, or any other bone lesion for that matter, should have pertinent clinical data, the radiologist's assessment of suitable roentgenograms, and a description of the surgeon's findings at the time of operation prior to his own gross and microscopic evaluation of the pathologic material. Because the author agrees with Jaffe's concept that each bone lesion should be considered as a clinicopathologic entity, each of the entities to be considered in the differential diagnosis will be presented as typical (or atypical) examples with a short clinical history, a roentgenogram, and one or more photomicrographs. The more precise details of roentgenographic interpretation of bone lesions are presented elsewhere in this monograph (Chapter 13); the x-rays are included in this presentation in order to reflect, in a general way, the gross pathology and to indicate to the surgical pathologist the precise localization in relation to the bone as a whole, *i.e.*, epiphyseal, diaphyseal, metaphyseal, central, eccentric and subperiosteal, and to indicate the presence or absence of extension to involve adjacent soft tissue. Relatively numerous photomicrographs are presented for the benefit of the surgical pathologist since, as Foote[6] has so aptly stated in his monograph on salivary gland tumors, "the many elaborate descriptions previously recorded in the literature scarcely require repetition and it is considered preferable to illustrate generously the microscopic features." This counsel seems especially apt in bone pathology since roentgenographic and histopathologic features can be considered together.

The opinions expressed with respect to the diagnosis of the lesions under discussion are based on the author's experience with more than 2000 cases collected from a variety of sources* into a Teaching File for Orthopaedic and Pathology residents. The cumulative experience acquired in categorizing these cases and in reviewing their clinical, radiographic, histopathologic, and follow-up data assessed in conjunction with the references cited in the bibliography form the basis for this review. The bibliography, which is incomplete, has been compiled as follows. Textbook references which have been consulted are included in the initial section under the term "Primary." Also included in this Primary section are several prior presentations on the subject of differential diagnoses of lesions of bone containing giant cells. The remaining references are cited under the specific title of the lesion to which they refer.

ULTRASTRUCTURE AND HISTOCHEMISTRY

The light-microscopic, histopathologic characteristics of the benign multinucleated giant cells occurring in the various lesions to be considered in the differential diagnosis of lesions containing giant cells show no distinctive features which would enable the pathologist to establish a specific diagnosis on this basis. Similarly, ultrastructural and histochemical studies by a variety of authors have failed to establish any significant and consistently demonstrable differences between the benign multinucleated giant cells found in benign giant cell tumor, benign chondroblastoma, aneurysmal bone cyst, nonossifying fibroma, eosinophilic granuloma, central and peripheral giant cell reparative granuloma of jaw bones, and pigmented villonodular tenosynovitis. Nor do they differ from the osteoclasts of either normal bone or bone affected by Paget's disease. Their histogenesis is likewise the subject of debate as Hanaoka, Friedman, and Mack[15] have indicated in their thorough review.

The stromal (or tumor) cell, on the other hand, is distinguishable in some of the lesions. For example, the stromal cell of giant cell tumor[22] is distinguishable by electron microscopy and histochemistry from the tumor cell of benign chondroblastoma.[16, 24] However, the stromal cells of these two tumors can more easily be distinguished on the basis of the light microscopic features, and for the most part distinction between the various tumors to be discussed is accomplished more readily on the basis of their clinical, radiographic, and histopathologic characteristics than by their histochemical or electron microscopic features.

DIFFERENTIAL DIAGNOSIS

As a convenience, the lesions to be considered have been divided into two major groups (Tables I and II). The first group includes the lesions which, in their differential diagnosis, are most likely to be confused with benign giant cell tumor. This confusion is the result of either their strong histopathologic resemblance to benign giant cell tumor or a moderately analogous histopathologic resemblance

* Memorial Center for Cancer and Allied Disease; New York City, the Los Angeles County-University of Southern California Medical Center, the Orthopaedic Hospital and the California Tumor Tissue Registry, all in Los Angeles; and from cases received in consultation.

TABLE I

Benign giant cell tumor of bone
Benign giant cell tumor of long tubular bone in nonepiphyseal location
Malignant giant cell tumor of bone
Benign giant cell tumor arising in Paget's disease of bone
Benign chondroblastoma
Benign chondroblastoma of long tubular bone in nonepiphyseal location
Malignant chondroblastoma
Giant cell reaction of hand and foot bones
Intraosseous (invasive, aggressive) pigmented villonodular synovitis and tenosynovitis
Brown tumor of hyperparathyroidism
Giant cell reparative granuloma of jawbones
Giant cell epulis of gingiva

TABLE II

Osteosarcoma with numerous benign multinucleated giant cells
Fibrous cortical defect (nonosteogenic fibroma)
Solitary and multifocal eosinophilic granuloma of bone
Aneurysmal bone cyst
Unicameral (solitary) bone cyst
Chondromyxoid fibroma
Gouty tophus in bone
Giant cell containing lesions not described in this presentation
Florid Paget's disease
Fibro-Osseous lesions (fibrous dysplasia, cherubism, cementifying and ossifying fibroma, osteoid osteoma and osteoblastoma)
Chronic granulomatous inflammation including sarcoid

coupled with their tendence to localize, when they occur in long tubular bones, at the epiphyseal end of the bone, which is the classical localization of benign giant cell tumor.

The remaining lesions (Table II) include those which contain benign multinucleated giant cells but whose histopathology is usually significantly different from that of benign giant cell tumor so that they can be differentiated on that basis alone. However, when they occur in long tubular bones, they tend to be located in either diaphyseal or metaphyseal areas rather than in the epiphyseal end. They require differentiation one from another rather than from giant cell tumor, *per se*.

Also appended to Table II are those lesions containing benign multinucleated giant cells which have been discussed elsewhere in this monograph. They are not considered in this presentation.

BENIGN GIANT CELL TUMOR OF BONE

The clinical history is that of a 29-year-old female with pain in the knee of 4 months duration. Laboratory data were within normal limits. Ninety per cent of giant cell tumors of bone occur in patients more than 20 years of age. The radiograph (Fig. 1–1) shows a slightly eccentric, radiolucent lesion with characteristic indistinct margins and located in the epiphyseal end of a major long tubular bone. More than 75% of giant cell tumors are located at or near the end of a major tubular bone.

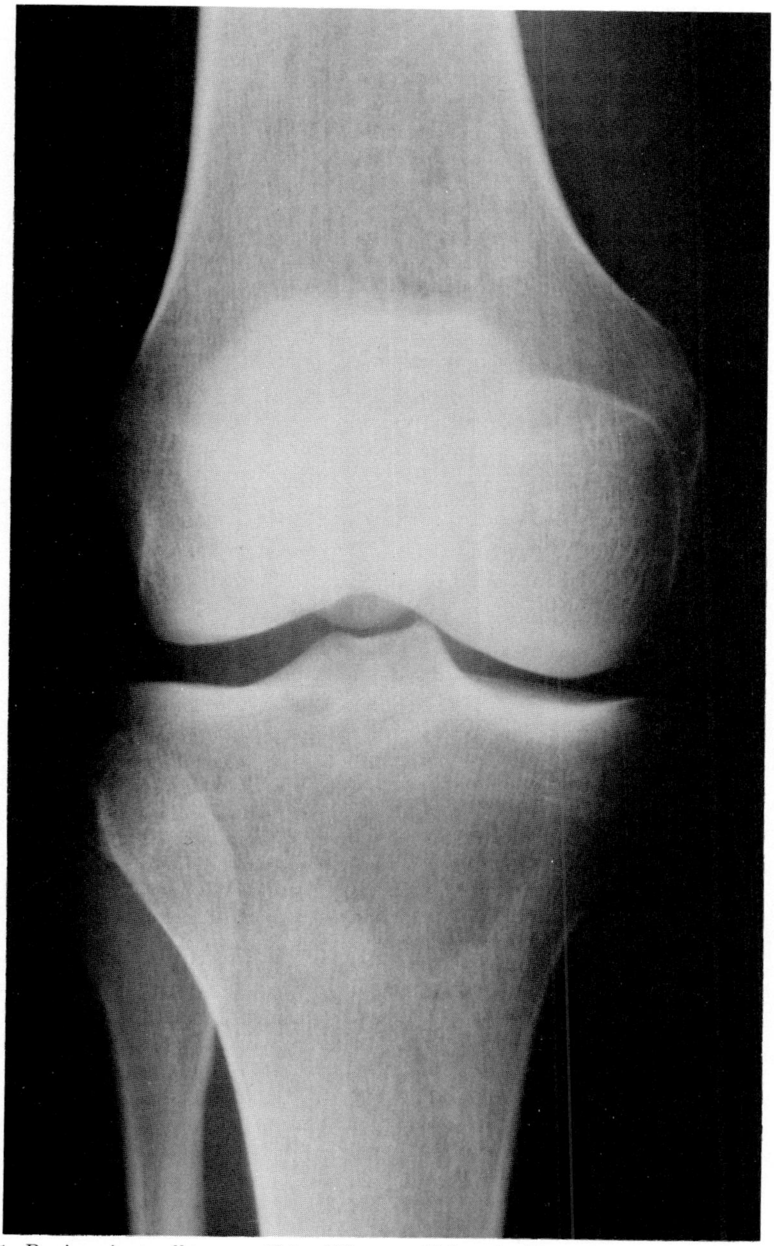

FIG. 1–1. Benign giant cell tumor; tibia of 29-year-old female. Characteristic eccentric localization in the epiphyseal end of a large long bone. The lesion is radiolucent and exhibits the more common pattern of poorly defined, indistinct peripheral margins.

Figure 1–2 is a composite of the radiograph and the gross specimen of a recurrent benign giant cell tumor of the radius in a 35-year-old male and illustrates a less common roentgenographic presentation with sclerotic, radio-opaque margins and a "soap bubble" appearance attributed to the ridging of the internal surfaces of either the expanded cortex or of reactive bone formation at

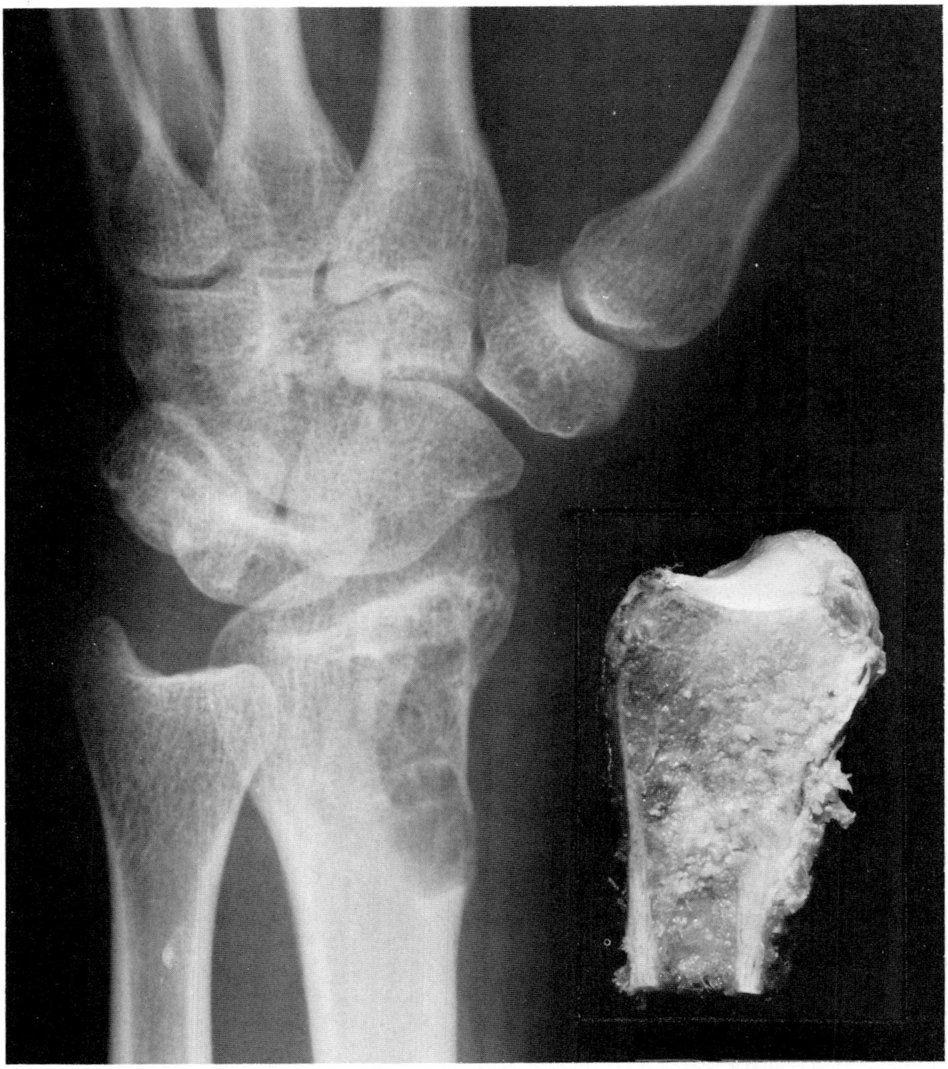

FIG. 1–2. Recurrent benign giant cell tumor, radius of 35-year-old male. Eccentric, radiolucent lesion in the epiphyseal end of a large long bone with less common "soap bubble" roentgenographic presentation. Superimposed photograph of the "block resected" gross specimen emphasizes the fact that the majority of the primary lesions to be discussed are solid rather than "cystic" as suggested by the x-ray.

the intramedullary margin of the tumor. The superimposed photograph of the transected specimen illustrates the solid nature of the lesion and belies the pseudocystic appearance of the x-ray. This is a practical point since nearly all of the lesions to be discussed in the differential diagnosis of giant cell tumor are solid; the two exceptions are unicameral bone cyst and aneurysmal bone cyst. This particular solid and fibrous-appearing tumor has transgressed the cortex and involves the adjacent soft tissues. Approximately 20% of benign giant cell tumors erode the cortex and involve the soft tissues.[33]

The "textbook" microscopic appearance of benign giant cell tumor of bone and the "standard" to which the other lesions to be discussed will be compared is shown in Figure 1–3. There are numerous, benign, multinucleated giant cells separated by tumor (or stromal) cells whose nuclei and cytoplasmic mass are of relatively uniform size and staining reaction. The cytoplasmic borders are quite frequently indistinct and little or no intercellular substance is produced. The nuclei of the stromal (tumor) cells resemble those of the multinucleated giant cells.

Actually, when multiple sections of a representative giant cell tumor of bone are examined, focal and sometimes considerable areas of the tumor will show significant variations from the textbook pattern. For example, there will be areas in most giant cell tumors in which the stromal cells are spindle-shaped (Fig. 1–4), and in some of these areas there will be collagen production. Less commonly, either focal or sometimes relatively extensive areas of a benign giant cell tumor may show evidence of more rapid growth; in such areas (Fig. 1–5) the stroma may appear more cellular, mitotic figures may be present in moderate numbers, and there may be some variation in nuclear and cytoplasmic staining and in nuclear

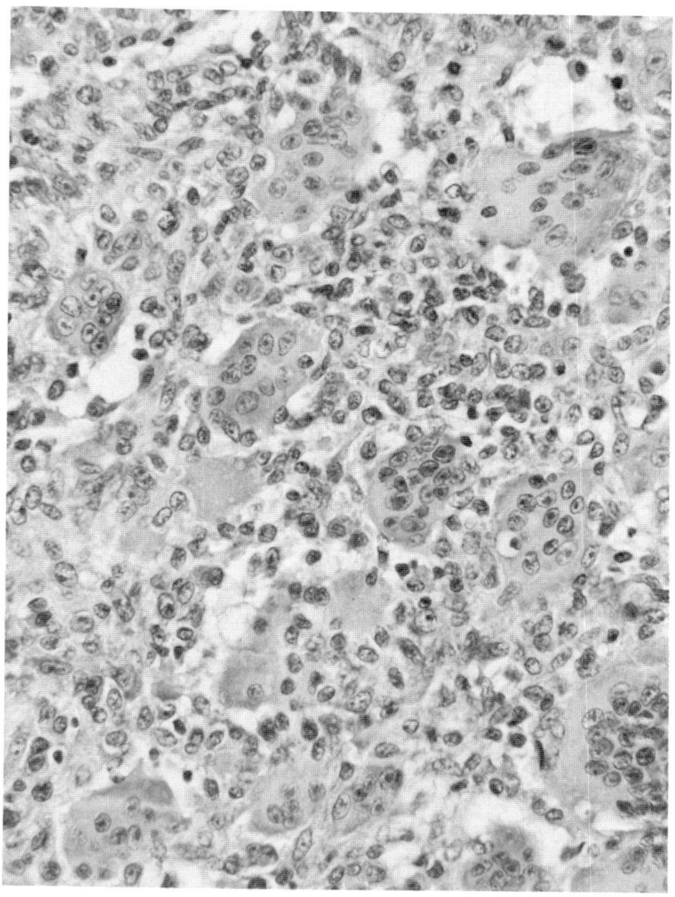

FIG. 1–3. Benign giant cell tumor of bone. Classical or "textbook" microscopic appearance. ×300.

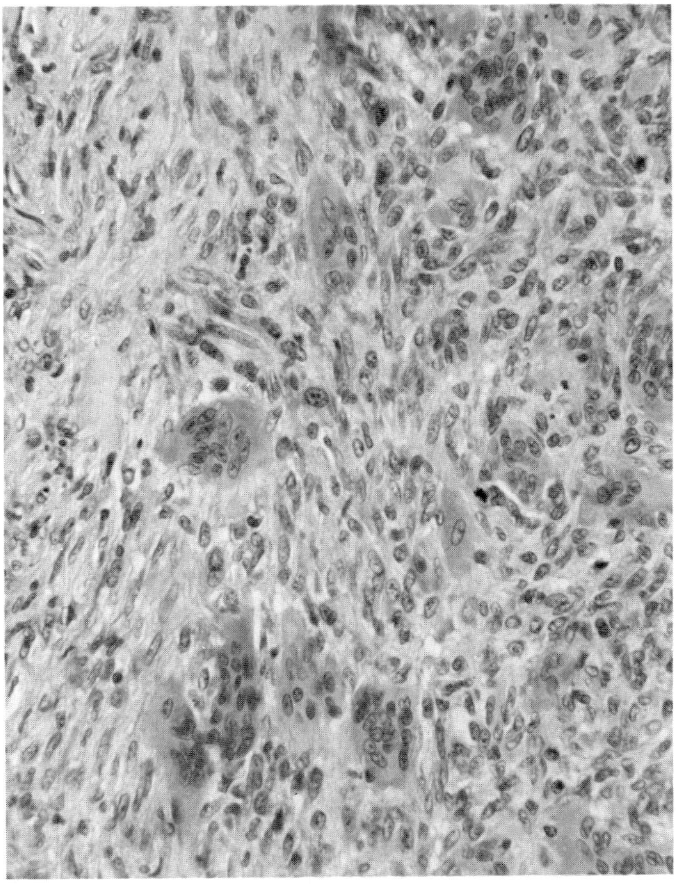

FIG. 1–4. Benign giant cell tumor of bone. Spindle-shaped tumor cells with focal collagen production (upper left). × 300.

cytoplasmic ratio. However, unless areas of definite sarcomatous degeneration, such as is illustrated in Figure 3–2 can be found, the lesion should be classified as a benign giant cell tumor.

Other variations in histopathology (not illustrated) include focal areas where multinucleated giant cells are sparse or absent, areas where collagen production is abundant, areas of hemosiderin deposition, and areas where lipid-laden macrophages are numerous. In our experience, occasional benign giant cell tumors will exhibit a predominance of one or another of these histopathologic features, and in these cases it is necessary to rely more heavily on the clinical and roentogenographic rather than the histopathologic features in arriving at the correct diagnosis.

Thirty to forty per cent of benign giant cell tumors have been reported as having focal areas of osteoid and bone production. This is practically never a dominant feature.

Finally, with respect to benign giant cell tumors, attempts to grade these lesions for prognostic purposes, *i.e.*, as predictive of likelihood of either

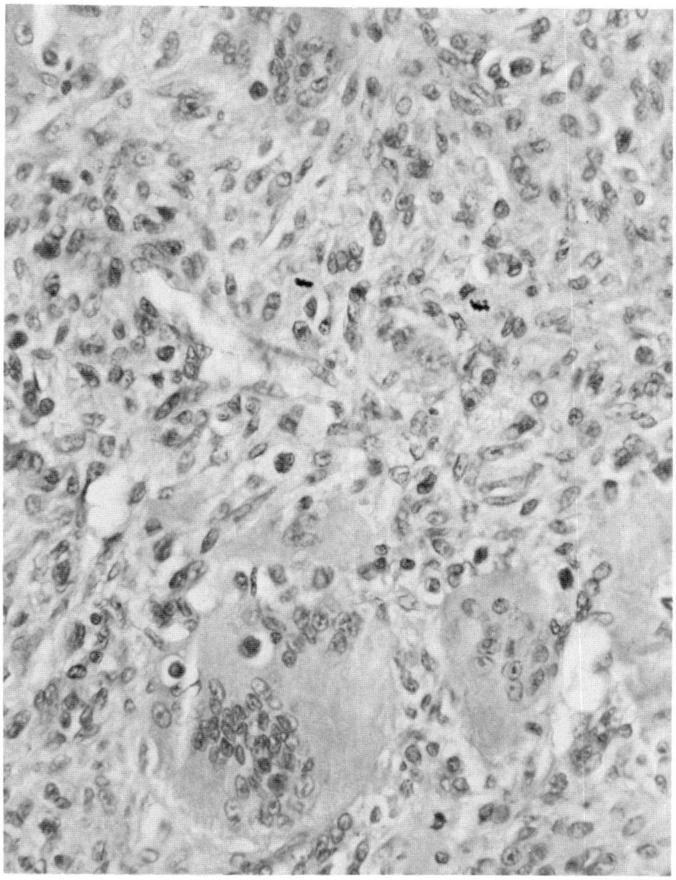

FIG. 1–5. Benign giant cell tumor of bone. Mitotic figures easily identified. Some variation in size, shape and staining reaction of cells and nuclei. Compare with malignant giant cell tumor in Figure 3–2. × 300.

recurrence or malignant transformation, on the basis of any of the histopathologic features presented above have been unsuccessful. It is important, therefore, in evaluating such lesions, to submit all of the tissue removed for microscopic examination to be certain that focal areas of malignant alteration are not missed.

BENIGN GIANT CELL TUMOR OF MAJOR LONG TUBULAR BONES IN NONEPIPHYSEAL LOCATION

Rarely, benign giant cell tumor of a long tubular bone occurs in either a diaphyseal or metaphyseal location (Fig. 2–1).[28, 42, 44, 48] The single case in our own files is a 27-year-old female admitted in January, 1963, with a complaint of pain in the lower thigh for one month. X-ray (Fig. 2–2) shows a diaphyseal lesion which was interpreted by the radiologist as "probably benign but rule out fibrosarcoma." At frozen section the lesion was interpreted as "probably benign giant cell tumor but await permanent sections." The diaphyseal localization obviously complicates the problem of correct diagnosis. The final diagnosis was benign giant

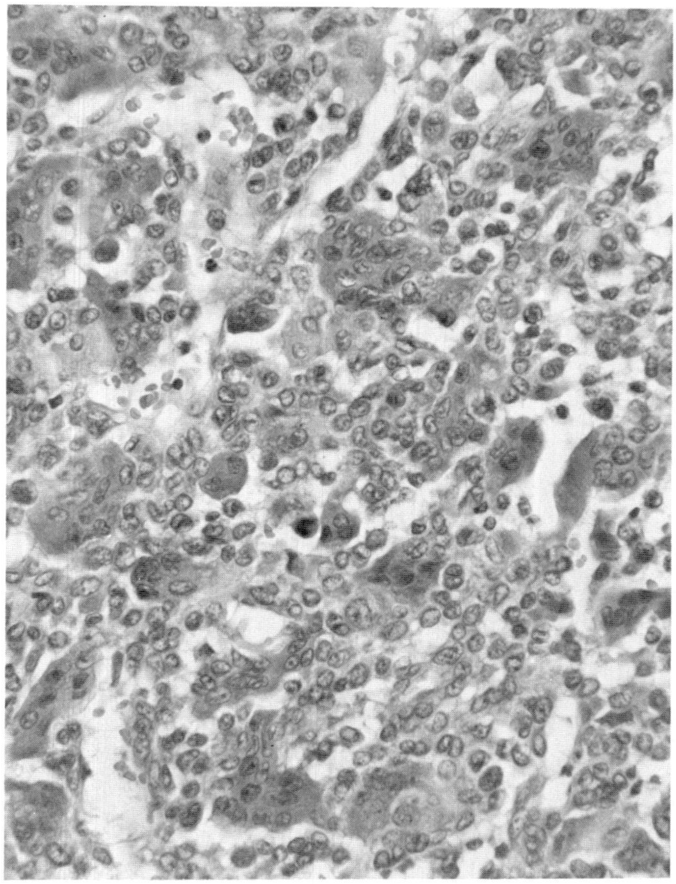

FIG. 2-1. Benign giant cell tumor in diaphysis. Note large number of endothelial-lined capillaries, a common feature of benign giant cell tumor. × 300.

cell tumor of bone and was confirmed in consultation by Drs. L. V. Ackerman, D. C. Dahlin, F. W. Stewart, and H. L. Jaffe. The patient was treated by thorough curettage and the defect packed with "bank" bone. The patient was well and without evidence of residual or recurrent tumor as of February, 1975, 12 years after treatment.

MALIGNANT GIANT CELL TUMOR OF BONE (SARCOMA OCCURRING IN, OR ARISING AT THE SITE OF PREVIOUSLY TREATED, BENIGN GIANT CELL TUMOR OF BONE)

It is important to distinguish benign giant cell tumor from the majority of the other benign lesions containing giant cells because it is a locally aggressive tumor with a significant recurrence rate and not infrequently undergoes malignant change. When benign giant cell tumor is treated by curettage, for instance, approximately 50% will recur. The histopathology of the recurrent tumor is ordinarily indistinguishable from that of the original lesion; the lesion is still benign and, if treated again by curettage, it is again at risk for 50% recurrence. If

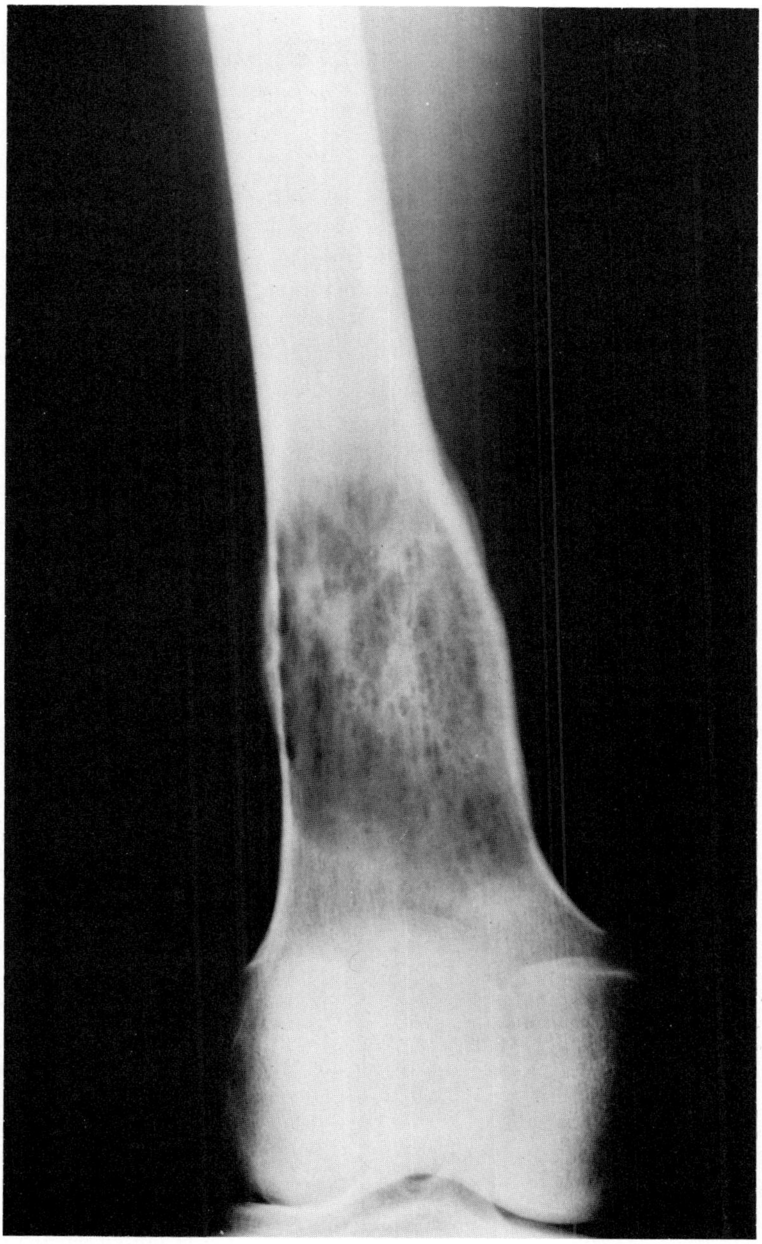

FIG. 2-2. Benign giant cell tumor in non-epiphyseal (diaphyseal) region of femur. Patient, a 27-year-old female.

treated by radical *en bloc* excision, nearly 100% of benign giant cell tumors can be cured,[28] but the size and localization of the majority of benign giant cell tumors render this solution impractical, *i.e.*, the *en bloc* excision would be tantamount to amputation.

Ten per cent of benign giant cell tumors undergo malignant transformation.

The most recent and probably the best definition of malignant giant cell tumor is Dahlin's[28] modification of that offered by Hutter, Worcester, Francis, Foote, and Stewart[31]: "To qualify as a malignant giant cell tumor, a tumor must have histologic evidence of the benign counterpart in the lesion under study or in material removed previously from the same area. Neoplasms in which stromal cells are malignant throughout, even though they may contain as many multinucleated benign cells as does a giant cell tumor, have the clinical features of osteogenic or fibrosarcomas and should be classed in the appropriate one of these groups. The problem is further confounded because a very few histologically benign giant cell tumors metastasize."

The composite x-rays (Fig. 3–1) are of the femur of a 44-year-old woman admitted to the hospital in October, 1961. The 1947 x-ray shows the site of a benign giant cell tumor which had been treated by curettage and packing with bone chips. The 1961 x-ray shows a malignant giant cell tumor (fibrosarcoma). In the interim between 1947 and 1961, the patient underwent two subsequent surgical operations and received two courses of radiation therapy. Sections of the

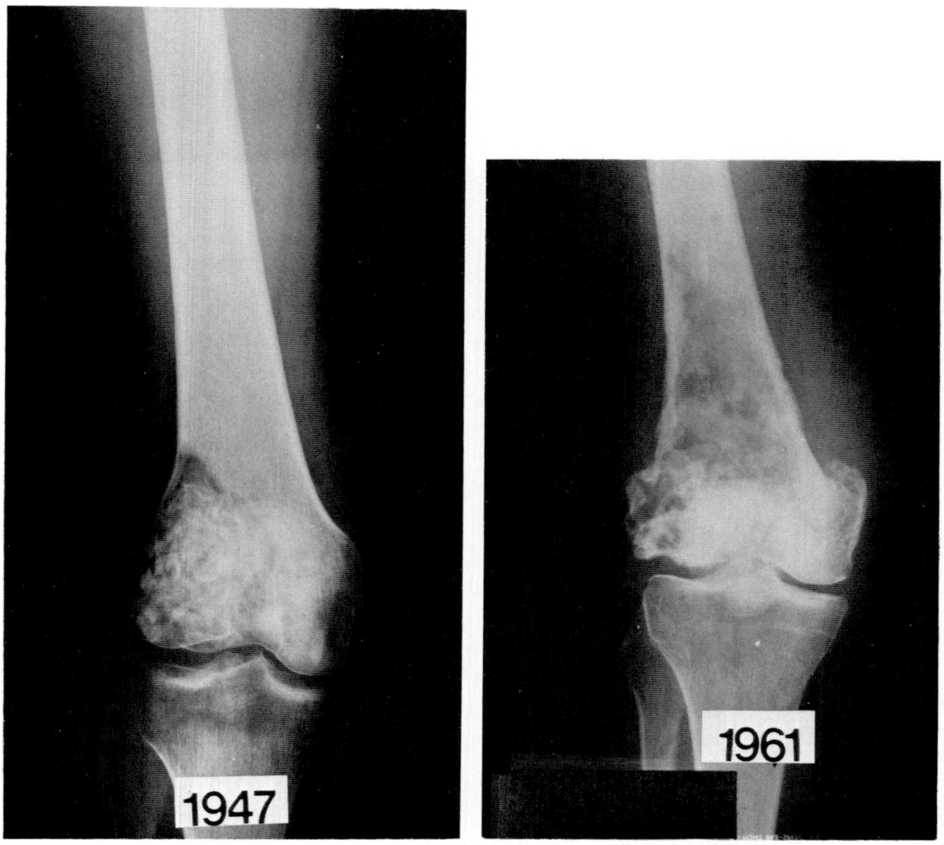

FIG. 3–1. X-rays of 1947 and 1961. Postoperative x-ray (1947) of benign giant cell tumor subsequent to curetting and packing with bone chips. X-ray (1961) just prior to amputation for malignant giant cell tumor of bone. Patient was 44-year-old woman when admitted for amputation in 1961.

amputation specimen (Fig. 3–2) show a fibrosarcoma. All of the cells illustrated are sarcomatous. The majority of malignant giant cell tumors are fibrosarcomas, a few osteosarcomas. Multinucleated giant cells were present in focal areas of this tumor but are not shown in the photomicrograph. Foci of clearly recognizable benign giant cell tumor were no longer present, however, and the diagnosis of malignant giant cell tumor was made because the sections of the originial lesion removed in 1947 showed a typical benign giant cell tumor. Nine out of ten patients who develop malignant giant cell tumor have had prior radiation therapy of their benign lesion.[28] Of the 1 in 10 who have no record of radiation therapy, the majority develop their malignant giant cell tumor after one or more attempts at surgical treatment. Rarely, foci of malignant change are found in the tissue removed at the initial surgical intervention.

Malignant giant cell tumor metastasizes as a sarcoma, *i.e.* the metastatic sarcoma is either a fibrosarcoma or an osteosarcoma. However, to further confuse our understanding of benign giant cell tumor, an occasional histopathologically benign giant cell tumor metastasizes, *i.e.*, the microscopic features of the

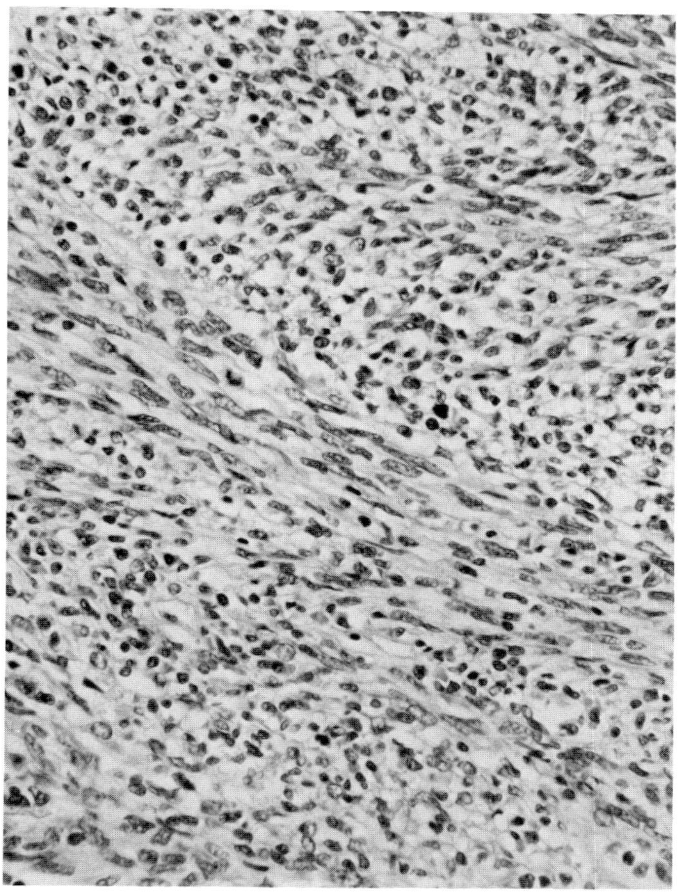

FIG. 3–2. Fibrosarcoma (malignant giant cell tumor) arising in benign giant cell tumor of bone. Same case as in Figure 3–1. × 300.

metastasis are the same as those seen in the initial benign giant cell tumor. Pan, Dahlin, Lipscomb, and Bernat[39] in 1964 reviewed the literature on this subject and were able to collect 16 cases. They were uncertain about the exact nature of some of these cases and cautioned that "accurate appraisal of the literature on the basis of histologic description or photomicrographs is impossible [because] in some of the reported cases there was rather rapid and widespread dissemination [which] makes one wonder if frankly sarcomatous change had occurred." They pointed out that in most of the cases where they felt fairly certain that the metastatic lesion had benign histopathology there was a remarkably protracted course, "more in line with what one might expect." Pan's own case was cured by lobectomy, and two similar cases subsequently reported by Goldenberg, Campbell, and Bonfiglio[30] were also cured by lobectomy. This knowledge, that a very rare histologically benign giant cell tumor may metastasize, is essential to the understanding of giant cell tumor behavior. Perhaps, as intimated by Pan *et al.*,[39] these "benign metastases" should be considered as "transplants." Two additional cases with multiple benign pulmonary "metastases" and long term survival have been recorded more recently.[34, 36]

BENIGN GIANT CELL TUMOR ARISING IN PAGET'S DISEASE OF BONE

Bone sarcoma is a rare but well-recognized complication of Paget's disease. Nevertheless, its occurrence is approximately 7 times more common than that of

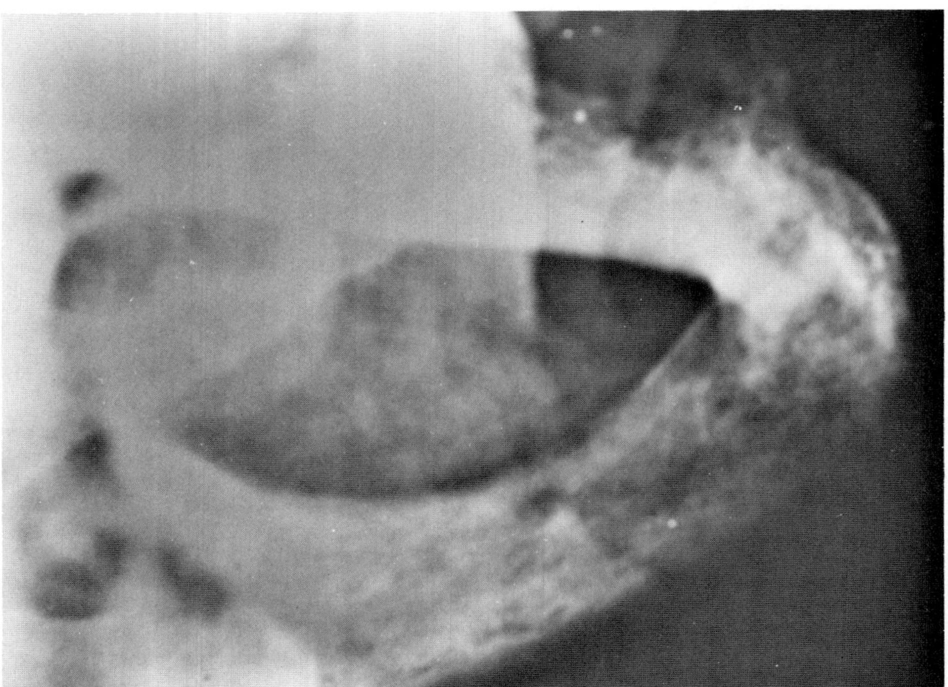

FIG. 4-1. Benign giant cell tumor arising in bone affected by Paget's disease. Tumor arose in mandible and extended into soft tissues anterior to mandible forming a 12.0-cm. mass. (Courtesy of Dr. James Taylor. Used with permission.)

benign giant cell tumor arising in Paget's disease. For practical purposes, patients with either benign giant cell tumor or sarcoma are more than 40 years of age, and most have a significantly elevated serum alkaline phosphatase. In contrast to ordinary benign giant cell tumor arising in bone unaffected by Paget's disease, the majority of those associated with Paget's disease are located in the skull and facial bones, and the rare case arising in a long bone does not involve the epiphyseal end of the bone.

Our illustrative case is that of a 65-year-old man who presented with a large tumor involving the soft tissues anterior to the mandible. X-ray (Fig. 4–1) revealed a destructive mass involving almost the entire mandible and extending anteriorly to involve the soft tissues of the chin. The roentgenologist noted that the mandible was also involved by Paget's disease. A biopsy of this lesion (Fig. 4–2) shows tumor histopathology indistinguishable from benign giant cell tumor arising in bone unaffected by Paget's disease. True, the stromal component appears to be more spindled, and there is more collagen production than in the average benign giant cell tumor, but these variations have already been described

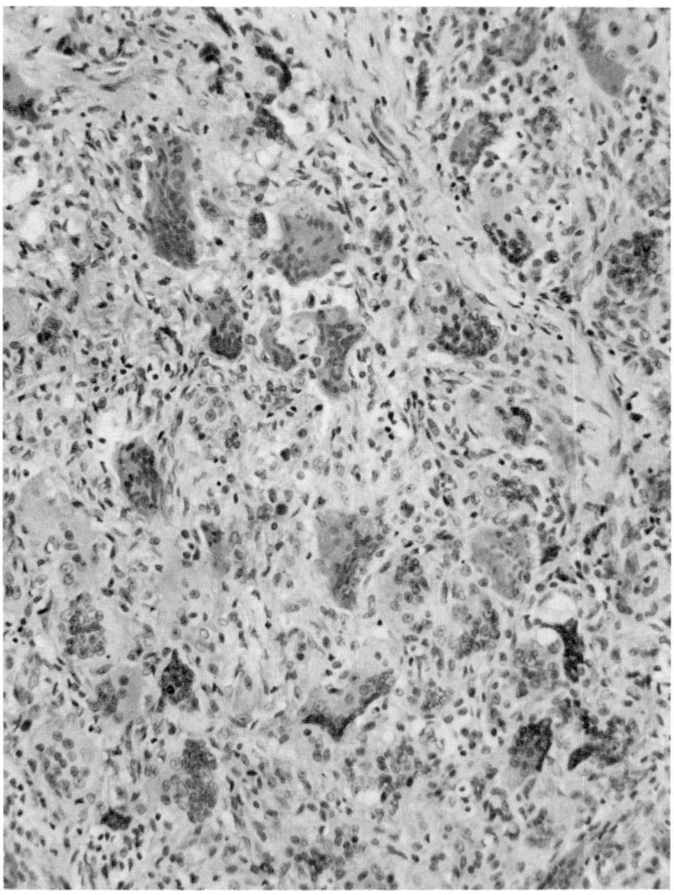

FIG. 4–2. Benign giant cell tumor arising in bone affected by Paget's disease. No evidence of malignant change. Compare with Figure 4–3. × 200.

as an occasional occurrence in ordinary benign giant cell tumor arising in patients without Paget's disease. This patient was treated by irradiation, and the tumor subsided. There was no recurrent or residual tumor present 3 years later when the patient died of other causes.

We[54] previously recorded 12 such cases of benign giant cell tumor arising in Paget's disease of bone (5 of our own and 7 collected from the literature). Five arose in the calvaria and 2 each from the maxilla and mandible—all distinctly unusual localizations for ordinary benign giant cell tumor of bone. The remaining 3 were 1 each in the ilium, humerus, and tibia, and none of these were in the epiphyseal end of the bone. A more recent report by Miller, Cuttina, Elzay, Levy, and Hardwick[55] describes 24 cases (16 in skull and facial bones, 5 in pelvic bones, and 3 in long bones). Patients with truly benign giant cell tumor arising in Paget's disease have an excellent prognosis.[50, 54, 55, 58] Virtually all of the patients are alive at 5 years without evidence of disease. Bone sarcomas arising in Paget's

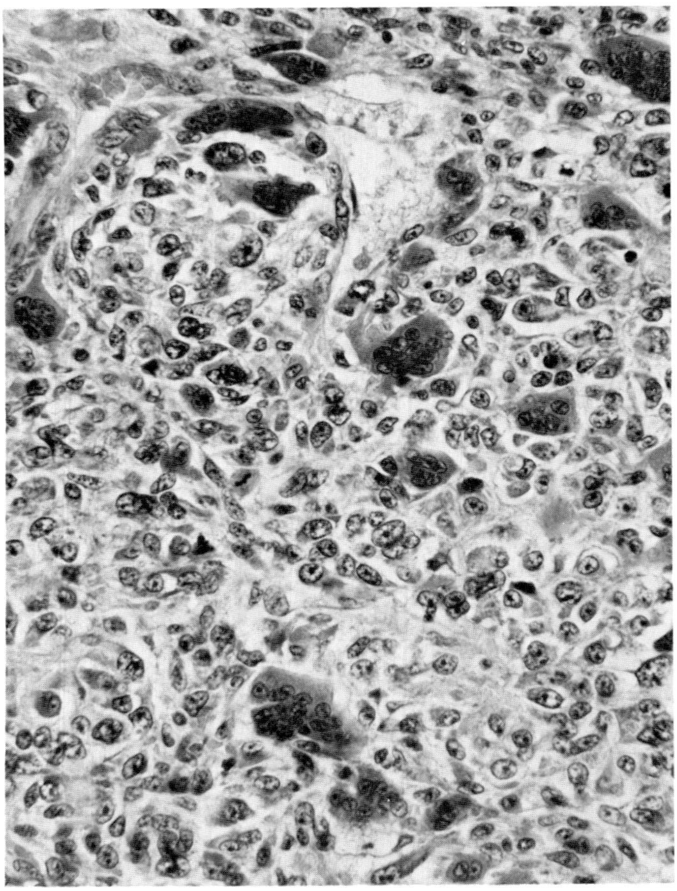

FIG. 4-3. Osteosarcoma with numerous benign-appearing multinucleated giant cells arising in Paget's disease of bone. Note nuclear pleomorphism of malignant "stromal" cells. × 300. Compare with Figures 4-2 (benign giant cell tumor in Paget's disease) and with Figures 1-3, 1-4, and 1-5 (benign giant cell tumor), and with Figure 3-2 (malignant giant cell tumor).

disease, on the other hand,[49, 55, 56] have a doleful prognosis. Some sarcomas arising in Paget's disease have large numbers of benign multinucleated giant cells and in occasional cases the differentiation from a benign giant cell tumor may be difficult unless particular attention is paid to the stromal cells. Figure 4–3 is a section from an osteosarcoma arising in Paget's disease of the tibial diaphysis of a 72-year-old man. Careful examination of the stromal cells in this tumor reveal considerable variation in size, shape, and staining reaction of their nuclei and relatively high nuclear to cytoplasmic ratios in many of the cells. Atypical mitoses and a few foci of osteoid were noted in other areas, and this tumor was properly classified as an osteosarcoma with numerous giant cells arising in Paget's disease of bone. This patient died within 1 year with widespread metastases.

BENIGN CHONDROBLASTOMA (EPIPHYSEAL CHONDROMATOUS GIANT CELL TUMOR, CODMAN TUMOR)

Benign chondroblastoma, like benign giant cell tumor, nearly always occurs in the epiphyseal end of a long bone, and more than 95% arise in sites that can be related to either primary or secondary centers of enchondral ossification and therefore could have been derived from cartilage growth plates. In contrast to benign giant cell tumor, more than 85% of the patients are less than 25 years of age. Our illustrative case is in a 16-year-old male who had noted pain in his shoulder for several months which was aggravated by playing football. The x-ray (Fig. 5–1) was taken at the end of the football season. Most chondroblastomas are smaller than the lesion illustrated, and, in fact, benign chondroblastomas are smaller on the average than benign giant cell tumors. The typical x-ray almost

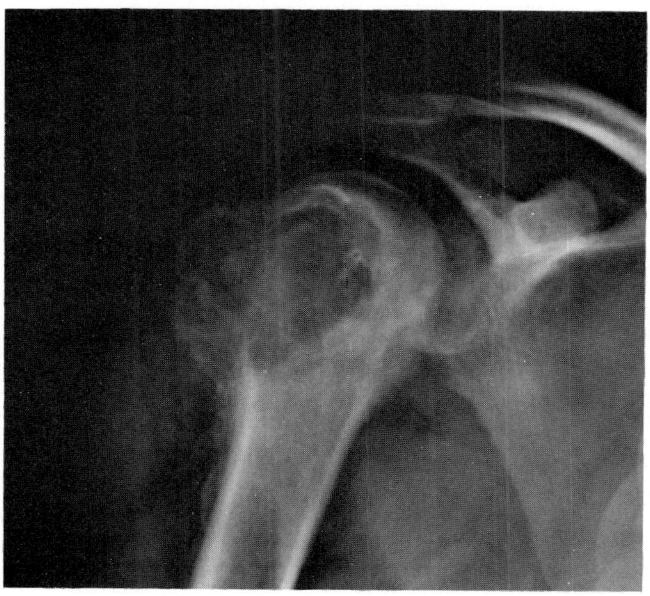

FIG. 5–1. Benign chondroblastoma. Eccentric lesion in epiphyseal end of humerus; 16-year-old male.

always exhibits a peripheral sclerotic rim surrounding the eccentric lesion and flocculent radio-opacities may be discernible within the lesion.

The composite photomicrograph (Fig. 5–2) shows sheets of chondroblasts which are "almost pathognomonic" of chondroblastoma. Where numerous these chondroblasts produce a relatively characteristic, somewhat monotonous pattern which is intensified by the orderly distribution of these relatively small, uniform-sized cells with hyperchromatic nuclei. Each cell appears to be isolated and equidistant from the next. Mitotic figures are present although seldom numerous. Benign multinucleated giant cells are variable in number; in some areas they are virtually absent (Fig. 5–2, upper half), and in other areas they may be moderate to abundant in number (Fig. 5–2, lower half). On the average they are seldom as numerous as in benign giant cell tumor. Some authors believe that, in addition to the chondroblasts, one must be able to demonstrate foci where chondroid matrix (Fig. 5–3, lower half), or calcification (Fig. 5–3, upper half) are present. These

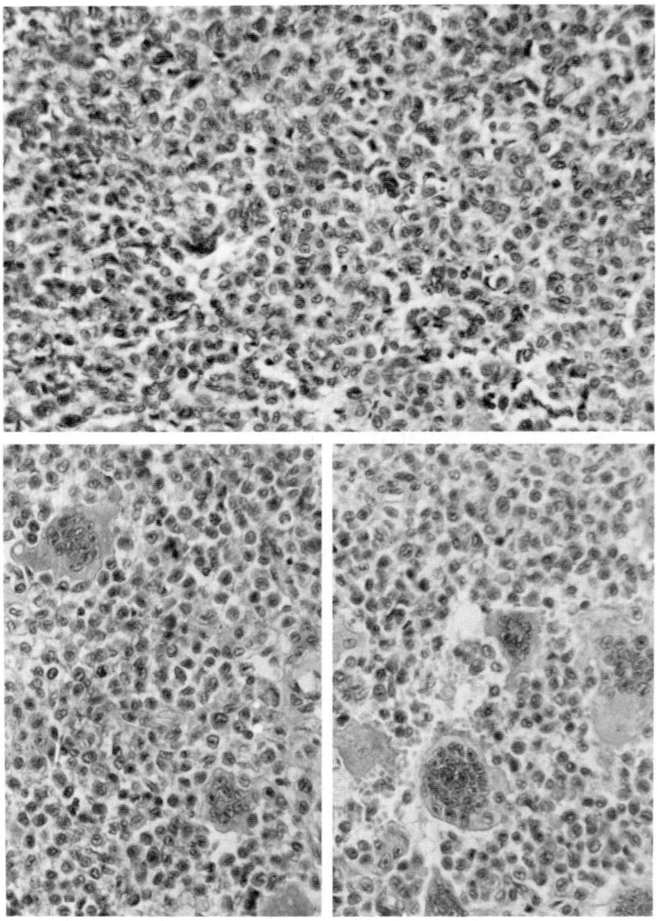

FIG. 5–2. Benign chondroblastoma. Sheets of highly characteristic, monotonous-appearing, uniform-staining chondroblasts (upper half) and benign multinucleated giant cells interspersed between chondroblasts (lower half). ×200. Compare stromal cells in Figure 5–2 with those in Figures 1–3 to 1–5.

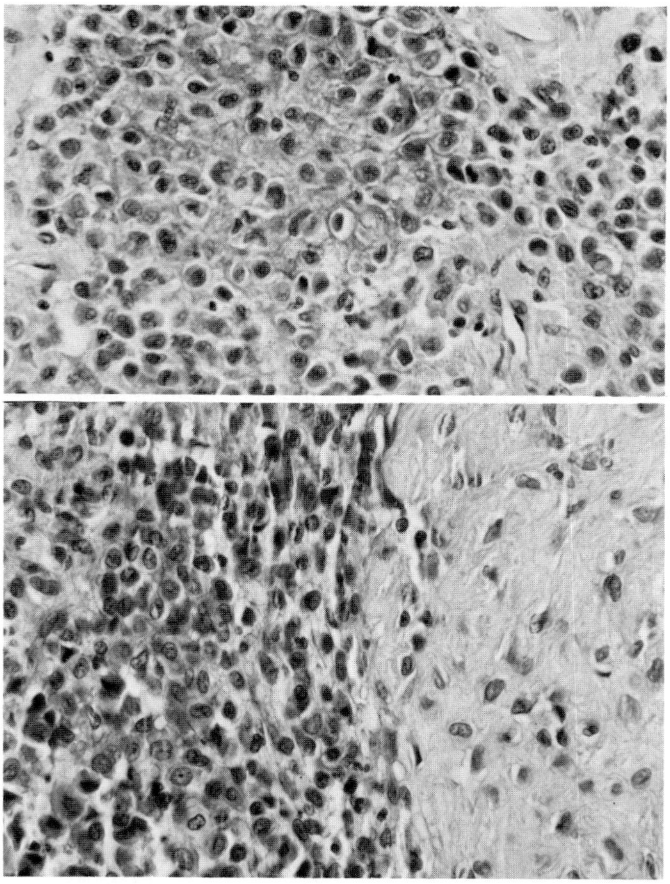

FIG. 5–3. Benign chondroblastoma. Skein-like focal calcification (upper half) and focal production of chondroid (lower half). × 300.

focal areas of either chondrification or calcification may be either sparse or they may dominate the histopathologic picture. Furthermore, in a significant number of cases the foci of solid matrix may more closely resemble collagen than cartilage, and in a few instances osteoid and bone production have been described.[62]

Cystic changes at the microscopic level have been described by Dahlin and Ivins[60] and by Schajowicz and Gallardo[67] in slightly more than 15% of cases, and we have noted similar changes. When these spaces contain blood the histopathology of these altered foci is similar to that of aneurysmal bone cyst. A few authors[118, 123] have included such lesions among their aneurysmal bone cysts. In the evaluation of such focal areas we strongly concur with the assessment of Dahlin and colleagues:[60, 120] "We have preferred to designate such lesions according to the well-established underlying process (in this case chondroblastoma) and merely make note of this secondary phenomena." Dahlin and colleagues[60, 120] further point out, and we agree, "that other lesions such as giant cell tumor, fibrous dysplasia, giant cell reparative granuloma, and simple cysts may contain zones which are indistinguishable from aneurysmal bone cyst."

BENIGN CHONDROBLASTOMA OF MAJOR LONG TUBULAR BONE IN NONEPIPHYSEAL LOCATION

Benign chondroblastoma, like benign giant cell tumor, occurs on rare occasions in a nonepiphyseal portion of a long tubular bone. The x-ray of an illustrative case (Fig. 6–1) shows a lesion in the diaphysis of the humerus of a 14-year-old boy. Fechner and Wilde[61] in 1974 reported a case occurring in the metaphysis of the femoral neck and reviewed the literature. Including their own case, they called

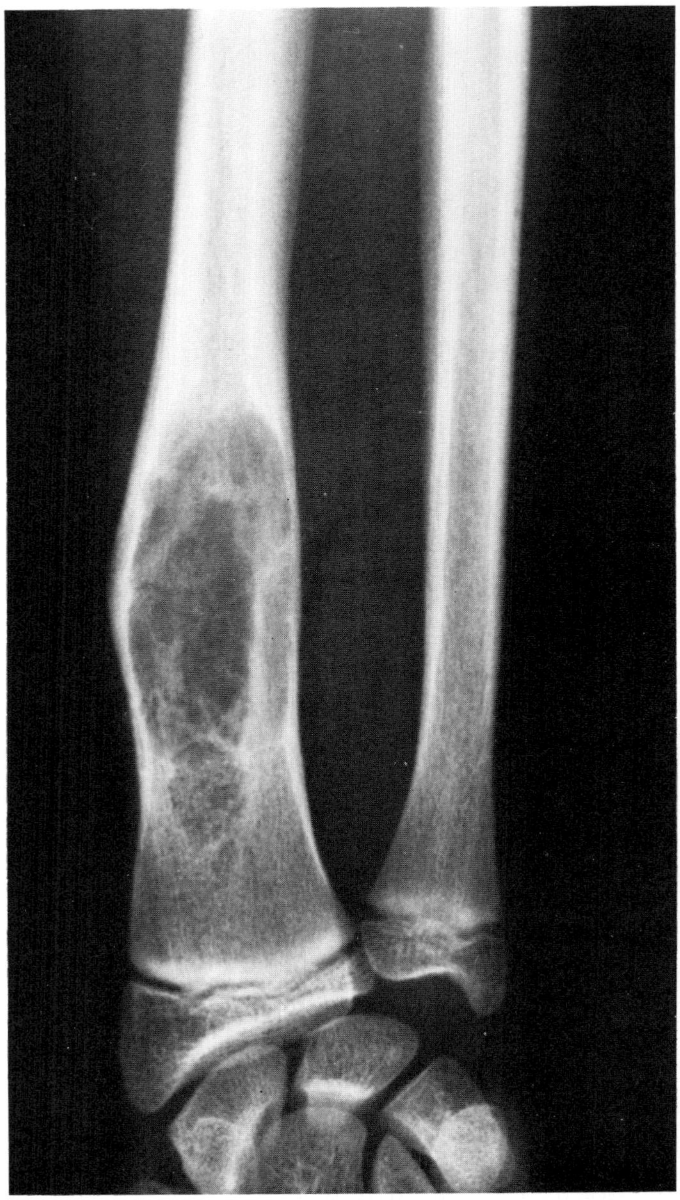

FIG. 6–1. Benign chondroblastoma, non-epiphyseal localization; 14-year-old male.

attention to 8 cases occurring in the metaphyses of the following bones: femoral neck, 2; distal femoral metaphysis, 3; distal tibial metaphysis, 2; and proximal tibial metaphysis, 1. Our case, presented here, is the first in the humerus.

MALIGNANT CHONDROBLASTOMA

Unlike benign giant cell tumor, benign chondroblastoma recurs in fewer than 10% of cases following meticulous curettage; furthermore, malignant change (except irradiation-induced osteogenic sarcoma) of benign chondroblastoma practically never occurs. In 1968, we[68] presented 22 cases of benign chondroblastoma and undertook a survey of the literature with respect to malignant chondroblastoma. In each case where the x-rays and photomicrographs left any doubt with respect to the correct diagnosis of malignant chondroblastoma, we attempted to obtain and review the microscopic sections. Many of the cases turned out to be sarcomas from their inception and were discarded; in other cases, sections were no longer available for review. The single case of chondroblastoma with metastasis which we were able to document was the one later reported in detail by Kahn, Wood, and Ackerman.[65] The metastases in this case were not sarcomatous in their microscopic appearance and did not differ appreciably from the initial benign chondroblastoma. Dahlin and Ivins[60] commented on this same case as follows, "Metastasis from benign chondroblastoma has been documented with autopsy findings and histologic evidence in one case. The death from metastasis occurred 15 years after the first of four ineffectual 'curettages and partial resections' of the primary tumor." A similar case of benign chondroblastoma with pulmonary metastasis has recently been reported by Green and Whittaker.[63] This patient remains well 3 years after biopsy of the pulmonary metastases which have shown no progression since the biopsy. Dahlin and Ivins[60] accepted 6 cases of chondroblastoma in which sarcomatous degeneration had occurred. One was from the Mayo Clinic and the other 5 were culled from the literature. Four had received radiation therapy and were considered to be irradiation-induced osteogenic sarcomas. Two other cases were considered to have undergone sarcomatous degeneration and had received no radiation therapy. One, a case from the Netherland's Committee on Bone Tumours, was a patient who developed metastasizing and fatal fibrosarcoma 14 years after curettage (personal communication from Dr. Van Rijssel to Dr. Dahlin), and the other was a case reported in detail by Sirsat and Doctor.[69]

In summary, metastasis from histopathologically benign chondroblastoma has been documented in two cases;[63, 65] sarcomatous transformation of a benign chondroblastoma without radiation therapy and with sarcomatous metastases has occurred in 2 instances,[60, 69] and 4 irradiation-induced osteogenic sarcomas at the site of benign chondroblastoma have been recorded.[60]

GIANT CELL REACTION OF HAND AND FOOT BONES

This 32-year-old school teacher complained of discomfort and swelling at the base of the left index finger with gradual enlargement following a "bump" two months earlier which first called her attention to the lesion. Serum calcium, phosphate, and alkaline phosphatase were normal. The x-ray (Fig. 7–1) shows an

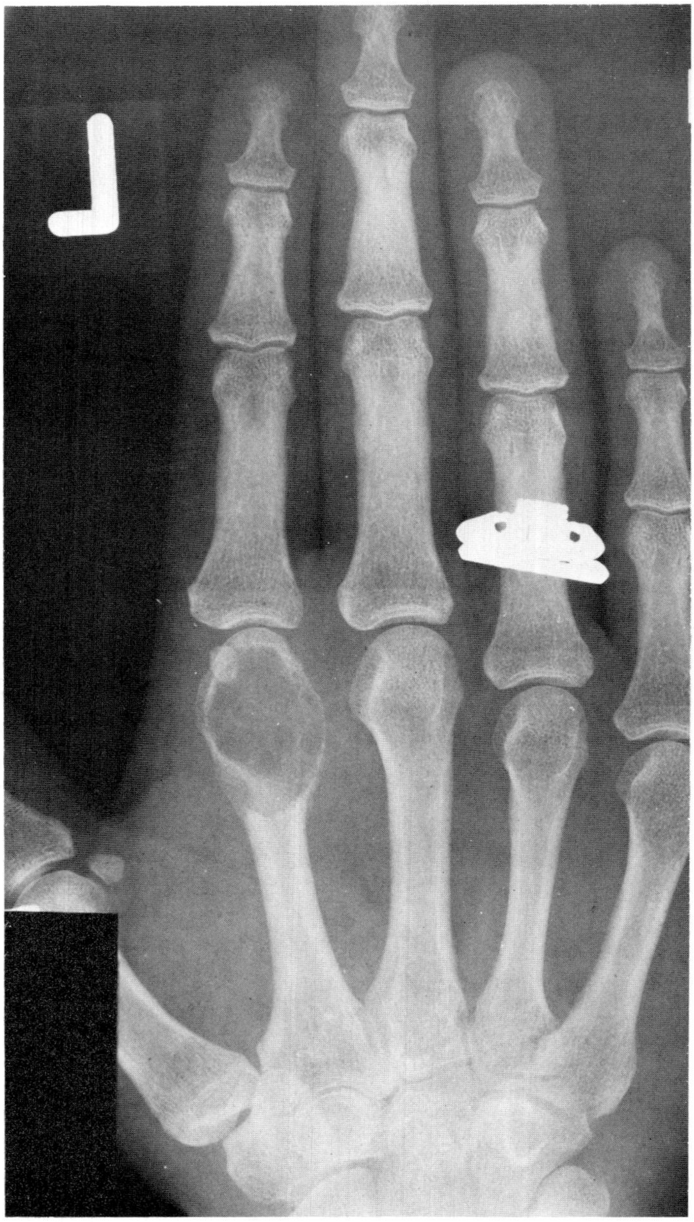

FIG. 7-1. Giant cell reaction of metacarpal, 32-year-old woman.

expansile, lytic lesion involving both metaphyseal and epiphyseal regions of a distal metacarpal bone. The characteristic microscopic features, present in all 7 of the cases in our files, are two in number. The first (Fig. 7-2) is a peculiar proliferation of spindle-shaped fibroblasts which produce large amounts of refractile collagen. Multinucleated giant cells are interspersed between the fibroblasts and may be sparse or numerous. The second pattern (Fig. 7-3) is quite

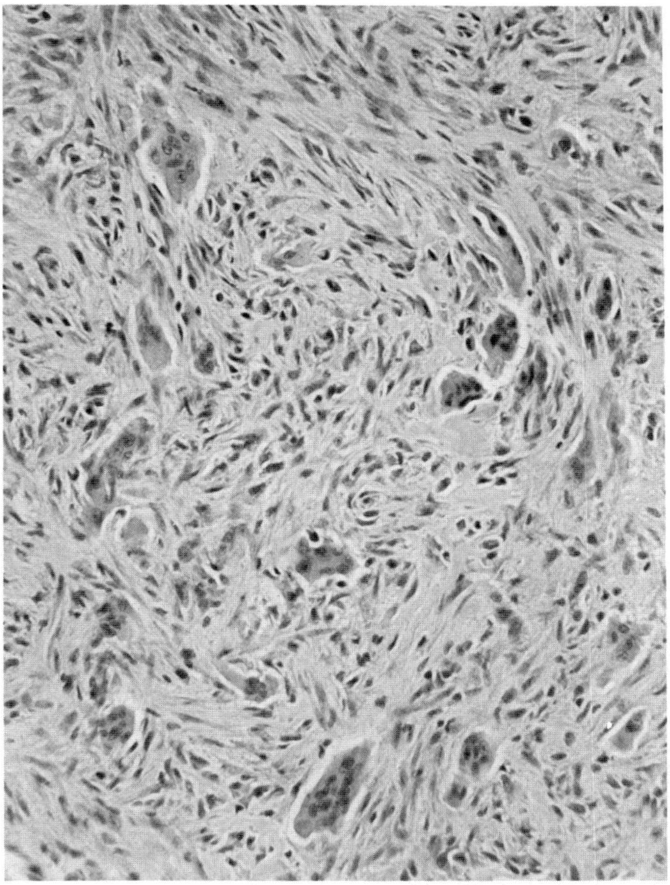

FIG. 7–2. Giant cell reaction of bone. Characteristic, spindle-shaped fibroblasts producing large amounts of refractile collagen. Moderate numbers of multinucleated giant cells. × 200.

similar to the first except that there is a considerable production of lesional osteoid and bone. The osteoid and bone production is quite extensive in some of the lesions. Lesser focal areas within these processes may resemble other lesions such as giant cell reparative granuloma of jaw bones, brown tumor of hyperparathyroidism, giant cell tumor, aneurysmal bone cyst, and even fibrous cortical defect, but the dominant pattern is that described above.

In our opinion, this is a distinctive lesion and deserves to be distinguished from other lesions containing giant cells. Giant cell reaction of bone was first mentioned by Ackerman and Spjut.[1] Two cases were described, both in finger phalanges and both in females, aged 35 and 10. A third case was added by Jernstrom and Stark,[71] occurring in the third metacarpal of a 21-year-old male. The fourth and fifth cases were reported by D'Alonzo, Pitcock, and Milford;[70] both were in middle finger phalanges of women 19 and 25 years of age. Jernstrom and Stark[71] showed us their case prior to publication and since that time we have accumulated 6 additional cases in our files. None of these 6 cases has been previously reported. They include 2 metacarpal lesions, 1 in a 32-year-old female

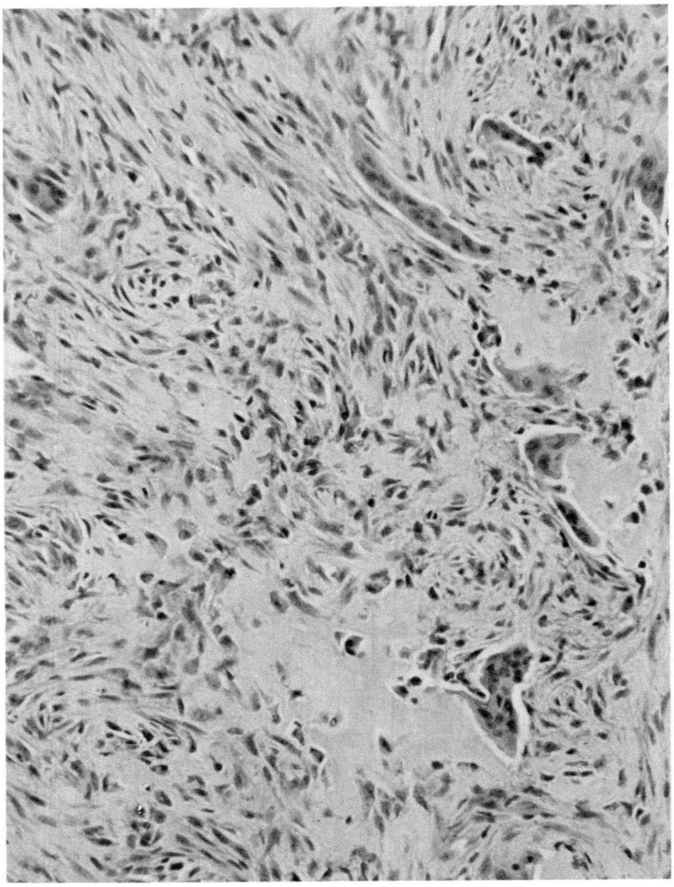

FIG. 7–3. Giant cell reaction of bone. Osteoid and bone production superimposed on spindle cell, collagen-producing stroma. × 200.

(Fig. 7–1, 7–2, and 7–3), the other in an 18-year-old female; 2 metatarsal lesions in 14- and 27-year-old females; 1 finger phalanx lesion in a 32-year-old female, and 1 of a toe phalanx in a 26-year-old female.

In summary, of these 11 lesions, 6 are in phalanges, 3 in metacarpals, and 2 in metatarsals; 3 patients are males and 8 females; and the ages ranged from 10 to 35 years. It is also worth noting that Schajowicz,[21] in his paper on giant cell tumors, commented that the "relative frequency of lesions in the phalanges, metacarpals, and metatarsals (seven cases) is quite remarkable, since these are considered rather rare locations." It seems probable that some of these cases are giant cell reaction rather than giant cell tumor.

In our opinion, giant cell reaction is a distinctive lesion with highly characteristic histopathologic findings which occurs in phalanges, metatarsals. and metacarpals and is usually curable by curettage. It is probably a more commonly occurring lesion than is now realized; it should be distinguished from other lesions containing giant cells.

INTRAOSSEOUS (INVASIVE, AGGRESSIVE) PIGMENTED VILLONODULAR SYNOVITIS AND TENOSYNOVITIS (GIANT CELL TUMOR OF TENDON SHEATH, FIBROUS XANTHOMA OF SYNOVIUM)

Jaffe[7] noted that, "it is of special interest that they [pigmented villonodular synovitis and tenosynovitis] sometimes erode the regional bone or bones in the course of their expansion. Indeed, the tenosynovial lesions, especially those developing in toes, in other parts of the foot, or at the ankle, not infrequently do this . . . [and] cases in which regional bone destruction has occurred often raise problems of clinical differential diagnosis." Aegerter and Kilpatrick[2] also suggested that involvement of bony structures was not uncommon and mentioned that they had accumulated 15 such cases in the prior 10 years. They suggested the name "intraosseous villonodular synovitis," to distinguish these cases from those of the usual type in which there was no bone involvement.

The patient whose x-ray is shown (Fig. 8–1) was a 51-year-old woman who complained of pain in the hip for 10 months. Invasion of both the acetabulum and femoral head is evident. The differential diagnosis is greatly simplified when the surgeon informs the pathologist that the lesion arose in either synovium or tenosynovium and appeared to be invading or eroding the bone rather than arising within it. The pathologist who then receives a gross specimen which is a relatively well-circumscribed mass of either red-brown or yellow-brown coloration should suspect that the lesion is a pigmented villonodular synovitis. Under these circumstances the pathologist is unlikely to confuse the histopathology of this lesion (Fig. 8–2) with either benign giant cell tumor or benign chondroblastoma. It is true that focal areas of pigmented villonodular synovitis may resemble

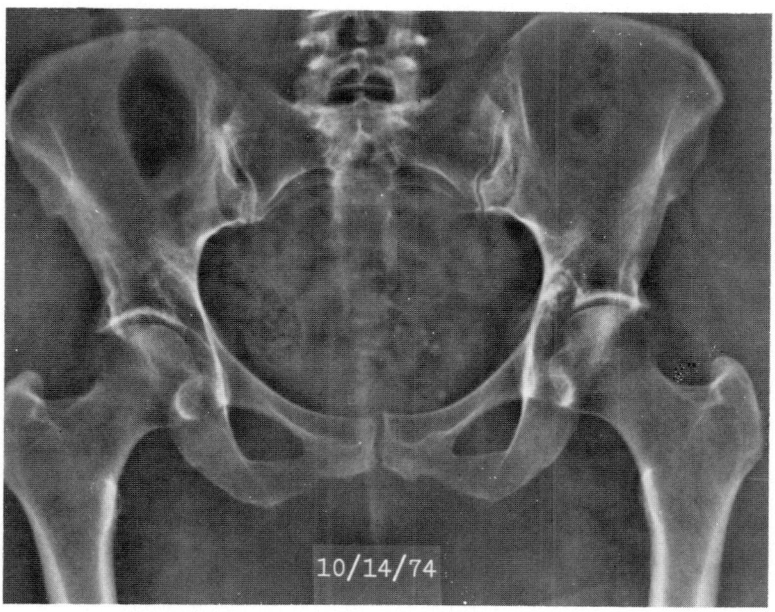

FIG. 8–1. Intraosseous (invasive) villonodular synovitis, left hip joint synovium, 51-year-old woman. Lesion is invading acetabulum and femoral head.

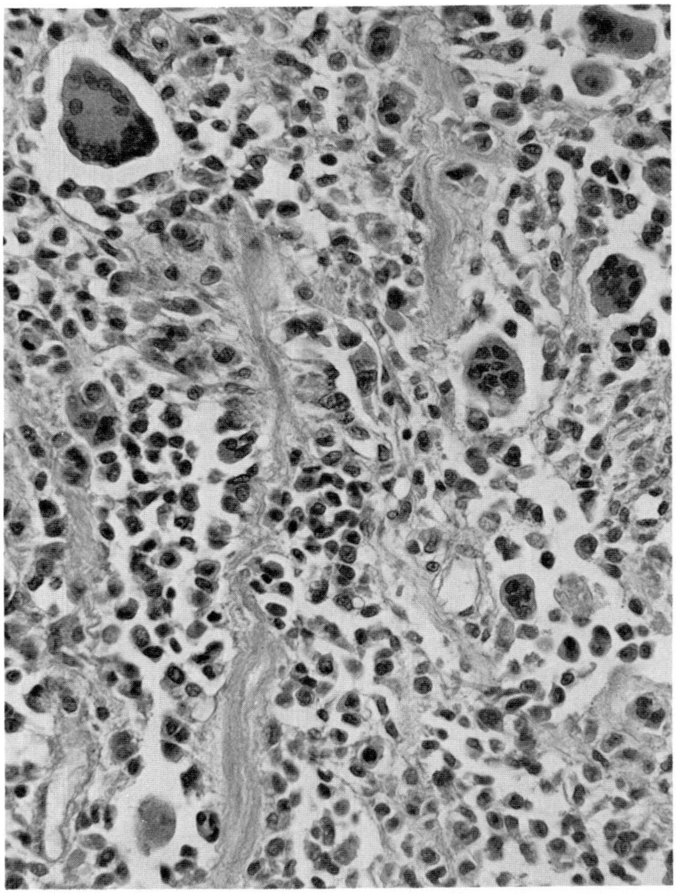

FIG. 8–2. Pigmented villonodular synovitis. Sheets of histiocytes and interspersed multinucleated giant cells. Bands of dense, hyalinized collagen are relatively characteristic. × 300.

microscopically benign chondroblastoma, but multiple sections will fail to show either chondroid, calcium deposition, or ossification. In the case of benign giant cell tumor, multiple sections will seldom show either wide bands or thin strands (Fig. 8–2) of dense, hyalinized, collagenous connective tissue which are nearly always present in pigmented villonodular synovitis. The histopathology of villonodular synovitis is discussed in greater detail elsewhere in this monograph (Chapter 11), and further description will not be undertaken.

BROWN TUMOR OF HYPERPARATHYROIDISM

Jaffe[8] has indicated that, "clinical complaints in primary hyperparathyroidism are referable in the main to: the hypercalcemia *per se*, renal and/or gastrointestinal disturbances, and the skeletal changes." The brown tumor of hyperparathyroidism is but one of the skeletal manifestations and, in more recently recorded large series of patients whose physicians are more aware of the early manifestations of hyperparathyroidism, the incidence of brown tumor as the presenting symptom appears to be slightly less than 5%. The classical biochemical findings are hypercalcemia, hypophosphatemia, elevated serum alkaline phosphatase activity, and increased urinary calcium and phosphorus excretion. Seldom, however, does a patient manifest all of these alterations, and it is generally agreed that the most significant, most constant, and most reliable finding is the presence of an elevated serum calcium (above 11.0 mg per 100 ml) for which other causes can be excluded. Serum protein should be determined along with the serum calcium, since approximately 70% of serum calcium is protein-bound calcium, and a normal calcium level in conjunction with a low protein level may mask an abnormally high calcium. McGeown and Morrison[88] have also emphasized the importance of repeating serum calcium determinations in patients suspected of having hyperparathyroidism since it fluctuates and intermittently may be normal.

The patient whose x-ray (Fig. 9–1) shows a lytic lesion in the crest of the ilium (conceivably an atypical localization for true giant cell tumor) was a 74-year-old physician whose chief complaints were pain in the left iliac crest, right hip, and heel, and 30-pound weight loss. Biopsy (Fig. 9–2) to rule out metastatic cancer reveals a lesion whose stromal cells are spindle-shaped and fibrogenic with moderate numbers of multinucleated giant cells. These features, as indicated previously, may occur in focal areas in a "true" giant cell tumor and occasionally may dominate the histopathologic findings. However, because of the atypical localization, the considerable spindle-cell component, and the more than average

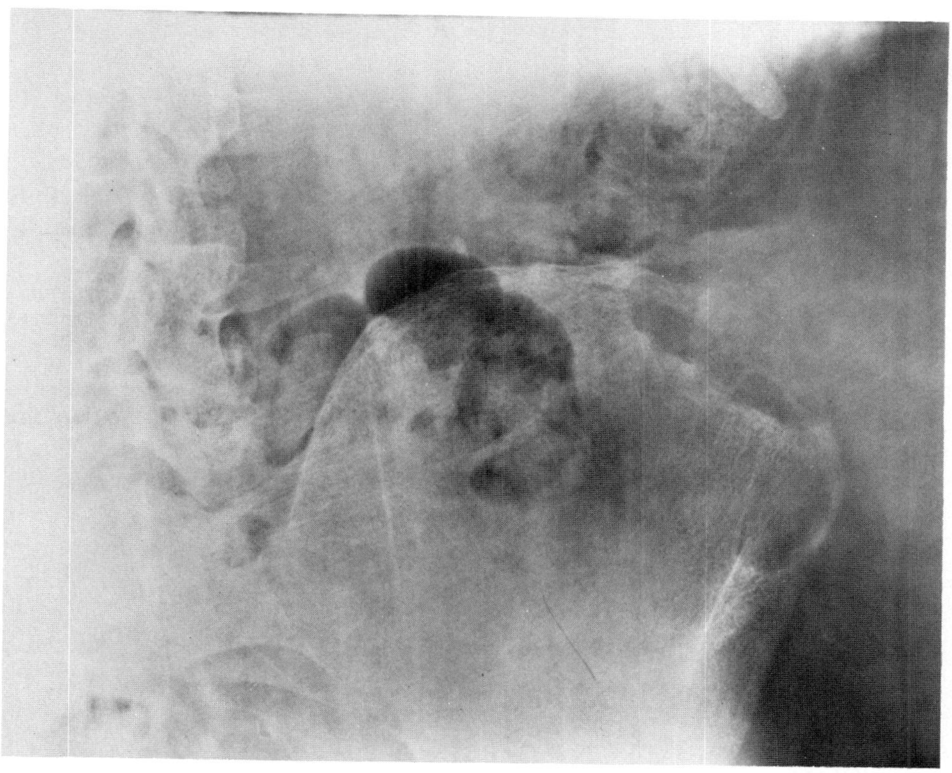

FIG. 9–1. Brown tumor of hyperparathyroidism in wing of ilium; 67-year-old physician.

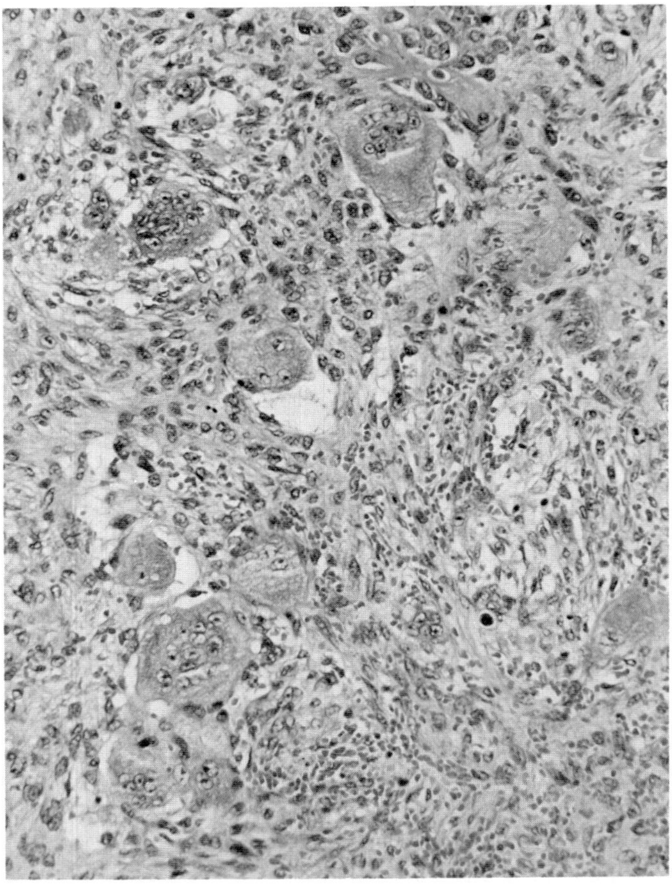

FIG. 9–2. Brown tumor of hyperparathyroidism. Same lesion as shown in Fig. 9–1. Compare with Figs. 1–2 through 1–5. Hematoxylin and eosin stain; × 200.

collagen production, it was suggested that serum calcium, phosphate, and alkaline phosphatase be determined. The serum calcium level was 13.9 mg per 100 ml, and at subsequent surgery a parathyroid adenoma was removed. In our files tumors from other patients whose initial symptoms were related to bone lesions and who subsequently were proven to have a brown tumor of hyperparathyroidism occurred in the following sites: jaws, metacarpal, rib, and clavicle. In addition, we have one case in whom a giant cell epulis arising in the soft tissues of the maxillary gingiva was the presenting symptom. Cases recorded in the literature with initial symptomatology related to a brown tumor are heavily weighted toward those occurring in the jaw and facial bones but also include examples in other sites most of which would be considered unusual localizations for a true giant cell tumor. Giant cell epulides of the gingival soft tissues have also been reported as the initial symptom. Furthermore, in the absence of Paget's disease of bone, true giant cell tumors practically never occur in the jaw or facial bones. For these reasons, whenever a bone lesion containing giant cells is encountered in the jaw or facial bones, in the bones of the hands and feet, or in a localization that would be considered atypical for true benign giant cell tumor, it is suggested that serum calcium, phosphate, and alkaline phosphatase be determined to rule out hyperparathyroidism.

As previously suggested, when dealing with lesions containing large numbers of giant cells, it is good practice to embed for microscopic examination, all of the tissue received. In this way, one may occasionally encounter fragments of bone originating peripheral to the brown tumor, and this bone may show the histopathologic alterations of osteitis fibrosa cystica (Fig. 9-3) and serve to confirm the diagnosis of hyperparathyroidism.

GIANT CELL REPARATIVE GRANULOMA OF JAWBONES

The term "giant cell reparative granuloma" was suggested by Jaffe[95] for lesions in the jaws which only mimic the true giant cell tumor of long bones and which have a number of histologic and clinical differences. The lesion arises in the bone and roentgenographically "appears as a roundish or oval area of increased radiolucency, which is sometimes faintly trabeculated. It thins and expands, but does not perforate the cortex of the affected jawbone." The lesion occurs

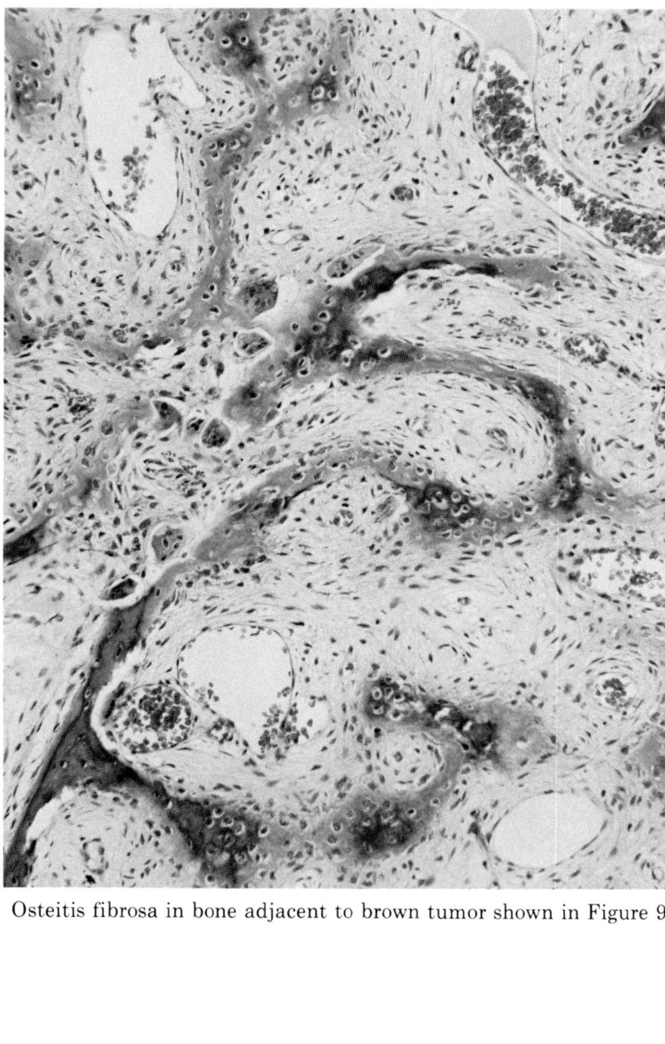

FIG. 9-3. Osteitis fibrosa in bone adjacent to brown tumor shown in Figure 9-2. × 120.

twice as often in females as in males. Approximately one-half of the patients are under 20 years of age, and the vast majority of cases occur prior to 40 years. The vast majority are cured by simple curettage.

The x-ray (Fig. 10–1) in our illustrative case shows a lesion in the maxilla of a 51-year-old man who complained of pain in the jaw of several weeks duration. There was swelling of the soft tissues of the gingiva. Curettage (Fig. 10–2) reveals

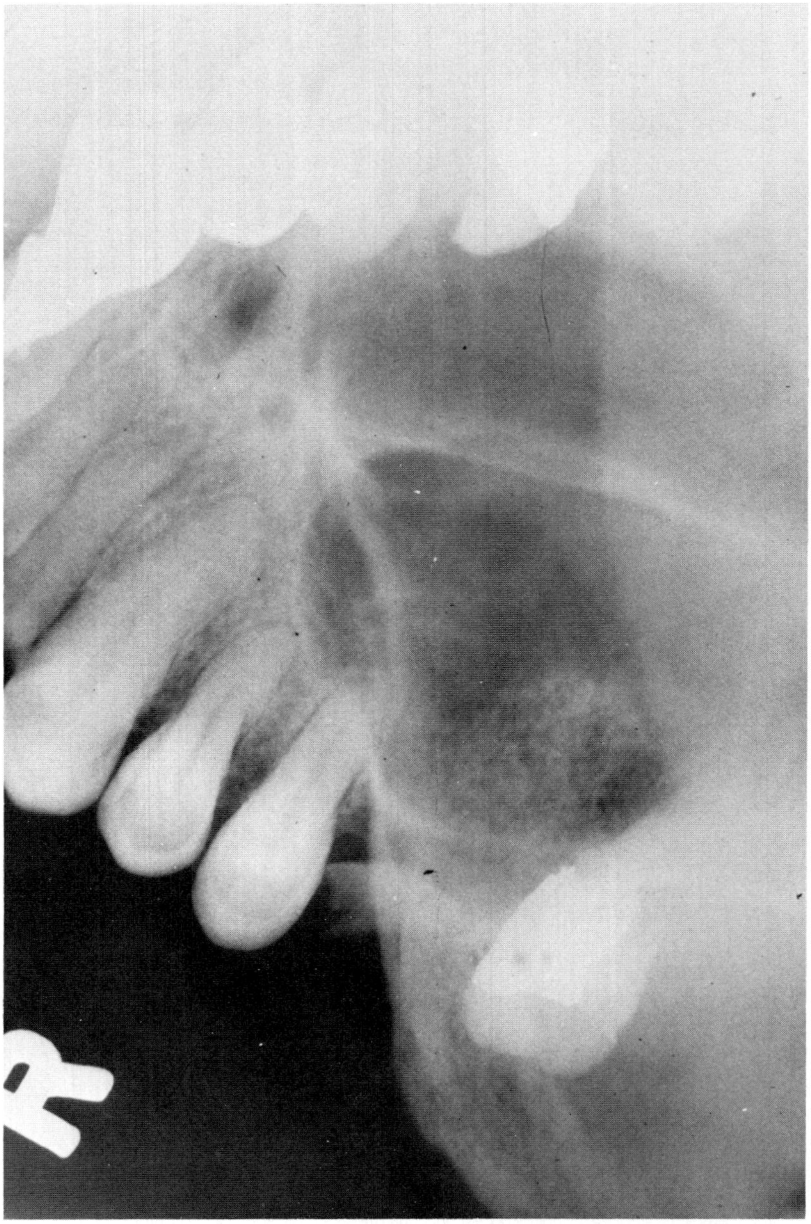

FIG. 10–1. Central giant cell reparative granuloma of jaw bone; 51-year old-male. This expansile lesion of the maxilla caused displacement of the teeth and a mass protruding into the hard palate.

a lesion in which the proliferating stromal cell is either oval or spindle-shaped and fibrogenic. Multinucleated giant cells are moderate in number, and there is a band of collagenized fibrous tissue separating adjacent lobules of lesional tissue. Austin, Dahlin, and Royer,[91] in commenting on the differences of giant cell reparative granuloma from true giant cell tumor noted that collagen was a prominent component in all of the giant cell reparative granulomas, whereas in giant cell tumors of bone large zones without collagen were constantly observed. They also noted that the average field of giant cell tumor contained 4 times as many benign multinucleated giant cells and more nuclei per cell on the average. Other features of giant cell reparative granuloma not illustrated in the photomicrograph include inclusions within the multinucleated giant cells of hemosiderin pigment, red blood cells, and large clear vacuoles whose nature is unknown,[97] osteoid and bone deposition,[7, 91, 97] and hemosiderin deposition and extravasated red blood cells in stromal areas.[7]

In connection with the osteoid and bone present in giant cell reparative granuloma, Waldron and Shafer[97] in many instances found "it difficult or impossible to determine whether the osteoid or bone occurred within the lesion as

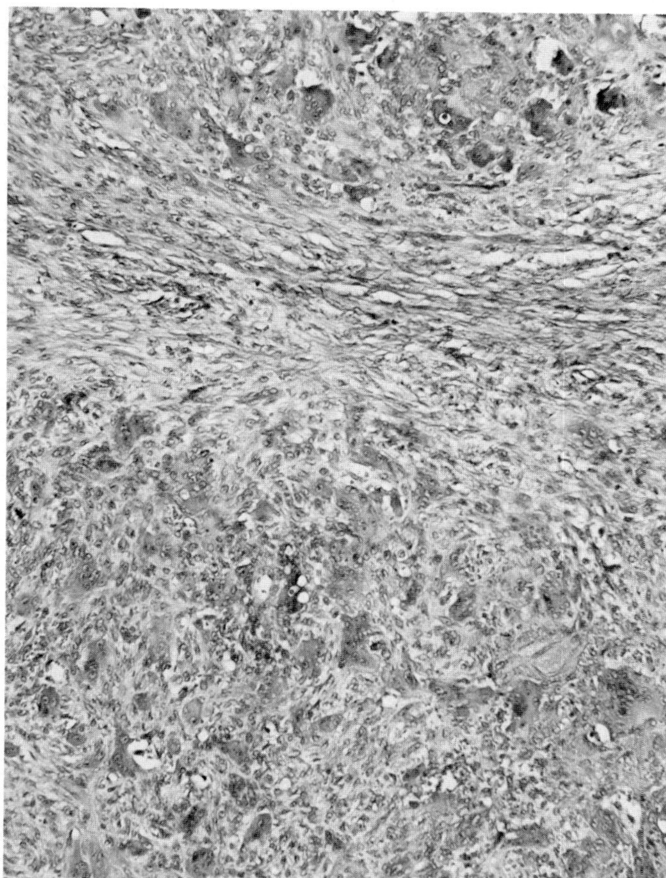

FIG. 10-2. Central giant cell reparative granuloma. × 120.

a result of plane of section, or whether it was an integral part of the lesion." However, osteoid or bone which was interpreted by them as being an integral component of the lesions was identified in more than three-fourths of the cases. Summarizing the histopathologic findings Austin *et al.*[91] noted that "this lesion in its typical form, rarely, if ever, occurs in bones other than those of the jaws. It is histologically distinct from giant cell tumor of bone in that its proliferating cells are basically fibrogenic and have a marked tendency to undergo metaplasia to a type of cell capable of producing osteoid and bone. Many of the lesions develop more or less parallel osseous trabeculae reminiscent of those seen in callus."

The differential diagnosis of giant cell reparative granuloma from other jaw bone lesions exhibiting multinucleated giant cells includes a large number of lesions. On the basis of histopathology the brown tumor of hyperparathyroidism (Fig. 9–2) is indistinguishable from giant cell reparative granuloma; the differential diagnosis must be based on the finding of an elevated serum calcium. The histopathologic differences from true giant cell tumor have already been discussed. Furthermore, for practical purposes true giant cell tumor does not occur in the jaw bone. Jaffe,[7] with all his experience, has encountered only 1 such lesion in a jaw bone. Austin *et al.*,[91] in 1959, felt that there were 2 lesions amongst their jaw bone lesions which might be true giant cell tumors, but Dahlin,[4] in 1967, in his monograph on bone tumors, states: "It was not possible to segregate any unequivocal giant cell tumors from the numerous giant cell reparative lesions of the jaw bones." Bhaskar, Bernier, and Godby[92] and Black and Ackerman[82] found no acceptable cases of true giant cell tumor in the jaw bone, and we have none in our own file. Benign giant cell tumor arising in Paget's disease of bone occurs in jaw bones. It can be differentiated on the basis of the elevated alkaline phosphatase values and by the roentgenographic evidence of Paget's disease in the adjacent bone. Dahlin and Ivins[60] have recorded 2 cases of benign chondroblastoma in the jaw bone, so this rare occurrence must be considered. Dehner, in the section on "Differential Diagnosis of Fibro-Osseous Lesions of Bone" elsewhere in this monograph (Chapter 14), discusses the fibro-osseous lesions which may occur in jawbones. Many of these contain multinucleated giant cells, including: fibrous dysplasia, cherubism, cementoblastoma, cementifying fibroma, ossifying fibroma, osteoid osteoma, and osteoblastoma. Florid Paget's disease of the jawbone contains numerous osteoclasts. Lesions still to be considered by us which do occur in jaw bones and which contain multinucleated giant cells are the following: osteosarcoma with numerous multinucleated giant cells, aneurysmal bone cyst, and eosinophilic granuloma. The giant cell epulis[7, 91, 97] (peripheral giant cell reparative granuloma) arising in the gingival soft tissues must be distinguished from the central giant cell reparative granuloma of jaw bones.

As indicated earlier, the lesions under consideration with respect to the differential diagnosis of lesions of bone containing giant cells have been divided into two groups. The first group (Table I) includes those lesions which are most likely to be confused with true benign giant cell tumor of bone. The second group (Table II) which we will now consider are those whose histopathology is usually sufficiently different from that of benign giant cell tumor that they can be differentiated on that basis alone in most cases. In addition, these lesions tend, when they occur in long tubular bones, to be localized either in the diaphyseal or metaphyseal regions rather than in the epiphyseal end. They are usually more difficult to differentiate one from another than from giant cell tumor or any of the other lesions so far discussed.

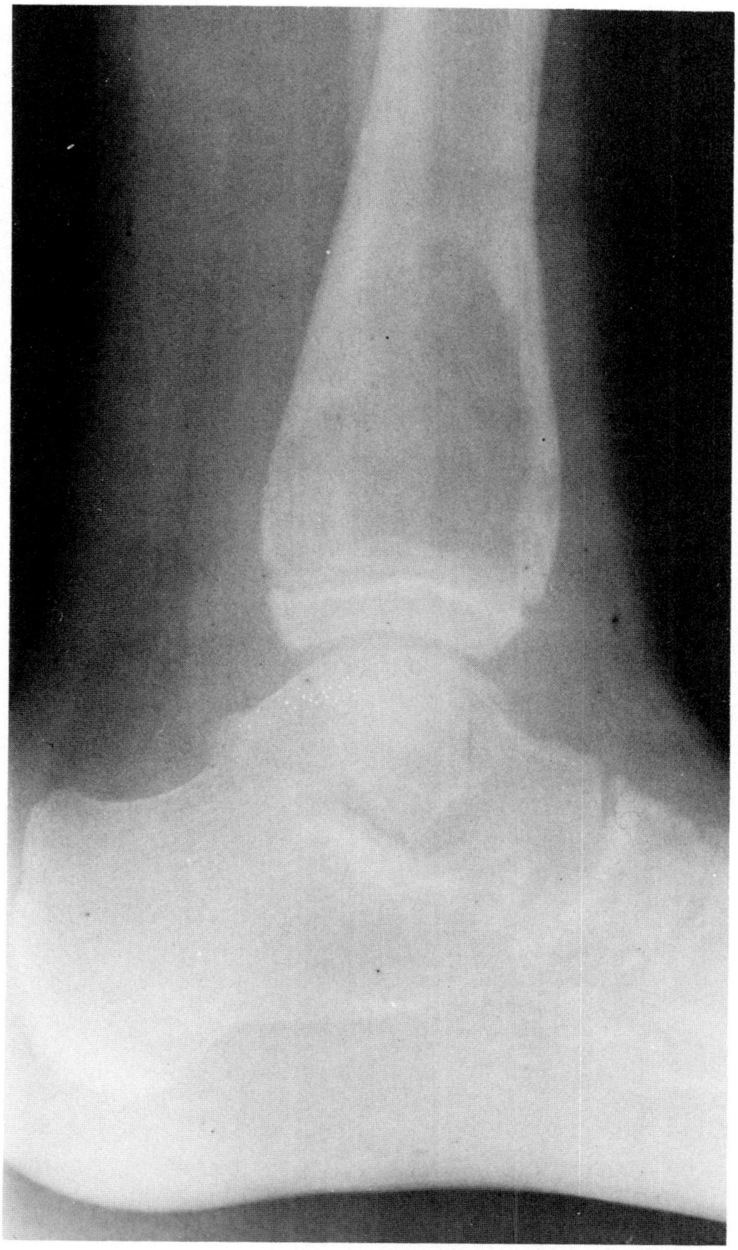

FIG. 11-1. Osteosarcoma with numerous benign multinucleated giant cells in tibial metaphysis of 15-year-old boy.

OSTEOSARCOMA WITH NUMEROUS BENIGN MULTINUCLEATED GIANT CELLS

Troup,[100] and later Troup, Dahlin, and Coventry,[101] made a special study of osteosarcomas which contained large numbers of benign multinucleated giant cells. Thirteen per cent of their osteosarcomas fit into this category. Because 8 of the 13 cases had an initial histologic diagnosis of giant cell tumor (none were so diagnosed in recent years), they compared the gross and roentgenographic features of their 53 cases of osteosarcoma with numerous giant cells with those expected to occur in benign giant cell tumor. They found that in only 3 of these osteosarcomas the involvement was restricted to or centered in the epiphysis. In the remainder, the epicenter of the osteosarcoma was in the metaphysis, and many were associated with elevation of the periosteum, extraosseous formation of new bone, and an identifiable Codman's angle. Many were radiolucent but in a majority of these the periosteum was perforated, and there was a considerable extraosseous mass. They concluded that they were unlike either benign or malignant giant cell tumor.

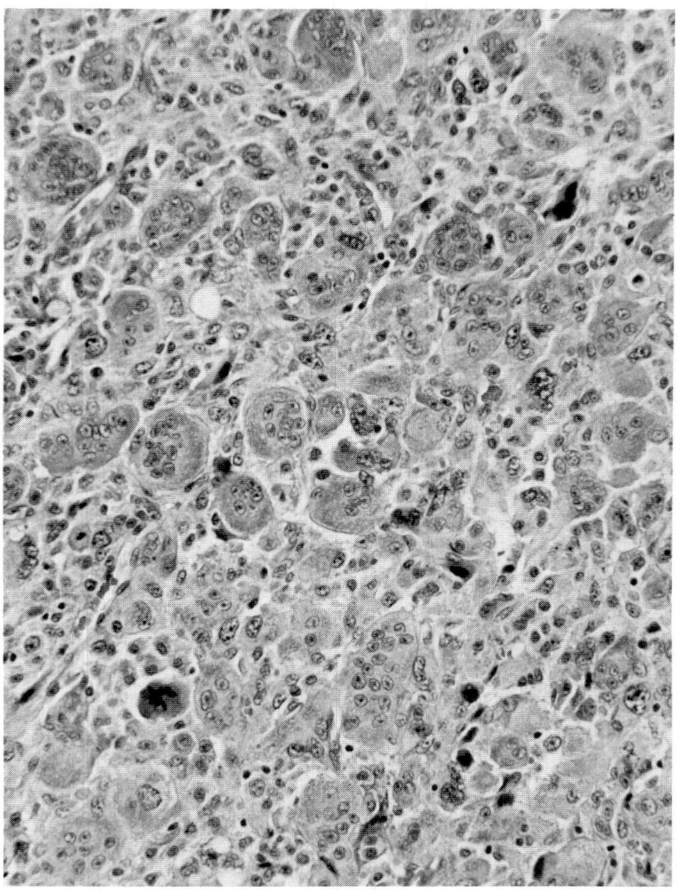

FIG. 11-2. Osteosarcoma with numerous benign multinucleated giant cells. Scattered malignant stromal cells. Compare with Figures 1-3, 1-4, 1-5, and 2-1. × 200.

A special group of osteosarcomas with numerous giant cells are the so-called telangiectatic osteosarcomas.[7, 12, 98, 99] These often exhibit numerous multinucleated giant cells, and with their cavernous, blood-filled spaces may resemble aneurysmal bone cyst in their histopathologic and sometimes their roentgenographic features.

These two types of osteosarcoma with numerous benign giant cells are best appreciated through illustrative examples. The x-ray (Fig. 11–1) shows a predominantly radiolucent area in the distal tibial metaphysis of a 15-year-old boy who complained of increasing pain and swelling subsequent to twisting his ankle 1 month earlier. Neither the localization of this osteosarcoma with benign multinucleated giant cells in the metaphysis nor the presence of an adjacent open epiphysis is compatible with a diagnosis of giant cell tumor, and the patient is younger than 90% of patients with giant cell tumor. For these reasons, when the initial sections showed large numbers of benign multinucleated giant cells and a relatively innocuous stromal component in a setting that was inappropriate for a diagnosis of giant cell tumor, numerous additional sections were prepared, and

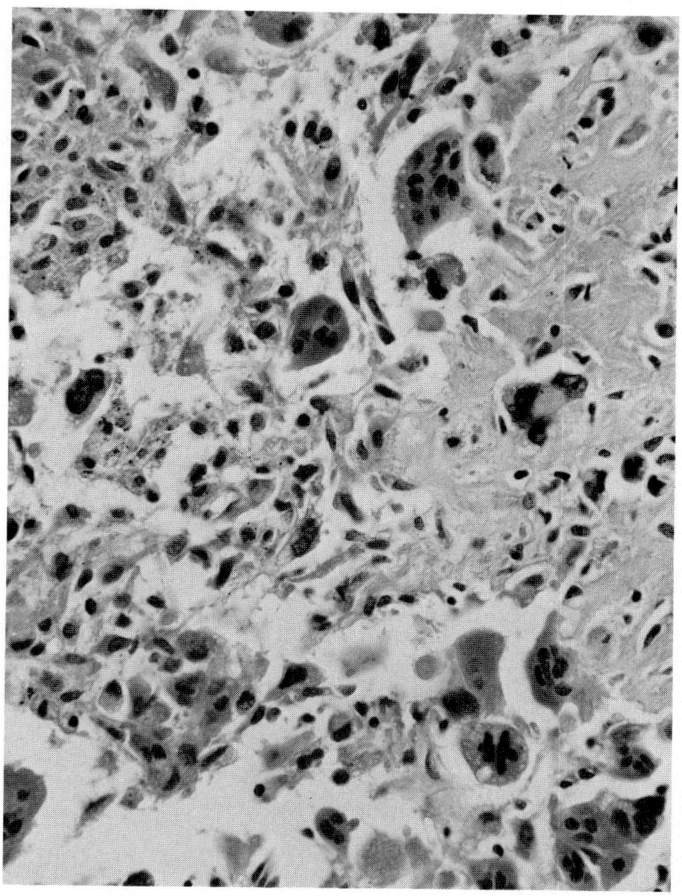

FIG. 11–3. Osteosarcoma with numerous benign multinucleated giant cells. Focus with tumor osteoid and tumor bone formation. × 300.

several foci were found (Fig. 11–2) where careful examination of the stromal cells revealed a significant number with large, hyperchromatic nuclei exhibiting variation in size, shape, and staining reaction, and with a considerable increase in nuclear-cytoplasmic ratio. In a few areas (Fig. 11–3) bizarre mitoses and foci of tumor osteoid and tumor bone were identified. This osteoid and bone were derived directly from the sarcomatous cells. (Compare Figs. 11–2 and 11–3 with 1–3, 1–4, 1–5, and 2–1.)

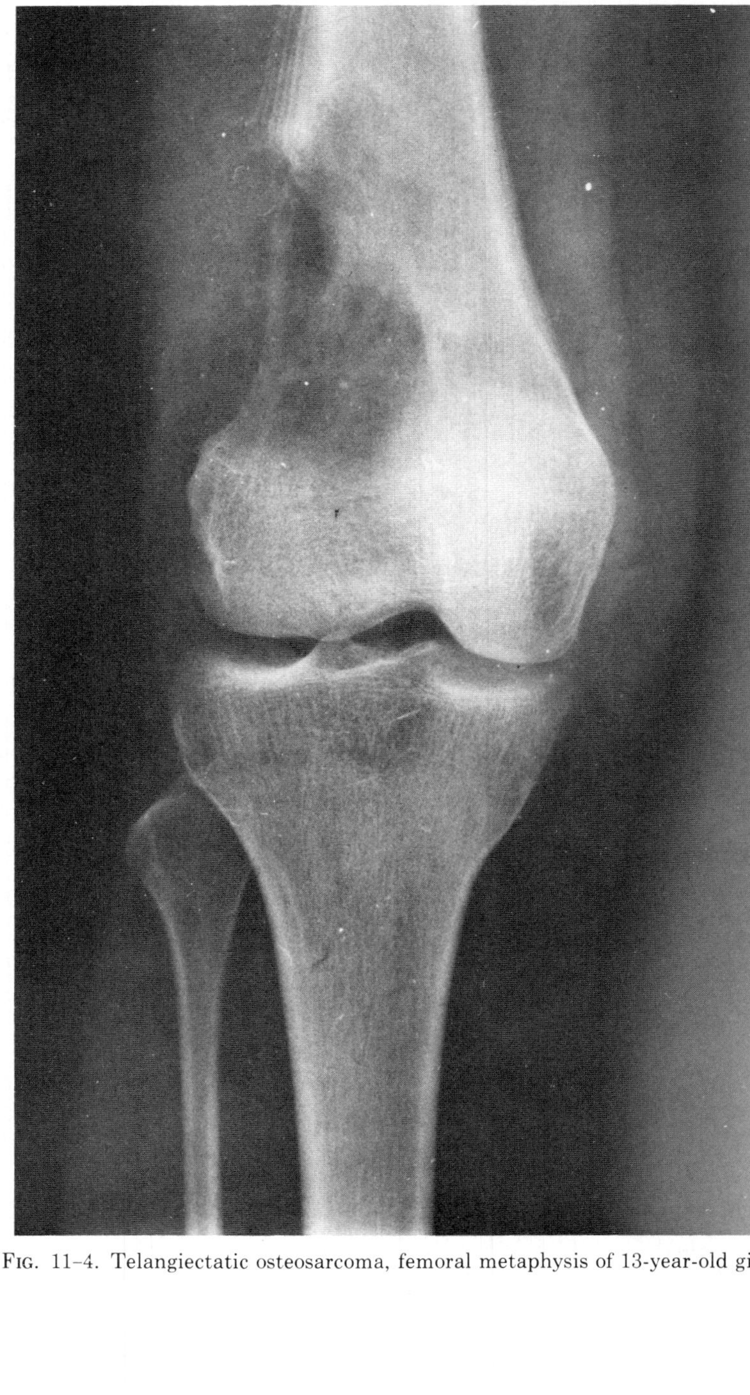

FIG. 11–4. Telangiectatic osteosarcoma, femoral metaphysis of 13-year-old girl.

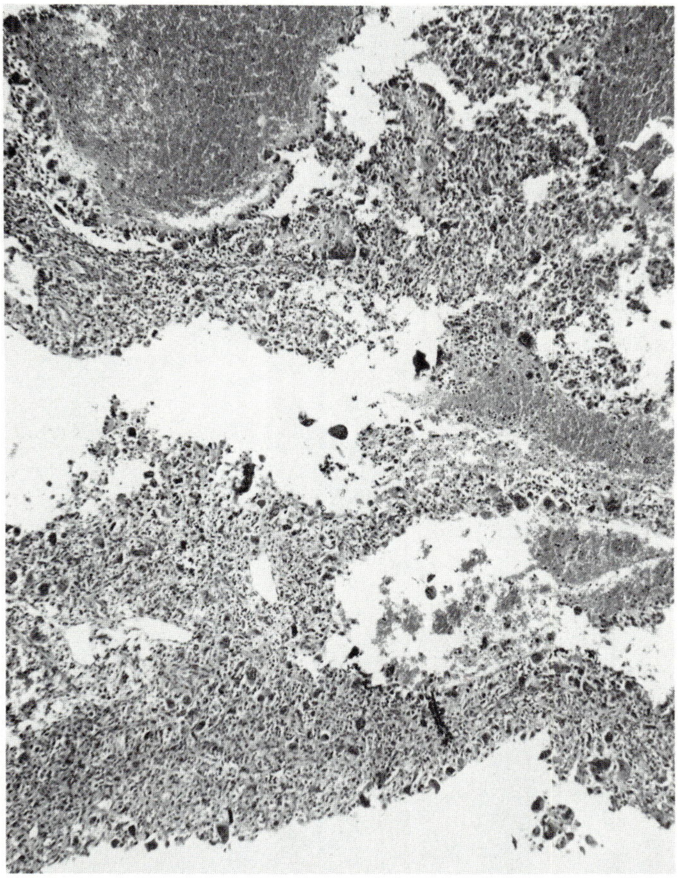

FIG. 11-5. Telangiectatic osteosarcoma with moderate numbers of benign multinucleated giant cells. Superficial resemblance to aneurysmal bone cyst. (Compare with Figure 14-3.) × 48.

The x-ray (Fig. 11-4) is of a telangiectatic osteosarcoma arising in the distal metaphysis of the femur of a 13-year-old girl whose chief complaint was a gradually enlarging mass on the lateral aspect of the right knee. Although the lesion is eccentric and there is a "blown-out" soft tissue extension (compare with Figure 14-1, aneurysmal bone cyst), the poorly defined peripheral, soft tissue margins, and the presence of Codman's angle are more in favor of a malignant tumor than an aneurysmal bone cyst. However, the lower power photomicrograph (Fig. 11-5) shows dilated and blood-filled cavernous spaces surrounded by a spindle cell, collagen-producing stroma in which numerous benign multinucleated giant cells are interspersed, and superficially resembles aneurysmal bone cyst (compare with Figure 14-3). Once again, however, careful microscopic study of multiple sections resulted in the identification of focal areas (Fig. 11-6) in which the oval- and spindle-shaped stromal cells are malignant. The malignant areas in this tumor were not extensive, and, possibly because of this, the correct diagnosis of this patient's tumor was delayed several months.

The importance of close cooperation between the surgeon, roentgenologist, and

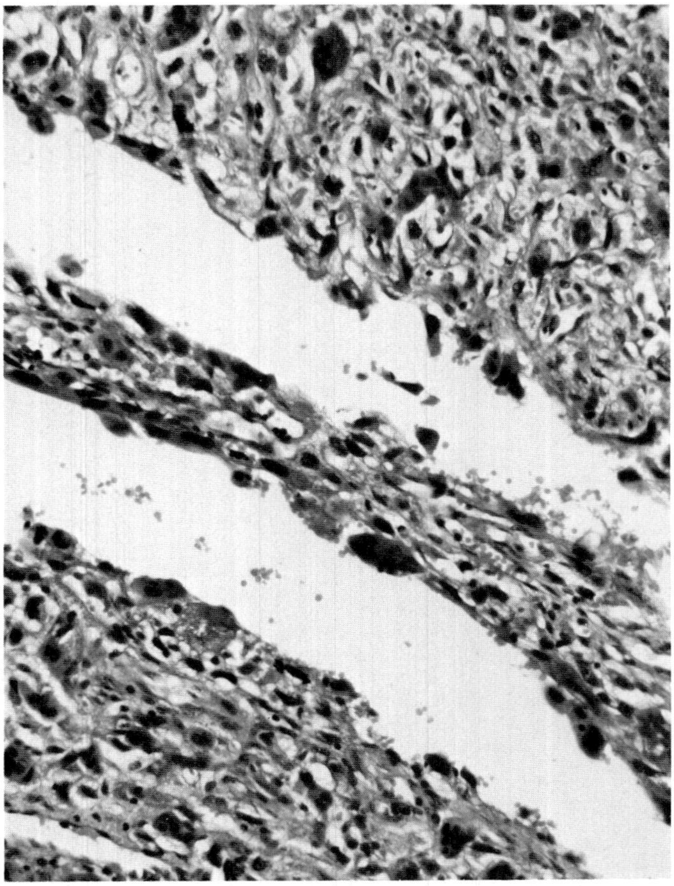

FIG. 11-6. Higher power of telangiectatic osteosarcoma shown in Figure 11-5, showing malignant oval- and spindle-shaped stromal cells. × 200.

pathologist in ascertaining the correct diagnosis is emphasized in cases such as these.

FIBROUS CORTICAL DEFECT (METAPHYSEAL FIBROUS DEFECT, METAPHYSEAL CORTICAL DEFECT, NONOSTEOGENIC FIBROMA, NONOSSIFYING FIBROMA)

The x-ray (Fig. 12-1) shows a relatively large fibrous cortical defect in the cortex of the tibial shaft of a 12-year-old male. Jaffe and Lichtenstein,[106] in 1941, described the clinical, radiographic, and pathologic findings in 10 cases of this distinctive entity. In this report, which concerned mostly relatively large lesions such as this one, they suggested the name nonosteogenic fibroma. Even when relatively large, the characteristic defect tends to be superficial, shallow, and located predominantly in relation to the cortex, and the edges of the defect are almost invariably sclerotic. Sontag and Pyle,[109] in 1941, subjected 101 healthy children to yearly roentgen examinations of their knees and described the roentgenographic findings in the 37 who had fibrous cortical defects. Caffey,[103] in

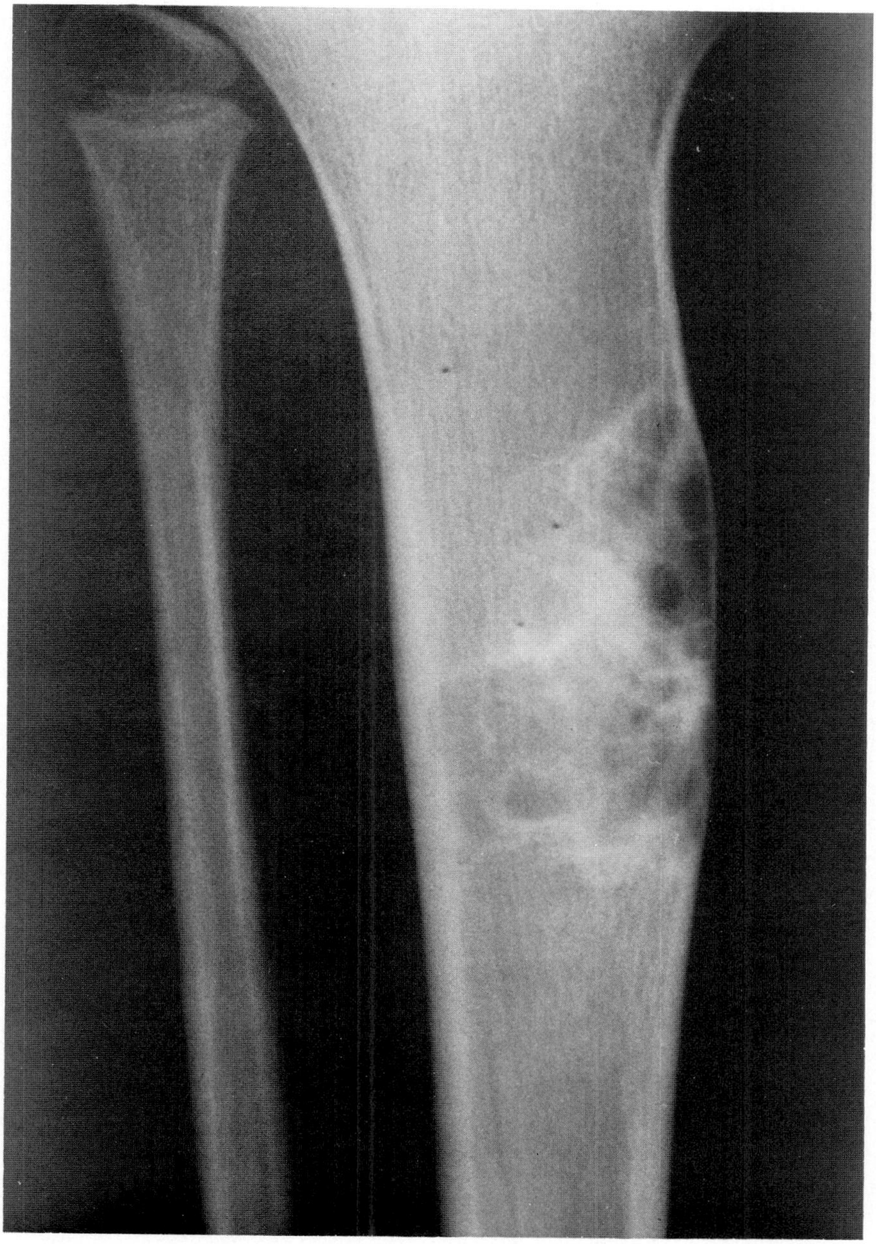

FIG. 12–1. Large fibrous cortical defect (nonosteogenic fibroma); tibial shaft of a 12-year-old boy.

1955, reported on a similar study, reviewed the literature, and commented extensively on the roentgenographic appearance, prevalence, and natural course. These two reports included a goodly number of smaller lesions such as the one illustrated in Figure 12–2. This lesion of the proximal tibia of a 13-year-old girl was an incidental finding in an x-ray taken because of knee pain following trauma. Caffey called attention to the fact that these defects, large and small,

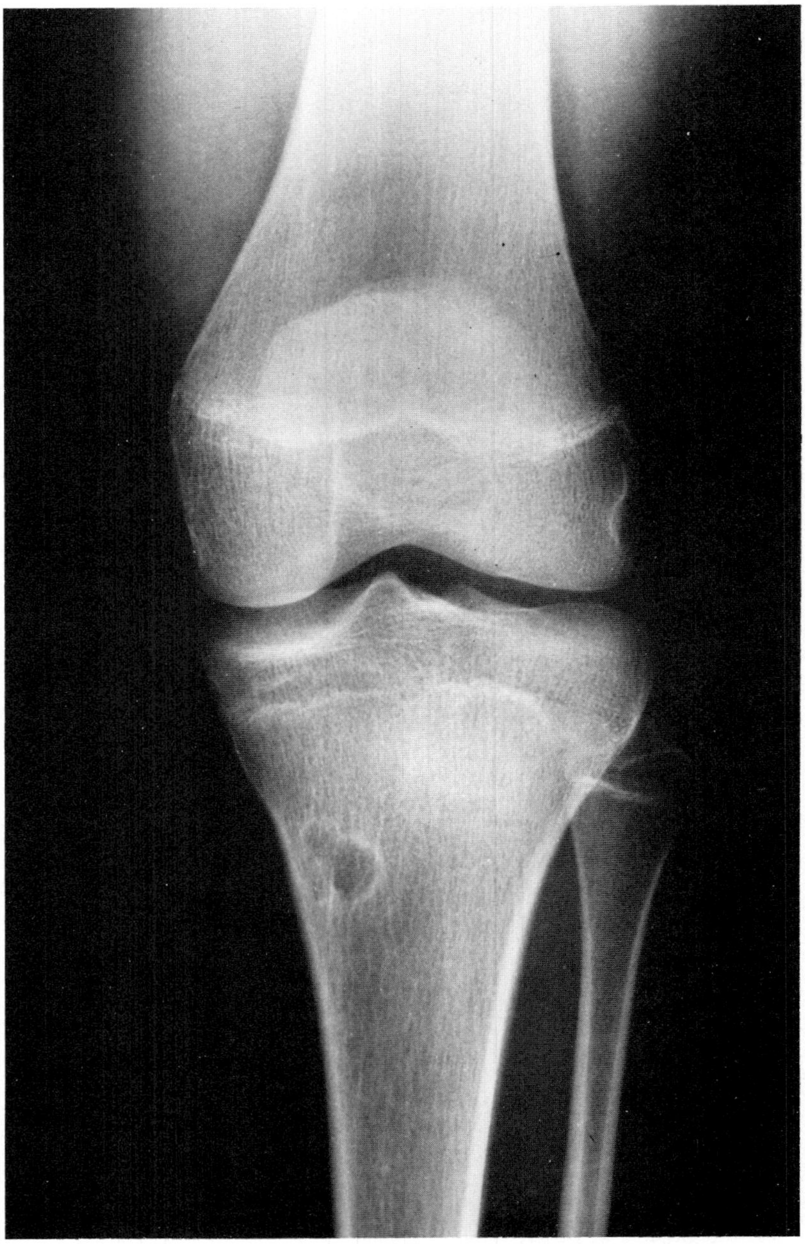

FIG. 12–2. A more average-sized metaphyseal fibrous defect; tibia of a 13-year-old girl. This patient was known to have a similar lesion in radius 4 years previously; it resolved without treatment.

can be demonstrated in 50% of boys and 25% of girls at one or more ages. He noted that they might be single or multiple, in a single bone or in several bones, that they are more frequently found on dorsal and medial aspects of the bone and, quite naturally. since they are of frequent occurrence, they are often encountered as an incidental finding in x-rays taken for other reasons.

Occasional cases are encountered in the 3rd and 4th decades but the majority of patients with this lesion are less than 20 years of age. When untreated, the vast majority of fibrous cortical defects will undergo spontaneous involution.

In cases where biopsy or curettage is undertaken, the microscopic findings are quite characteristic. The basic proliferating stromal element can be categorized in currently fashionable terminology as "fibrous histiocytic;" some of the fibroblasts appear to be transforming into histiocytes, and there is a prominent storiform pattern (Fig. 12-3). Accumulations of lymphocytes are seen in focal areas, and multinucleated giant cells, which may be few or numerous, are present in moderate numbers. Also, in some of the cases, for no known reason, it is technically difficult to cut "thin" sections, and the relative thickness of the section imparts a pseudocellular appearance (Fig. 12-3). Ordinarily (Fig. 12-4) there are focal areas in which few or many lipid-laden histiocytes are present. Focal accumulations of hemosiderin-containing histiocytes are also frequently seen. Finally, neither osteoid nor bone formation is present within the lesion unless there has been a complicating fracture or infraction.

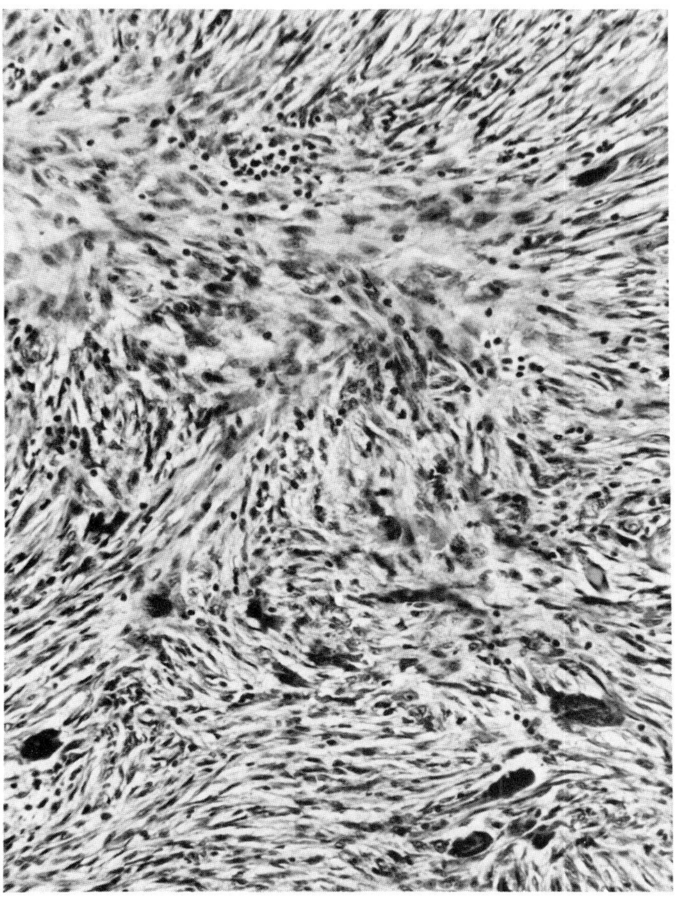

FIG. 12-3. Fibrous cortical defect. Note storiform configuration and focal accumulations of lymphocytes. × 200.

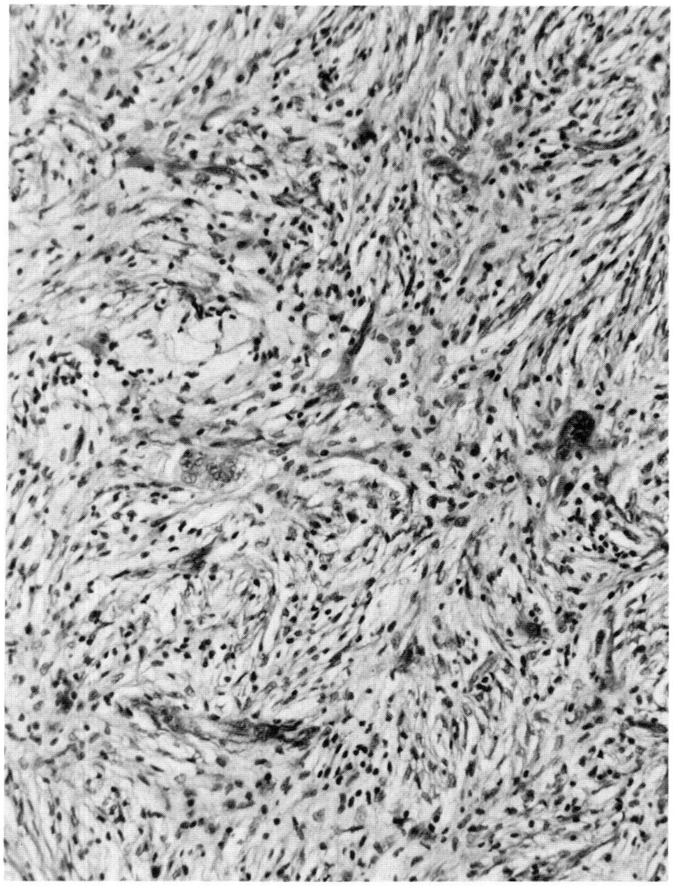

FIG. 12-4. Metaphyseal fibrous defect. Lipid-laden histiocytes apparently derived from fibroblasts. × 200.

Schrieber (1976), radiologist at Los Angeles Orthopaedic Hospital, has assured the author that the roentgenographic findings in the vast majority of fibrous cortical defects are sufficiently characteristic to be virtually pathognomonic. He further states that the average radiologist appreciates these roentgenographic characteristics and will make the correct diagnosis in the vast majority of cases. This is fortunate, since the lesion is so commonly encountered and because it requires no therapy and will undergo spontaneous involution. It is also important to the pathologist, since the majority of the cases in which he is likely to see microscopic sections are likely to be either atypical in their roentogenographic findings, or unusually large, or complicated by a pathologic fracture.

SOLITARY AND MULTIFOCAL EOSINOPHILIC GRANULOMA OF BONE

My own views on solitary and multifocal eosinophilic granuloma are essentially identical with those expressed by Lieberman, Jones, Dargeon, and Begg[112] in their masterful reappraisal of eosinophilic granuloma of bone, Hand-Schüller-

Christian syndrome, and Letterer-Siwe syndrome. I am reproducing their summary since I am unable to express it more succinctly. "An analysis of 82 personally followed cases reveals no justification for the current theory that eosinophilic granuloma of bone, Hand-Schüller-Christian disease and Letterer-Siwe disease represent component parts of a single nosologic entity. The following conclusions are reached: 1. Eosinophilic granuloma of bone is a benign disorder but may, in the multifocal form, be responsible for considerable morbidity. 2. The Hand-Schüller-Christian triad is nonspecific. Foam cells are of no help in diagnosis and are usually found in areas of nonspecific reaction. 3. There is no purpose in using the term 'Hand-Schüller-Christian disease' as a synonym for multifocal eosinophilic granuloma. 4. "Letterer-Siwe-Disease" is a clinical term which has been used to characterize various malignant histiocytic lymphomas and occasional infectious processes. 5. The term 'histiocytosis-X' is

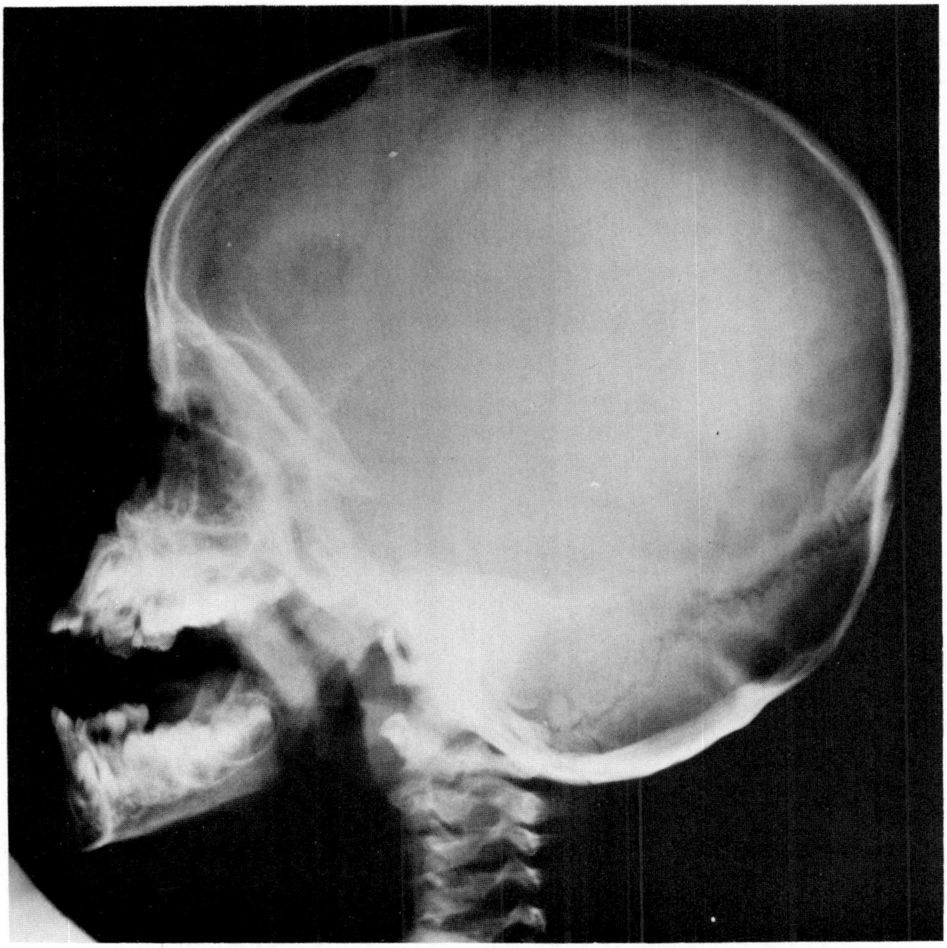

FIG. 13-1. Eosinophilic granuloma, 3-year-old male with multifocal disease. "Classical" punched-out lytic defect near midline, right parietal bone. A second lesion in the lateral aspect of the left parietal bone is faintly visible.

unnecessary and may lead to therapeutic errors." Otani,[115] McGavran and Spady,[113] and Spjut, Dorfman, Fechner, and Ackerman[12] are in accord with this view; whereas Dahlin, Ghormley, and Pugh,[5] Enriquez, Dahlin, Hayles, and Henderson,[110] Jaffe,[8] Lichtenstein,[111] and Schajowicz and Slullitel[116] still adhere to the "multiple-manifestations-of-the-same-disease" or "histiocytosis-X" concept.

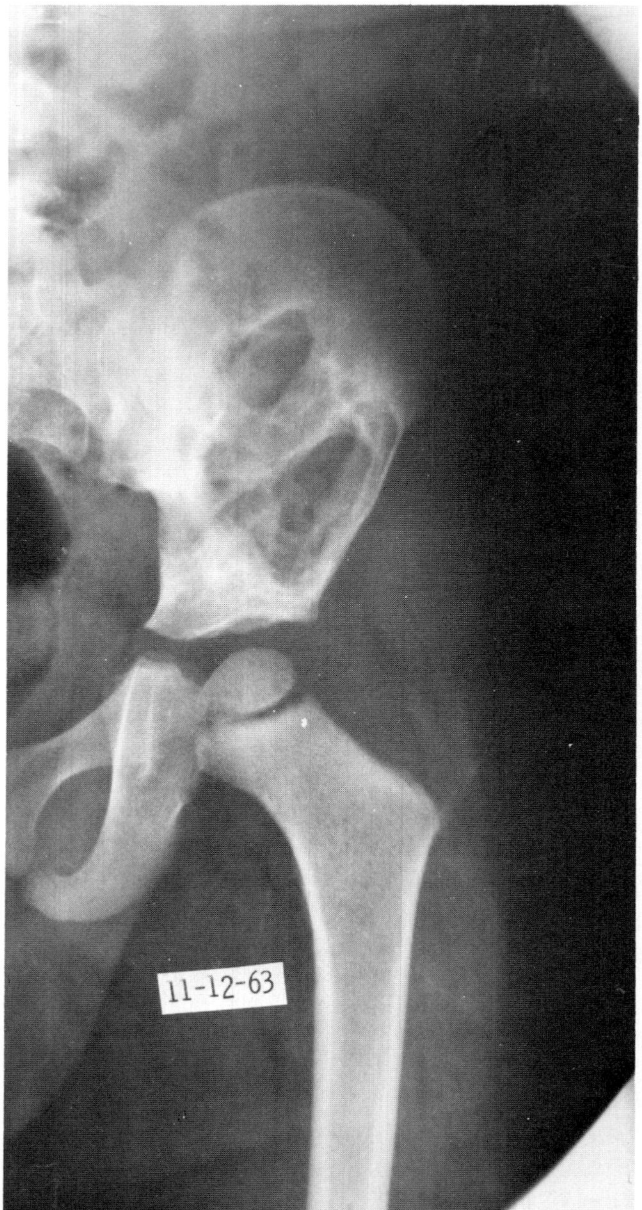

FIG. 13-2. Eosinophilic granuloma, ilium. Same patient as in Figure 13-1.

The classical reontgenographic presentation (Fig. 13–1) is a "punched-out," lytic defect similar to the one illustrated here arising near the midline of the parietal bone. This patient was a 3-year-old boy with multifocal eosinophilic granuloma. In fact, a second punched-out defect can be seen in the lateral aspect of the opposite parietal bone. Eosinophilic granuloma may occur in practically any bone in the body; when in long bones, its usual localization is in the diaphysis or metaphysis, but rare instances of epiphyseal involvement have been recorded.[8, 114, 116] Occasionally the roentgenographic findings are more bizarre (Fig. 13–2), as illustrated in this ilial lesion from the same patient whose skull x-ray is shown. Furthermore, when eosinophilic granuloma extends to involve the cortex and periosteum,[8, 114, 117] periosteal new bone production may produce a "pseudomalignant" appearance, and the x-ray findings may be misinterpreted as indicative of either reticulum cell sarcoma, Ewing's sarcoma, plasma cell myeloma, or metastatic cancer.

The typical microscopic picture of eosinophilic granuloma (Fig. 13–3) is characterized by the presence of sheets of histiocytes. These histiocytes may dominate the histopathologic picture, or there may be an intermingling of eosinophils, lymphocytes, and polymorphonuclear leukocytes. The eosinophils, which are nearly always present (and which are not easily recognized in the black and white photograph) in at least a few foci, may be quite numerous and may dominate the histologic picture in selected fields. Multinucleated benign giant cells may be virtually absent, or may be quite numerous as seen in the lower half of the composite photomicrograph (Fig. 13–3). When the surgical pathologist is faced with a frozen section from an eosinophilic granuloma accompanied by a pseudomalignant roentgenogram, these multinucleated giant cells and/or eosinophils, even though few in number, can be very helpful since neither is found with significant frequency in either reticulum cell sarcoma, Ewing's sarcoma, or multiple myeloma.

Clinical features are usually not helpful in the differential diagnosis. There are seldom alterations in serum chemical determinations, and although the majority of patients have the first manifestations of their disease prior to 20 years of age, the range in patients with unifocal disease is 16 months to 61 years and in multifocal disease from 1 month to 57 years.[112]

ANEURYSMAL BONE CYST

The x-ray (Fig. 14–1) shows a lesion involving the metaphyseal region of the femur of a 7-year-old boy who was admitted with a chief complaint of pain in the distal left thigh for 1 month. This x-ray is best appreciated when Jaffe's[121] original descriptive terminology is applied: "The term 'aneurysmal' in the name relates to a sort of 'blowout' distention of part of the contour of the cavity . . . [and] what characterizes the lesion roentgenographically is a ballooned-out distention of the periosteum, usually outlined by a paper-thin subperiosteal bone shell . . . the position of the lesion in relation to the shaft is eccentric, that is, the lesion does not traverse the entire diameter of the bone." Tillman, Dahlin, Lipscomb, and Stewart[127] further noted in their 48 cases involving long tubular bones that, although the x-rays in three-quarters of the cases did show the lesion

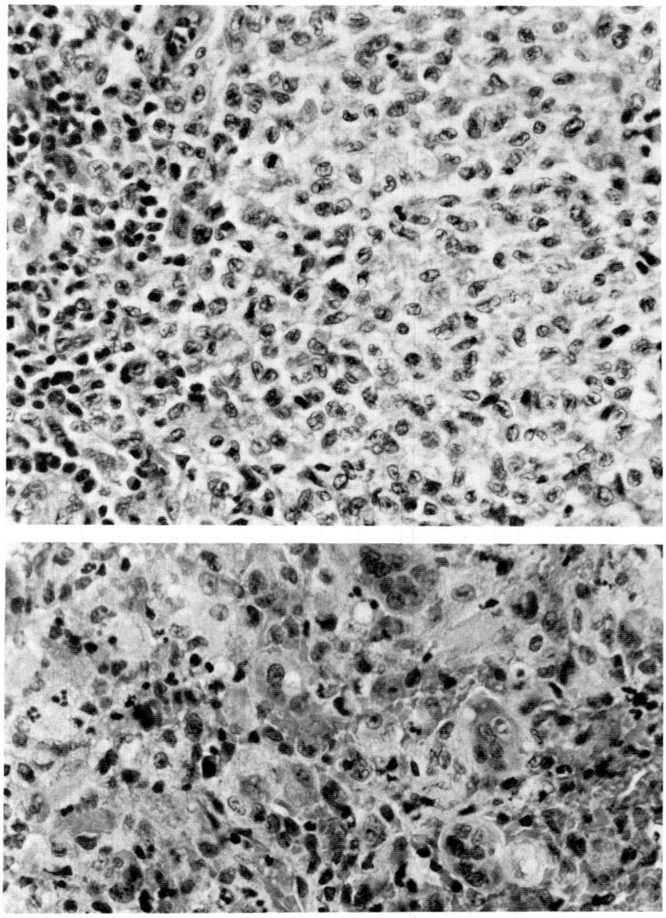

FIG. 13–3. Eosinophilic granuloma. Upper portion of composite photomicrograph shows sheets of histiocytes and interspersed lymphocytes, plasma cells, and eosinophils (the latter poorly delineated in this black and white photograph). Lower half shows a focus in which benign multinucleated giant cells are fairly numerous. × 300.

to be eccentric, one-quarter were not eccentric and caused a symmetrical and circumferential expansion of the bone. They also made special mention of the roentgenographic aspect of the inner margin of the eccentric lesions; they found this inner margin abrupt but ill-defined rather than sharp or punched-out and without marginal sclerosis as one expects to see in chondromyxoid fibroma. All but 5 of their 48 lesions in long tubular bones were metaphyseal, and the 5 exceptions were diaphyseal in location. None occurred in the epiphyseal end.

The gross pathologic features of aneurysmal bone cyst, when the expanded periosteal shell of bone has been removed, and the lesion transected (Fig. 14–2), are those of a spongy fibrous tissue mass honeycombed by spaces of varying size. This should be contrasted with the mostly solid appearance of the majority of the lesions previously discussed (compare Figs. 14–2 and 1–2). The thickness of the walls separating the channels varies from lesion to lesion, as do the size and the number of the spaces.

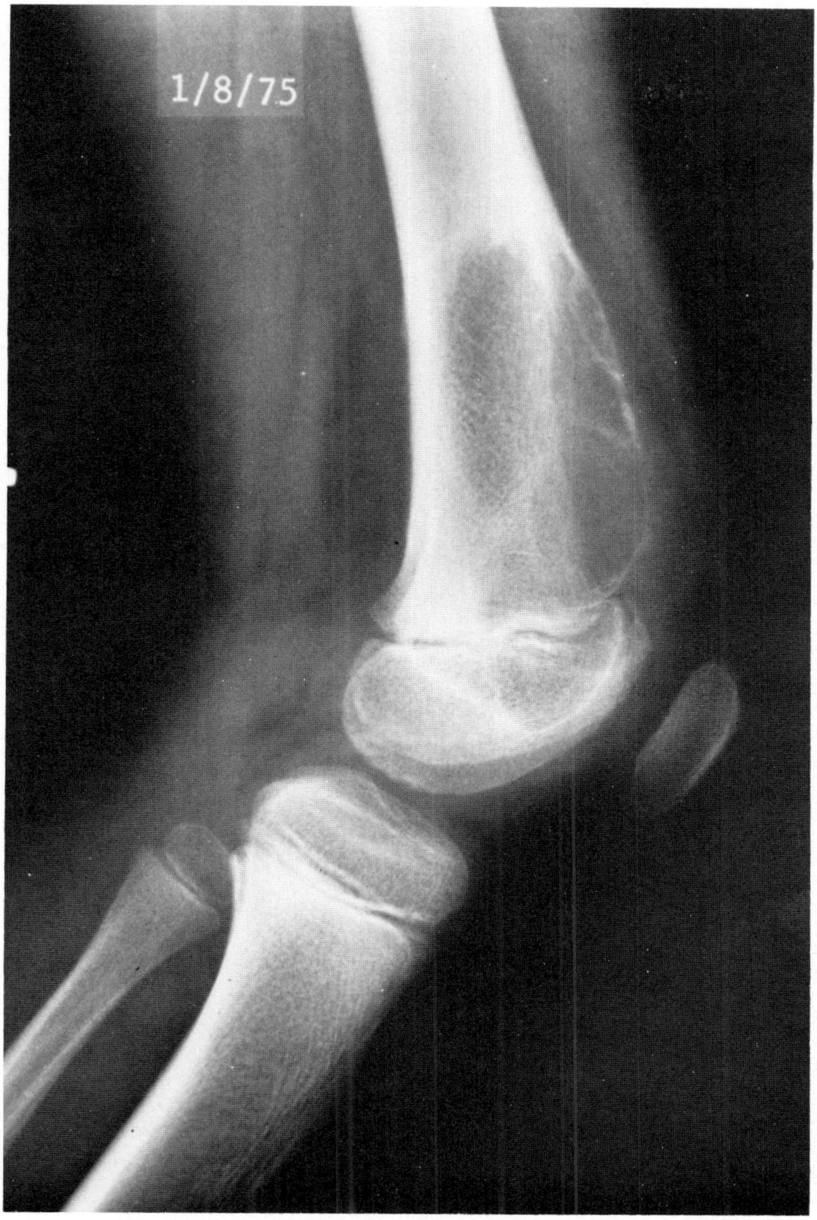

FIG. 14-1. Aneurysmal bone cyst, distal metaphysis of left femur of 7-year-old boy.

Microscopic examination (Fig. 14-3) shows the tissue between the spaces of this lesion to be, for the most part, collagen-producing fibrous tissue. Multinucleated giant cells vary from sparse to numerous. The spaces may be lined by either multinucleated giant cells, by endothelium-like cells, or by fibroblasts. Osteoid deposition can be seen in the upper half (*A*) of the composite photomicrograph (Fig. 14-3). Other constituents which may be present in the solid areas of the tumor include bony trabeculae and foci of tissue with a chondroid aura which mostly were associated with bony metaplasia.

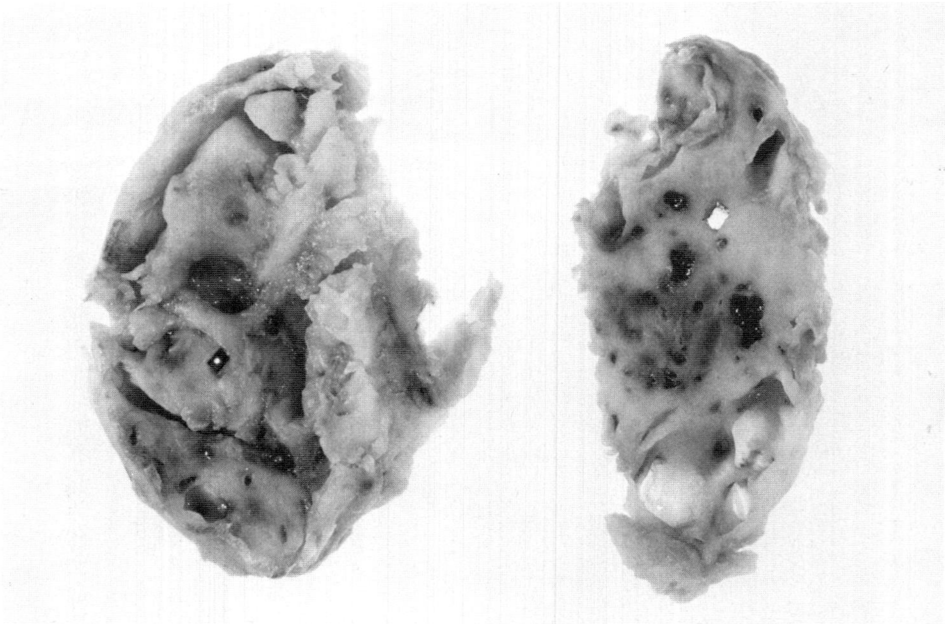

FIG. 14–2. Gross specimen. Resected and bisected aneurysmal bone cyst from radial metaphysis of 15-year-old girl. Compare with Figure 1–2.

Because it has been suggested that aneurysmal bone cyst may represent a complication of some preexisting process,[118, 119, 122, 123] Tillman *et al.*[127] studied thoroughly all of the tissue removed in their 95 cases. They concluded that, "Although fibrous portions in some of them [aneurysmal bone cysts] were somewhat like nonosteogenic fibromas and others had zones reminiscent of fibrous dysplasia, the histologic features were not typical of these lesions [and] no acceptable evidence of a precursor was found in any of them" Our own experience is similar. The overall features of an eccentric, metaphyseal lesion with unique gross and microscopic pathologic features occurring most often in patients less than 20 years of age affords recognition of this distinctive bone process.

UNICAMERAL (SOLITARY) BONE CYST

Boseker, Bickel, and Dahlin[129] have furnished the following statistics from their 145 cases of unicameral bone cyst: 10% of unicameral bone cysts occur in long tubular bones, and 90% of these arise either in the humerus or the femur (nearly twice as often in the humerus as the femur). The average age of patients with lesions in the long tubular bones is 9 years, and the range is 2 to 42 years. For the 10% that occur in flat bones, the average age is 30 years and the range from 2 to 72 years. Males are affected 3 times as often as females.

The x-ray (Fig. 15–1) from our illustrative case shows a lytic lesion arising in the metaphysis of the fibula of a 13-year-old female. The lesion abuts the epiphyseal plate and causes a uniform expansion of the bone for a distance of several centimeters. Ordinarily, this expansion does not exceed the width of the epiphyseal plate, although Lodwick[135] claims it is not an infrequent occurrence.

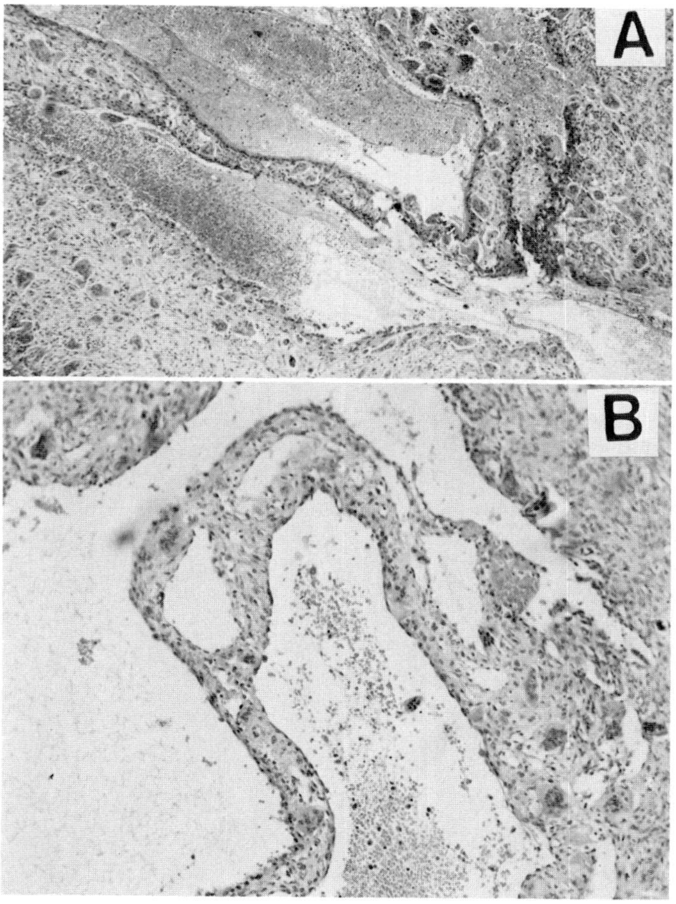

FIG. 14-3. Aneurysmal bone cyst. Compare with telangiectatic osteosarcoma, Figure 11-5. *A*, × 48; *B*, × 75.

Lesions such as this one in which the x-ray shows the lesion abutting on the epiphyseal plate are considered "active." Lesions in which the x-ray shows a zone of normal-appearing bone separating the lesion from the epiphyseal plate are considered "inactive" or "latent." Extension through the epiphyseal plate almost never occurs.

At operation, the surgeon ordinarily encounters a thin-walled, solitary (unicameral) cystic structure which contains either clear serous or blood-tinged serous fluid. All but 3 of the 145 cysts reported by Boseker *et al.*[129] contained such fluid which was not under pressure. It is important in the differential diagnosis of this lesion from aneurysmal bone cyst that the pathologist be aware of the surgeon's findings since, as Boseker *et al.*[129] have so aptly stated: The finding "of a fluid-filled cyst in a young person, in a typical location, with a thin glistening lining should convince the surgeon almost without regard to the microscopic appearance that he is dealing with a simple cyst."

The semitranslucent, cystic structure (which contained clear serous fluid)

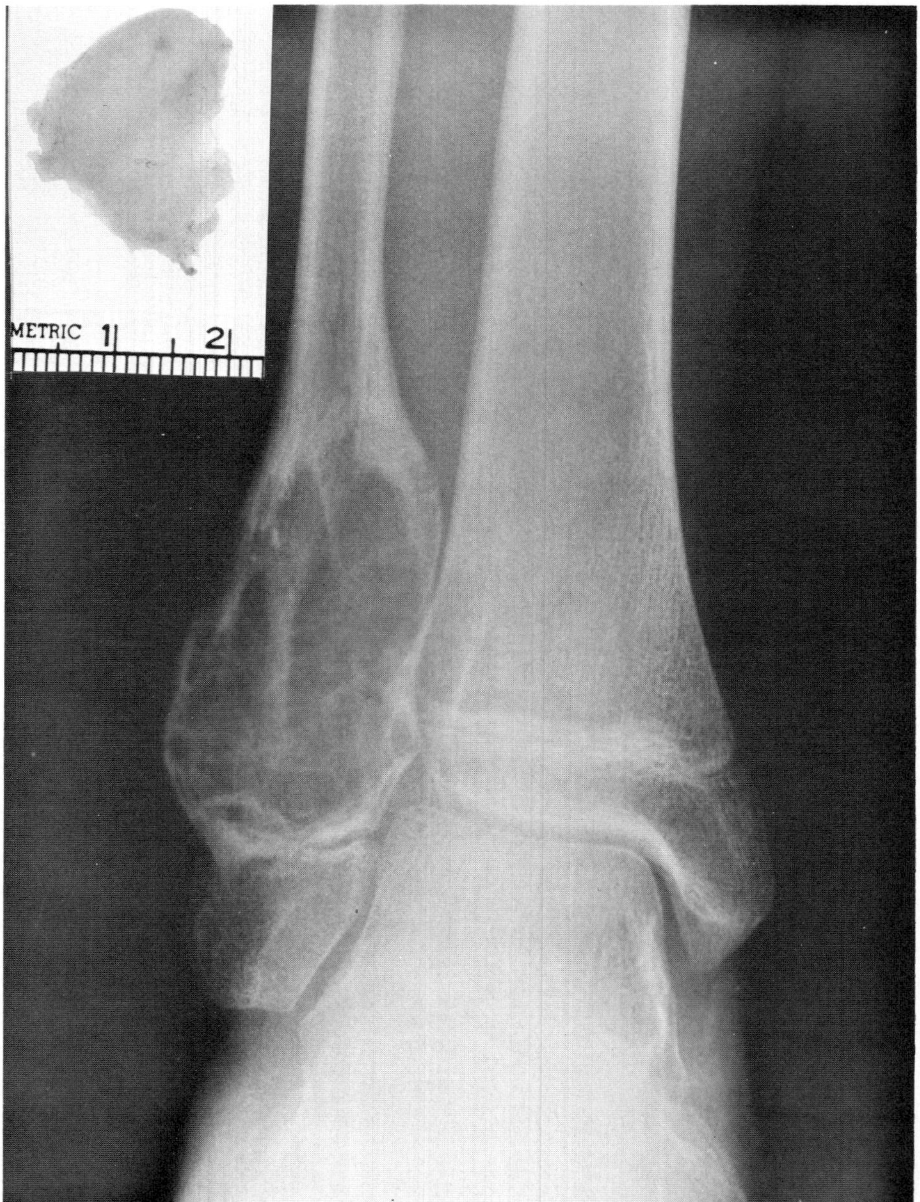

FIG. 15-1. X-ray and gross specimen (inset). Unicameral bone cyst, recurrent; 13-year-old girl.

removed from our patient is shown in the inset of (Figure 15-1). This lesion, incidentally, is a recurrent one, this patient having had a curettage 2 years earlier. Recurrence rates vary greatly depending on whether the lesion arises in a long tubular bone or in a flat bone. The majority of flat bone cysts are easily cured whereas those occurring in long tubular bones have recurrence rates varying from 8 to 40%. The lesser recurrence rates have resulted from more radical extirpative procedures undertaken in more recent years.[129, 131] Latent or inactive cysts of long bone are considered more amenable to therapy than active cysts by the majority of authors.

Microscopically (Fig. 15–2), the lining of a typical and uncomplicated solitary cyst is well-vascularized, fibrogenic connective tissue, and the fibroblasts lining the actual cavity are usually more plump and active appearing. More peripherally, they produce considerable collagen, and there are considerable areas where osteoid and coarse fiber, reactive type of subperiosteal new bone is being laid down. Multinucleated giant cells may be sparse or numerous. In less typical material and especially in cases where there has been prior infraction or fracture with hemorrhage and either resolution or organization of clot, and particularly in recurrent lesions which have been previously either curetted or curetted and packed with bone chips, there may be areas in which there are cholesterol clefts and pigment deposition, areas of calcification and ossification, and areas which resemble aneurysmal bone cyst. In fact, peculiar areas of ossification, such as those illustrated in Jaffe and Lichtenstein's original paper (Fig. 6, page 1014)[134] occur not infrequently in "complicated" cases and, in our opinion, 2 cases have

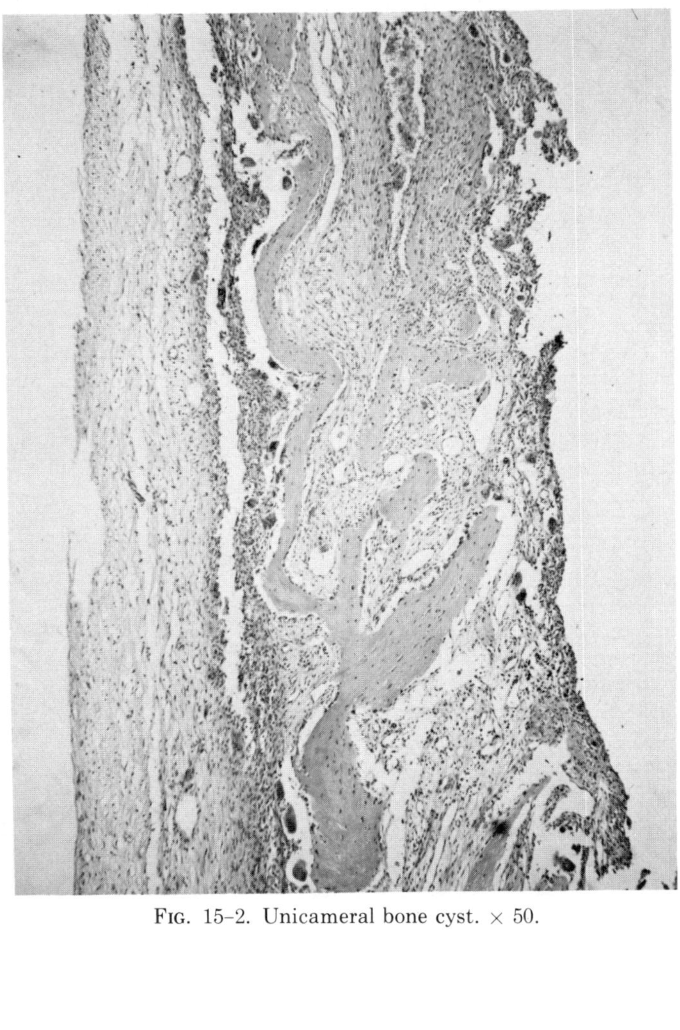

FIG. 15–2. Unicameral bone cyst. × 50.

been reported[132] as, "Cementoma of long bones. An extragnathic odontogenic tumor."

On the basis of the histopathologic finding alone the differentiation of "complicated" unicameral bone cyst from aneurysmal bone cyst may be difficult in occasional cases. This is because the curetted material is received as multiple fragments, and anatomic reconstruction is difficult. In such cases it is essential in

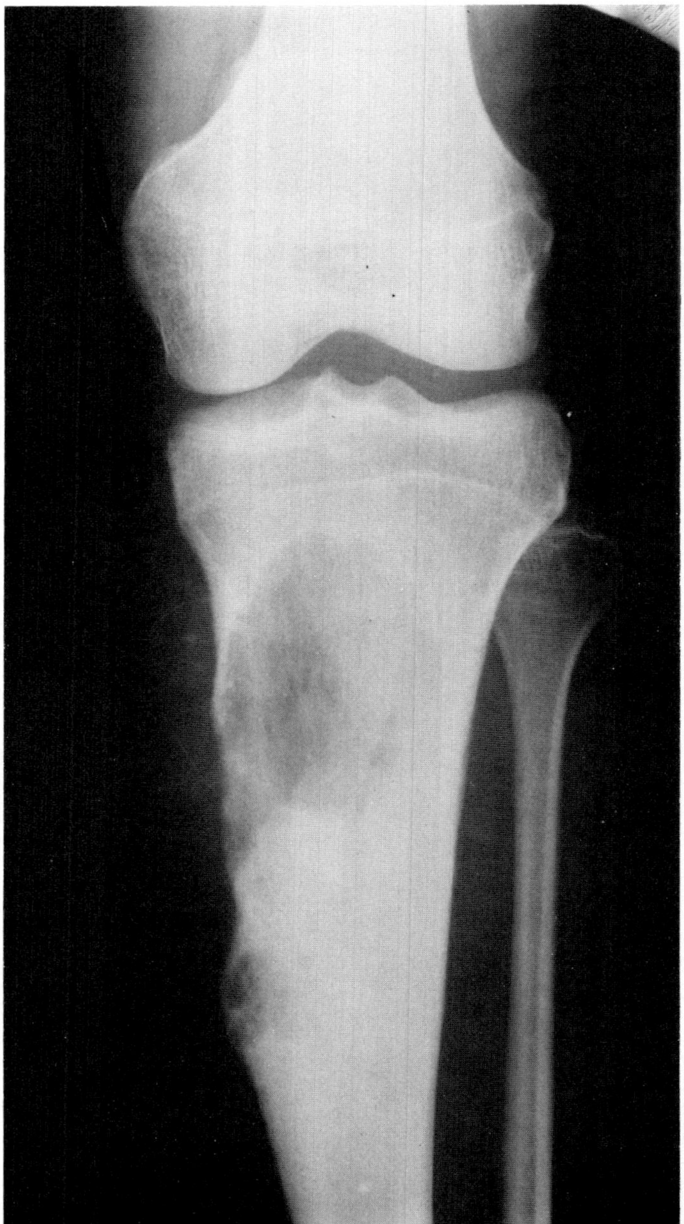

FIG. 16–1. Chondromyxoid fibroma, tibia; 21-year-old man.

establishing the correct diagnosis that the surgical pathologist have the advantage of the clinical history (prior fracture or infraction, previous therapy), roentgenographic interpretation, and the surgeon's description of the findings at the time of surgery prior to microscopic evaluation of the curetted material.

CHONDROMYXOID FIBROMA OF BONE

Chondromyxoid fibroma is a distinctly uncommon tumor. In fact, Rahimi, Beabout, Ivins, and Dahlin were able to collect only 76 examples[144] prior to 1972, at which time Dahlin and Ivins had accumulated 125 cases of chondroblastoma[60] and Dahlin has reported the incidence of benign chondroblastoma to be less than 1% of all tumor and tumor-like lesions of bone. Pertinent to this discussion of lesions containing giant cells, and of some interest, is the finding of Rahimi *et al.*[144] that they were able to identify "osteoclast-like" giant cells in only 40% of their 76 chondromyxoid fibromas; Schajowicz and Gallardo,[146] on the other hand, found such giant cells in all but 3 of their 32 cases.

The patients with chondromyxoid fibroma are slightly older, on the average, than those with benign chondroblastoma; the peak incidence is in the 2nd and

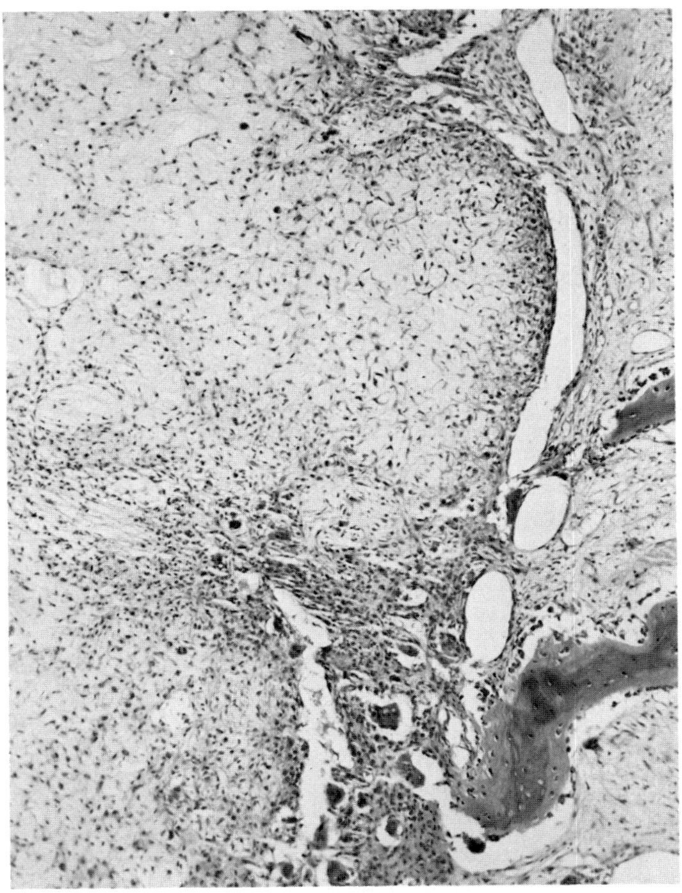

FIG. 16–2. Chondromyxoid fibroma. × 60.

3rd decades, and between 55 and 60% of the lesions occur in patients less than 30 years of age. Rahimi *et al.*[144] in their review of the literature ascertained that chondromyxoid fibroma has occurred in all but the carpal bones. When located in the long tubular bones, as it is in more than 75% of cases, it is invariably in the metaphysis and practically never violates the epiphyseal plate which it occasionally abuts.

The illustrative x-ray (Fig. 16–1) shows a large, somewhat eccentric, predominantly lytic metaphyseal lesion with well-demarcated, somewhat sclerotic borders except in relation to the cortex. This lesion presented in the tibia of a 21-year-old man who was struck below the knee by a baseball at the age of 9 years and has had persistent swelling ever since and in recent years intermittent sharp pain with activity. Feldman, Hecht, and Johnston[140] have described the more classical x-ray appearance of chondromyxoid fibroma occurring in a long tubular bone as, "a circumscribed, eccentrically situated, round or oval metaphyseal defect with its long axis directed along the long axis of the bone. Its size has ranged from 1.0 to 10.0 cm. in length and from 4.0 to 7.0 cm. in width, averaging 3.0 × 2.0 × 2.0 cm. Although the lesion may appear trabeculated, in most

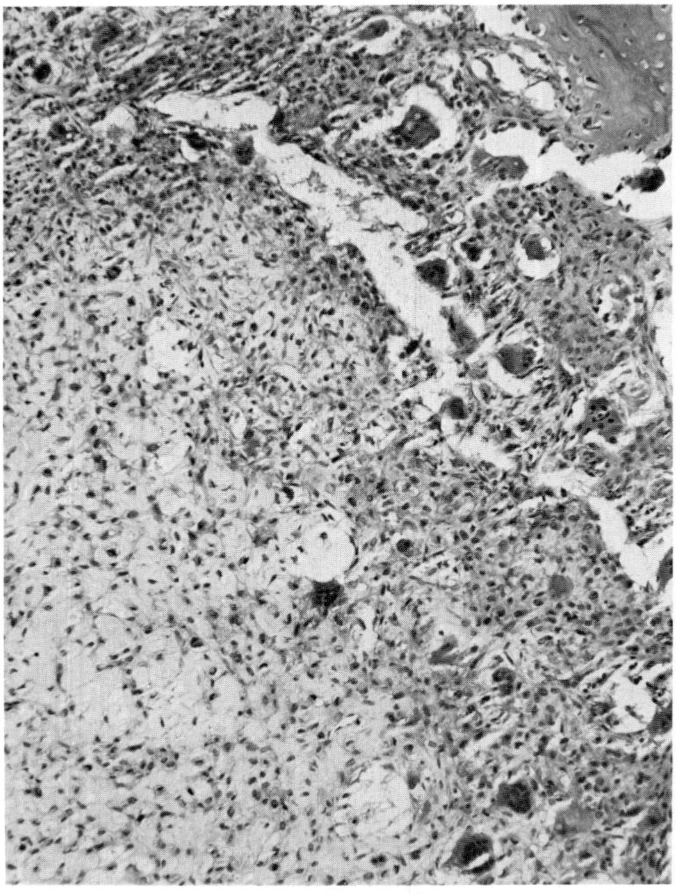

FIG. 16–3. Chondromyxoid fibroma. × 120.

instances these are 'pseudotrabeculae' and a reflection of the corrugation or grooving of adjacent bone by the lobulated periphery of the tumor. The inner boundary of the defect is usually well-demarcated by a sclerotic scalloped margin. The external contour tends to be expanded as the tumor grows, with resultant thinning and total or partial erosion of the overlying subperiosteal bone. Although rigorous periosteal reaction is unusual, the mass may occasionally be externally demarcated by a thin or thick shell of periosteal bone."

The cut surfaces have been described[142, 144, 146] as lobulated, solid, firm, rubber and resilient, gray-white, somewhat translucent, and as resembling fibrocartilage or fibrous tissue. Microscopic examination (Fig. 16–2) shows characteristic lobules of "chondromyxoid" composition, varying in size and fusing with neighboring lobules. Rahimi *et al.*[144] have described, "between the lobules of tumor, (Fig. 16–3) . . . a very loose, richly vascularized, connective tissue . . . which is usually fibroblastic with spindle-shaped cells . . . but sometimes [the cells] are round or polygonal and resemble the cells seen in benign chondroblastoma." When benign multinucleated giant cells are present, they are usually found in these areas. Such chondroblastoma-like areas were found by Rahimi *et al.* in one-fourth of their cases.[144] In the central portions of the myxoid lobules, the cells are either spindled or stellate; some of these cells may be contained in abortive lacunae and impart a chondroid appearance. Cells toward the periphery of the myxoid lobules may be slightly larger, more numerous, more variable in size and, since mitotic figures are not uncommon, such areas (Fig. 16–3) may arouse a suspicion of malignancy. Hyaline type tumor cartilage is not found in chondromyxoid fibroma. Other metaphyseal tumors containing giant cells (Table II) are not likely to be confused with chondromyxoid fibroma on the basis of their histopathologic characteristics. The significant differential diagnosis of chondromyxoid fibroma is from chondrosarcoma, and the false diagnosis of chondrosarcoma can be avoided by careful evaluation of the radiographic, gross, and microscopic pathologic features. Perhaps appropirate to our present day "medicolegal climate," Rahimi *et al.*[144] have noted that, "Paradoxically, because of the fear of unnecessarily radical treatment of benign tumors, pathologists have often considered or made the diagnosis of chondromyxoid fibroma when the lesion in question was actually a chondrosarcoma."

The question of malignant transformation has been critically evaluated by Dahlin *et al.*[4, 144] and they found no case in which malignant change had been convincingly documented. They did not include irradiation-induced osteogenic sarcomas arising at the site of previously treated chondromyxoid fibromas.

GOUTY TOPHUS EPIPHYSEAL END OF LONG TUBULAR BONE

This final case is presented as a cautionary note. In a given case, the pathologist may receive from the orthopaedic surgeon a detailed and even voluminous summary of the medical findings, and he may have reviewed at length the x-rays with the roentgenologist, and he may have undertaken profound deliberations with respect to the differential diagnostic alternatives and be caught unawares when presented with the microscopic sections.

The x-ray in this "just-such-a-case" (Fig. 17–1) reveals a small, slightly eccentric, radiolucent defect with a well-demarcated, scalloped, and slightly sclerotic margin. Schrieber, the radiologist at Los Angeles Orthopaedic Hospital, assures me that no experienced radiologist, even with special expertise in skeletal diagnostic radiology would be likely to consider gouty tophus amongst the differential diagnostic alternatives in this case.

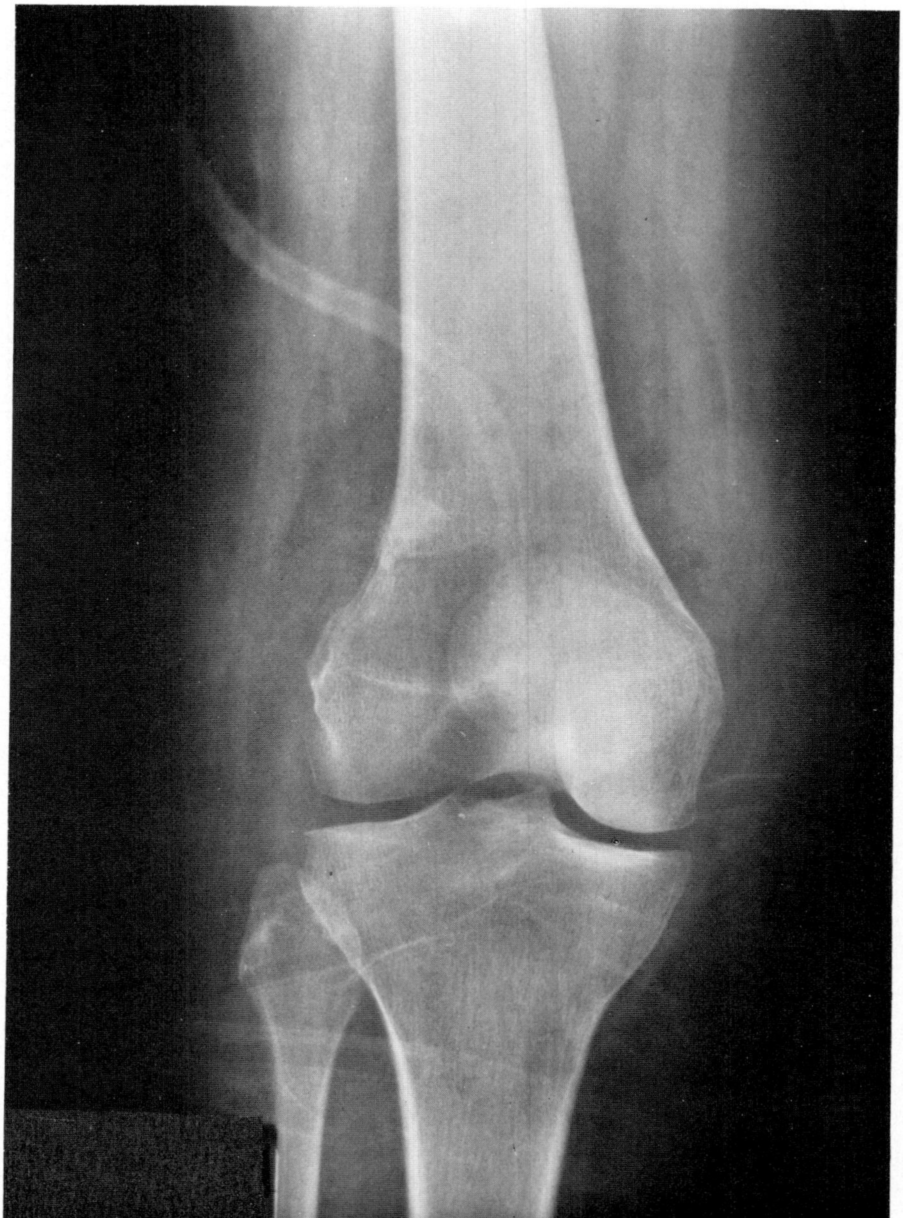

FIG. 17–1. Gouty tophus presenting in distal epiphysis of femur; 66-year-old woman.

The patient, a 66-year-old woman, had twisted her foot a few days earlier, and this had caused considerable pain in the foot and the popliteal area. The pain became progressively worse and was followed by swelling of the knee. Following several days of conservative treatment for possible thrombophlebitis with symptomatic improvement but without subsidence of the swelling in the knee, an x-ray was taken. The lesion was soon curetted.

Microscopic examination of the curetted tissue (Fig. 17–2) shows a gouty tophus. As might be expected there was also involvement of the adjacent synovium, but this was minimal compared to the bony involvement. Because the tissue had been fixed in formalin (a watery solution), the sodium urate crystals have been dissolved out of the tissue, and the area they formerly occupied is seen as an amorphous, eosinophilic zone which is surrounded by multinucleated foreign body giant cells, histiocytes, lymphocytes, and desmoplastic connective tissue. These findings are characteristic of gouty tophus. Deeper sections from the blocks, apparently from an area where the formalin had failed to penetrate (Fig. 17–3), show the needle-shaped, yellow-brown, sodium urate crystals. If one

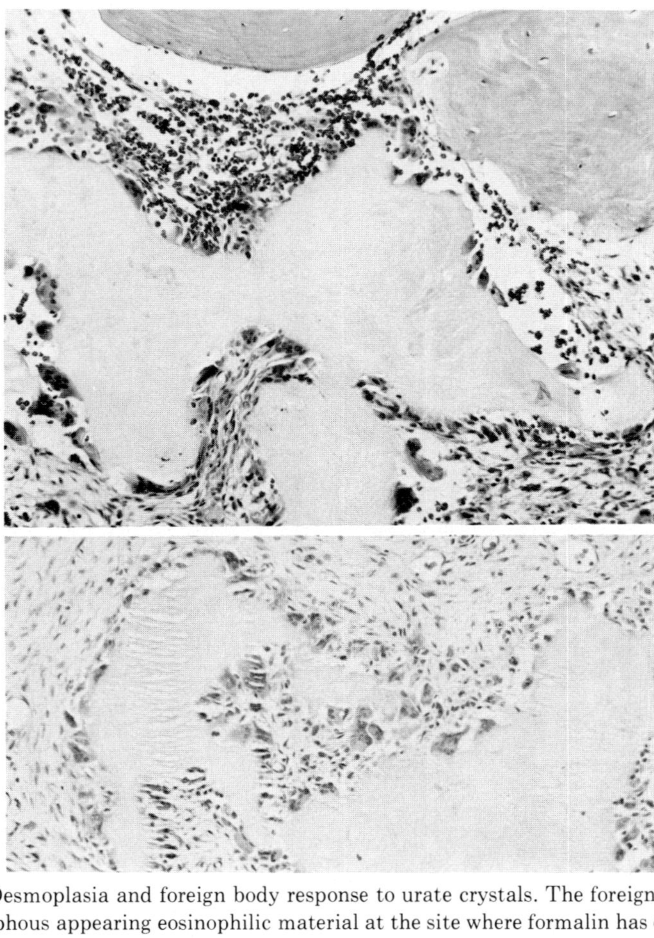

FIG. 17–2. Desmoplasia and foreign body response to urate crystals. The foreign body giant cells surround amorphous appearing eosinophilic material at the site where formalin has dissolved out the urate crystals. × 120.

suspects gout at the time the surgical specimen is taken, it should be fixed in absolute alcohol so that the sodium urate crystals will not dissolve.

After the diagnosis of gouty tophus was made, this woman had several serum uric acid determinations which were only slightly elevated above high normal values. She has, to date, no other symptoms referable to gout, and evidence of other tophi has not been found.

Tophi in bone[8, 149] are, of course, well known but ordinarily occur only late in the evolution of the disease; a gouty tophus in bone as the initial manifestation is virtually unknown.

PRIMARY GIANT CELL TUMORS OF SOFT SOMATIC TISSUES AND TUMORAL CALCINOSIS

Two lesions which arise in soft somatic tissues and which do not invade the skeletal tissues occasionally cause confusion in the differential diagnosis of lesions of bone containing giant cells and should be mentioned briefly. These are giant cell tumor of soft parts[150, 151] and tumoral calcinosis.[153]

Primary giant cell tumors of soft somatic tissues bearing a striking histopatho-

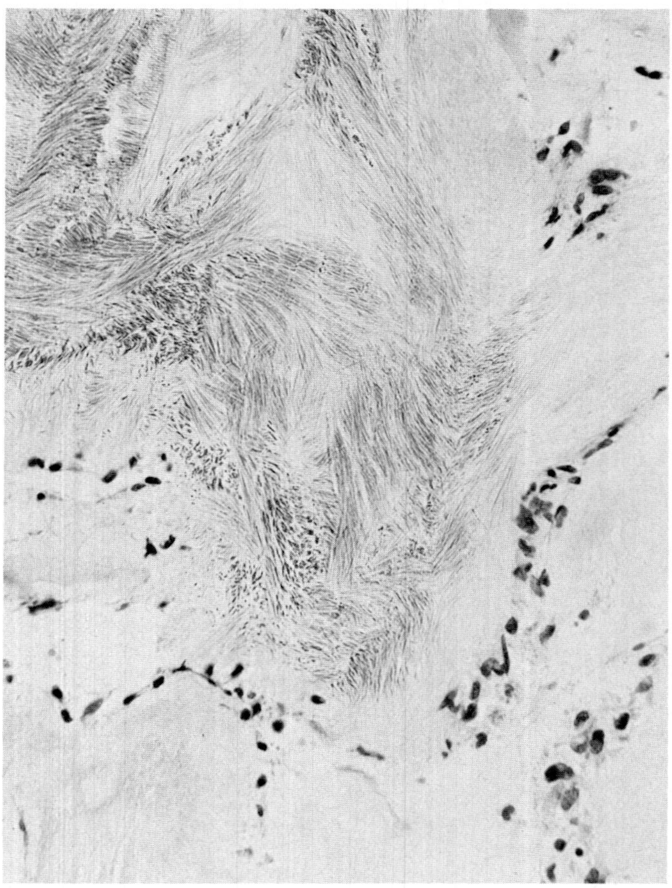

FIG. 17–3. Needle-shaped urate crystals from a deeper section of the same paraffin block shown in Figure 17–2. The formalin had apparently not penetrated sufficiently to dissolve the crystals. × 300.

logic resemblance to giant cell tumor of bone have been described. Salm and Sissons[151] reported 14 such tumors, none of which metastasized, and which they considered to be benign. Guccion and Enzinger[150] recorded 32 cases, 12 of which were described as superficial and 20 as deep. Fourteen of their 20 deeply situated tumors metastasized, and 2 of the superficial tumors metastasized, and they considered the tumor to be a malignant giant cell tumor of soft parts.

Harkess and Peters,[153] in 1967, collected 27 cases of tumoral calcinosis from the literature, to which they added 6 of their own. They concluded that the following were the criteria for the diagnosis of tumoral calcinosis: "The presence of large, painless, calcified masses in juxta-articular sites; the absence of abnormal values of serum calcium and phosphate (similar soft tissue calcifications can be seen with vitamin-D intoxication, Burnett's syndrome, and secondary hyperparathyroidism and must be excluded); no associated renal disease, metabolic disorder or collagen disease; the disease manifests itself before the age of 20; there be evidence of familial or racial predisposition." The histopathology of the tumor is reminiscent of gouty tophus except that the reactive proliferation of foreign body giant cells, histiocytes, lymphocytes and desmoplastic connective tissue is a reaction to the calcium deposition rather than to the urate crystals. The interested reader is directed to the paper by Harkess and Peters[153] for additional details.

REFERENCES

Primary

1. Ackerman, L. V., and Spjut, H. J.: *Tumors of Bone and Cartilage. Atlas of Tumor Pathology*, Section II, Fascicle 4. Armed Forces Institute of Pathology, Washington, D.C. 1962.
2. Aegerter, E., and Kirkpatrick, J. A., Jr.: *Orthopedic Diseases: Physiology, Pathology, Radiology*. 3rd ed. Philadelphia, W. B. Saunders Co., 1968.
3. Cohen, D. M., Dahlin, D. C. MacCarty, C. S.: Vertebral giant cell tumor and variants. *Cancer 17:* 461–472, 1964.
4. Dahlin, D. C.: *Bone Tumors: General Aspects and Data on 3,987 Cases*. 2nd ed. Springfield, Ill., Charles C Thomas, 1967.
5. Dahlin, D. C., Ghormley, R. K., and Pugh, D. G.: Giant cell tumor of bone; differential diagnosis. *Proc. Staff Meet. Mayo Clin. 31:* 31–42, 1956.
6. Foote, F. W., and Frazell, E. L.: Tumors of the major salivary glands. *Cancer 6:* 1065–1133, 1953.
7. Jaffe, H. L.: *Tumors and Tumorous Conditions of Bones and Joints*. Philadelphia, Lea & Febiger, 1958.
8. Jaffe, H. L.: *Metabolic, Degenerative, and Inflammatory Diseases of Bones and Joints*. Philadelphia, Lea & Febiger, 1972.
9. Lichtenstein, L.: *Bone Tumors*. 3rd ed. St. Louis, C. V. Mosby Company, 1965.
10. Lichtenstein, L.: *Diseases of Bone and Joints*. St. Louis, C. V. Mosby Company, 1970.
11. Sissons, H. A.: Discussion. Giant cell tumour of bone and related conditions; giant cell tumour variants. *Proc. R. Soc. Med. 49:* 416–422, 1956.
12. Spjut, H. J., Dorfman, H. D., Fechner, R. E., and Ackerman, L. V.: *Tumors of Bone and Cartilage. Atlas of Tumor Pathology*, Section II, Fascicle 5. Armed Forces Institute of Pathology, Washington, D.C., 1971.

Ultrastructure and Histochemistry of Multinucleated Giant Cells in Bone Lesions

13. Adkins, K. F., Martinez, M. G., and Romaniuk, K.: Ultrastructure of giant-cell lesions; mononuclear cells in peripheral giant-cell granulomas. *Oral Surg. 33:* 775–786, 1972.
14. Gallardo, H., De Lustig, E. S., and Schajowicz, F.: Growth and maintenance of human

giant-cell bone tumors (Osteoclastomas) in continuous culture. *Oncology 24:* 146–159, 1970.

15. Hanaoka, H., Friedman, B., and Mack, R. P.: Ultrastructure and histogenesis of giant cell tumor of bone. *Cancer 25:* 1408–1423, 1970.
16. Huvos, A. G., Marcove, R. C., Erlandson, R. A., and Miké, V.: Chondroblastoma of bone; a clinicopathologic and electron microscopic study. *Cancer 29:* 760–771, 1972.
17. Kuhlman, R. E., and McNamee, M. J.: Quantitative microchemical studies of chondroblastoma, giant cell tumor, chondromyxoid fibroma and desmoplastic fibroma. *Clin. Orthop. 69:* 264–270, 1970.
18. Ores, R., Rosen, P., and Ortiz, J.: Localization of acid phosphatase activity in a giant cell tumor of bone. *Arch. Pathol. 88:* 54–57, 1969.
19. Pepler, W. J.; The histochemistry of giant cell tumours (osteoclastoma and giant cell epulis). *J. Pathol. Bacteriol. 76:* 505–510, 1958.
20. Sapp, J. P.: Ultrastructure and histogenesis of peripheral giant cell reparative granuloma of the jaws. *Cancer 30:* 1119–1129, 1972.
21. Schajowicz, F.: Giant-cell tumors of bone (osteoclastoma); a pathological and histochemical study. *J. Bone Joint Surg. 43-A:* 1–29, 1961.
22. Steiner, G. C., Ghosh, L., and Dorfman, H. D.: Ultrastructure of giant cell tumors of bone. *Hum. Pathol. 3:* 569–586, 1972.
23. Welsh, R. A., and Meyer, A. T.: A histogenetic study of chondroblastoma. *Cancer 17:* 578–589, 1964.
24. Welsh, R. A., and Meyer, A. T.: Nuclear fragmentations and associated fibrils in giant cell tumor of bone. *Lab. Invest. 22:* 63–72, 1970.
25. Wertheimer, F. W.: Enzyme histochemistry of giant cell reparative granulomas. *Oral Surg., Oral Med., Oral Pathol. 23:* 464–469, 1967.

Benign and Malignant Giant Cell Tumor of Bone

26. Barnes, R.: Giant-cell tumour of bone; editorials. *J. Bone Joint Surg. 54-B:* 213–215, 1972.
27. Cares, H. L., and Bakay, L.: Giant cell lesions of the skull. *Acta Neurochir. 25:* 1–18, 1971.
28. Dahlin, D. C., Cupps, R. E., and Johnson, E. W.: Giant-cell tumor; a study of 195 cases. *Cancer 25:* 1061–1070, 1970.
29. Frangakis, E. K.: Soft-tissue spread of giant-cell tumor; a case report. *J. Bone Joint Surg. 53-A:* 994–998, 1971.
30. Goldenberg, R. R., Campbell, C. J., and Bonfiglio, M.: Giant-cell tumor of bone; an analysis of two hundred and eighteen cases. *J. Bone Joint Surg. 52-A:* 619–664, 1970.
31. Hutter, R. V. P., Worcester, J. N., Francis, K. C., Foote, F. W., and Stewart, F. W.: Benign and malignant giant cell tumors of bone; a clinicopathological analysis of the natural history of the disease. *Cancer 15:* 653–690, 1962.
32. Jacobs, P.: The diagnosis of osteoclastoma (giant-cell tumour); a radiological and pathological correlation. *Br. J. Radiol. 45:* 121–136, 1972.
33. Johnson, E. W.: Adjacent and distant spread of giant cell tumours. *Am. J. Surg. 109:* 163–166, 1965.
34. Kutchemeshgi, A. D., Wright, J. R., and Humphrey, R. L.: Pulmonary metastases from a well-differentiated giant cell tumor of bone; report of a patient with apparent response to cyclophosphamide therapy. *Johns Hopkins Med. J. 134:* 237–245, 1974.
35. Larsson, S.-E., Lorentzon, R., and Boquist, L.: Giant-cell tumor of bone; a demographic, clinical and histopathological study of all cases recorded in the Swedish cancer registry for the years 1958 through 1968. *J. Bone Joint Surg. 57-A:* 167–173, 1975.
36. McGrath, P. J.: Giant-cell tumors of bone; an analysis of fifty-two cases. *J. Bone Joint Surg. 54-B:* 216–229, 1972.
37. Mnaymneh, W. A., Dudley, H. R., and Mnaymneh, L. G.: Giant cell tumor of bone; an analysis and follow-up study of the forty-one cases observed at the Massachusetts General Hospital between 1925 and 1960. *J. Bone Joint Surg. 46-A:* 63–75, 1964.
38. Morton, J. J.: Giant cell tumor of bone. *Cancer 9:* 1012–1026, 1956.
39. Pan, P., Dahlin, D. C., Lipscomb, P. R., and Bernatz, P. E.: "Benign" giant cell tumor of the radius with pulmonary metastasis. *Mayo Clin. Proc. 39:* 344–349, 1964.

40. Potter, G. D., and McClennan, B. L.: Malignant giant cell tumor of the sphenoid bone and its differential diagnosis. *Cancer 25:* 167–170, 1970.
41. Riley, L. H., Hartmann, W. H., and Robinson, R. A.: Soft-tissue recurrence of giant-cell tumor of bone after irradiation and excision. *J. Bone Joint Surg. 49-A:* 365–368, 1967.
42. Schajowicz, F.: Giant cell tumor of bone; a pathological and histochemical study. *J. Bone Joint Surg. 43-A:* 1–29, 1961.
43. Schwinn, C. P.: Benign giant cell tumor of bone. Anatomic Pathology No. AP-4. CCE Council on Anatomic Pathology of the American Society of Clinical Pathologists. 1973.
44. Sherman, M., and Fabricius, R.: Giant-cell tumor in the metaphysis in a child; report of an unusual case. *J. Bone Joint Surg. 43-A:* 1225–1229, 1961.
45. Shifrin, L. Z.: Giant cell tumor of bone. *Clin. Orthop. 82:* 59–66, 1972.
46. Stargardter, F. L., and Cooperman, L. R.: Case reports; giant-cell tumour of sacrum with multiple pulmonary metastases and long-term survival. *Br. J. Radiol. 44:* 976–979, 1971.
47. Sybrandy, S., De La Fuente, A. A.: Multiple giant-cell tumour of bone; report of a case. *J. Bone Joint Surg. 55-B:* 350–356, 1973.
48. Wilkerson, J. A., and Cracchiolo, A.: Giant cell tumor of the tibial diaphysis. *J. Bone Joint Surg. 51-A:* 1205–1209, 1969.

Benign Giant Cell Tumor Arising in Paget's Disease of Bone

49. Barry, H. C.: Sarcoma in Paget's disease of bone in Australia. *J. Bone Joint Surg. 43-A:* 1122–1134, 1961.
50. Brooke, R. I.: Giant-cell tumor in patients with Paget's disease. *Oral Surg., Oral Med., Oral Pathol. 30:* 230–241, 1970.
51. Foote, F. W., Jr.: Case 10. *Seminar on Diseases of Maxillofacial Region Including Salivary Gland,* edited by Foote, F. W., Jr., and Horn, R. C., Jr. *Proceedings of the Twenty-Sixth Seminar of the American Society of Clinical Pathologists, 1960,* pp. 31–33. Chicago, American Society of Clinical Pathologists, 1961.
52. Griffey, L. E., and Tedeschi, L. G.: Giant cell tumor of ethmoid; complication of Paget's disease of bone. *Arch. Otolaryngol. 87:* 615–617, 1968.
53. Hutter, R. V. P., Foote, F. W., Jr., Frazell, E. L., and Francis, K. C.: Giant cell tumors complicating Paget's disease of bone. *Cancer 16:* 1044–1056, 1963.
54. McKenna, R. J., Schwinn, C. P., Soong, K. Y., and Higinbotham, N. L.: Osteogenic sarcoma arising in Paget's disease. *Cancer 17:* 42–66, 1964.
55. Miller, A. S., Cuttino, C. L., Elzay, R. P., Levy, W. M., and Harwick, R. D.: Giant cell tumor of the jaws associated with Paget disease of bone; report of two cases and review of the literature. *Arch. Otolaryngol. 100:* 233–236, 1974.
56. Porretta, C. A., Dahlin, D. C., and Janes, J. M.: Sarcoma in Paget's disease of bone. *J. Bone Joint Surg. 39-A:* 1314–1329, 1957.
57. Russell, D. S.: Malignant osteoblastoma and the association of malignant osteoclastoma with Paget's ostetitis deformans. *J. Bone Joint Surg. 31-B:* 281–290, 1949.
58. Schajowicz, F., and Slullitel, I.: Giant cell tumor associated with Paget's disease of bone; a case report. *J. Bone Joint Surg. 48-A:* 1340–1349, 1966.

Benign and Malignant Chondroblastoma of Bone

59. Cares, H. L., and Terplan, K.: Chondroblastoma of the skull; case report. *J. Neurosurg. 35:* 614–618, 1971.
60. Dahlin, D. C., and Ivins, J. C.: Benign chondroblastoma; a study of 125 cases. *Cancer 30:* 401–413, 1972.
61. Fechner, R. E., and Wilde, H. D.: Chondroblastoma in the metaphysis of the femoral neck; a case report and review of the literature. *J. Bone Joint Surg. 56-A:* 413–415, 1974.
62. Gravanis, M. B., and Giansanti, J. S.: Benign chondroblastoma; report of four cases with a discussion of the presence of ossification. *Am. J. Clin. Pathol. 55:* 624–631, 1971.
63. Green, P., and Whittaker, R. P.: Benign chondroblastoma. Case report with pulmonary metastasis. *J. Bone Joint Surg. 57-A:* 418–420, 1975.
64. Jaffe, H. L., and Lichtenstein, L.: Benign chondroblastoma of bone. A reinterpretation of the

so-called calcifying or chondromatous giant cell tumor. *Am. J. Pathol. 18:* 969–991, 1942.

65. Kahn, L. B., Wood, F. M., and Ackerman, L. V.: Malignant chondroblastoma; report of two cases and review of the literature. *Arch. Pathol. 88:* 371–376, 1969.
66. Neviaser, R. J., and Wilson, J. N.: Benign chondroblastoma in the finger. *J. Bone Joint Surg. 54-A:* 389–392, 1972.
67. Schajowicz, F., and Gallardo, H.: Epiphysial chondroblastoma of bone; a clinicopathological study of sixty-nine cases. *J. Bone Joint Surg. 52-B:* 205–226, 1970.
68. Schwinn, C. P., and Spiegel, P. G.: Chondroblastoma of bone, benign and malignant. Presented at the Annual Meeting of the American Society of Clinical Pathologists. Miami Beach, Florida. October, 1968.
69. Sirsat, M. V., and Doctor, V. M.: Benign chondroblastoma of bone; report of a case of malignant transformation. *J. Bone Joint Surg. 52-B:* 741–745, 1970.

Giant Cell Reaction of Hand and Foot Bones

70. D'Alonzo, R. T., Pitcock, J. A., and Milford, L. W.: Giant-cell reaction of bone; report of two cases. *J. Bone Joint Surg. 54-A:* 1267–1271, 1972.
71. Jernstrom, P., and Stark, H. H.: Giant cell reaction of a metacarpal. *Am. J. Clin. Pathol. 55:* 77–81, 1971.

Intraosseous (Invasive, Aggressive) Pigmented Villonodular Synovitis and Tenosynovitis. (Giant Cell Tumor of Tendon Sheath, Fibrous Xanthoma of Synovium)

72. Breimer, C. W., and Freiberger, R. H.: Bone lesions associated with villonodular synovitis. *Am. J. Roentgenol. 79:* 618–629, 1958.
73. Carr, C. R., Berley, F. V., and Davis, W. C.: Pigmented villonodular synovitis of the hip joint; a case report. *J. Bone Joint Surg. 36-A:* 1007–1013, 1954.
74. Chung, S. M., and Janes, J. M.: Diffuse pigmented villonodular synovitis of the hip joint; review of the literature and report of four cases. *J. Bone Joint Surg. 47-A:* 293–303, 1965.
75. Decker, J. P., and Owen, B. J.: An invasive giant cell tumor of tendon sheath in the foot. *Bull. Ayer Clin. Lab. 4:* 43–53, 1954.
76. Fletcher, A. G., Jr., and Horn, R. C., Jr.: Giant cell tumors of tendon sheath origin; a consideration of bone involvement and report of two cases with extensive bone destruction. *Ann. Surg. 113:* 374–385, 1951.
77. Jones, F. E., Soule, E. H., and Coventry, M. B.: Fibrous xanthoma of synovium (giant-cell tumor of tendon sheath, pigmented nodular synovitis); a study of one hundred and eighteen cases. *J. Bone Joint Surg. 51-A:* 76–86, 1969.
78. McMaster, P. E.: Pigmented vellonodular synovitis with invasion of bone; report of six cases. *J. Bone Joint Surg. 42-A:* 1170–1183, 1960.
79. Phalen, G. S., McCormack, L. J., and Gazale, W. J.: Giant cell tumor of tendon sheath (benign synovioma) in the hand; evaluation of 56 cases. *Clin. Orthop. 15:* 140–151, 1959.
80. Scott, P. M.: Bone lesions in pigmented villonodular synovitis. *J. Bone Joint Sur. 50-B:* 306–311, 1968.
81. Schajowicz, F., and Blumenfeld, I.: Pigmented villonodular synovitis of the wrist with penetration into bone. *J. Bone Joint Surg. 50-B:* 312–317, 1968.

Brown Tumor of Hyperparathyroidism

82. Black, B. K., and Ackerman, L. V.: Tumors of the parathyroid; a review of twenty-three cases. *Cancer 3:* 415–444, 1950.
83. Carlotti, A. E., Camitta, F. D., and Connor, T. B.: Primary hyperparathyroidism with giant cell tumors of the maxilla; report of case. *J. Oral. Surg. 27:* 722–727, 1969.
84. Clark, O. H., and Taylor, S.: Osteoclastoma of the jaw and multiple parathyroid tumors. *Surg. Gynecol. Obstet. 135:* 188–192, 1972.
85. Hellström, J., and Ivemark, B. I.: Primary hyperparathyroidism; clinical and structural findings in 138 cases. *Acta Chir. Scand.* [*Suppl.*] *294:* 1–113, 1962.
86. Kleinfeld, G.: A clinical and pathological study of 63 functioning parathyroid tumors. *Cancer 12:* 902–911, 1959.

87. Males, J. L., Howard, W. J., Mask, D. R., Townsend, J. L., Snow, J. B., and McPherson, H. T.: Primary hyperparathyroidism presenting as a giant cell tumor of the maxilla. *Arch. Intern. Med. 132:* 107–111, 1973.
88. McGeown, M. G., and Morrison, E.: Hyperparathyroidism. *Postgrad. Med. J. 35:* 330–337, 1959.
89. Rosenberg, E. H.,. and Guralnick, W. C.: Hyperparathyroidism. A review of 220 proved cases with special emphasis on findings in the jaws. *Oral Surg., Oral Med., Oral Pathol.* (*Supplement 2*) *15:* 84–94, 1962.
90. Shanon, E., and Rapoport, Y.: Giant cell tumor of the palate in hyperparathyroidism. *Laryngoscope 82:* 425–429, 1972.

Giant Cell Reparative Granuloma of Jawbones

91. Austin, L. T., Dahlin, D. C., and Royer, R. Q.: Giant-cell Reparative granuloma and related conditions affecting the jawbones. *Oral Surg., Oral Med., Oral Pathol. 12:* 1285–1295, 1959.
92. Bhaskar, S. N., Bernier, J. L., and Godby, F.: Aneurysmal bone cyst and other giant cell lesions of the jaws; report of 104 cases. *J. Oral Surg. 17:* 30–41, 1959.
93. Curtis, M. L., Hatfield, C. G., and Pierce, J. M.: A destructive giant cell lesion of the mandible. *J. Oral Surg. 31:* 705–709, 1973.
94. Dehner, L. P.: Tumors of the mandible and maxilla in children. I. Clinicopathologic study of 46 histologically benign lesions. *Cancer 31:* 364–384, 1973.
95. Jaffe, H. L.: Giant cell reparative granuloma, traumatic bone cyst and fibrous (fibro-osseous) dysplasia of the jaw bones. *Oral Surg., Oral Med., Oral Pathol. 6:* 159–175, 1953.
96. Seldin, H. M., Seldin, S. D., Rakower, W., and Selman, A. J.: Giant cell tumor of the jaws. *J. Am. Dent. Assoc. 55:* 210–222, 1957.
97. Waldron, C. A., and Shafer, W. G.: The central giant cell reparative granuloma of the jaws; an analysis of 38 cases. *Am. J. Clin. Pathol. 45:* 437–447, 1966.

Osteosarcoma with Numerous Benign Multinucleated Giant Cells

98. Farr, G. H., Huvos, A. G., Marcove, R. C., Higinbotham, N. L., and Foote, F. W.: Telangiectatic osteogenic sarcoma; a review of twenty-eight cases. *Cancer 34:* 1150–1158, 1974.
99. McKenna, R. J., Schwinn, C. P., Soong, K. Y., and Higinbotham, N. L.: Sarcomata of the osteogenic series (Osteosarcoma, fibrosarcoma, chondrosarcoma, parosteal osteogenic sarcoma, and sarcomata arising in abnormal bone); an analysis of 552 cases. *J. Bone Joint Surg. 48-A:* 1–26, 1966.
100. Troup, J. B.: The significance of benign giant cells in osteogenic sarcoma. M.S. thesis, University of Minnesota, Minneapolis, 1958.
101. Troup, J. B., Dahlin, D. C., and Coventry, M. B.: The significance of giant cells in osteogenic sarcoma; Do they indicate a relationship between osteogenic sarcoma and giant cell tumor of bone? *Proc. Staff Meet. Mayo Clin. 35:* 179–186, 1960.

Fibrous Cortical Defect (*Metaphyseal Fibrous Defect, Nonossifying Fibroma, Nonosteogenic Fibroma*)

102. Berkin, C. R.: Non-ossifying fibroma of bone. *Br. J. Radiol. 39:* 469–471, 1966.
103. Caffey, J.: On fibrous defects in cortical walls of growing tubular bones; their radiologic appearance, structure, prevalence, natural course, and diagnostic significance. *Adv. Pediatr. 7:* 13–51, 1955.
104. Cunningham, J. B., and Ackerman, L. V.: Metaphyseal fibrous defects. *J. Bone Joint Surg. 38-A:* 797–808, 1956.
105. Hatcher, C. H.: The pathogenesis of localized fibrous lesions in the metaphyses of long bones. *Ann. Surg. 122:* 1016–1030, 1945.
106. Jaffe, H. L., and Lichtenstein, L.: Non-osteogenic fibroma of bone. *Am. J. Pathol. 18:* 205–221, 1942.
107. Schrieber, R. L.: Personal communication.
108. Selby, S.: Metaphyseal cortical defects in the tubular bones of growing children. *J. Bone Joint Surg. 43-A:* 395–400, 1961.
109. Sontag, L. W., and Pyle, S. I.: The appearance and nature of cyst-like areas in the distal femoral metaphyses of children. *Am. J. Roentgenol. 46:* 185–188, 1941.

Solitary and Multifocal Eosinophilic Granuloma of Bone

110. Enriquez, P., Dahlin, D. C., Hayles, A. B., and Henderson, E. D.: Histiocytosis X; a clinical study. *Mayo Clin. Proc. 42:* 88–99.
111. Lichtenstein, L.: Histiocytosis X (eosinophilic granuloma of bone, Letterer-Siwe disease, and Schuller-Christian disease). Further observations of pathological and clinical importance. *J. Bone Joint Surg. 46-A*: 76–90, 1964.
112. Lieberman, P. H., Jones, C. R., Dargeon, H. W. K., and Begg, C. F.: A reappraisal of eosinophilic granuloma of bone, Hand-Schuller-Christian syndrome and Letterer-Siwe syndrome. *Medicine 48:* 375–400, 1969.
113. McGavran, M. H., and Spady, H. A.: Eosinophilic granuloma of bone; a study of twenty-eight cases. *J. Bone Joint Surg. 42-A:* 979–992, 1960.
114. Ochsner, S. F.: Eosinophilic granuloma of bone; experience with 20 cases. *Am. J. Roentgenol. Radium Ther. Nucl. Med. 97:* 719–726, 1966
115. Otani, S.: A discussion on eosinophilic granuloma of bone, Letterer-Siwe disease and Schuller-Christian disease. *J. Mt. Sinai Hosp. 24:* 1079–1092, 1957.
116. Schajowicz, F., and Slullitel, J.: Eosinophilic granuloma of bone and its relationship to Hand-Schuller-Christian and Letterer-Siwe syndromes. *J. Bone Joint Surg. 55-B:* 545–565, 1973.
117. Schrieber, R. L.: Personal communication.

Aneurysmal Bone Cyst

118. Biesecker, J. L., Marcove, R. C., Huvos, A. G., Mikė, V.: Aneurysmal bone cysts. *Cancer 26:* 615–625, 1970.
119. Buraczewski, J., and Dabska, M.: Pathogenesis of aneurysmal bone cyst; relationship between the aneurysmal bone cyst and fibrous dysplasia of bone. *Cancer 28:* 597–604, 1971.
120. Dahlin, D. C., Besse, B. E., Pugh, D. G., and Ghormley, R. K.: Aneurysmal bone cysts. *Radiology 64:* 56–65, 1955.
121. Jaffe, H. L. Aneurysmal bone cyst. *Bull. Hosp. Joint Dis. 11:* 3–13, 1950.
122. Jaffe, H. L.: Discussion following a paper by Donaldson, W. F., Jr.; aneurysmal bone cyst. *J. Bone Joint Surg. 44-A:* 40, 1962.
123. Levy, W. M., Miller, A. S., Bonakdarpour, A., and Aegerter, E.: Aneurysmal bone cyst secondary to other osseous lesions. Report of 57 cases. *Am. J. Clin. Pathol. 63:* 1–8, 1975.
124. Lichtenstein, L.: Aneurysmal bone cyst; a pathological entity commonly mistaken for giant-cell tumor and occasionally for hemangioma and osteogenic sarcoma. *Cancer 3:* 279–289, 1950.
125. Lichtenstein, L.: Aneurysmal bone cyst; further observations. *Cancer 6:* 1228–1237, 1953.
126. Lindbom, A., Soderberg, G., Spjut, H. J., and Sunnqvist, O.: Angiography of aneurysmal bone cyst. *Acta Radiol. 55:* 12–16, 1961.
127. Tillman, B. P., Dahlin, D. C., Lipscomb, P. R., and Stewart, J. R.: Aneurysmal bone cyst; an analysis of ninety-five cases. *Mayo Clin. Proc. 43:* 478–495, 1968.

Unicameral (Solitary) Bone Cyst

128. Baker, D. M.: Benign unicameral bone cyst; a study of forty-five cases with long-term follow up. *Clin. Orthop. 71:* 140–151, 1970.
129. Boseker, E. H., Bickel, W. H., and Dahlin, D. C.: A clinicopathologic study of simple unicameral bone cysts. *Surg. Gynecol. Obstet. 127:* 550–560, 1968.
130. Cohen, J.: Simple bone cysts; studies of cyst fluid in six cases with a theory of pathogenesis. *J. Bone Joint Surg. 42-A:* 609–616, 1960.
131. Fahey, J. J., and O'Brien, E. T.: Subtotal resection and grafting in selected cases of solitary unicameral bone cyst. *J. Bone Joint Surg. 55-A:* 59–68, 1973.
132. Friedman, N. B., and Goldman, R. L.: Cementoma of long bones; an extragnathic odontogenic tumor. *Clin. Orthop. 67:* 243–248, 1969.
133. Hagberg, S., and Mansfeld, L.: The solitary bone cyst; a follow-up study of 24 cases. *Acta Chir. Scand. 133:* 25–29, 1967.
134. Jaffe, H. L., and Lichtenstein, L.: Solitary unicameral bone cyst; with emphasis on the roentgen picture, the pathologic appearance and the pathogenesis. *Arch. Surg. 44:* 1004–1025, 1942.
135. Lodwick, G. S.: Juvenile unicameral bone cyst; a roentgen reappraisal. *Am. J. Roentgenol. 80:*

495–504, 1958.

136. Neer, C. S., Francis, K. C., Marcove, R. C., Terz, J., and Carbonara, P. N.: Treatment of unicameral bone cyst; a follow-up study of one hundred and seventy-five cases. *J. Bone Joint Surg. 48-A:* 731–745, 1966.
137. Smith, R. W., and Smith, C. F.: Solitary unicameral bone cyst of the calcaneus; a review of twenty cases. *J. Bone Joint Surg. 56-A:* 49–56, 1974.
138. Spence, K. F., Sell, K. W., and Brown, R. H.: Solitary bone cyst; treatment with freeze-dried cancellous bone allograft; a study of one hundred seventy-seven cases. *J. Bone Joint Surg. 51-A:* 87–96, 1969.

Chondromyxoid Fibroma

139. Dahlin, D. C.: Chondromyxoid fibroma of bone, with emphasis on its morphological relationship to benign chondroblastoma. *Cancer 9:* 195–203, 1956.
140. Feldman, F., Hecht, H. L., and Johnston, A. D.: Chondromyxoid fibroma of bone. *Radiology 94:* 249–260, 1970.
141. Iwata, S., and Coley, B. L.: Report of six cases of chondromyxoid fibroma of bone. *Surg. Gynecol. Obstet. 107:* 571–576, 1958.
142. Jaffe, H. L., and Lichtenstein, L.: Chondromyxoid fibroma of bone; a distinctive benign tumor likely to be mistaken especially for chondrosarcoma. *Arch. Pathol. 45:* 541–551, 1948.
143. Marcove, R. C., Kambolis, C., Bullough, P. G., and Jaffe, H. L.: Fibromyxoma of bone; a report of 3 cases. *Cancer 17:* 1209–1213, 1964.
144. Rahimi, A., Beamout, J. W., Ivins, J. C., and Dahlin, D. C.: Chondromyxoid fibroma; a clinicopathologic study of 76 cases. *Cancer 30:* 726–736, 1972.
145. Ralph, L. L.: Chondromyxoid fibroma of bone. *J. Bone Joint Surg. 44-B:* 7–24, 1962.
146. Schajowicz, F., and Gallardo, H.: Chondromyxoid fibroma (fibromyxoid chondroma) of bone; a clinico-pathological study of thirty-two cases. *J. Bone Joint Surg. 53-B:* 198–216, 1971.
147. Schutt, P. G., and Frost, H. M.: Chondromyxoid fibroma. *Clin. Orthop. 78:* 323–329, 1971.

Gout

148. Schrieber, R. L.: Personal communication.
149. Talbot, J. H.: *Gout*, 3rd ed. New York, Grune & Stratton, Inc., 1967.

Giant Cell Tumors of Soft Somatic Tissues

150. Guccion, J. G., and Enzinger, F. M.: Malignant giant cell tumor of soft parts; an analysis of 32 cases. *Cancer 29:* 1518–1529, 1972.
151. Salm, R., and Sissons, H. A.: Giant cell tumours of soft tissues. *J. Pathol. 107:* 27–39, 1972.
152. Soule, E. H., and Enriquez, P.: Atypical fibrous histiocytoma, malignant fibrous histiocytoma, malignant histiocytoma and epithelioid sarcoma; a comparative study of 65 tumors. *Cancer 30:* 128–143, 1972.

Tumoral Calcinosis

153. Harkess, J. W., and Peters, H. J.: Tumoral calcinosis; a report of six cases. *J. Bone Joint Surg. 49-A:* 721–731, 1967.

Chapter 16

Chondrosarcoma and Its "Variants"

DAVID C. DAHLIN

CHONDROSARCOMA

Chondrosarcoma is a malignant neoplasm whose cells produce hyaline cartilage that is usually lobulated.[7] The cytologic features of the common well-differentiated sarcomas are only subtly different from those of benign neoplasms of hyaline cartilage, and they include somewhat hyperchromatic and enlarged nuclei as well as an increased number of multinucleated, usually binucleated, forms.[9] For those relatively rare chondrosarcomas of borderline histologic malignancy, it is necessary to use, in addition to the microscopic abnormalities, information indicating aggressiveness, usually afforded by the roentgenogram in the form of large size and bony destruction by the tumor. Often this lesion is accompanied by pain.

The patient's age is an important factor. Malignant neoplasms of hyaline cartilage without highly anaplastic elements are predominantly tumors of adulthood and old age. Such tumors are uncommon in the 3rd decade of life and distinctly unusual in patients less than 20 years old.

The location of the tumor in the skeleton provides an important bias. For instance, neoplasms of cartilage occurring in the axial skeleton or in the major bones of the appendicular skeleton near the body are usually malignant, whereas those of distal skeletal parts, especially in the hands and feet, are usually benign. Further, chondrosarcomas with ample histologic evidence for malignancy but originating in the cartilaginous cap of an exostosis are more amenable to successful wide surgical resection than are those that begin centrally in a bone.

Also, certain tumorous masses of hyaline cartilage, such as those that develop in synovial chondromatosis or in the cartilage of the larynx, are nearly always benign in that they do not metastasize. In fact, any cartilaginous lesion not originating in the skeleton has an unpredictable but usually benign clinical course. The pathologist must determine the exact site of origin of a cartilaginous neoplasm before attempting to predict its malignant capability from its histologic appearance.

Metastasis from chondrosarcoma is usually hematogenous and hence to the lungs. Spread to regional nodes occurs, but is much less common. The usual chondrosarcoma is well-differentiated, and metastasis occurs in less than one-half of them; the greatest threat is local recurrence. Local recurrence may be delayed, even developing more than 10 years after the primary surgery. Local recurrence can be obviated only by wide local resection. Such wide resection is often provided only by hindquarter or forequarter amputation because of the common location of such tumors near the hip or shoulder joint.

Most chondrosarcomas are well-differentiated and composed of lobules of hyaline cartilage, which may be myxoid or liquefied. Calcification secondary to degeneration or actual bone production often occurs in chondrosarcomas. Hence a transition type of sarcoma exists in which it is difficult to know whether osteoid is being produced by malignant cells and the tumor is a chondroblastic osteosarcoma or whether the osteoid or bone is in reality formed from an alteration of malignant cartilage. It is not always possible to state with certainty whether a problem tumor such as this should be designated as merely chondrosarcoma.

The gross pathologic features of chondrosarcoma reflect its hyaline cartilage quality. Soft or myxoid lesions are usually aggressive. Large size and invasiveness are important features of malignancy. Small or large chondrosarcomas frequently contain mineral as calcific foci in degenerating neoplastic lobules or in bony trabeculae formed in the tumors. Large lobules of chondrosarcoma tend to become centrally gelatinous or cystic.

Roentgenographically, chondrosarcoma often produces strongly suggestive features.[12] Large size and permeative aggressiveness are usually shown. The practically diagnostic calcific islands in chrondrosarcoma are common and indicate its basically cartilaginous nature. When chondrosarcoma begins within a major tubular bone, it may distend the outline of the bone even though the bony cortices are thickened. The chondrosarcoma that occurs in the cap of an osteochondroma may produce a mass that is difficult to see on the roentgenogram unless it is large. Often, though, this mass shows evidence of irregular calcification. Whenever the cartilaginous cap of an exostosis is irregular and more than a few millimeters thick, it should be suspected of having histologic features of chondrosarcoma. Severe destruction of the nearby cortex is especially likely to be produced by tumors that have dedifferentiated highly malignant zones.

VARIANTS

Mesenchymal chondrosarcoma.[13] This lesion is a relative newcomer among malignant tumors, but one that is now recognized as an entity by the World Health Organization. It is characterized by a variable component of cartilaginous islands, the cells of which are likely to be well-differentiated, and, paradoxically, by a second component of small undifferentiated cells so closely packed as to mimic the pattern of Ewing's sarcoma (Fig. 1, *A* and *B*). In these zones of small cells, the vascular arrangement is often like that of hemangiopericytoma. The cartilaginous islands may show partial or prominent calcification and, apparently later, ossification. Such mineralized zones produce radiodensity that is usually manifested on the roentgenogram, which shows the overall destructive quality of a chondrosarcoma (Fig. 1 *C*). Nearly one-third of such tumors arise in somatic soft tissue, but histologically they are similar to tumors of bony origin. The available evidence suggests that these neoplasms are radioresistant and that, even after radical removal, metastasis often occurs. Radical removal similar to that

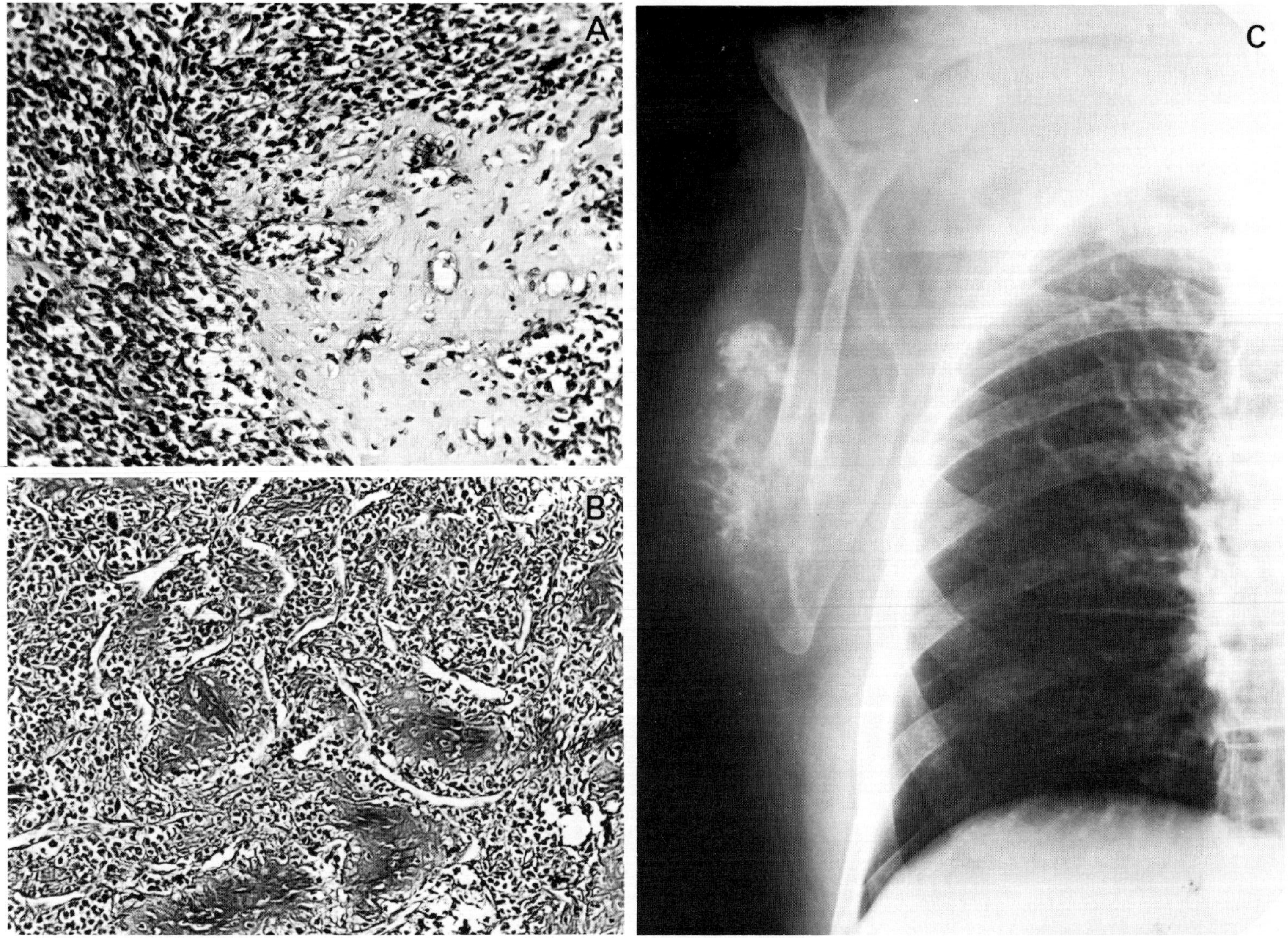

FIG. 1. Mesenchymal chondrosarcoma. *A*, with chondroid zone and its prominent component of small round to oval cells. Hematoxylin and eosin stain; × 200. *B*, although many mesenchymal chondrosarcomas contain large islands of cartilaginous material in this area, they are small but

for osteosarcoma seems imperative. Metastasis may develop more than 5 years after removal of the primary lesion. These tumors have been found in many skeletal sites; several of them have arisen in the jaw.

Dedifferentiated cartilaginous tumors. Dedifferentiation of the average low grade or well-differentiated and clinically indolent cartilaginous tumor has now become recognized as a significant problem.[2] Many smoldering cartilaginous tumors have changed rather suddenly into aggressive anaplastic sarcomas (Fig. 2*A*). Statistically, in our own material, such conversion occurred in 33 of 370 cases. When chondrosarcomas recur they usually do so in the same well-differentiated form of the original tumor. Sometimes the recurrent lesion has a slightly increased cellular activity. In lesions that were considered to be dedifferentiated, however, the second element was highly anaplastic and often had nearly completely overrun the indolent cartilaginous tumor of origin. The engrafted new tumor was a spindle cell sarcoma (fibrosarcoma) in 22 cases and an osteosarcoma (Fig. 2, *B* and *C*) in the remaining 11 cases. Surgical intervention had been performed for the low grade chondrosarcoma in only 7 of the 33 cases. Hence, such dedifferentiation is an expected development in the evolution of some chondrosarcomas. When the anaplastic sarcoma has supervened, the prognosis is poor. Radical surgery is obviously mandatory at the earliest practicable time. Twenty-three of the 28 patients treated prior to 1969 were dead at the time of study in 1970.

Roentgenographic features often gave evidence of the slowly growing chondrosarcoma, thus abetting the clinical evaluation suggesting this. In a few recent cases, extensive lysis in part of a chondrosarcomatous zone has been suggestive of such dedifferentiation. Generally, however, the radiologist knows only that the lesion has produced the type of alteration suggestive of chondrosarcoma.

The feature of dedifferentiation introduces two problems. If a surgeon elects to treat a suspected cartilaginous lesion of the skeleton conservatively, by observation or by some form of limited surgery, he must recognize that change to a more active form of tumor may occur. The frequency of such change is not known, but the risk is probably small. The second problem is that any unusual portions of a tumor of hyaline cartilage must be sampled histologically to ascertain such change. Further, the pathologist must be alert to the possibility of an underlying cartilaginous tumor when fibrosarcoma or osteosarcoma is seen in an older patient.

Chondrosarcomas of skeleton of hands and feet.[3] These are unusual lesions that emphasize the need for consultation between the histopathologist and the roentgenologist in assessing chondrosarcomas (Fig. 3). Only 10 chondrosarcomas of these distally located bones have been noted in the files of the Mayo Clinic before 1974. Twenty such malignant tumors were sent to this clinic for diagnosis. Overt histologic evidence or roentgenographic or surgical evidence of aggressiveness was necessary in judging these tumors to be malignant. The problem is complicated because adequate removal (such as by amputation of a digit, of the affected ray, or of part or all of a hand or foot), as indicated by the location and extent of the tumor, affords a good chance for cure. Only 4 of the 30 tumors studied produced unequivocal evidence of metastasis, but 3 patients died of un-

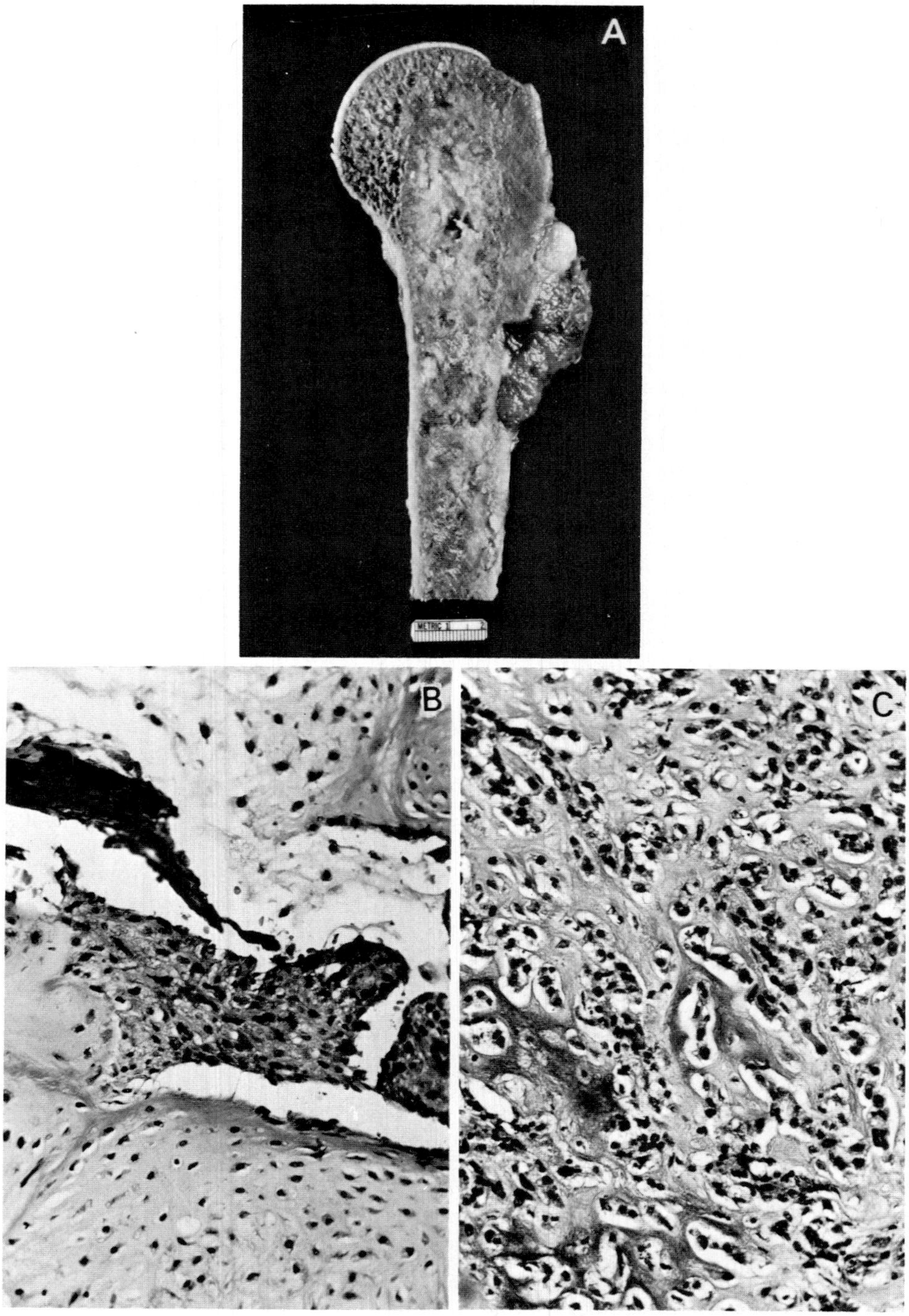

FIG. 2. *A*, grade 1 chondrosarcoma filling head and adjacent shaft of humerus. Extraosseous softer component of this lesion from a 71-year-old man is grade 4 osteosarcoma. *B*, grade 1 chondrosarcoma lobules separated by highly cellular dedifferentiated zone. Hematoxylin and eosin stain; × 200. *C*, larger zone, grade 4 osteosarcoma, in dedifferentiated grade 1 chondrosarcoma of Figure 2*B*. Hematoxylin and eosin stain; × 200.

known cause. Curettage or subtotal removal of these sarcomas by any procedure less than total resection was unsuccessful.

Cartilaginous tumors of soft tissues of hands and feet. Although only 11 such tumors of hyaline cartilage were found in the Mayo Clinic files,[4] 59 others had been sent in for a diagnostic opinion before 1974. Most of these were sent because the original pathologist was concerned by the histologic evidence of activity in these tumors. Paradoxically, although most of these tumors had multinucleation and other features suggestive of chondrosarcoma (Fig. 4), none produced proved or even suspected metastasis. Recurrence developed in 12 of the total of 70 cases, but such recurrence did not indicate increased aggressiveness. Histologic appearances and sometimes a distinct relationship with tendon sheaths indicated that most of these tumors were probably derived from synovium. Three were multicentric when first seen. Nine of the 70 tumors contained fibrous histiocytic (xanthoma-like) zones, further evidence of their tenosynovial origin. All had the gross appearance of hyaline cartilage, at least in part. Roentgenologic or surgical evidence that they were soft tissue tumors was essential in their interpretation. More than half of those studied roentgenologically contained mineralized material.

Articular synovial chondromatosis.[11] In a study of 32 cases of this condition, our group found that it is a primary monarticular affection; two-thirds of the lesions occurred in the knee joint. Any major articulation can be the site of syno-

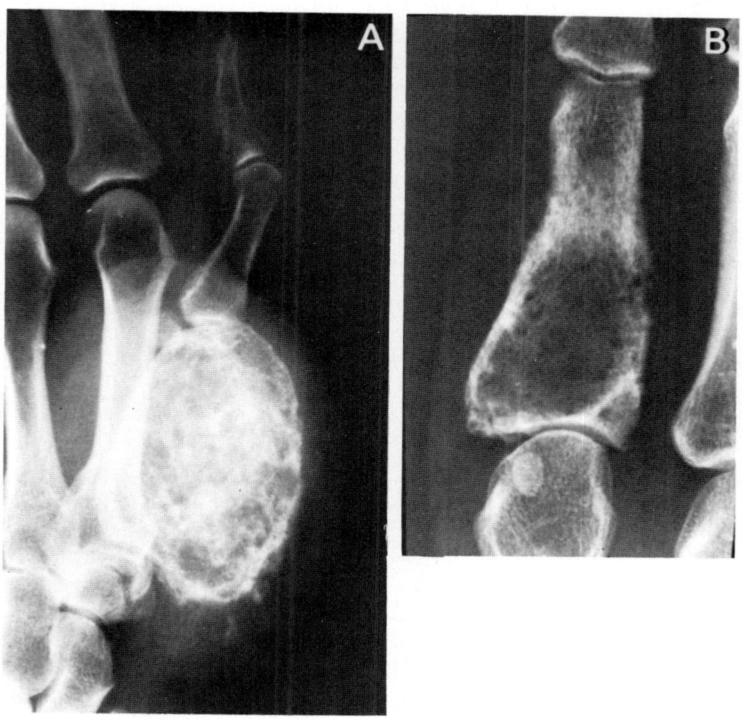

FIG. 3. Chondrosarcoma. *A*, first metacarpal. Its large size is indicated, as is perforation through "expanded" shell of bone. *B*, phalanx. Poor delimitation and perforation through altered cortex are apparent by roentgenogram.

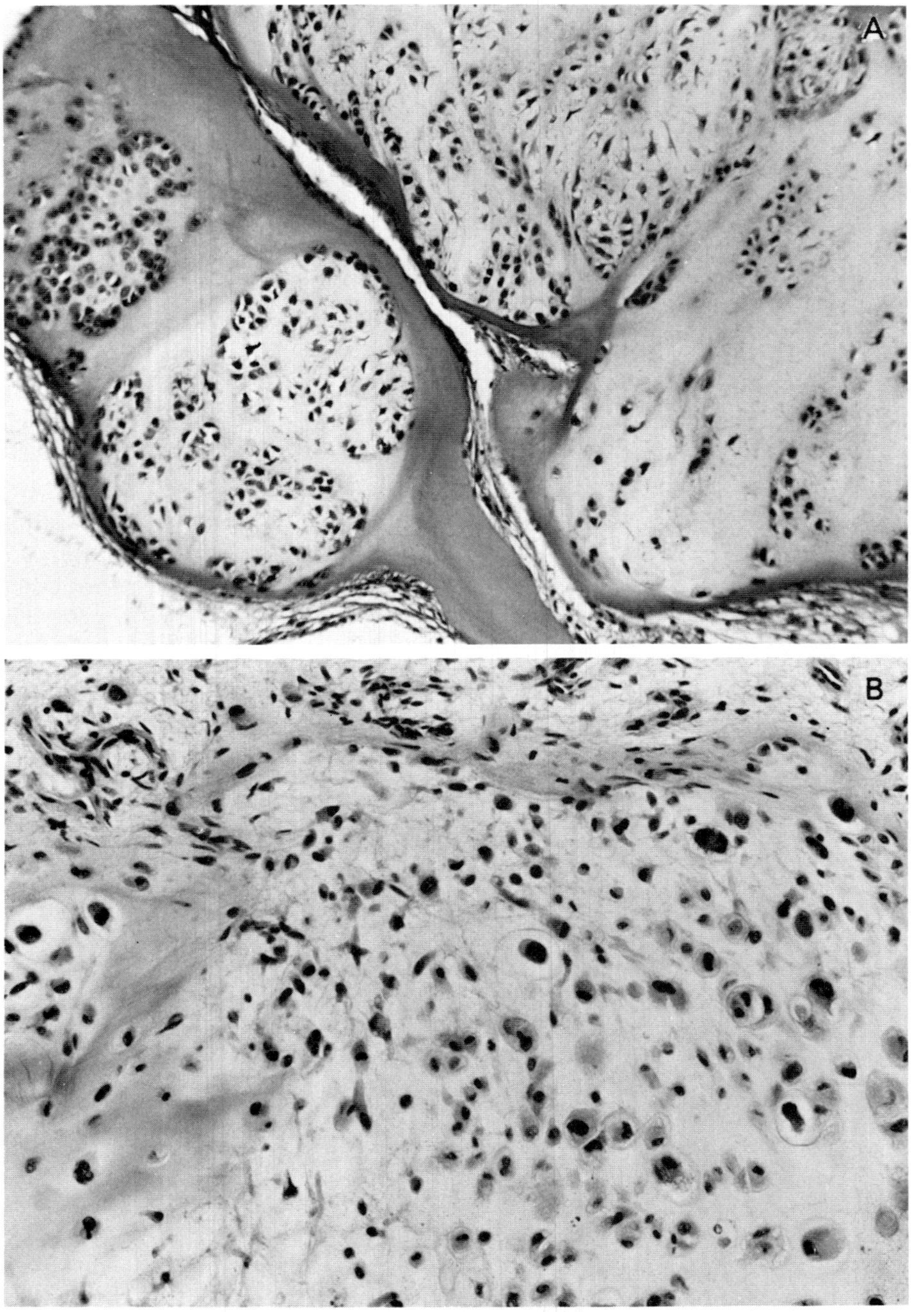

FIG. 4. *A*, lobules of chondroma of soft tissues of hand. Hematoxylin and eosin stain; × 100. *B*, higher magnification of probably tenosynovial cartilaginous benign tumor of soft tissues of hand, illustrating nuclear variation in size and shape, features erroneously suggestive of sarcoma. Hematoxylin and eosin stain; × 160.

vial chondromatosis, and even the temporomandibular joint has been the source of several lesions.[1] Characteristically, small or large masses of cartilage develop, apparently by a process of metaplasia, in the synovium. These usually become pedunculated and may become loose bodies in the joint. When the condition is chronic or neglected, the cartilaginous tumors may become confluent and huge. Calcific foci are common but usually are small and within the lobules of this lesion (Fig. 5*A*). The importance of synovial chondromatosis is that in about two-thirds of the cases, the cartilaginous islands contain enlarged nuclei and show multinucleation (Fig. 5*B*). These features taken out of context suggest that the lesion is malignant. By contrast, however, the process is nearly always benign. Our group at the Mayo Clinic has never seen malignant change in synovial chondromatosis, even when the condition has been neglected. In very rare instances, however, such change has been reported.[10] It is far more common, in our experience, to suspect or to diagnose erroneously chondrosarcoma in such cases if the pathologist fails to assure himself that the problem lesion is synovial and, hence, almost certainly benign.

Cartilaginous tumors of larynx.[5] These tumors pose a problem in that often their histologic appearance (Fig. 6) does not reflect their clinical behavior. In a study of 22 pertinent lesions of this organ, we found that, microscopically, no less than 18 contained either areas of chondrosarcoma or areas suggestive of chondrosarcoma. None of the cartilaginous tumors in our series has metasta-

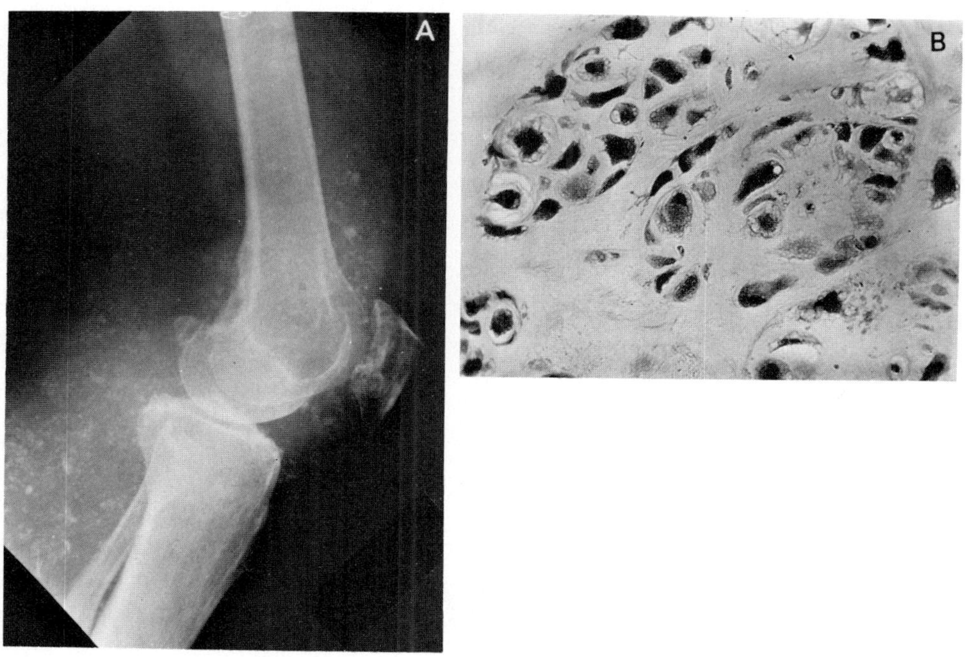

FIG. 5. *A*, knee area with marked enlargement of joint and generally small foci of calcification in synovial chondromatosis. *B*, enlarged nuclei and multinucleation in cellular zone of synovial chondromatosis of a knee. Hematoxylin and eosin stain; $\times$ 300.

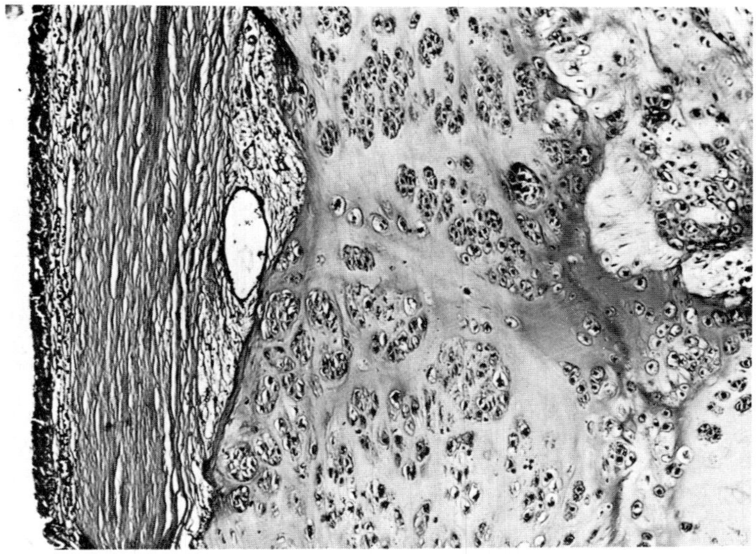

FIG. 6. Cellular cartilaginous tumor of larynx, with enough nuclear variation in size and binucleation to predict that tumor, if in large bone, should be chordoma and have an aggressive, malignant course. Hematoxylin and eosin stain; × 75.

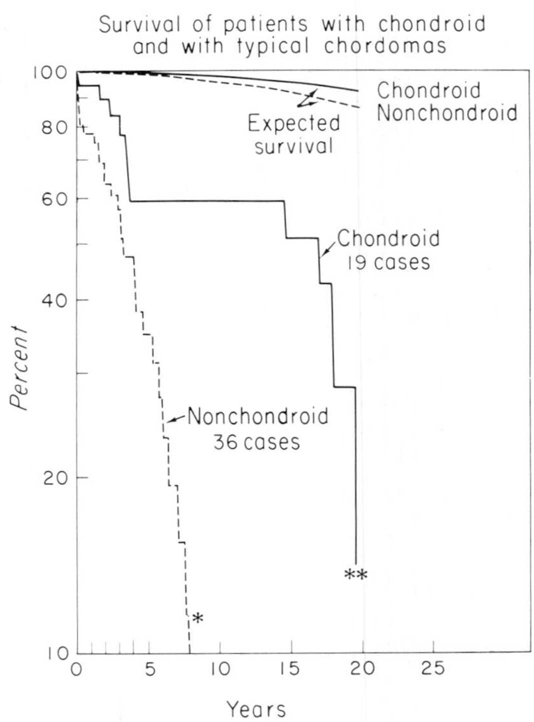

FIG. 7. Paradoxically, chordomas that resembled chondrosarcoma had better prognosis, as indicated, than did the nonchondroid or ordinary chondrosarcomas.

sized. Control of the local lesion and even of its occasional recurrence has been achieved by modest surgical means. Although metastasis of chondrosarcomas of this organ has been reported, such cases are oddities and unexpected.[14]

Chondroid chordoma.[6] Knowledge of the site of origin of the chondroid chordoma is mandatory if its clinical behavior is to be predicted. A recent study of 55 spheno-occipital chordomas revealed that 19 contained foci remarkably similar to those seen in chondrosarcoma or, less commonly, in chondroma. Paradoxically, subtotal removal, often with adjunctive radiation therapy, produced a prolonged symptom-free period in more cases of this mixture of chordoma and ordinary "cartilaginous" tumor than in cases of classic chordoma (Fig. 7). The general postoperative behavior was remarkably better than would have been predicted.

Periosteal Chondroma.[8] Tumors with benign clinical evolution in this peripheral location with respect to the bone of origin may be several centimeters in

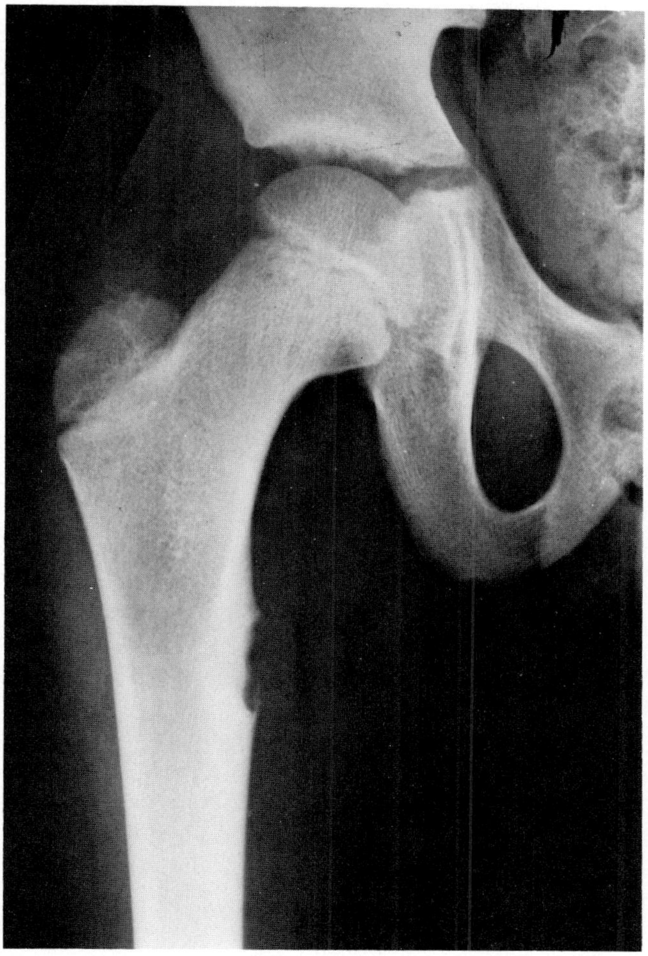

FIG. 8. Periosteal chondroma in its typically eccentric location. Such peripherally situated cartilaginous tumors, though clinically benign, may have ominous cytologic irregularities.

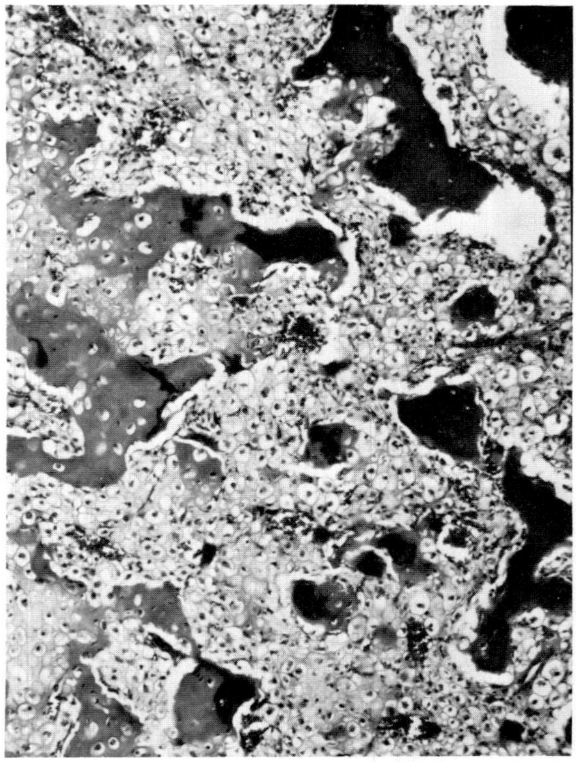

FIG. 9. Clear cell chondrosarcoma. Tumor is characterized by prominent component of osteoid and bony trabeculae separated by relatively large, clear neoplastic cells which betray their cartilage-forming capability only in areas. Hematoxylin and eosin stain; × 100.

largest diameter. Characteristically, they produce a rounded or somewhat scalloped defect in the subjacent cortical bone, and often this defect has a sclerotic margin (Fig. 8). Sometimes a cartilaginous tumor in such a location contains plumper nuclei than average and even fairly numerous binucleated forms. These cytologic features are not to be construed as indications of aggressiveness or malignancy.

"Clear-cell" chondrosarcoma. This lesion has abundant young bony trabeculae that have caused it to be confused with osteoblastoma. Its sprinkling of benign multinucleated forms spuriously suggests atypical chondroblastoma as a designation. The tumor may even contain prominent aneurysmal bone cyst-like areas. The background and sometimes sparse component of truly cartilaginous cells indicate its true nature, although the most prominent cell of the tumor is rounded and contains clear cytoplasm (Fig. 9). The details of this lesion are currently under investigation. Tumors of this type tend to be slow-growing, but eventual metastasis can occur.

SUMMARY

Although the general pathologic features of skeletal chondrosarcoma may be known, the exact localization of the cartilaginous tumors in unusual sites is mandatory if the clinical behavior is to be predicted. Chondrosarcomas in extraskeletal sites not discussed herein are very rare and can be expected to behave in a relatively indolent but malignant clinical fashion.

REFERENCES

1. Ballard, R., and Weiland, L. H.: Synovial chondromatosis of the temporomandibular joint. *Cancer 30:* 791–795, 1972.
2. Dahlin, D. C., and Beabout, J. W.: Dedifferentiation of low-grade chondrosarcomas. *Cancer 28:* 461–466, 1971.
3. Dahlin, D. C., and Salvador, A. H.: Chondrosarcomas of bones of the hands and feet; a study of 30 cases. *Cancer 34:* 755–760, 1974.
4. Dahlin, D. C., and Salvador, A. H.: Cartilaginous tumors of the soft tissues of the hands and feet. *Mayo Clin. Proc. 49:* 721–726, 1974.
5. Goethals, P. L., Dahlin, D. C., and Devine, K. D.: Cartilaginous tumors of the larynx. *Surg. Gynecol. Obstet. 117:* 77–82, 1963.
6. Heffelfinger, M. J., Dahlin, D. C., MacCarty, C. S., and Beabout, J. W.: Chordomas and cartilaginous tumors at the skull base. *Cancer 32:* 410–420, 1973.
7. Henderson, E. D., and Dahlin, D. C.: Chondrosarcoma of bone; a study of two hundred eighty-eight cases. *J. Bone Joint Surg. (Am.) 45A:* 1450–1458, 1963.
8. Lichtenstein, L., and Hall, J. E.: Periosteal chondroma; a distinctive benign cartilage tumor. *J. Bone Joint Surg. (Am.) 34A:* 691–697, 1952.
9. Lichtenstein, L., and Jaffe, H. L.: Chondrosarcoma of bone. *Am. J. Pathol. 19:* 553–589, 1943.
10. Mullins, F., Berard, C. W., and Eisenberg, S. H.: Chondrosarcoma following synovial chondromatosis; a case study. *Cancer 18:* 1180–1188, 1965.
11. Murphy, F. P., Dahlin, D. C., and Sullivan, C. R.: Articular synovial chondromatosis. *J. Bone Joint Surg. (Am.) 44A:* 77–86, 1962.
12. Reiter, F. B., Ackerman, L. V., and Staple, T. W.: Central chondrosarcoma of the appendicular skeleton. *Radiology 105:* 525–530, 1972.
13. Salvador, A. H., Beabout, J. W., and Dahlin, D. C.: Mesenchymal chondrosarcoma; observations on 30 new cases. *Cancer 28:* 605–615, 1971.
14. Swerdlow, R. S., Som, M. L., and Biller, H. F.: Cartilaginous tumors of the larynx. *Arch. Otolaryngol. 100:* 269–272, 1974.

Chapter 17

Small Round Cell Tumors of Bone

WALTER M. LEVY, M.D.

Neoplasms that arise from the bone marrow components are logically classified as myelogenic tumors on the basis of the assumption that they originate from the marrow cells. Included in this category and occurring in the following order of frequency are: plasma cell myeloma, Ewing's sarcoma, reticulum cell sarcoma, and Hodgkin's disease of bone. Bone marrow infiltrates, which usually occur in the various types of leukemia, may also produce obvious bony changes and might well be included in the myelogenic group of neoplasms but, for practical purposes, are excluded. They are usually classified along with the hematological disorders and will not be discussed in this chapter. All of these neoplasms are strikingly similar histologically in size and shape of cells and are therefore colloquially designated as small cell tumors. However, because of obvious clinical differences between the various entities, it is mandatory that they be accurately classified as to cell type, despite the histologic similarities, in order to understand better their biologic nature and institute appropriate treatment.

EWING'S SARCOMA

Ewing's sarcoma, a malignant neoplasm of the marrow reticulum, was first delineated as an entity by James Ewing in 1921. It arises from immature reticulum cells of the medullary cavity and accounts for 7% of all malignant neoplasms of bone. It is a tumor of childhood and adolescence and is especially encountered between 10 and 30 years of age. Fifty per cent of the neoplasms occur prior to 20 years of age, and 90% before 30 years of age. In the series reported by Aegerter and Kirkpatrick[1] 40 of 132 cases occurred under 10 years of age, whereas only 4 occurred after 30 years of age. The lower extremity (particularly the femur and tibia) and the pelvic girdle are common sites of involvement with occurrence being almost as frequent in the ribs. In our series, approximately two-thirds of the neoplasms occurred in cylindrical bones, and the younger the patient, the more apt is this to be true. In patients under 20 years of age, 54 tumors occurred in cylindrical bones, and 31 were in flat bones. In 25 patients over 20 years of age, a flat bone was the primary site of involvement in all but 6 cases. This strongly suggests that Ewing's sarcoma arises in the hematopoietic tissue, for after the age of skeletal maturity, most of the red marrow is found within flat bones. The striking clinical symptom of Ewing's sarcoma is pain of progressive severity, which, like many pains associated with tumefaction, is worse at night. The pain is usually of 1 to several months duration when the patient first seeks aid, a helpful differential feature permitting the lesion to be distinguished from pyogenic osteomyelitis, which usually has a shorter history of no longer than 2 weeks.[3] Tenderness and the presence of a soft tissue mass are also prominent findings with an accompanying impaired function of the part. In addition to the local signs of an apparent inflammatory process, constitutional symptoms are frequently encountered in the nature of anemia, leukocytosis (up to 20,000 white blood cells per cm^2 and rarely as high as 40,000) with an increased sedimintation rate, and fever. The fever is usually of low grade, varying from 100°F to 101°F, but on rare occasions it may rise to 105°F. Constitutional symptoms make it mandatory that Ewing's sarcoma be differentiated from osteomyelitis. Significantly, patients affected by Ewing's sarcoma with constitutional symptoms have a poorer prognosis and shorter survival time than those without symptoms. Frequently there are soft tissue masses before the underlying cortex gives radiographic evidence of penetration. This is due to the fact that Ewing's sarcoma readily grows through the nutrient canals of the cortex to reach extraosseous sites.

Usually Ewing's sarcoma presents with the characteristic roentgenographic lytic lesion in the shaft of a long bone with a laminated periosteal reaction parallel to the shaft (the onion skin pattern of subperiosteal bone formation) (Fig. 1). However, the appearance is frequently variable, and the classical pattern is seen in a minority of cases[3]. Many cases are entirely osteolytic, whereas others show minimal bone production, and in a small percentage of cases a striking bone production and sclerosis is an outstanding feature. It has been pointed out that two types of reactive bone formation may be seen: (1) periosteal reaction, and (2) reactive proliferation of cortical and medullary bone. From the roentgenographic standpoint, Ewing's sarcoma of the flat bones has no specific characteristic, for some lesions are osteolytic, others sclerotic, and still others exhibit a mixture of the two patterns.

Grossly, the neoplasm may be soft or fibrous and grey-white, while in other instances it is gelatinous. Foci of hemorrhage and necrosis are conspicuous in many tumors. Microscopically, Ewing's sarcoma is usually composed of small, round, tightly packed cells arranged in cords or nests with individual cells varying from two to three times the size of a lymphocyte (Fig. 2). The pattern is usually one of monotonously uniform appearing cells composed of moderately basophilic nuclei with well-defined nuclear membranes. Few nucleoli are noted, and these few are generally inconspicuous. The cytoplasm is scant, and cytoplasmic borders are indistinct. The neoplastic cells have a tendency to aggregate around blood vessels in a pseudorosette pattern, while intervening bands of fibrous tissue irregulatly isolate islands of tumor cells. Foci of hemorrhage and necrosis complete the histologic picture. As first emphasized by Schajowicz,[4] the periodic acid-Schiff reaction (PAS) may be used to distinguish Ewing's sarcoma from primary reticulum cell sarcoma of bone. With this stain, glycogen granules are readily demonstrated in the cytoplasm of Ewing's sarcoma

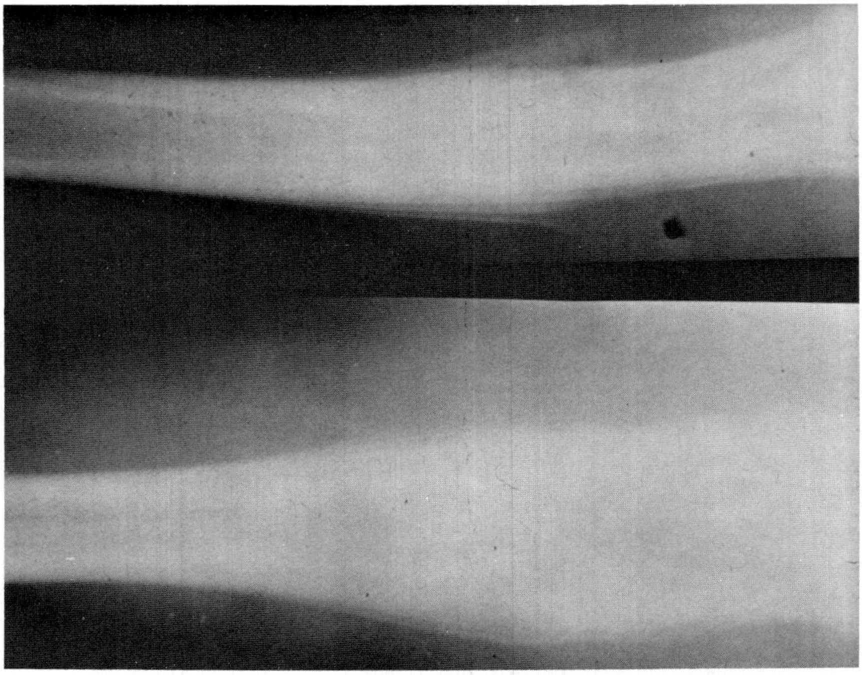

FIG. 1. Roentgenogram of Ewing's sarcoma. Note the layers of periosteal new bone formation, resulting in the onion skin appearance characteristic of Ewing's tumor of cylindrical bones.

cells, but are not seen in the cells of reticulum cell sarcoma. This differential stain, although very useful, is not to the best of the author's knowledge specific. More recently, electron microscopic examination of Ewing's sarcoma tissue by Friedman and Gold[5] has served to delineate ultrastructural differences between these two neoplasms. In their study, Ewing's sarcoma cells were noted to have very few intracytoplasmic organelles and single-layered plasma membranes. The cytoplasmic pallor of the cells when viewed by light microscopy is probably explained by the relative paucity of organelles, whereas the single-layered plasma membrane contrasts sharply with the trilaminar structure of most plasma membranes. They also determined that the cytoplasmic constituents of Ewing's sarcoma cells are mainly organelles, (mitochondria) concerned with aerobic metabolism of the cell, whereas the presence of a few membranes of endoplasmic reticulum and Golgi apparatus indicates that the cell probably secretes protein to a limited degree. In addition, Friedman and Gold[5] noted a transition from immature cells to cells showing increased nuclear and cytoplasmic density, which they interpreted as evidence of maturation, inferring that Ewing's sarcoma has its origin from immature reticulum cells.

The differential diagnosis of Ewing's sarcoma includes metastatic neuroblastoma, reticulum cell sarcoma, metastatic anaplastic carcinoma from various sites, as well as osteomyelitis and eosinophilic granuloma. Neuroblastoma may be distinguished by the clinical demonstration of an adrenal or retroperitoneal tumor, particularly with calcification, and the histologic formation in neuroblastoma of lobules associated with focal areas of calcification with stippling,

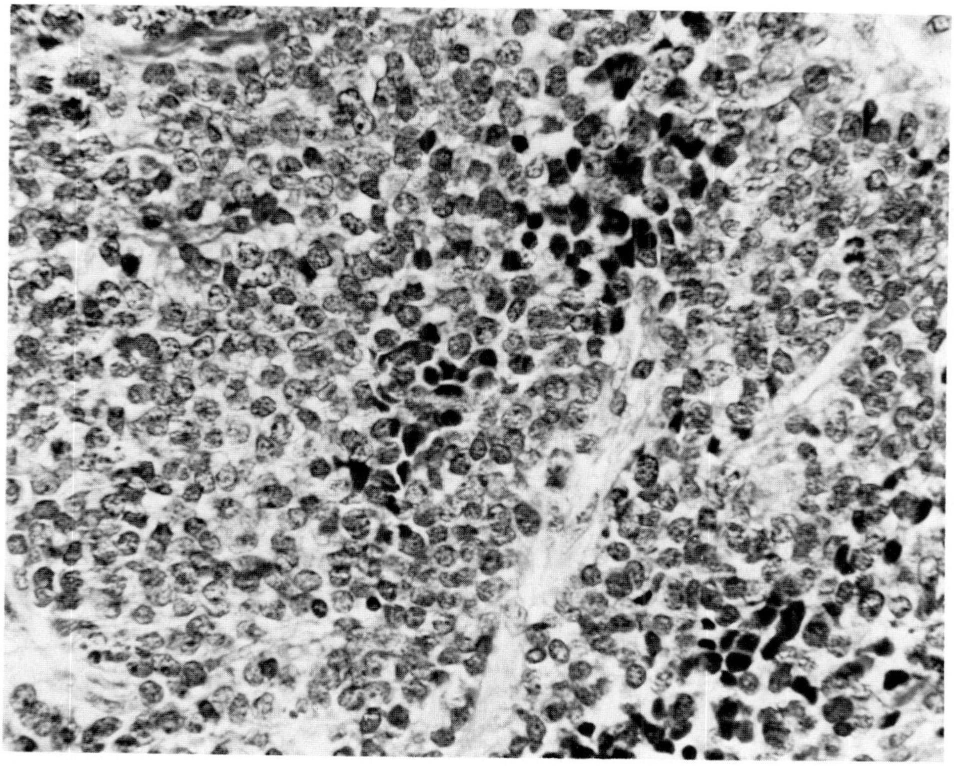

FIG. 2. Ewing's sarcoma. Sheets of tightly packed, small, round cells with scant pale cytoplasm and indistinct cell borders. Hematoxylin and eosin stain × 400.

pink-staining fibrillar background, and pseudorosettes. The cells also are PAS-negative. Anaplastic or oat cell carcinoma of the lung metastatic to bone can mimic Ewing's sarcoma to a certain degree but the different shape of the cells and the dense nuclei, together with the difference in age, roentgenograph appearance, and frequently positive sputum cytology should readily allow one to distinguish it from Ewing's sarcoma. Primary reticulum cell sarcoma can create a problem in differential diagnosis. However, the negative PAS stain for glycogen granules within the cytoplasm of the reticulum cells, together with the subtle but distinctly different appearance of the cell on hematoxylin and eosin stain, and the roentgenographic appearance should lead to separation of the two entities. Osteomyelitis may mimic Ewing's sarcoma from the standpoint of the roentgenographic appearance, but the heterogeneous mixture of various types of inflammatory cells make distinction fairly easy. Lesions of the histiocytosis group usually produce radiographic changes of a solid rather than a laminated periosteal reaction and careful assessment of the cellular features permits their diagnosis.

RETICULUM CELL SARCOMA (MALIGNANT LYMPHOMA) OF BONE

Primary reticulum cell sarcoma was described by Parker and Jackson in 1939.[6] They reported 17 cases and emphasized that the tumor occurred in all age groups in both cylindrical and flat bones, caused extensive destruction of bones, and was often associated with extensive soft tissue growth. They stated that reticulum cell sarcoma of bone had a much better prognosis than Ewing's sarcoma.

Reticulum cell sarcoma of bone is relatively rare and comprises no more than 3 to 5% of primary bone neoplasms. To date, approximately 200 cases have been reported in the literature. The neoplasm, which involves males more than females in a 2:1 ratio, appears to be evenly distributed throughout the life span and, although there is a widespread impression that the tumor involves primarily patients more than 40 years of age, such is actually not the case, for in Parker and Jackson's original series,[6] 70% of the patients were under 40 years of age, and 45% of the neoplasms occurred under 30 years of age. The skeletal distribution of the lesions is very much like that of Ewing's sarcoma. Approximately 50% of the cases involved the femur and tibia, 20% the bones of the upper extremity, and the remaining 30% involve flat bones of the trunk. Unlike patients with Ewing's sarcoma, those with primary reticulum cell sarcoma feel relatively well and frequently do not seek medical attention until a year or more after the initial manifestations. As Parker and Jackson[6] so aptly stated in their article, "in no other bone tumor is the apparent well-being of the patient and the size of the tumor so markedly contrasted". Patients with reticulum cell sarcoma frequently have large radiographic lesions and yet feel well in contrast to those with Ewing's sarcoma, who feel ill despite the small size of their lesions. Eventually the neoplasms are recognized by the appearance of pain, tumor mass, and impaired function of the part. Constitutional symptoms in the form of fever and leukocytosis are less marked than in patients with Ewing's sarcoma. Pathologic features are encountered in approximately 20% of patients, and the lesions located near the ends of the bones frequently cause a low grade inflammation of the adjacent synovium with joint effusion. Radiologically, reticulum cell sarcoma usually produces a destructive, lytic defect of bone with far less periosteal reaction than is encountered in Ewing's sarcoma. The neoplasms characteristically appear as coalescent lytic areas within the cancellous bone, and eventually they extend to the cortex and produce a focal sclerotic reaction, the result of a moderate degree of reactive new bone formation. Rather enigmatically, reticulum cell sarcoma will produce large soft tissue masses contiguous to an involved bone, while the bone itself exhibits very little destructive change.

Grossly the tumor is pinkish grey, solid and of fish-fresh consistency, as is typical of malignant lymphoma. Microscopically, the tumor cells are identical with the neoplastic reticulum cells identified in primary sarcoma of lymph nodes. Individual tumor cells exhibit indistinct boundaries and moderately acidophilic or basophilic cytoplasm with numerous irregular processes arising from cytoplasmic cell membranes that have been likened to pseudopods. The nuclei of the tumor cells are lobulated or reniform in shape, or frankly indented, and exhibit large, prominent, bright red nucleoli (Fig. 3). The cells of reticulum cell sarcoma vary considerably in size, and on occasion many giant cell forms are encountered which resemble Reed-Sternberg cells. Invariably, reticulum cell sarcoma exhibits a mixed cell population with numerous lymphocytes, and seldom is it comprised

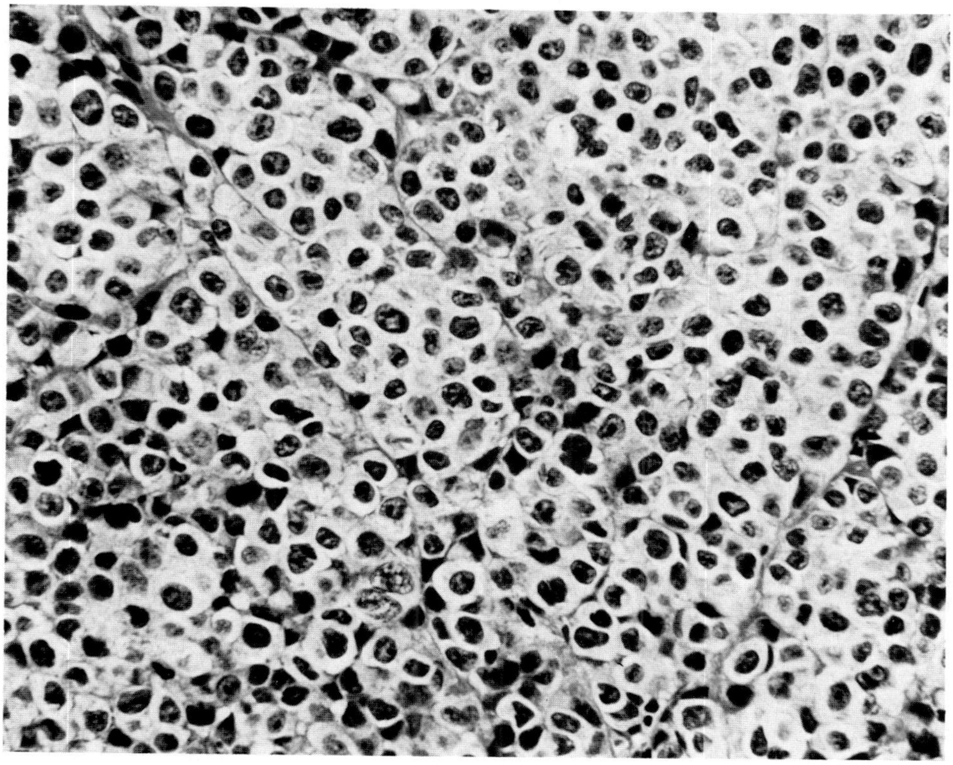

FIG. 3. Reticulum cell sarcoma (malignant lymphoma). Reticulum and histiocyte-appearing cells with moderately large and irregular nuclei. Some cells have prominent nucleoli. Hematoxylin and eosin stain × 400.

of a pure culture of reticulum cells. In addition to occasional foci of hemorrhage and necrosis, reticulum cell sarcoma frequently exhibits a fibrous tissue stroma, and on reticulum stain, fine reticular fibers are seen to envelop individual tumor cells, a feature not appreciated in Ewing's sarcoma. Also in contrast with Ewing's sarcoma, the PAS stain fails to reveal any significant number of cytoplasmic glycogen granules.

Metastases from reticulum cell sarcoma occur in approximately one-half of the cases and usually involve regional lymph nodes (22% of cases), but may also involve other bones (15% of cases) and lungs (10% of cases). The five-year survival rate approaches 50%.

PLASMA CELL MYELOMA

Plasma cell myeloma is a malignant neoplasm of plasma cells that involves the skeletal system in a solitary, multiple, or diffuse pattern. It is the most commonly encountered primary malignant neoplasm of bone except in patients under 30 years of age. Only rarely is it seen prior to 40 years of age. In most series, the disease is seen more frequently in males than females (3:2 ratio), but the sex difference is not significant. Infrequently the disease first manifests itself in extraosseous sites such as the oronasopharynx, gastrointestinal tract, spleen, and lymph nodes, but almost invariably extraosseous myleoma disseminates to other sites including the skeletal system. The disorder is characterized by the elaboration of excessive amounts of immunoglobulins of all five major classes that are indistinguishable biochemically and electrophoretically from normal globulins, and the total serum proteins are usually elevated from 5 to 15% in myelomatosis. In addition, light-chain subunits of the immunoglobulin fractions are also elaborated in the form of Bence Jones proteins. Only one specific type of immunoglobulin (or fragment thereof) is elaborated in any individual patient and remains constant throughout the course of the disease. Apparently, all of the neoplastic cells represent the clone of a single progenitor and these disorders are, therefore, referred to as monoclonal gammopathies. On extremely rare occasions, more than one type of immunoglobulin may be produced (polyclonal gammopathy). Although the etiology of the disorder, like that of most malignant neoplasms, is not known, recent studies with laboratory animals suggest that these neoplasms may be induced by a long-standing chronic inflammation.[7] Injections of foreign materials such as plastics and mineral oil intraperitoneally into a specific strain of mice has produced marked reactive reticuloendothelial cell proliferation followed by granuloma formation and subsequent neoplastic alteration. That the condition might represent a perverted end-stage immunologic response to chronic antigenic stimulation, however, is still speculative and not substantiated. Radiographically, multiple myeloma presents as punched-out lytic lesions of the skeleton with involvement in descending order of frequency of

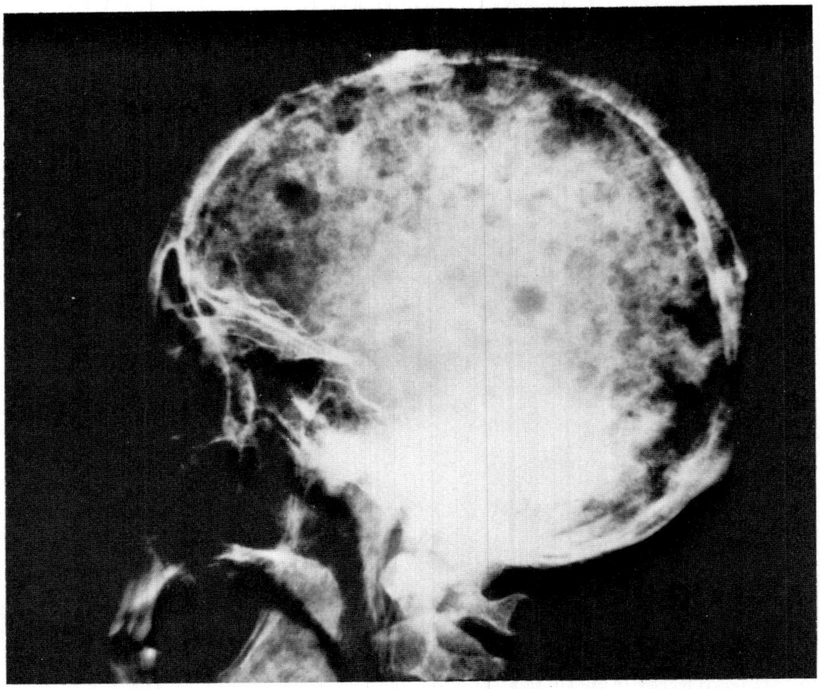

FIG. 4. Roentgenogram of plasmacytoma: multiple lytic lesions of the skull with no bone reaction.

the vertebrae, ribs, skull, pelvis, femur, clavicle, and scapula (Fig. 4). Flat bones are usually involved, and pain owing to vertebral fractures with pressure on nerve roots is a frequent symptom.

Grossly, the solitary as well as the diffuse lesions within the skeletal system present as reddish grey, gelatinous areas of tumefaction, while microscopically the neoplastic plasma cells are usually readily identified. On occasion, the plasma cells are rather poorly differentiated with both multinucleated and giant cell forms. Amyloid deposits throughout the body, usually of a primary distribution type, may be encountered. So-called "myeloma nephrosis" caused by obstructive tubular disease is also established as a feature of the disorder. Hematologic manifestations in the form of bleeding tendencies, sludging of blood, and anoxia owing to hyperviscosity are also well-known features. The differential diagnosis on histologic appraisal involves distinguishing plasma cell neoplasm from chronic inflammation. In an inflammatory process, the cellular infiltrate is usually of a mixed type and associated with an increased fibrous stroma and increased vascularity. The survival time following establishment of the diagnosis of multiple or diffuse myeloma is usually no more than 1 to 2 years, and death usually is the result of infection, anemia, or intercurrent renal failure, a reflection of myeloma nephrosis. Recent therapy with Cytoxan and other chemotherapeutic agents has promised increased survival rates, but at present the long-term prognosis for this malignant neoplasm is poor.

HODGKIN'S DISEASE OF BONE

Hodgkin's disease frequently involves the skeletal system as part of a generalized systemic involvement, but on rare occasions it may be discovered on biopsy of a radiographically detected lesion, and in such cases it is thought to be the initial process. The author has encountered five such cases in his material.

Hodgkin's disease of bone appears to be no different from that of soft tissue. The lesion is noted especially in young adults and histologically is identical to the disease of lymph nodes.

Like most of the round cell tumors, the radiographic findings are usually those of a lytic bone lesion with ill-defined borders and a varying degree of periosteal reaction. The prognosis for the disease varies according to the histologic type.

REFERENCES

1. Aegerter, E., and Kirkpatrick, J. A.: Orthopedic Diseases. 4th ed. Philadelphia, W. B. Saunders Co., 1975.
2. Dahlin, D. C.: Bone Tumors. 2nd ed. Springfield, Charles C. Thomas Publishers, 1967.
3. Edeiken, J., and Hodes, P. J.: Roentgen Diagnosis of Disease of Bone. 2nd ed., vol. 2. Baltimore, Williams & Wilkins Co., 1973.
4. Schajowicz, F.: Ewing's sarcoma and reticulum cell sarcoma of bone. *J. Bone Joint Sorg. 41A:* 349–356, 1959.
5. Friedman, B., and Gold, H.: Ultrastructure of Ewing's sarcoma of bone. *Cancer 22:* 307–322, 1968.
6. Parker, F., Jr., and Jackson, H., Jr.: Primary reticulum cell sarcoma of bone. *Surg. Gynec. Obstet. 68:* 45–53, 1939.
7. Potter, M.: A resume of the current status of the development of plasma cell tumors in mice. *Cancer Res. 28:* 1891–1896, 1968.

Index

Page references in *italic* type refer to illustrations.

Abscess
  paravertebral, associated with osteomyelitis, 45, 46
  subperiosteal, in adult osteomyelitis, 44
  tuberculous, differentiation from ankylosing spondylitis, 105
Achilles tendon
  clear cell sarcoma, 177
  rheumatoid arthritis, 136
Actinomyces israelii, actinomycosis, 55
Actinomycetes, maduromycosis, 56
Actinomycosis, 55–56
  characteristics, 55–56
  periostitis, 55
  sites, 55, 56, *56*
  with sulphur granules, 55, 56
Aerobacter, osteomyelitis, 40
Aging
  joints, 110–114
  systemic factor in determining osteoarthritis, 124
Alcoholism
  associated with aseptic necrosis, 62
  similarity to idiopathic aseptic necrosis, 83
Alkaline phosphatase
  in idiopathic osteoporosis, 29
  in osteomalacia, 29
American Rheumatism Association, 140
  rheumatoid arthritis diagnostic criteria, 131
Amianthoid degeneration, 112
Amyloidosis
  associated with ankylosing spondylitis, 140
  complicating primary osteomyelitis, 48
Anaplastic neoplasm, in sarcomatous transformation of fibrous dysplasia, 230
Anemia, sickle cell (*see* Sickle cell anemia)
Aneurysmal cyst (*see* Cyst)
Ankle
  extraarticular localized nodular synovitis, 168
  hemangioma, 172
  pigmented villonodular synovitis, 165
  Reiter's syndrome, 141
  rheumatoid arthritis, 131
  synovial chondromatosis, 160
  tenosynovitis, 259
  viral osteomyelitis, 50
Ankylosis
  and infant osteomyelitis, 42
  in hyperostotic spondylosis, 126
  in osteoarthritis of finger, 126
  in viral osteomyelitis, 50
  incidence, 126
Antibody
  anti-deoxyribonucleic acid, measurements of, 92
  antinuclear
    positive tests for, 89, 91
    relationship to renal disease, 91, 92
    staining pattern in scleroderma, 90
    test, 93
  anti-ribonucleoprotein, 93
  antistreptococcal, in rheumatic fever, 88–89
  distribution to sarcoma-associated antigen, 189
  fluorescence antinuclear test, 89–92
  positive antinuclear tests, associated with scleroderma, 89
  ribonucleoprotein, 90, 92, 93
Anti-deoxyribonucleic acid
  antibodies against, 92
  trypanosome in measurements of, 92
Anti-deoxyribonucleic acid binding (Farr technique), 90, 91
Anti-deoxyribonucleac acid test, 93
  and *Crithidia luciliae*, 92, 93
Antigen
  human skeletal and soft tissue sarcomas, 188
  multiple streptococcal, as test for rheumatic fever, 89
  sarcoma-associated, antibody distribution to, 189
Antigen HL-A W27
  associated with ankylosing spondylitis, 133
  histocompatibility
    and bowel disease, 133
    and juvenile chronic polyarthritis, 133
    and spondylitis, 133
    associated with ankylosing spondylitis, 140
    associated with psoriatic spondylitis, 141
    associated with Reiter's syndrome, 133
    associated with sacroiliitis, 133
  rheumatoid arthritis, 133
Antigen of human sarcoma
  common tumor-associated
    immunofluorescence, 188–189
    immunology, 188–192
Anti-ribonucleoprotein, antibodies against, 93
Aortitis
  ankylosing spondylitis, 140
  in Reiter's syndrome, 142
Arm
  epithelioid sarcoma, 176
  synovial sarcoma, 173
Arteritis,
  coronary, rheumatoid arthritis, 138
  renal, rheumatoid arthritis, 138
Arthralgia
  associated with mixed connective tissue disease, 92
  in enteric arthritis, 142

Arthritis
and variola osteomyelitis, *51*
associated with
gout, 98, 99, 101, 103, *104*
hemophilia, 98, 99, 101
psoriasis, 98, 99, *141*
Reiter's syndrome, 141
rheumatic disease, 88–97
rheumatism, 98–101, *102*, *103*
synovitis, 130
tuberculosis, 98, *101*, 103
bacterial, radiologic diagnosis, 98
clinical, 99–103
clinical approach, differentiation from radiologic approach, 98–99
degenerative
radiologic diagnosis, 99
similarity to stage VI of idiopathic aseptic necrosis, 73
differentiation from synovial sarcoma, 174
early rheumatoid, *109*
sites, 108, *109*
enteric, 142
associated with ankylosing spondylitis, 142
associated with arthralgia, 142
associated with intermittent migratory arthritis, 143
associated with migratory polyarthritis, 142
associated with regional ileitis, 143
associated with sarcoiliitis, 142
associated with spondylitis, 142, 143
colitis in, 142
differentiation from adult rheumatoid arthritis, 130
histology, 143–144
radiologic findings, 142, 144
ulcerative colitis in, 143
gouty, radiologic diagnosis, 99, 101, 103, *104*
hemophiliac
radiologic diagnosis, 98, 99, 101
site, 101
hypertrophic, associated with erosive osteoarthritis, 106
immunology, 88–97
inflammatory, 130
cartilage loss in, 130
etiology, 130
hyperemia in, 130
morphologic changes, 130
synovial, 130
intermittent migratory
associated with enteric arthritis, 143
associated with Whipple's disease, 143
juvenile rheumatoid, 138–139
and dermatitis, 139
chronic, iridocyclitis in, 139
histology, 139
differentiation from adult rheumatoid arthritis, 130
differentiation from rheumatoid arthritis, 133
hepatosplenomegaly in, 139
keratopathy in, 139
lymphadenopathy in, 139
pericarditis in, 139
site, 139
termed Still's disease, 139
mono-articular, 138
neuropathic, and ankylosing spondylitis, 105
post-*Shigella*, and HL-A W27, 133
psoriatic, *141*
and histocompatibility antigen HL-A W27, 133
and rheumatoid arthritis, 140–141
differentiation from adult rheumatoid arthritis, 130
differentiation from ankylosing spondylitis, 140
differentiation from rheumatoid arthritis, 133
differentiation from spondylitis in Reiter's syndrome, 141
HL-A W27 in, 141
"pencil in cup" deformity, *141*
radiologic diagnosis, 98, 99
sites, *141*
psoriatic and rheumatoid, sites, 140
pyogenic, 99
etiology, 99, 100
radiologic approach, differentiation from clinical approach, 98–99
radiologic findings, 103–108
reactive
and genitourinary infections, 133
and intestinal infections, 133
and rheumatic fever, 133
and *Salmonella*, 133
and *Shigella*, 133
and streptococcal infection, 133
and *Yersinia*, 133
rheumatoid, 131–138
adult, differentiation from ankylosing spondylitis, 130
adult, differentiation from Reiter's syndrome, 130
adult, differentiation from related arthritides, 130
advanced, radiologic diagnosis, 98, 100, 101
advanced, site, 100
and ischemia, 138
and multinucleated histiocytic giant cell, 138
and Newcastle disease viruses, 132
and psoriatic arthritis, 140–141
and pulmonary parenchyma, 136
and Reiter's syndrome, 141–142
and related arthritides, 130–145
and renal arteritis, 138
and synovial multinucleated giant cell, 134
antigen HL-A W27, 133
associated with juvenile chronic polyarthritis, 139
associated with *Mycoplasma*, 131
associated with secondary osteoarthritis, 122, 134

associated with vasculitis, 138
Baker's cyst, 138
characteristics, 131, 132, 134, 136
coronary arteritis, 138
diagnosis, 131
differentiation from ankylosing spondylitis, 133, 140
differentiation from "erosive" osteoarthritis, 126
differentiation from gout, 136
differentiation from gouty synovitis, 133
differentiation from juvenile rheumatoid arthritis, 133
differentiation from pigmented villonodular synovitis, 164
differentiation from psoriatic arthritis, 133
differentiation from Reiter's syndrome, 133, 142
differentiation from systemic lupus erythematosus, 90, 93, 133, 142
etiology and pathogenesis, 131–132
fibrosarcoma mistaken for, 101
genetic factors, 133
histology, 136
immune abnormality in patients, 95
inflammatory pannus in, 134
lymphocytes T and B in, 132
micrology, 136–138
mistaken for thrombophlebitis, 101
more than one disease?, 95
nodules, 136, 138, *138*
pathologic change, 133, 134, *134–138*, 136, 138
pathologic change in edema of the sublining layer of synovium, 133
pathologic change in hyperemia of sublining layer of synovium, 133
pathologic change in hyperplasia of lining cells of synovium, 133
pathologic change in hypertrophic villous synovitis, 133
patients with positive antinuclear antibody test, 89
phagocytosis in, 132
radiologic diagnosis, 98, 99, *102*, *103*, 108
radiologic findings, 131
rheumatoid factor produced in, 132
sites, 100, 131, *134*, *136*, 136–138
"variants," genetic factors in, 133
rubella virus of rheumatic synovial cells in, 132
septic, in childhood osteomyelitis, 44
tuberculous, 100
radiologic diagnosis, 98, *101*, 103
yersinia-reactive, and HL-A W27, 133
Arthropathy
neurotrophic
associated with arthritis, 98, 103
characteristics, 103
radiologic diagnosis, 98, 103
Arthroplasty, hip, 110
Articular processes, chondrification, 7–8
Articular synovial chondromatosis (*see* chondromatosis)
Articular zones, epiphysis, 2
Aseptic necrosis (*see* necrosis)
Atrophy, disuse, 25

Bacterial infection (*see* name of disease or site)
Bacteriodes, osteomyelitis, 40
Baker's cyst, rheumatoid arthritis, 138
Balanitis, circinate, associated with Reiter's disease, 141
Basophilic cytoplasm, bone structure, 18
Basophilic ribosomes, and endoplasmic reticulum, 18
Blastomyces dermatidis, blastomycosis, 54
Bedsonia viruses, etiology of Reiter's syndrome, 142
Blastema, embryology, 1, 2, 9
Blastomycosis, 54
differentiation from
coccidioidomycosis, 54
paracoccidioidomycosis, 54
sites, 54
Blennorrhagicum, keratodermia, associated with Reiter's syndrome, 141
Bone collar, primary, embryology, 5
Bone matrix
neurovascular canal, 22
osteoblasts, 18
osteomalacia, 29
Bone structure, 16–24
canal, 22–23
capillaries, 22–23
Bone tissue
osteoblast, 18
osteoclast, 18
osteocyte, 18
primary, 20
Bowel disease, and histocompatibility antigen HL-A W27, 133
Brachium, neuralgia of, and osteoarthritis, 122
Brain
and staging system in human embryo, 7
embryology, 2
Brodie's abscess, and primary osteomyelitis, 47
Brown tumor
in osteomalacia, 35
of hyperparathyroidism, 225, 257 260–263, *262*, 266
differentiation from giant cell granuloma, 225
differentiation from giant cell reaction, 257
differentiation from giant cell reparative granuloma, 266
etiology, 261
incidence, 260
site, 261, 262
Brucella abortus, osteomyelitis, 49
Brucella melitensis, ostemyelitis, 49
Brucella suis, osteomyelitis, 49
Brucella osteomyelitis, 49
etiology, 49
histology, 49

Brucella osteomyelitis—*continued*
  Langhans' giant cells in, 49
  similarity to tuberculosis, 49
  sites, 49
Brucellosis, 49
Buccal mucosa, ulcerations, associated with Reiter's syndrome, 141
Bud
  limb, embryology, 9
  periosteal, replaces cartilage, 5
  upper limb, apical ectodermal ridge, 13
Burnett's syndrome, associated with tumoral calcinosis, 293

Café-au-lait spots, fibrous dysplasia, 209
Caffey's disease, similarity to viral osteomyelitis, 50
Caisson disease, 82
  associated with aseptic necrosis, 62
  similarity to idiopathic aseptic necrosis, 82
  site, 82
Calcaneus, embryology, 2
Calcar, in osteoarthritis, 114
Calcification, 1
  chondroblastoma, 205
  chondrosarcoma, 205
  lesional, differentiation from ossification, 205–208
  matrix, 6, 19
Calcinosis
  soft somatic tissues and tumoral
    primary giant cell tumor of, histology, 292–293
  tumoral
    associated with Brunett's syndrome, 293
    associated with secondary hyperparathyroidism, 293
    differentiation from gouty tophus, 293
    etiology, 293
Calcium
  in disuse osteoporosis, 25
  in idiopathic osteoporosis, 29
  in osteomalacia, 29, 32
"Calcium front," in osteomalacia, 32
Calcium phosphate, bone structure, 17
Calf, rheumatoid arthritis, 138
Calvaria
  benign giant cell tumor arising in Paget's disease, 250
  embryology, 1
  fibrous dysplasia, 209, 211, *215*, 216, *216*
  Paget's disease, 250
Calvarium (*see* calvaria)
Canaliculi, bone structure, 19
Cancellous bone, idiopathic osteoporosis, 25, *26*, 27, 29
Cancer
  metastatic
    destruction of bone, 199
    differentiation from eosinophilic granuloma, 279
Carcinoma
  metastatic, differentiation from epithelioid sarcoma, 176
  metastatic anaplastic, differentiation from Ewing's sarcoma, 314, 315
  site, 187
Carnegie system, stages of human embryo, 1, 7
Carpus
  coccidioidomycosis, 52
  embryology, 2
  idiopathic aseptic necrosis, 61
  site of synovial chondromatosis, 160
Carpal lunate, idiopathic aseptic necrosis, 61
Carpal synovium, coccidioidal granulomas in, *53*
Cartilage
  adult articular, chondrocytes in, 124
  articular
    embryology, 2
    growth zones, 2
  calcification, 2
  destruction, 5
  developmental phases, *4*
    embryology, 1, 5
  hyaline
    benign neoplasms of, differentiated from well-differentiated sarcoma, 300
    rings, 2
    tumorous masses, 300
    tumorous masses in larynx, 300
    well differentiated sarcoma differentiated from benign neoplasm of, 300
  loss of, in inflammatory arthritis, 130
  malignant, differentiation from chondroblastic osteosarcoma, 301
  metacarpal, 13–14
  metatarsal, 13
  ossification (*see* Ossification, endochondral)
  osteoarthritis, 110
  phalanges, 14
  "secondary," 2
    sites, 2
  sites, 14
  surface
    degeneration, 114, 116
    necrobiotic chondrocyte in degeneration of, 114
Cartilage cells, *5*
  hypertrophied, 5
    appearance, 6
  vacuolization, 3
Cartilaginous model
  replaced, 2
Cartilaginous rings
  hyaline, of vertebral centra, 2
Cartilaginous tumor
  and chondrosarcoma, 307, 310, 311
  dedifferentiated, 303
    associated with fibrosarcoma, 303
    associated with osteosarcoma, 303
    etiology, 303
    radiologic findings, 303

therapy, 303
dedifferentiation into anaplastic sarcoma, 303
dedifferentiation into spindle cell sarcoma, 303
of soft tissue, 305
differentiation from chondrosarcoma, 305, *305*
etiology, 305
incidence, 305
recurrence, 305
site, 305
sites, 305
Cavitation, articulations, 10
Cell aging
in osteoarthritis, 112–116
Cementoblastoma
diagnosis, 221
differentiation from cementifying fibroma, 221
differentiation from osteoblastoma, 222
differentiation from osteoid osteoma, 222
differentiation from periapical cemental dysplasia, 221
mandible, *223*
pathology, 222
radiology, 222
Cementoma, 230
differentiation from unicameral cyst, 286
sites, 227, 230, 286
Cementum, differentiation from osteoid, 218
Centra
chondrification, 7–8
embryology, 7
Cervix, carcinoma of, 187
Cherubism, 225
site, 225
Chondrific center
embryology, 10
site, 10, 13
Chondrification, 1
articular processes, 7–8
sites, 7, 8, 11, 13
stages, *13*
Chondroblastoma, 287
benign
differentiation from chondromyxoid fibroma of bone, 287–289
differentiation from pigmented villonodular synovitis, 259, 260
histologic characteristics, 252, 253
sites, 254, 255
differentiated from osteogenic sarcoma, 255
with sarcomatous degeneration, 255
Chondrocranium, embryology, 9
Chondrocyte, necrobiotic, in degeneration of cartilage surface, 114
Chondroid chordoma, 309
Chondroma
differentiation from spheno-occipital chordoma, 309
periosteal, 309, *309*, 310
Chondroblastoma
benign, 251–253, *251*, *252*
differential diagnosis, 237
differentiation from benign giant cell tumor, 251
differentiation from chondromyxoid fibroma of bone, 289
differentiation from giant cell tumor, 255
differentiation from pigmented villonodular synovitis, 259, 260
incidence, 251
lack of malignant change, 255
multinucleated giant cell in, 252
of major long bone in nonepiphyseal location, 254
of major long bone, sites, 254, 255
sarcomatous transformation of, 255
sites, 251, 254, 255
calcification, 205
differentiation from clear cell chondrosarcoma, 310
malignant, 255
metastasis in, 255
osteogenic sarcoma in, 255
sarcomatous degeneration in, diagnosed as irradiation-induced osteogenic sarcomas, 255
sites, 198, 202
Chondrocalcinosis
and degenerative joint disease in osteoarthritis, 125
radiologic diagnosis, 99
Chondrocytes
and osteoarthritis, 124
articular, in osteoarthritis, 112–113
in retardation of degradation from osteoarthritis, 124
replication
in adult articular cartilage, 124
osteoarthritis, 113
Chondroma
formed in synovial chondrosarcoma, 179
juxtacortical, 202
periosteal, 309–310
Chondromalacia
differentiation from osteoarthritic fibrillation, 117
of patella, 117, 124
Chondromalacia patellae
osteotomy for, 124
Chondromatosis
articular synovial, 305–307
appearance of malignancy, 307
diagnosis, 307
sites, 305–307
characteristics, 159–160
differentiation from tenosynovial osteochondroma, 160
synovial, 159–162, *307*
cytology, 161
diagnosis, *159*
etiology, 160
radiology, 160
sites, 160, *307*
therapy, 162

Chondromatosis—*continued*
  synovial, 159-162, *307*
    tumorous masses of hyaline cartilage in, 300
Chondrosarcoma, 300–301
  and cartilaginous tumor, 307
  association with osteochondroma, 301
  clear cell, *310*, 310
    cytology, 310
    differentiation from chonodroblastoma, 310
    differentiation from osteoblastoma, 310
  cytology, 300, 301
  diagnosis, 300
  differentiation between lesional calcification and ossification, 205
  differentiation
    from cartilaginous tumors of larynx, 307
    from cartilaginous tumors of soft tissues of foot, 305, *305*
    from cartilaginous tumors of soft tissues of hands, 305, *305*
    from chondromyxoid fibroma, 289
    from spheno-occipital chordoma, 309
  etiology, 230
  from sarcomatous transformation of fibrous dysplasia, 230
  importance of localization of cartilaginous tumors, 310–311
  in Paget's disease, 152
  incidence, 198, 300, 303
  mesenchymal, 301–303, *302*
    associated with hemangiopericytoma, 311
    cytology, 301
    differentiation from Ewing's sarcoma, 301
    etiology, 301
    therapy, 301, 303
  metastasis of, 309
  ossification, 205
  sites, *231*, 300, 303, *304*, 305, *305*
  synovial, 157, 179–181, *180*
    characterization, 179, 181
    chondroma formed in, 179
    etiology, 180
    histology, 181
    incidence, 180
    osteochondroma formed in, 179
    primary malignant tumor from synovium, 173
    prognosis, 181
    sites, 180
    therapy, 180, 300, 301, 303
  variants, 300–311
Chordoma
  chondroid, 309
    clinical behavior, 309
  sacrum, 199
  spheno-occipital, 309
    differentiation from chondroma, 309
    differentiation from chondrosarcoma, 309
Cisterna, bone structure, 18
Clavicle
  brown tumor of hyperparathyroidism, 262
  embryology, 1, 2
  "secondary" cartilage in, 2
Clear cell sarcoma (*see* Sarcoma)
Cleidocranial dysostosis (*see* Dysostosis)
Clone, osteoarthritis, 113
Coccidioidal granuloma, *53*
  in carpal synovium, *53*
  in os pisiforme, *53*
Coccidioidomycosis, 52–54
  characteristics, 52
  incidence, 54
  long bones, 52
  lytic foci, 54
  of os pisiforme, *52*
  of os triquetrum, *52*
  similarity to blastomycosis, 54
  sites, 52, 54
Codman triangle
  bone destruction, 199, *200*
  in osteosarcoma, *205*
Codman tumor, 251–253
Codman's angle
  associated with osteosarcoma with benign multinucleated giant cells, 268
  diagnosis, 271
Colitis
  in enteric arthritis, 142
  ulcerative
    differentiation from ankylosing spondylitis, 140
    enteric arthritis, 143
Collagen, bone structure, 16, 20
Collagen fibril, bone structure, 16, *17*, 22
Collagen "unmasking," sites, 112
Collagenous fiber, and trabecula, 5
Condensations
  mesenchyme, 1
Conjunctivitis
  a component of Reiter's syndrome, 141
Connective tissue (*see* Mixed connective tissue disease)
Coronary arteritis, rheumatoid arthritis, 138
Cortical bone
  disuse osteoporosis, 25
  idiopathic osteoporosis, *28*
Cortical defect (*see* Fibrous cortical defect)
Cortico-steroid therapy, associated with aseptic necrosis, 62
Costochondral juntions, salmonella osteomyelitis, 48
Coxa vara, osteoarthritis, 122
Cranial skeletal system, extragnathic, fibrous dysplasia, 226–227
Cranial vault
  coccidioidomycosis, 52
  phycomycosis, 54
Craniofacial bones
  fibrous dysplasia, 210–220, *214–217*, 226
  polyostotic fibrous dysplasia, 232
Crithidia luciliae, and anti-deoxyribonucleic acid test, 92, 93
Crural elements, embryology, 11

Cryptococcosis, 54
associated with Hodgkin's disease, 54
associated with lymphoma, 54
Cylindrical bones
Ewing's sarcoma, 312, *314*
reticulum cell sarcoma, 316
Cyst
aneurysmal, 279–282, *282*, *283*
characteristics, 279–281
differential diagnosis, 237
differentiation from fibro-osseous lesions of periodontal membrane, 210
differentiation from fibrous dysplasia, 253
differentiation from giant cell reaction, 257
differentiation from giant cell reparative granuloma, 253
differentiation from giant cell tumor, 253
differentiation from osteosarcoma with benign multinucleated giant cells, 269
differentiation from unicameral bone cyst, 285, 286
sites, 199, 279, *281*, *282*
ganglion, wrist, 171
ganglion and synovial, 171–172
characteristics, 171
pathology, 171
popliteal, synovial cyst, 171
rheumatoid, site of rheumatoid arthritis, 101
sites, 198
subchondral (*see* Ganglion cyst)
synovial, histology, 171–172
unicameral, 282–287, *284*
associated with multinucleated giant cell, 285
characteristics, 282–285
diagnosis, 287
differentiation from aneurysmal bone cyst, 285, 286
differentiation from cementoma of long bones, 286
recurrence rates, 284
sites, 282
Cystic cavities, coccidioidomycosis, 54
Cytoplasm
basophilic
bone structure, 18
staining, 18
endoplasmic reticulum, bone structure, 18
intercellular matrix, 3
ribosomes, 20
Cytoplasmic folds, active osteoclast, 20
Cytotoxic tests
differentiation between rheumatoid and nonrheumatoid lymphocytes, 95
differentiation between rheumatoid and nonrheumatoid synovial cells, 95

Deossification, periarticular, site, 103
Deoxyribonucleic acid, antibodies to, 90
Deoxyribonucleoprotein, antibodies to, 90
Deposition, matrix, 1
Dermatitis
hyperkeratotic, associated with Reiter's syndrome, 141
in juvenile rheumatoid arthritis, 139
Dermatomyositis, differentiation from mixed connective tissue disease, 92
Destruction of bone
geographic, 199, 202–205
Osteosarcoma, *202*
Diabetes
associated with ankylosing spondylosis, 122
associated with phycomycosis, 54
Diaphysis
adult osteomyelitis, 44
and typhoid salmonella osteomyelitis, 48
site of salmonella osteomyelitis, 49
Disc, intervertebral, and vertebral osteomyelitis, 45
Dura mater, site of rheumatoid arthritis, 136
Dysostosis, cleidocranial, 2
Dysphagia, associated with mixed connective tissue disease, 92
Dysplasia
congenital, cause of osteoarthritis of hip, 122
craniofacial fibrous, sites, 211
epiphyseal, possible etiologic agent for osteoarthritis, 125
fibrous, 226–230
anaplastic neoplasm in, 230
and café-au-lait spots, 209
and fibro-osseous lesion, 209–220
and Graves' disease, 209
and myositis ossificans progressiva, 209
as monostotic lesion, 227
associated with hyperparathyroidism, 210
associated with precocious puberty, 210
characteristics, 209, 226
diagnosis, 216, 218–220
diagnosis as monostotic lesion, 227
differentiation between recurrent and nonrecurrent tumor, 226
differentiation from aneurysmal bone cyst, 253
differentiation from cementifying fibroma, 210
differentiation from desmoplastic fibroma, 230
differentiation from fibro-osseous lesion, 232
differentiation from fibro-osseous lesion of periodontal membrane, 210
differentiation from fibrosarcoma, 230
differentiation from mixed fibro-osseous lesions, 225
differentiation from nonosteogenic fibroma, 282
differentiation from ossifying fibroma, 210, 222, 230
differentiation from other fibro-osseous lesions, 232
differentiation from periapical cemental dysplasia, 209–210
differentiated from Von Recklinghausen's

Dysplasia—*continued*
fibrous, 226–230
neurofibromatosis, 210
etiology, 209–210
fibro-osseous lesion of bone, 209–220
fibro-osseous lesions of, differentiation from fibro-osseous lesions of periodontal membrane, 210
fibrosarcoma developed in, 209
histology, 216, 228
hyperostosis in, 216
incidence, 211, 218
incidence as monostotic lesion, 227
irradiation therapy as cause of sarcoma in, 226
malignant potential, 225–226
radiologic findings, 211
sarcomatous transformation of, 230
sarcomatous transformation of, prognosis, 230
sarcomatous transformation of, sites, 230
sites, 209, 210–220, *212–217*, 226, 227, *228*, 230, 232
sphenoid lesion in, 216
therapy, 226
transformation into chondrosarcoma, 230
transformation into osteosarcoma, 230
monostotic fibrous, sites, 232
overt, incidence, 122
periapical cemental
differentiation from cementoblastoma, 221
differentiation from fibrous dysplasia, 221
polyostitic fibrous, 209, 227, *229*, 232
characteristics, 232
"Shepherd's crook" with, *229*
sites, 227, 232
precocious puberty, 209

Eburnation, with arthritis, 130
Ectoderm, apical, embryology, 9
Ectodermal ridge, apical, upper limb bud, 13
Edema, in childhood osteomyelitis, 43
Elbow
hemangioma, 172
pigmented villonodular synovitis, 165
rheumatoid arthritis, 131
synovial chondromatosis, 160
synovial sarcoma, 173
viral osteomyelitis, 50
Embryo, stages, 1
Embryology, 1–15
Embryopathy, thalidomide, 11
Enchondroma, *206*
differentiation between lesional calcification and ossification, 205
Endoplasm
reticulum, 20
Endoplasmic reticulum, and basophilic ribosomes, 18
Epiphyseal center, embryology, 10
Epiphyseal palate, closure, in aseptic necrosis, 61
Epiphysial regions, endochondral ossification, 6
Epiphysis
and adult osteomyelitis, 44
and childhood osteomyelitis, 43
and infantile osteomyelitis, 42
and salmonella osteomyelitis, 49
articular zones, 2
embryology, 2
ossification, 6
Epithelioid cells
fungal osteomyelitis, 52
Epithelioid sarcoma (*see* Sarcoma)
Erythematosus
systemic lupus
deficiency of thymosin in, 95
differentiated from rheumatoid arthritis, 90, 93, 133, 142
differentiation from scleroderma, 90
joint involvement, differentiation from adult rheumatoid arthritis, 130
T cell in, 95, 132
Escherichia coli, bacteriology of osteomyelitis, 40
Estrogens, idiopathic osteoporosis, 29
Ethmoid bone, craniofacial fibrous dysplasia, 211
Ewing's sarcoma, *204*, 312–315, *315*
bone destruction, etiology of human skeletal and soft tissue sarcomas, 199
cytology, 313
diagnosis, 313
differentiation from eosinophilic granuloma, 279
differentiation from mesenchymal chondrosarcoma, 301
differentiation from metastatic anaplastic carcinoma, 314, 315
differentiation from metastatic neuroblastoma, 314, 315
differentiation from osteomyelitis, 313–315
differentiation from primary reticulum cell sarcoma, 313
differentiation from pyogenic osteomyelitis, 313
differentiation from reticulum cell sarcoma, 314–317
etiology, 312
gross characteristics, 313
incidence, 312
radiology, 313, *314*
sites, 312, *314*
small round cell tumors of bone, 312
types of reactive bone formation, 313
Ewing's tumor, long bones, 198
Extragnathic and long bones, fibro-osseous lesions, 226–230
Extragnathic sites
fibro-osseous lesion, 226–230

Facial bones
benign giant cell tumor arising in Paget's disease, 249, 250
brown tumor of hyperparathyroidism, 262
Coccidioidomycosis, 52
Paget's disease, 250
Fanconi's disease, 32
Farr technique

(anti-deoxyribonucleic acid binding), 90, 91
in measurements of anti-deoxyribonucleic acid, 92
Femoral head
aseptic necrosis, 118, 119
associated with osteoarthritis, 117
associated with synovial retinaculum, 119
Gaucher's disease, 82
in idiopathic aseptic necrosis, 61–87, *66–68*, *70*, *72*
intraosseous villonodular synovitis, 259
ischemia, 62
osteoarthritis, 114, *115*, 116, *118*
osteophytes on, 123
Femoral head cartilage, collagen "unmasking" in aging, 112
Femoral neck
benign chondroblastoma, 254, 255
fractures, and osteoarthritis, 117
osteophyte, 121
Femur
and salmonella osteomyelitis, 48
aneurysmal bone cyst, 279, *281*
benign chondroblastoma, 254, 255
benign giant cell tumor, *245*, *246*
bone cyst, 198
cementoma, 230
childhood osteomyelitis, 42
embryology, 2, 11
endochondral ossification, 2
Ewing's sarcoma, 312
fibrous dysplasia, 209, 230
fibrous dysplasia as monostotic lesion, 227
giant cell tumor, 198
gouty tophus, *290*
idiopathic osteoporosis, 29
osteomalacia, 29, *31*, 33, 34
osteomyelitis, *46*
Paget's disease, 148, *149–153*, 154
parosteal osteosarcoma, 198
polyostotic fibrous dysplasia, 227
reticulum cell sarcoma, 316
sarcomatous transformation of fibrous dysplasia, 230
"Shepherd's crook," *229*
telangiectatic osteosarcoma, 271
unicameral bone cyst, 282
Fiber (*see* Collagenous fiber)
Fibril, bone formation, 16
Fibrillation, relationship to osteoarthritis, 110, 111
Fibrocartilage, bone structure, *18*
Fibroma
ameloblastic, characteristics, 225
cementifying, 220–224, 226
characteristics, 232
differentiation from cementoblastoma, 221
differentiation from fibrous dysplasia, 210
differentiation from focal chronic osteomyelitis, 220
differentiation from ossifying fibroma, 220–221
recurrence in children, 210
site, 210, 220, 226
cemento-ossifying
diagnosis, 232
differentiation from fibro-osseous lesion, 232
central, 225
differentiation from desmoplastic fibroma, 225
incidence, 225
radiology, 225
site, 225
chondromyxoid, *203*, *286–288*, 287–289
associated with benign multinucleated giant cell, 289
calcification, 205–208
differentiation from benign chondroblastoma, 287, 289
differentiation from chondrosarcoma, 289
histology and gross characteristics, 289
incidence, 287–288
radiological findings, 288, 289
sites, 288
desmoplastic
destruction of bone, 199
differentiation from central fibroma, 225
differentiation from fibro-osseous lesion, 210, 218, 219
differentiation from fibrous dysplasia, 230
nonossifying, 272–276
differential diagnosis, 237
sites, 198
nonosteogenic, 272–276
differentiation from fibrous dysplasia, 282
ossifying, *203*, 220–224, 230
differentiation from cementifying fibroma, 220–222
differentiation from fibromatosis, 222, 224
differentiation from fibrous dysplasia, 210, 222, 230
differentiation from focal chronic osteomyelitis, 220
differentiation from osteoblastoma, 226
differentiation from osteosarcoma, 224
sites, *203*, 220, 222, 226, 227, 230
ossifying and cementifying, diagnosis, 220
Fibromatosis
differentiation from fibro-osseous lesion, 218
differentiation from ossifying fibroma, 222, 224
Fibro-osseous lesion (*see* Lesion)
Fibrosarcoma, 247
associated with dedifferentiated cartilaginous tumor, 303
developed in fibrous dysplasia, 209
differentiation from fibrous dysplasia, 230
from metastasis of malignant giant cell tumor, 247
in benign giant cell tumor, *247*
in Paget's disease, 152
incidence by age, 198
mistaken for rheumatoid arthritis, 101
Fibrosis

Fibrosis—*continued*
in plasma cell osteomyelitis, 48
in viral osteomyelitis, 50
reactive, differentiation from fibro-osseous lesions, 219
Fibrous cortical defect, 272–276
characteristics, 272
differentiation from giant cell reaction, 257
incidence, 275
metaphyseal, 272–276
site, 272, *272–274*, 273
therapy, 275–276, *275*
Fibrous defect
metaphyseal, 272–276, *276*
Fibrous dysplasia (*see* Dysplasia)
Fibrous neoplasms
jaw masses resembling
differentiation from odontogenic myxoma, 225
Fibula
associated with teratogen, 11
chondrification, 11
fibrous dysplasia, 209
ossification, 11
polyostotic fibrous dysplasia, 227
unicameral bone cyst, 282
Finger
ankylosis occurring in osteoarthritis of, 126
coronal section, *6*, *7*
epithelioid sarcoma, 176
extraarticular localized nodular synovitis, 168, 170
osteoarthritis, 121, 126
sagittal section, *4*
synovial chondromatosis, 160
Finger phalanges
giant cell reaction, 257
Fistula
associated with actinomycosis, 56
fungal osteomyelitis, 51
in adult osteomyelitis, 44
in primary osteomyelitis, 47
Fistula-carcinoma
complication of primary osteomyelitis, 48
Flat bones
Ewing's sarcoma, 312
reticulum cell sarcoma, 316
unicameral bone cyst, 282
Foam cells
extraarticular localized nodular synovitis, 168
in pigmented villonodular synovitis, 162
Foot
blastomycosis, 54
cartilaginous tumors of soft tissues, 305
differentiation from chondrosarcoma, 305, *305*
etiology, 305
incidence, 305
recurrence, 305
chondrific center, 10, *13*
chondrosarcoma
incidence, 303
therapy, 303
chondrosarcoma of skeleton of, 303, 305
coccidioidomycosis, 52
embryology, 10
extraarticular localized nodular synovitis, 168
giant cell reaction, 255–258
gouty tophus of epiphyseal end of long tubular bone, 291
histoplasmosis, 54
idiopathic osteoporosis, *26*
maduromycosis, 56
periarticular deossification, 103
pigmented villonodular synovitis, 165
Reiter's syndrome, 141
rheumatoid arthritis, 131
salmonella osteomelitis, 49
sporotrichosis, 55
synovial sarcoma, 173
tenosynovitis, 259
viral osteomyelitis, 50
Foot-plate
embryology, 11
Fracture
associated with Paget's disease, 151
cause of osteoarthritis, 124
femoral neck, 117
in idiopathic aseptic necrosis caused by trauma, 75–77, 79
metacarpal in idiopathic osteoporosis, 29
pathologic
in adult osteomyelitis, 44
in stage III of idiopathic aseptic necrosis, 69
site of traumatic aseptic necrosis, 83
sites, *31*, 37, 117
subchondral
cause of necrosis, 116
onset in idiopathic aseptic necrosis, 84
Fracture callus
differentiation from osteomalacia, 32
Freiberg's disease
idiopathic aseptic necrosis, 61
Frontal bone
craniofacial fibrous dysplasia, 211
embryology, 2

Gammopathies
monoclonal, associated with plasma cell myeloma, 318
polyclonal, associated with plasma cell myeloma, 318
Ganglia, similarity to subchondral pseudocysts, 119
Gangrene, differentiation from osteomyelitis, 40
Garré, sclerosing osteomyelitis of, 47
Gastrectomy, in osteomalacia, 29
Gastrocnemius muscle, site of rheumatoid arthritis, 100
Gastrointestinal tract, plasma cell myeloma, 318
Gaucher cell, in Gaucher's disease, 83
Gaucher's disease
associated with aseptic necrosis, 62

destruction of bone, 199
similarity to idiopathic aseptic necrosis, 82–83
sites, 82
Genes
contributing factor in degenerative joint disease, 125
factor determining osteoarthritis, 124
Genitourinary infections
and reactive arthritis, 133
Giant cell
benign multinucleated, *252*
associated with chondromyxoid fibroma of bone, 289
associated with solitary and multifocal eosinophilic granuloma of bone, 279
differential diagnosis, 237
differentiation from giant cell lesion of bone, 238
differentiation from stroma (tumor) cells, 241
in osteosarcoma, *267*, 268–271, *269*
in extraarticular localized nodular synovitis, 168
in fungal osteomyelitis, 52
multinucleated
and pigmented villonodular synovitis, 162
associated with unicameral bone cyst, 285
in benign chondroblastoma, 252
multinucleated histiocytic, and rheumatoid arthritis, 138
soft tissue malignant, tumor, 179
synovial multinucleated, and rheumatoid arthritis, 134
Giant cell granuloma, 225
differentiation from "brown tumor" of hyperparathyroidism, 225
differentiation from fibro-osseous lesion, 219
differentiated from fibro-osseous lesion of periodontal membrane, 210
Giant cell lesion
differential diagnosis, 236–299
radiologic investigation, 236
differentiation from benign giant cell tumor, 237
differentiation from benign multinucleated giant cell, 238
histochemistry, 237
site, 238
ultrastructure, 237
Giant cell reaction, *257*, *258*
differentiation from aneurysmal cyst, 257
differentiation from brown tumor of hyperparathyroidism, 257
differentiation from fibrous cortical defect, 257
differentiation from giant cell tumor, 257, 258
site, 255–258, *256*
Giant cell reparative granuloma of jaw
differential diagnosis, 237
Giant cell tumor
arising in Paget's disease, prognosis, 250
benign, *242–245*
diagnosis, 241–243
differentiation from benign chondroblastoma, 251
differentiation from giant cell lesions of bone, 237
differentiation from giant cell reparative granuloma, 266
differentiation from pigmented villonodular synovitis, 259
differentiation from sarcoma in Paget's disease, 251
fibrosarcoma in, *247*
in Paget's disease, 248–251, *248*, *249*, 266
in Paget's disease, differentiation from giant cell reparative granuloma, 266
in Paget's disease, incidence, 249
in Paget's disease, sites, 249, 250
of major long bone in nonepiphyseal location, 243–244
pathology, 242
radiologic findings, 240
sites, 238, 239, *239*, *240*, 243, 244, *245*, *246*, 249, 250
therapy, 245
benign and metastasizing, therapy, 248
differentiation from aneurysmal cyst, 253
differentiation from benign chondroblastoma, 255
differentiation from giant cell reaction, 257, 258
differentiation from giant cell reparative granuloma, 265, 266
differentiation from primary giant cell tumors of soft somatic tissues, 292, 293
epiphyseal chondromatous, 251–253
in Paget's disease
prognosis, 250
malignant, 244–248
and fibrosarcoma, 247
associated with radiation therapy of benign lesion, 247
definition, 246
differentiated from extraarticular localized nodular synovitis, 171
fibrosarcoma from metastasis of, 247
recurrence, 244
therapy, 246, 247
metastasis of, 247, 248
primary
of soft tissues and tumoral calcinosis, 292–293
of soft somatic tissues, differentiation from giant cell tumor, 292, 293
sites, 198, 199
true, differentiation from giant cell reparative granuloma, 265, 266
Giant cell tumor of tendon sheath (*see* Extraarticular localized nodular synovitis)
Giant cell tumor of tendon sheath (*see* Tenosynovitis)
Giant cell tumor of tendon sheath
malignant (*see* Malignant neoplasms of synovium)
Golgi apparatus, osteocyte, 18
Golgi zone, bone structure, 18
Gonococcal organisms, etiology of Reiter's syndrome, 142

Gout
associated with arthritis, 98, 99, 101, 103, *104*
associated with aseptic necrosis, 62
differentiation from rheumatoid arthritis, 136
hemostasis in, 83
similarity with idiopathic aseptic necrosis, 83
Gouty synovitis
differentiated from rheumatoid arthritic synovitis, 133
Gouty tophus
differentiation from tumoral calcinosis, 293
sites, 289–292, *290*
Grafting
as a cause of osteomyelitis, 40
Granulation tissue
in plasma cell osteomyelitis, 48
Granuloma
coccidioidal, *53*
in os pisiforme, *53*
eosinophilic, *277*, *280*
destruction of bone, 199
differential diagnosis, 237
differentiation from Ewing's sarcoma, 279, 314
differentiation from metastatic cancer, 279
differentiation from plasma cell myeloma, 279
differentiation from reticulum cell sarcoma, 279
giant cell
differentiation from "brown tumor" of hyperparathyroidism, 225
differentiation from fibro-osseous lesion, 210, 219
site, 225
giant cell reparative
differential diagnosis, 237
differentiation from aneurysmal bone cyst, 253
differentiation from benign giant cell tumor, 266
differentiation from brown tumor of hyperparathyroidism, 266
differentiation from true giant cell tumor, 265, 266
histology, 263
incidence, 264
site, 257, 263–267, *264*
giant cell tumor, differentiation from giant cell reaction, 257
solitary and multifocal eosinophilic, 276
associated with "histiocytosis-X," 278
associated with multinucleated benign giant cells, 279
characteristics, 277–279
Hand-Schüller-Christian disease in, 277
in parietal bone, *277*, 279
incidence, 279
terminology, 277–278
tissue response in histoplasmosis, 54
Granuloma of jawbones, giant cell reparative, 263–267
Granuloma tissue, response in histoplasmosis, 54
Granulomatous process, inflammatory, differentiation from epithelioik sarcoma, 176
Graves' disease, and fibrous dysplasia, 209
Growth zone
articular cartilage, 2
cartilaginous, 2
embryology, 2

Hand
advanced rheumatoid arthritis, 100
blastomycosis, 54
cartilaginous tissue, 305, *305*
chondrific center, *13*
chondrosarcoma, 303, 305
coccidioidomycosis, 52
coronal section, *3*
degenerative changes, 125
related to osteoarthritis, 125
embryology, 10
epithelioid sarcoma, 176
erosive osteoarthritis, 105
extraarticular localized nodular synovitis, 168
giant cell reaction, 255–258
histoplasma duboisii, *55*
histoplasmosis, 54
lipoma, 173
pigmented villonodular synovitis, 165
Reiter's syndrome, 141
rheumatoid arthritis, 131
salmonella osteomyelitis, 49
synovial sarcoma, 173
Hand-Schüller-Christian disease, in solitary and multifocal eosinophilic granuloma of bone, 277
Haversian system, 22
Head
fibro-osseous lesion, 210–225
fibrous dysplasia, 211
monostotic fibrous dysplasia, 227, 232
Heart
failure, associated with Paget's disease, 151
rheumatoid arthritis, 136
surgery, and osteomyelitis, 39
Heberden's nodes
and soft tissues in osteoarthritis, 121
in osteoarthritis
characteristics, 125
relationship to factors determining osteoarthritis, 125
similarity to subchondral pseudocysts, 119
Heel, brown tumor of hyperparathyroidism in, 261
Hemangioma
characteristics, 172
histology, 172
incidence, 172
neoplasms and neoplasm-like lesions, 159
of the synovium, 172
sites, 172
synovial, differentiation from pigmented villonodular synovitis, 164
therapy, 172
Hemangiopericytoma, associated with mesenchy-

mal chondrosarcoma, 311
Hematogenous osteomyelitis, 39–41
Hemimelia
paraxial, 10–11, 14
associated with polydactyly, 13
radial, 13
and thalidomide, 13
defective or absent thumb, 13
unilateral intercalary, 14
tibial, 11, 13, 14
thalidomide-associated, 13
unilateral, 14
Hemochromatosis, differentiation from pigmented villonodular synovitis, 164
Hemoglobinopathies
and sickle cell anemia, 80, 82
associated with salmonella osteomyelitis, 49
related to sickle cell anemia
differentiation from idiopathic aseptic necrosis, 82
Hemophilia
associated with arthritis, 98, 99, 101
differentiation from ankylosing spondylitis, 105
differentiation from pigmented villonodular synovitis, 164
Hemosiderin-laden cell in pigmented villonodular synovitis, 162
Hemostasis
altered, associated with aseptic necrosis, 62
in gout, 83
Hepatosplenomegaly, in juvenile rheumatoid arthritis, 139
Hip
arthroplasty, 110
aseptic necrosis, 117–118
brown tumor of hyperparathyroidism in, 261
caisson disease, 82
coxa vara, 122
idiopathic aseptic necrosis, 64, 68, 71, 84
intraarticular localized nodular synovitis, 167
intraosseous villonodular synovitis, 259
locking, in stage IV of idiopathic aseptic necrosis, 71
osteoarthritic degeneration, 123
osteoarthritis, 117, 122–123, 125
osteophyte, 121
pigmented villonodular synovitis, 164
rheumatoid arthritis, 131
subchondral pseudocyst, 119
synovial chondromatosis, 160
synovial chondrosarcoma, 180
synovitis, 84
Hip joint
childhood osteomyelitis, 44
pigmented villonodular synovitis, 165
Histiocytoma
fibrous
(*see* also Synovitis, extraarticular localized nodular)
differentiation from extraarticular localized nodular synovitis, 167
differentiation from fibro-osseous lesions, 219, 220
"histiocytosis-X" concept, associated with solitary and multifocal eosinophilic granuloma, 278
Histocompatibility antigen HL-A W27 (*see* Antigen HL-A W27)
Histoplasma duboisii, 55
associated with histoplasmosis, 54
sites, *55*
Histoplasmosis, 54
associated with *Histoplasma duboisii*, 54
granuloma tissue response in, 54
sites, 54
Hodgkin's disease, 312, 319
associated with cryptococcosis, 54
etiology, 319
incidence, 319
prognosis, 319
radiologic findings, 319
"Hole zone," 16, 17
Hormone, factor determining osteoarthritis, 124
Humerus
and salmonella osteomyelitis, 48
benign chondroblastoma, 254
benign giant cell tumor arising in Paget's disease, 250
bone cyst, 198
caisson disease, 82
cementoma, 230
childhood osteomyelitis, 43
chondroblastoma, 198
chondrosarcoma, *304*
embryology, 2, 4, 6
endochondral ossification, 2
fibrous dysplasia, 209
idiopathic aseptic necrosis, 61
osteosarcoma, *304*
Paget's disease, 250
polyostotic fibrous dysplasia, 227
unicameral bone cyst, 282
viral osteomyelitis, 50
Humerus head
coronal section, *12*
Hydroxyapatite crystals, 17
Hypercalcemia
associated with disuse osteoporosis, 25
cause of hyperparathyroidism, 260, 261
in Paget's disease, 151
Hypercortisonism
associated with osteoporosis, 82
cause of aseptic necrosis, 82
etiology, 82
gross characteristics, 82
histology, 82
Hyperemia, in inflammatory arthritis, 130
Hyperostosis, in fibrous dysplasia, 216
Hyperparathyroidism
associated with fibrous dysplasia, 210
brown tumor of, 225, 257, 260–263, *262*, 266
differentiation from giant cell granuloma, 225
differentiation from giant cell reaction, 257
differentiation from giant cell reparative granuloma, 266

Hyperparthyroidism—*continued*
associated with fibrous dysplasia, 210
etiology, 261
incidence, 260
sites, 261, 262
etiology, 260, 261
in osteomalacia, 32
primary, etiology, 260
secondary, associated with tumoral calcinosis, 293
"Hyperphosphatasia," defined, 146
Hypophosphatasia, in osteomalacia, 29
Hypophosphatemia, cause of brown tumor of hyperparathyroidism, 261

Idiopathic asceptic necrosis (*see* Necrosis)
Idiopathic osteoporosis (*see* Osteoporosis)
Ileitis, regional, associated with enteric arthritis, 143
Iliac crest
idiopathic osteoporosis, *26*, 27
osteomalacia, 31, 32, 34
Ilium
benign giant cell tumor arising in Paget's disease, 250
brown tumor of hyperparathyroidism in, 261
chondrosarcoma, *231*
Paget's disease, 250
polyostotic fibrous dysplasia, 227
Infarction
differentiation from salmonella osteomyelitis, 49
in osteomyelitis, 40
in sickle cell anemia, 49
Inflammatory arthritis (*see* Arthritis)
Intestinal absorption
associated with osteomalacia, 29
in osteomalacia, 29
Intestinal infection, associated with reactive arthritis, 133
Involucrum
childhood osteomyelitis, 43
formation in viral osteomyelitis, 50
in infantile osteomyelitis, 41
Iridocyclitis, in juvenile chronic rheumatoid arthritis, 139
Iritis, associated with Reiter's syndrome, 141
Ischemia
and rheumatoid arthritis, 138
femoral head, 62
Ischium, chondrosarcoma, *231*

Jaw
actinomycosis, 55
brown tumor of hyperparathyroidism, 262
cementoma, 230
cherubism, 225
fibro-osseous lesion, 209, 210, 225
in children, 222
fibrous dysplasia, 210, 211, *212*, *213*, 226
focal chronic osteomyelitis, 220
giant cell granuloma, 225
giant cell reparative granuloma, 257, 263–267
masses resembling fibrous neoplasms, 225
ossifying fibroma, 222
polyostotic fibrous dysplasia, 232
primary osteomyelitis, 47
tumor-like lesions, 209
Joint
aging, 110–114
cartilaginous growth zone, 2
diarthrodial, rheumatoid arthritis, 138
interphalangeal, Reiter's syndrome, 141
interzone, embryology, 2
Luschka, osteoarthritis, 122
Joint detritis, in osteoarthritis, 121
Joint disease
degenerative
and osteotomy, 125
differentiation from pigmented villonodular synovitis, 164
etiology, 125
genes as contributing factor in, 125
in osteoarthritis, 125
incidence, 125
genetic contributions to, 125
radiologic diagnosis, 98–109
Joint fibrillation, systemic factor determining osteoarthritis, 124

Keratopathy, in juvenile rheumatoid arthritis, 139
Kienböck's disease, and idiopathic aseptic necrosis, 61
Klebsiella, bacteriology of osteomyelitis, 40
Knee
articular synovial chondromatosis, 305–307
aseptic necrosis, 119
benign giant cell tumor of bone, 238
chondromyxoid fibroma, 288
extraarticular localized nodular synovitis, 168
fibrous cortical defects, 272
hemangioma, 172
hemophiliac arthritis, 101
intraarticular localized nodular synovitis, 167
lipoma, 173
nonossifying fibroma, 198
osteocartilaginous exostoses, 198
osteophyte, 121
pigmented villonodular synovitis, 164, 165
Reiter's syndrome, 141
rheumatoid arthritis, 131, *134*
synovial chondromatosis, 160, *307*
synovial chondrosarcoma, 180
synovial sarcoma, 173, 174
synovium of, *135*

Lamina
chondrification, 7–8
Lamina splandens
osteoarthritis, 114, 115
Langhans' giant cells

in Brucella osteomyelitis, 49
Larynx
cartilaginous tumor, 307, 309
differentiation from chondrosarcoma, 307
therapy, 309
tumorous masses of hyaline cartilage in, 300
Leg
blastomycosis, 54
epithelioid sarcoma, 176
synovial sarcoma, 173
Legg-Calve-Perthes disease, and idiopathic aseptic necrosis, 61
Legg-Perthes disease
and idiopathic aseptic necrosis, 63, 83, 84
and osteoarthritis, 123
Lesion
benign neoplasm and neoplasm-like, 159–173
benign, radiation therapy of, associated with giant cell tumor, 247
fibro-osseous, 209–235
and fibrous dysplasia, 209–220
clinicopathologic correlation and prognosis, 225–226
diagnosis, 209, 232
differentiation from aneurysmal cyst, 210
differentiation from cemento-ossifying fibroma, 232
differentiation from chronic osteomyelitis, 225
differentiation from desmoplastic fibroma, 210, 218, 219
differentiation from fibromatosis, 218
differentiation from fibrous dysplasia, 232
differentiation from fibrous histiocytoma, 219, 220
differentiation from giant cell granuloma, 219
differentiation from odontogenic myxoma, 219
differentiation from osteoblastoma, 210
differentiation from reactive fibrosis, 219
differentiation from tumor-like lesion, 209
etiology, 230
of periodontal membrane, differentiation from desmoplastic fibroma, 210
of periodontal membrane, differentiation from osteoblastoma, 210
problem of terminology, 209
sites, 209–230
giant cell (*see* Giant cell lesion)
mixed fibro-osseous, differentiation from fibrous dysplasia, 225
tumor-like
differentiation from fibro-osseous lesions of bone, 209
site, 209
Letterer-Siwe disease, definition of, 277
Leukemia
lymphocytic, destruction of bone, *201*
murine, virus, RNA-related, contained in human sarcoma, 190–191
possible etiologic agent of human skeletal and soft tissue sarcomas, 187
Leukocyte
neutrophilic
in fungal osteomyelitis, 52
Ligamentum teres, osteoarthritis, 121
Lining cells, mature osteon, 23
Lipoma
arborescent, in neoplasms and neoplasm-like lesions of the synovium, 172
characteristics, 172–173
incidence, 172, 173
neoplasms and neoplasm-like lesions, 159
of the synovium, 172–173
sites, 173
synovium, adipose tissue tumor in, 172, 173
Lobectomy, therapy for metastasizing benign giant cell tumor, 248
Long bones
and salmonella osteomyelitis, 48
aneurysmal bone cyst, 279
benign chondroblastoma, 251, 254, 255
benign giant cell tumor, 243–244, 249, 250
Brucella osteomyelitis, 49
cementoma, 227
childhood osteomyelitis, 42–44
chondroblastoma, 198
chondromyxoid fibroma, 288
coccidioidomycosis, 52
Ewing's tumor, 198
fibro-osseous lesion, 210, 226–230
fibrous dysplasia, 230
giant cell lesion, 238
giant cell tumor, 198
gouty tophus, 289–292
radiologic findings, 290–291
nonossifying fibroma, 198
ossifying fibroma, 227
and cementifying fibroma, 220
osteocartilaginous exostoses, 198
Paget's disease, 249, 250
salmonella osteomyelitis, 49
sarcomatous transformation of fibrous dysplasia, 230
tumors of Paget's disease, 152
Long tubular bone, gouty tophus, 291
Looser zone, in osteomalacia, 29
Lung
actinomycosis, 55
epithelioid sarcoma, 177
extraarticular localized nodular synovitis, 170
metastasis in, 248, 255
Lupus erythematosus
characteristics, 93
discoid, 91
staining pattern from antinuclear antibodies, 90
systemic, 89–92
characteristics, 94–95
differentiation from rheumatism, 90, 93
immunologic reactions in, 89–92
Lymph node
epithelioid sarcoma, 177
plasma cell myeloma in, 318

Lymph node—*continued*
primary sarcoma of, differentiation from reticulum cell sarcoma, 316
regional, metatasis in synovial sarcoma, 174
Lymphadenopathy, in juvenile rheumatoid arthritis, 139
Lymphocyte
and rheumatic disorder, 132
and sporotrichosis, 55
and therapy in rheumatic disorders, 132
in fungal osteomyelitis, 52
nonrheumatoid, differentiation from rheumatoid, 95
production of lymphotoxin, 95
rheumatoid, differentiation from nonrheumatoid, 95
sporotrichosis, 55
Lymphocytes T and B, in rheumatoid arthritis, 132
Lymphogranuloma venereum, associated with questionable viral osteomyelitis, 51
Lymphoma
associated with cryptococcosis, 54
Burkitt's, possible etiologic agent of human skeletal and soft tissue sarcoma, 187
in vertebra, 199
malignant (*see* Reticulum cell sarcoma)
bone destruction, 199
differentiation from reticulum cell sarcoma, 316
site, 199
Lymphotoxin
produced by lymphocytes, 95
Lytic foci
coccidioidomycosis, 54

Maduromycosis, 56–57
characteristics, 56
sites, 56
Malformations, thalidomide syndrome, 11
Mandible
actinomycosis, 55, *56*
benign giant cell tumor arising in Paget's disease, 249, 250
cementifying fibroma, 210, 220
cementoblastoma, *223*
embryology, 1, 2
fibro-osseous lesion in children, 210
fibrous dysplasia, 209, 211, 226, 232
ossification, 9
ossifying fibroma, 220, 222, 230
Paget's disease, 250
"secondary" cartilage in, 2
viral osteomyelitis, 50
Marrow
cavity, embryology, 5
formation, 5
Matrix
calcification, 6, 19
changes, osteoarthritis, 111–112
characteristics, 112
deposition, 1
embryology, 1
in woven bone, 22
intercellular
bone cells, 16
embryology, 2, 3
of polysaccharides, 16
separates cells, 2
osteocytes, 18, 19
perilacunar, bone formation, 19
protein polysaccharides, 18
unmineralized, bone structure, 16
Matrix production, 19
osteocyte, 19
Maxilla
actinomycosis, 55
benign giant cell tumor arising in Paget's disease, 250
brown tumor of hyperparathyroidism, 262
cementifying fibroma, 210, 226
fibro-osseous lesion in children, 210
fibrous dysplasia, 209, 211, 212, *217*, 232
giant cell reparative granuloma, 264, *264*
ossification, 9
ossifying fibroma, 230
in children, 222
Paget's disease, 250
Meninges, embryology, 2
Mesenchymal cell, embryology, 2
Mesenchymal chondrosarcoma (*see* Chondrosarcoma)
Mesenchymal condensation, 1
limb, 9
Mesenchymal tissue, embryology, 1
Mesenchyme
definition, 1
in infantile osteomyelitis, 41
Mesoblast, embryology, 1
Mesoderm, embryology, 1, 9
Metacarpal cartilage, 13–14
Metacarpal shaft, *5*
Metacarpophalangeal joint, rheumatoid arthritis, 100
Metacarpus
brown tumor of hyperparathyroidism, 262
chondrosarcoma, *305*
coronal section, *8*, *9*
early rheumatoid arthritis, 108
embryology, 13–14
extraarticular localized nodular synovitis, 169
giant cell reaction, *256*, 256, 257
idiopathic osteoporosis, 27, *28*, 29
longitudinal section, *11*
polyostotic fibrous dysplasia, 227
transverse section, *10*
Metaphyseal cortical defect, 272–276
Metaphyseal fibrous defect (*see* Fibrous defect)
Metaphysis, embryology, 6
Metastatic tumor (*see* site or specific disease)
Metatarsal cartilage, 13
Metatarsal head, idiopathic aseptic necrosis, 61

Metatarsophalangeal joint, periarticular deossification, 103
Metatarsus
coccidioidomycosis, 52
embryology, 13–14
giant cell reaction, 258
polyostotic fibrous dysplasia, 227
Microscopy, light and electron, 16–24
Mineral content, in woven bone, 22
Mineralization, bone structure, 18
Mitochondrium, bone structure, 18–20
Mixed connective tissue disease
associated diseases
arthralgia, 92
dysphagia, 92
muscle weakness, 92
Raynaud's phenomenon, 92
renal disease, 92
sclerodactyly, 92
associated with ribonucleoprotein antibodies, 92–93
differentiation from dermatomyositis, 92
differentiation from scleroderma, 92
Mixed fibro-osseous lesion (*see* Fibro-osseous lesions)
Molars, ossifying fibroma and cementifying fibroma, 220
Mucor, in phycomycosis, 54
Mucor osteomyelitis, in phycomycosis, 54
Muscle weakness, associated with mixed connective tissue disease, 92
Mycobacterial synovitis, differentiation from rheumatoid arthritic synovitis, 133
Mycoplasma
possible etiologic agent of Reiter's syndrome, 142
possible etiologic agent of rheumatoid arthritis, 131
Myeloma
in vertebra, 199
plasma cell, 317–319
and small round cell tumor, 312
associated with monoclonal gammopathies, 318
associated with myeloma nephrosis, 319
associated with polyclonal gammopathies, 318
cytology, 319
differential diagnosis, 319
differentiation from eosinophilic granuloma, 279
etiology, 318
gross characteristics, 319
hematology, 319
histology, 319
in lymph nodes, 318
prognosis, 319
sites, 199, 318
small round cell tumors of bone, 312
therapy, 319
Myocarditis, in Reiter's syndrome, 142
Myositis ossificans progressiva, abnormality of fibrous dysplasia, 209
Myxoma
odontogenic
differentiation from fibro-osseous lesions, 219
differentiation from jaw masses resembling fibrous neoplasms, 225

Nasal cavity, paracoccidioidomycosis, 54
Neck
fibro-osseous lesion, 209–225
monostotic fibrous dysplasia, 232
synovial sarcoma, 173
Necrosis
aseptic
associated with altered hemostasis, 62
associated with cortico-steroid therapy, 62
associated with Gaucher's disease, 62
associated with gout, 62
differentiation from osteoarthritis, 117–119
etiology, 82, 117
evolution, 118
following dislocation, similarity to idiopathic aseptic necrosis, 79–80
following united femoral neck fracture, similarity to idiopathic asceptic necrosis, 77–79
nontraumatic, 62
of femoral head, associated with osteoarthritis, 117
of femoral head, associated with synovial retinaculum, 119
post-traumatic, 62
radiology, 118, *118*
site, 117–119
etiology, 116
idiopathic aseptic, 61–87
anatomic considerations, 62–63
and Legg-Calve-Perthes disease, 61, 63, 83, 84
and osteochondritis dissecans, 61
and trauma, 61
caisson disease, 82
clinical diagnosis, 75
diagnosis, radiology, 84–85
differential diagnosis, 75, 77, 79, 80, 82, 83
differentiation from osteoarthritis, 75
differentiation from sickle cell anemia and related hemoglobinopathies, 82
etiology, 83–84
Freiberg's disease, 61
gross characteristics, 61
gross pathology, 85
healing, 83
histology, 61, 63–64
historical background, 62
in Kienböck's disease, 61
pathology, 63–75
prosthesis, 85
similarity to alcoholism, 83
similarity to aseptic necrosis following dislocation, 79–80
similarity to aseptic necrosis following united femoral neck fracture, 77–79

Necrosis—*continued*
  idiopathic aseptic, 61–87
    similarity to Gaucher's disease, 82–83
    similarity to gout, 83
    similarity to primary osteoarthritis, 84
    sites, 61–87, *66–68*, *70*, *72*
    stage I, 64–65
    stage I, site, 64
    stage II, 65–68
    stage II, histology, 65, 67
    stage II, pathology, 67, 68
    stage II, radiology, 65
    stage III, 68–71, *74*
    stage III, histology, 69
    stage III, pathologic fracture, 69
    stage III, radiology, 68, 69
    stage IV, 71, 73, *77*, *78*
    stage IV, characteristics, 71
    stage IV, histology, 71
    stage IV, osteoporosis in, 71
    stage IV, radiology, 71–73
    stage IV, site, 71
    stage IV, synovitis in, 71
    stage V, 73, *79*
    stage V, gross characteristics, 73
    stage V, histology, 73
    stage V, radiology, 73
    stage VI, 73, 75, *81*
    stage VI, characteristics, 73
    stage VI, histology, 75
    stage VI, radiology, 73
    stage VI, similarity to degenerative arthritis, 73
    stages, 64–75
    subchondral fracture, 84
    synovitis in, 84
    therapy, 85
  ischemic, differentiation from, in osteomyelitis, 40
  physiological, 9
  traumatic aseptic, 83
    and osteochondritis dissecans, 83
    fracture site, 83
    sites, 83
Neoplasm (*see* site or specific disease)
Neoplasm, fibrous (*see* Fibrous)
Neoplasm
  benign and neoplasm-like lesions, 159–173
Nephrosis, myeloma, associated with plasma cell myeloma, 319
Neural arch
  embryology, 2
  ossification, 8
  vertebra
    embryology, 2
  vertebral osteomyelitis, 45
Neural processes, chondrification, 7–8
Neuralgia, brachial, osteoarthritis, 122
Neuroblastoma, metastatic, differentiation from Ewing's sarcoma, 314, 315
Neurofibroma, intraosseous, differentiation from jaw masses resembling fibrous neoplasms, 225
Neurovascular canal
  bone matrix, 22
  osteon, 22
New York, rheumatoid arthritis diagnostic criteria, 131
Newcastle disease viruses, rheumatoid arthritis, 132
Nocardia asteroides, cause of nocardiosis, 56
Nocardia osteomyelitis, of pubic bone, *57*
Nocardiosis, 56
  etiology, 56
Nodules, rheumatoid arthritis, 136, 138, *138*
Notochord, embryology, 7

Occipital region, embryology, 9
Occiput, site of rheumatoid arthritis, 136
Ochronosis
  radiologic diagnosis, 99, 106, 107, *108*
  spine, 108
Oral cavity
  paracoccidioidomycosis, 54
  site of actinomycosis, 55
Oronasopharynx, plasma cell myeloma, 318
Os pisiforme
  coccidioidal granuloma in, *53*
  coccidioidomycosis of, *52*
Os triquetrum, coccidioidomycosis of, 52
Osseous metastasis, synovial neoplasms secondary to, 181
Ossific center
  definition, 2
  embryology, 2
Ossification, 1–6, 10
  cartilage, 2
  chondrosarcoma, 205
  differentiation from lesional calcification, 205–208
  embryonic period, 2
  endochondral, 1–6
    site, 2
  epiphysial centers, 6
  fetal period, 8
  intramembranous, 1–2, 5
    site, 1, 2
  sites, 4, 8, 9, 11
Osteitis deformans, 146
Osteitis pubis
  characteristics, 46
  cultures of proteus in, 46
  cultures of pseudomonas in, 46
Osteoarthritic change, secondary, subchondral pseudocyst in, 118
Osteoarthritic degeneration, sites, 123
Osteoarthritic fibrillation, differentiation from chondromalacia of the patella, 117
Osteoarthritis, 110–129
  anatomic basis for symptoms in, 125
  and chondrocytes, 124
  and fibrillation, 110, 111

and Heberden's nodes, 125
and Legg-Perthes disease, 123
and neuralgia of brachium, 122
and vertebral osteophyte, 122
articular chondrocytes in, 112–113
asbestoid degeneration, 112
associated with aseptic necrosis of femoral head, 117
associated with coxa vara, 122
associated with epiphyseal dysplasia, 125
associated with subchondral pseudocysts, 119, 120
biochemistry, a determining factor in, 124
brachial neuralgia, 122
calcar in, 114
cartilage surface degeneration in, 114, 116
caused by coxa vara, 122
cell aging in, 112–116
cellular proliferation in, differentiation from rheumatoid pannus, 114
characteristics, 110
chondrocalcinosis and degenerative joint disease in, 125
chondrocytes in, 113
clones, 113
determinants
mechanical factors as, 124
systemic factors as, 124–125
determined by hormone, 124
differentiation from aseptic necrosis, 117–119
differentiation from idiopathic aseptic necrosis, 75
erosive
differentiation from psoriasis, 105
differentiation from rheumatoid arthritis, 126
radiologic diagnosis, 99, 105, 106, *106*
sites, 105
etiology, 112, 122, 124
genes as determining factor, 124
Heberden's nodes in, characteristics, 125
hip, associated with aseptic necrosis of femoral head, 117
incidence, 110
joint detritis in, 121
lamina splandens, 114, 115
mechanical factors in pathogenesis of, 122–124
necrosis of bone, 116–117
not a single disease, 126
osteophytes of, site, 122
pathogenesis of, mechanical factors, 122–124
pathologic anatomy, 114–116, *115*
radiology, 114
primary
differentiated from secondary osteoarthritis, 123
similarity to idiopathic aseptic necrosis, 84
pseudocysts, 118
radiology, 122–123
related to degenerative changes of the hand, 125
repair or reversal of, 124
secondary
associated with rheumatoid arthritis, 122, 134
differentiation from primary osteoarthritis, 123
sites, 110, 114, *115*, 116, 117, *118*, 121, 122
soft tissues in, 121
and Heberden's nodes, 121
sources of pain, 125
spinal, differentiation from spondylosis, 121
subchondral bone changes in, 117
subchondral bone necrosis in, 116
symptoms, anatomic basis for, 125
synovial mucin in, 116
systemic influences in, 124–125
terminology, 111
Osteoblast
bone matrix, 18
bone structure, 18, 19, *19*, 23
bone tissue, 18
embryology, 1, 2, 5
Osteoblastic metastases, destruction of bone, 202
Osteoblastoma
differentiation
between lesional calcification and ossification, 207
from cementoblastoma, 222
from clear cell chondrosarcoma, 310
from fibro-osseous lesions of periodontal membrane, 210
from ossifying fibroma, 226
from osteosarcoma, 224
radiology, 207
site, 199
Osteocartilaginous exostoses, sites, 198
Osteochondritis dissecans
and idiopathic aseptic necrosis, 61
in traumatic aseptic necrosis, 83
Osteochondroma
association with chondrosarcoma, 301
formed in synovial chondrosarcoma, 179
tenosynovial, differentiation from chondromatosis, 160
Osteochondromatosis (*see* Synovial chondromatosis)
synovial, 121
Osteoclast
active, 20
cytoplasmic folds, 20
bone structure, 19, 20, *21*
bone tissue, 18
embryology, 6
in buds, 5
resorption compartment, *21*
Osteocyte
bone structure, 18–20, *20*, 23
embryology, 2
Golgi, 18
matrix, 18
matrix production, 19
mature, bone structure, 18, 19
osteolysis, 19
Osteocyte lacunae, in osteomalacia, 32

Osteocyte organelle, bone structure, 19
Osteodystrophy, renal, 33
Osteogenesis, review, 1
Osteoid
  bone structure, 18, 23
  definition, 2
  differentiation from cementum, 218
  embryology, 4
  produced in extraarticular localized nodular synovitis, 169
  unmineralized, 23
Osteoid osteoma, in vertebra, 199
Osteoid tissue, osteomalacia, 29, 32
Osteolysis
  in bone production, 19
  in osteocyte, 19
Osteolytic lesion, tibia, 35
Osteoma
  fibrous (*see* Ossifying fibroma)
  osteoid
    confused with sclerosing osteomyelitis, 47
    differentiation from cementoblastoma, 222
    site, 199
Osteomalacia, 25–38
  and Fanconi's disease, 32
  associated with pseudofracture, *31*
  associated with renal disorders, 29, 32, 33
  associated with vitamin D, 32–33
  bone matrix, 29
  "brown tumor" in, 35
  "calcium front" in, 32
  calcium in, 29
  differentiation from fracture callus, 32
  differentiation from Paget's disease, 32
  etiology, 29
  gastrectomy in, 29
  histologic diagnosis, 29–32
  hyperparathyroidism in, 32
  hypophosphatasia in, 29
  illustrative cases, 33
  intestinal absorption, 29
  looser zone, 29
  osteocyte lacunae in, 32
  osteoid tissue in, 29, 32
  parathyroid overactivity in, 32
  sites, 29, *31*, 31–34,
  treatment, 32–33
  "umbauzonen" in, 29
  vitamin D-resistant, 32, 33
Osteomyelitis, 39–60
  adult, 44
    pathologic fracture in, 44
    sequestrum in, 44
    site, 44, 45
    subperiosteal abscess, 44
  and metastatic neoplasm, 40
  and *Salmonella*, 40
  as problem of surgical pathology, 40–41
  associated with paratyphoid B, 49
  associated with paravertebral abscess, 45–46
  associated with *Salmonella cholerasuis*, 49
  Bacteriodes as etiologic agent, 40
  bacteriological etiology, 40
  bacteriology, 39–40
  Brucella, 49
    etiology, 49
    histology, 49
    Langhans' giant cells in, 49
    sites, 49
  childhood, 42–44
    associated with septic arthritis, 44
    continuation of secondary chronic osteomyelitis, 48
    sites, 42–44
  childhood septic, 48
  chronic, 225
    differentiation from fibro-osseous lesion, 225
    in childhood, 43
  destruction of bone, 199
  diagnosis, 39
  differentiation from Ewing's sarcoma, 313–315
  differentiation from gangrene, 40
  differentiation from ischemic necrosis, 40
  etiology, 39–41, 49, 50, *57*
  focal chronic
    differentiation from ossifying fibroma and cementifying fibroma, 220
    site, 220
  fungal, 51–52
    diagnosis, 52
    giant cell in, 52
    histologic characteristics, 52
    lymphocyte in, 52
    neutrophilic leukocyte in, 52
    sites, 51, 52
    symptoms like those of tuberculosis, 52
  hematogenous, 39–41, *45*
  histology, 40–41
  incidence, 39
  infantile, 41–42
    and sequela, 42
    and staphylococcus, 42
    etiology, 42
    involucrum in, 41
    mesenchyme in, 41
    periosteum, 41
    pyarthrosis in, 42
    sequestration in, 43
  infarction in, 40
  mortality, 39
  plasma cell, 47, 48
    fibrosis in, 48
    granulation tissue in, 48
  primary, 46–48
    amyloidosis, complication of, 48
    and Brodie's abscess, 47
    and fistula-carcinoma, 48
    etiology, 46–47
    incidence, 46–47
      site, 47
    purulent, 40
    pyogenic, differentiation from Ewing's sarcoma, 313
    salmonella, 48–49

and perichondritis, 48
and pyarthrosis, 49
and sequestrum, 49
associated with hemoglobinopathies, 49
differentiation from infarction, 49
sites, 48–49
sclerosing
confused with osteoid osteoma, 47
of Garré, 47
secondary chronic, continuation of childhood osteomyelitis, 48
sequestrum, 40, 41, *41*
sites, 39, 40, 45, 46, *46*, 51, 57
surgical pathology associated with, 40
thorax, 39
typhoid salmonella
periosteum, 48
vaccinial, smallpox, 50, 51
variola, and arthritis, *51*
vertebral, 45–46
differentiation from other diseases, 46
neural arches, 45
site, 45
thorax, 45
viral, 49–51
associated with lymphogranuloma venereum, 51
concurrence with smallpox, 49
fibrosis in, 50
histology, 50
involucrum formation in, 50
similarity to Caffey's disease, 50
sites, 50
virus variola in, 50
Osteon
and pericytes, 23
bone structure, 22, 23
developing, *22*, 23
mature, 23, *23*
lining cells, 23
nerves, 23
pericytes, 23
resorbing, 23
smooth muscle cell, 23
Osteonecrosis, 61–87
Osteophyte
formation, 130
function, 121
radiology, 121
sites, 119–121, 123
structure, 119–121
vertebral, osteoarthritis, 122
Osteophytosis, posterior cervical, etiology, 122
Osteoplasis, bone structure, 19
Osteoplastic phase, bone structure, 19
Osteoporosis, 25–38
calcium in, 25
disuse, 25
associated with hypercalcemia, 25
idiopathic, *26*
idiopathic, 25–29
biochemical abnormalities, 29
calcium in, 29
etiology, 29
in metacarpal fracture, 29
sites, 25, *26*, 27, *28*, 29
in stage IV of idiopathic aseptic necrosis, 71
senile, not associated with osteoarthritis, 125
symptom of hypercortisonism, 82
"Osteoporosis circumscripta," in Paget's disease, 149
Osteosarcoma, *205*
associated with dedifferentiated cartilaginous tumor, 303
associated with fibrous dysplasia, 226
benign multinucleated giant cell in, 268–271
chondroblastic, differentiation from malignant cartilage, 301
destruction of bone, *200*, *202*
developed in fibrous dysplasia, 209
diagnosis, 199
differentiation from ossifying fibroma, 224
differentiation from osteoblastoma, 224
from dedifferentiated cartilaginous tumor, 303
in Paget's disease, 152, 251
incidence by age, 198
metastasis of malignant giant cell tumor into, 247
parosteal, in femur, 198
sclerotic foci of, *207*
sites, *304*
telangiectatic, *270–272*
sites, 271
transformation of fibrous dysplasia into, 230
with benign giant cell tumor of tibia, 269
with benign multinucleated giant cells, *267*, 268–271, *269*
associated with Codman's angle, 268
differentiation from aneurysmal cyst, 269
sites, 268
with giant cells, differentiation from aneurysmal cyst, 269
Osteotomy
anatomic material from 124
and degenerative joint disease, 125
for chondromalacia patellae, 124

Paget, J., 146, 152
Paget's disease, 146–156
and fibrosarcoma, 152
and tumor, 152
associated with cardiac failure, 151
associated with fracture, 151
associated with "osteoporosis circumscripta," 149
associated with paraplegia, 155
benign giant cell tumor in, 248–251, *248*, *249*, 266
differentiation from giant cell reparative granuloma, 266
incidence, 249
sites, 249, 250
chondrosarcoma in, 152

Paget's disease—*continued*
  differentiation from osteomalacia, 32
  etiology, 146
  giant cell tumor in
    prognosis, 250
  histology, 146, *147*, *148*
  hypercalcemia in, 151
  illustrative cases, 152–155
  incidence, 146, 148, 152
  osteosarcoma in, 152, 251
  pathology, 146, 148–151
  platybasia, 149
  radiological findings, 148, *150–153*
  sarcoma in, 251
    cytology, 251
    differentiation from benign giant cell tumor, 251
    prognosis, 251
  sites, 148, *149–154*, 152, 154, 155, 249, 250
  therapy, 151
Palate
  ulcerations of, associated with Reiter's syndrome, 141
Panarteritis, in vasculitis, 138
Pannus, inflammatory, in rheumatoid arthritis, 134
Panner's disease, 61
Parachordal area, embryology, 9
Paracoccidioides brasiliensis, 54
Paracoccidioidomycosis, 54
  differentiation from balstomycosis, 54
  site, 54
Paranasal sinuses, ossifying fibroma, 230
Paraplegia, associated with Paget's disease, 155
Paratyphoid B, associated with sickle cell anemia 49
Parathyroid overactivity, in osteomalacia, 32
Parietal bone
  embryology, 2
  solitary and multifocal eosinophilic granuloma of bone, *277*, 279
Patella
  chondromalacia, 117
    osteotomy for, 124
Pelvic bone
  benign giant cell tumor, 250
  Paget's disease, 250
Pelvic girdle
  Ewing's sarcoma, 312
Pelvis
  as route in spread of vertebral osteomyelitis, 45
  fibrous dysplasia, 209
  fracture, *31*
  idiopathic osteoporosis, 29
  Paget's disease, 148
  tumors in Paget's disease, 152
Periapical cemental dysplasia (*see* Dysplasia)
Pericarditis
  in juvenile rheumatoid arthritis, 139
  in Reiter's syndrome, 142
Perichondritis, and salmonella osteomyelitis, 48
Perichondrium
  embryology, 2, 4, 5
  function, 2
Pericytes, osteon, 23
Periodontal membrane
  fibro-osseous lesions, 210
  ossifying fibroma and cementifying fibroma, 220
  site of origin for ossifying and cementifying fibromas, 210
Pseriosteal bone
  embryology, 2
Periosteal shell
  embryology, 5
Periosteum
  and adult osteomyelitis, 44
  and osteomyelitis, 40
  and typhoid salmonella osteomyelitis, 48
  childhood osteomyelitis, 43
  embryology, 2, 5
  in infantile osteomyelitis, 41
Periostitis, caused by actinomycosis, 55
Phagocytosis, in rheumatoid arthritis, 132
Phalanges
  cartilage, 14
  chondrosarcoma, 305
  coccidioidomycosis, 52
  embryology, 4, *4*
  extraarticular localized nodular synovitis, 168, 169
  psoriatic and rheumatoid arthritis, 140
  psoriatic arthritis, *141*
  tuberosity, 4
Phycomycosis, 54
  associated with diabetes, 54
  caused by mucor, 54
  site, 54
  staphylococcal osteomyelitis in, 54
Plasma cell
  fungal osteomyelitis, 52
  sporotrichosis, 55
Plasma cell osteomyelitis, 47, 48
Platybasia, in Paget's disease, 149
Pleura
  actinomycosis, 55
  rheumatoid arthritis, 136
Pneumococcus
  etiology of osteomyelitis, 40
Poliomyelitis, immobilization of a limb, 25
Polyarthritis
  acute, associated with rheumatic fever, 88
  juvenile chronic
    and histocompatibility antigen HL-A W27, 133
  rheumatoid arthritis, 139
  migratory, in enteric arthritis, 142
Polydactyly
  appearance, 14
  associated with paraxial hemimelia, 13
Polysaccharides
  bone structure, *18*
  intercellular matrix with, 16

Precartilage stage, 2
Premolar
  cementifying fibroma, 220
  ossifying fibroma, 220
Prostheses, cause of osteomeylitis, 40
Protein polysaccharides, embryology, 18
Proteus
  cultures of, in osteitis pubis, 46
  etiology of osteomyelitis, 40
Pseudocyst
  subchondral
    associated with osteoarthritis, 119, 120
    histology, 119
    in secondary osteoarthritic change, 118
    similarity to ganglia, 119
    similarity to Heberden's nodes, 119
    site, 119
Pseudofracture, associated with osteomalacia, *31*
Pseudomonas
  cultures of, in osteitis pubis, 46
  etiology of osteomyelitis, 40
Psoriasis
  associated with arthritis, 98, 99, *141*
  differentiation from ankylosing spondylitis, 105
  differentiation from erosive osteoarthritis, 105
Psoriatic arthritis (*see* Arthritis)
Puberty, precocious, associated with fibrous dysplasia, 210
Pubic bone, nocardia osteomyelitis of, *57*
Pubis, chondrosarcoma, *231*
Pulmonary parenchyma, site of rheumatoid arthritis, 136
Pyarthrosis, and salmonella osteomyelitis, 49
  in infantile osteomyelitis, 42

Radius
  aneurysmal bone cyst, *282*
  benign giant cell tumor, 239, *240*
  giant cell tumor, 198
  viral osteomyelitis, 50
Raynaud's phenomenon
  associated with mixed connective tissue disease, 92
Reed-Sternberg cells, differentiation from cells of reticulum cell sarcoma, 316
Reiter's disease
  characteristics, 103, 141
  differentiation from ankylosing spondylitis, 105
  radiologic diagnosis, 108
Reiter's syndrome
  ankylosing spondylitis, 140
  aortitis, 142
  associated with arthritis, 141
  associated with bedsonia viruses, 142
  associated with blennorrhagicum keratodermia, 141
  associated with circinate balantitis, 141
  association with conjunctivitis, 141
  associated with histocompatibility antigen HL-A W27, 133
  associated with hyperkeratotic dermatitis, 141
  associated with iritis, 141
  associated with *mycoplasma*, 142
  associated with myocarditis, 142
  associated with ulcerations of buccal mucosa, 141
  associated with ulcerations of Palate, 141
  associated with uveitis, 141
  differentiation from adult rheumatoid arthritis, 130
  differentiated from rheumatoid arthritis, 133, 142
  etiology, 142
    and gonococcal organisms, 142
    and *Shigella* organisms, 142
  HL-A W27 in patients, 142
  pericarditis in, 142
  radiology, 141
  rheumatoid arthritis, 141–142
  sites, 141
  spondylitis in, 141
  urethritis, a component of, 141
Renal arteritis
  associated with rheumatoid arthritis, 138
Renal disease
  associated with mixed connective tissue disease, 92
  relationship to antinuclear antibody, 91, 92
Renal disorder
  associated with osteomalacia, 29, 32, 33
Renal osteodystrophy, 33
Resorption compartment
  osteoclast, *21*
Reticulum
  endoplasmic, 18, 20
    bone structure, 23
    free ribosome, 18
  endoplasmic cytoplasm, bone structure, 18
Reticulum cell sarcoma (*see* Sarcoma)
Retinaculum, site of osteoarthritis, 121
Retroperitoneum, site of synovial sarcoma, 173
Rheumatic disease
  arthritis as aid in diagnosis and prognosis of, 88–97
  cell-mediated immune reactions in, 93–95
  diagnosis and prognosis, 88–97
  Immunologic aspects, 88–97
  pathogenesis, 94
  tests for, 94
Rheumatic disorder
  and lymphocyte, 132
  therapy, 132
Rheumatic fever
  and multiple streptococcal antigens, 89
  and reactive arthritis, 133
  antistreptococcal antibody in, 88–89
  associated with acute polyarthritis, 88
  preceded by group A streptococcus, 88
Rheumatism, associated with arthritis, 98–101, *102, 103*
Rheumatoid disease, malignant, 138

Rheumatoid factor, produced in rheumatoid arthritis, 132
Rheumatoid pannus, differentiation from cellular proliferation in osteoarthritis, 114
Rheumatoid synvoial cell, differentiation from nonrheumatoid synovial cell, 95
Rib
  actinomycosis, 55
  brown tumor of hyperparathyroidism, 262
  cartilage
    Osteoarthritis, 110
  chondrification, 7–8
  coccidioidomycosis, 52
  Ewing's sarcoma, 312
  fibrous dysplasia, 209
    as monostotic lesion, 227
  osteomyelitis, 39
  polyostotic fibrous dysplasia, 227
  salmonella osteomyelitis, 48
Ribonucleoprotein
  antibody, 90, 92, 93
    associated with mixed connective tissue disease, 92–93
Ribosome
  bone structure, 18
  cytoplasm, 20
  free, endoplasmic reticulum, 18
Rickets, 29
  vitamin D-resistant, *30*
Rous, P., 187
Rubella virus
  of rheumatic arthritis, in synovial cells, 132

Sacroiliac
  ankylosing spondylitis, 105, 139
Sacroiliitis
  associated with enteric arthritis, 142
  associated with histocompatibility antigen HL-A W27, 133
Sacroiliac, Reiter's syndrome, 141
Sacrum
  Paget's disease, 148
  sarcoma, 199
Salmonella, and reactive arthritis, 133
Salmonella cholerasuis, in sickle cell anemia with osteomyelitis, 49
Salmonella osteomyelitis, 40
  associated with sickle cell anemia, 49, *50*
  etiology in patients with sickle cell anemia, 49
Salmonella typhimurium, in osteomyelitis with sickle cell anemia, 49
Sarcoma (*see* Sarcomatous transformation of fibrous dysplasia)
  anaplastic, from dedifferentiation of cartilaginous tumor, 303
  antigen, 189
  associated with antigen, antibody distribution to, 189
  clear cell, 177, *178*
    characteristics, 177–178
    cytology, 178
    histology, 157
    tendon sheaths, associated with the synovium, 173
    therapy, 179
  cytologic features, 300
  epidemiology, 191
  epithelioid, 176–177, *177*
    differentiation from inflammatory granulomatous process, 176
    differentiation from metastatic carcinoma, 176
    differentiation from synovial sarcoma, 176–177
    histology, 176–177
    incidence, 176
    primary malignant, from synovium, 173
    sites, 176, 177
    therapy, 177
  from benign chondroblastoma, 255
  from fibrous dysplasia, 230
  human
    antigen, 188–192
    common tumor-associated, 188–192
    containing a filterable substance, 190
    containing RNA related to murine leukemia virus, 190–191
    cytology, 190, 191
    etiology, 187, 190
    extract from, 190
    extract from, cytology, 190
    extract from, etiology, 190
    immunofluorescence of common tumor-associated antigen of, 188–189
    immunology, 187, 188
    immunology of common tumor-associated antigen of, 188–192
    RNA-related murine leukemia virus contained in, 190–191
  human skeletal and soft tissue
    Burkitt's lymphoma, a possible etiologic agent in, 187
    etiology, 187–195
    leukemia as possible etiologic agent of, 187
  in fibrous dysplasia, 226
  in Paget's disease
    classified as osteosarcoma, 251
    cytology, 251
    differentiation from benign giant cell tumor, 251
    prognosis, 251
  neoplastic cell and stroma of synovial, differentiation from normal synovium, 175
  of lymph node, primary, differentiation from reticulum cell, 316
  of reticulum cell, differentiation from Reed-Sternberg cell, 316
  osteogenic
    diagnosed as chondroblastoma, 255
    in chondroblastoma, 255
    irradiation-induced, 255
    irradiation-induced, malignant change in, 255

parosteal osteogenic, incidence by age, 198
primary malignant epithelioid, from synovium, 173
primary, of lymph nodes, differentiation from reticulum cell sarcoma, 316
primary reticulum cell, differentiation from Ewing's sarcoma, 313
reticulum cell, 312, 315–317
cytology, 316
differentiation from eosinophilic granuloma, 279
differentiation from Ewing's sarcoma, 314–317
differentiation from malignant lymphoma, 316
differentiation from primary sarcoma of lymph nodes, 316
histologic findings, 316, 317
incidence, 316
prognosis, 316, 317
radiologic findings, 316
sites, 316, 317
sites, 36, 198, 199, 230
spindle cell, from dedifferentiated cartilaginous tumor, 303
synovial, 173–176
characteristics, 174
differentiation from arthritis, 174
differentiation from epithelioid sarcoma, 176–177
differentiation from nodular synovitis, 174
differentiation from normal synovium, 175
histology, 157, 174–175
incidence, 173
regional lymph node metastasis in, 174
sites, 173, 174
therapy, 175–176
with extraarticular localized nodular synovitis, 169
transformation from fibrous dysplasia, 230
viruses, interspecies transmission of, 191–192
well-differentiated, differentiation from benign neoplasm of hyaline cartilage, 300
Sarcoma of soft tissue (*see* Soft tissue)
Sarcomatous transformation of fibrous dysplasia, sites, 230
Scalp, epithelioid sarcoma, 177
Scapula
embryology, 2
endochondral ossification, 2
osteomalacia, 33, 34
viral osteomyelitis, 50
Schmorl, G., 146
Sclerodactyly, associated with mixed connective tissue disease, 92
Scleroderma
associated with positive antinuclear antibody tests, 89
differentiation from mixed connective tissue disease, 92
differentiation from systemic lupus erythematosus, 90
staining pattern from antinuclear antibodies, 90
Sequestrum
and adult osteomyelitis, 44
and salmonella osteomyelitis, 49
Sequela, and infantile osteomyelitis, 42
Sequestration, in childhood osteomyelitis, 43
"Shepherd's crook"
diagnosis, 227
sites, *229*
with polyostotic fibrous dysplasia, *229*
Shigella
and reactive arthritis, 133
Shigella organisms, etiology of Reiter's syndrome, 142
Shoulder
and childhood osteomyelitis, 44
aseptic necrosis, 119
pigmented villonodular synovitis, 165
synovial chondromatosis, 160
Sickle cell anemia
and hemoglobinopathies, 80, 82
and related hemoglobinopathies
differentiation from idiopathic aseptic necrosis, 82
sites, 82
associated with
osteomyelitis, 49
paratyphoid B, 49
Salmonella cholerasuis, 49
salmonella osteomyelitis, 49, *50*
Salmonella typhimurium, 49
etiology of salmonella osteomyelitis in, 49
infarction in, 49
Sinus
paranasal, ossifying fibroma and cementifying fibroma, 220
phycomycosis, 54
Sinusoids, in childhood osteomyelitis, 43
Skeletal development, timing of events, 7
Skeletal elements
embryology, 2
stages, *12*
Skeletal reconstruction, 6
Skeletal sarcoma, 187–195
Skeleton
facial
embryology, 1
function, 16
staging of developmental events, 7
Skull
benign giant cell tumor arising in Paget's disease, 249, 250
blastomycosis, 54
diploë, embryology, 2
embryology, 9
fibrous dysplasia, 211
histoplasmosis, 54
ossifying fibroma and cementifying fibroma, 220
Paget's disease, 148, 149, 152, 250
sporotrichosis, 55

Skull—*continued*
  suture, embryology, 1
  vault, embryology, 2
Small bones, osteomyelitis, 51
Smallpox
  concurrence with viral osteomyelitis, 49
  etiologic agent of vaccinial osteomyelitis, 50, 51
Soft tissue, cartilaginous tumors of, recurrence, 305
Soft tissue sarcoma, 187–195
Somatic tissues and tumoral calcinosis
  primary
    giant cell tumor of, 292–293
    giant cell tumor of, histology, 292–293
Somites, 7
Sphenoid bone, craniofacial fibrous dysplasia, 211
Sphenoid lesion, in fibrous dysplasia, 216
Sphenoid ridge, fibrous dysplasia, *214*
Spheno-occipital chordoma, 309
Spine
  actinomycosis, 55
  ankylosing spondylitis, 105, 122, 140
  blastomycosis, 54
  Brucella osteomyelitis, 49
  cervical, osteoarthritis, 122
  coccidioidomycosis, 52
  degenerative disease of, 121–122
    radiology, 122
  hyperostotic ankylosing spondylosis, 122
  idiopathic osteoporosis, 29
  juvenile rheumatoid arthritis, 139
  ochronosis, 108
  osteoarthritis, 110, 121, 122
  osteomyelitis, 39
  Paget's disease, *154*, 155
  roots, site of pain in osteoarthritis, 125
  sarcoma, 198–199
  spondylitis, 140
  typhoid salmonella osteomyelitis, 48
  vertebral osteomyelitis, 45
Spleen
  plasma cell myeloma, 318
  salmonella osteomyelitis, 49
Spondylitis
  and histocompatibility antigen HL-A W27, 133
  ankylosing, 105, 139, 140
    and neuropathic arthritis, 105
    aortitis, 140
    associated with amyloidosis, 140
    associated with antigen HL-A W27, 133
    associated with enteric arthritides, 142
    associated with histocompatibility antigen HL-A W27, 133, 140
    associated with Reiter's syndrome, 140
    characteristics, 140
    differentiation from adult rheumatoid arthritis, 130
    differentiation from hemophilia, 105
    differentiation from psoriasis, 105
    differentiation from psoriatic arthritis, 140
    differentiation from Reiter's disease, 105
    differentiation from Reiter's syndrome, 105, 140
    differentiation from rheumatoid arthritis, 133, 140
    differentiation from spondylitis in psoriasis, 141
    differentiation from tuberculous abscess, 105
    differentiation from ulcerative colitis, 140
    histology, 140
    radiologic diagnosis, 99, 105, *105*
    sites, 105, 122, 139, 140
    syndesmophyte in, 140
  associated with enteric arthritides, 142, 143
  differentiation from spinal osteoarthritis, 121
  in psoriasis, differentiated from ankylosing spondylitis, 141
  in Reiter's syndrome, 141
    differentiated from psoriatic arthritis, 141
  psoriatic, histocompatibility antigen HL-A W27 in, 141
  sites, 140
Spondylosis
  ankylosing
    associated with diabetes, 122
    associated with diabetes mellitus, 122
  differentiation from spinal osteoarthritis, 121
  hyperostotic, ankylosis occurring in, 126
  hyperostotic ankylosing, spine, 122
Sporothrix schenckii, 54
Sporotrichosis, 54–55
  and lymphocyte, 55
  sites, 55
  staphylococcus in, 55
Stages, human embryo, 1
Staging, developmental events in skeleton, 7
Staging in human embryos, Carnegie system, 7
Staphylococcal osteomyelitis, in phycomycosis, 54
Staphylococcus
  and infantile osteomyelitis, 42
  cause of osteomyelitis in patients with sickle cell anemia, 49
  cause of pyogenic arthritis, 99, 100
  etiologic agent in osteomyelitis, 39, 40
  in sporotrichosis, 55
Sternum
  and osteomyelitis, 39
  site of Paget's disease, 148
Still's disease, 139
Streeter, G. L., staging in human embryos, 7
Streptococcal antigens, multiple, as test for rheumatic fever, 89
Streptococcal infection, and reactive arthritis, 133
Streptococcus, group A, precedes rheumatic fever, 88
Stroma (tumor) cell, differentiation from benign multinucleated giant cell, 241
Structure of bone, normal, 16–24
Subchondral bone
  changes, in osteoarthritis, 117
  fracture, cause of necrosis, 116
  necrosis, in osteoarthritis, 116

Subchondral pseudocysts (*see* Pseudocysts)
Subperiosteal abscess, in adult osteomyelitis, 44
Sulphur granules, with actinomycosis, 55, 56
Surgical pathology, associated with osteomyelitis, 40
Syndesmophyte, in ankylosing spondylitis, 140
Synovial cell
  nonrheumatoid, differentiation from rheumatoid cell, 95
  pigmented villonodular synovitis, 162
  rheumatoid
    differentiation from nonrheumatoid synovial cell, 95
    rubella virus in, 132
Synovial chondromatosis (*see* Chondromatosis)
Synovial fluid, complement in, 93
Synovial inflammation, chronicity, 134
Synovial inflammatory process, in inflammatory arthritis, 130
Synovial joints, embryology, 10
Synovial mucin, in osteoarthritis, 116
Synovial neoplasm, secondary to osseous metastasis, 181
Synovial retinaculum, associated with aseptic necrosis of femoral head, 119
Synovial sarcoma (*see* Sarcoma)
Synovioma, benign (*see* Extraarticular localized nodular synovitis)
Synovitis
  associated with arthritis, 130
  detritic
    associated with osteoarthritis, 126
    cause of pain, 125
  differentiation from synovial hemangioma, 164
  extraarticular localized nodular, 167–171
    characteristics, 167–169
    diagnosis, 168
    differentiation from fibrous histiocytoma, 167
    differentiation from malignant giant cell tumor, 171
    giant cell in, 168
    histology, 168–170
    osteoid produced in, 169
    sites, 168–170
    therapy, 169, 170
  gouty, differentiated from rheumatoid arthritis, 133
  histology, 133
  hypertrophic villous, pathologic change in rheumatoidal arthritis, 133
  in idiopathic aseptic necrosis, 84
  in stage IV of idiopathic aseptic necrosis, 71
  intraarticular localized nodular, 167
    characteristics, 167
    etiology, 167
    histology, 167
    incidence, 167, 168
    sites, 167
    therapy, 167
  intraosseous pigmented villonodular, 259–260
  intraosseous villonodular, sites, 259
  localized nodular, differentiation from pigmented villonodular synovitis, 162
  neoplasms and neoplasm-like lesions of pigmented villonodular, and the synovium, 162–167
  nodular, 159
    differentiation from synovial sarcoma, 174
  pigmented villonodular, 162–167, *260*
    and multinucleated giant cell, 162
    characteristics, 162–165
    cytology, 165–166
    diagnosis, 259
    differentiation from benign chondroblastoma, 259, 260
    differentiation from benign giant cell tumor, 259
    differentiation from degenerative joint disease, 164
    differentiation from hemochromatosis, 164
    differentiation from hemophilia, 164
    differentiation from localized nodular synovitis, 162
    differentiation from rheumatoid arthritis, 164
    etiology, 164
    foam cells in, 162
    hemosiderin-laden cell in, 162
    histology, 163–165
    incidence, 164
    prognosis, 166–167
    radiologic findings, 259, *259*
    sites, 162, 164–165
    therapy, 166–167
  rheumatoid
    differentiated from gouty syonvitis, 133
    differentiated from mycobacterial synovitis, 133
  villonodular, radiologic diagnosis, 99, 106, *107*
Synovium
  adipose tissue tumor in, lipoma, 172–173
  associated with clear cell sarcoma of tendon sheaths, 173
  benign, differentiation from malignant metastasizing synovioma, 168
  chondrosarcoma, 179–181
  edema of the sublining layer of, pathologic change in rheumatoid arthritis, 133
  fibrous xanthoma of, (*see* Tenosynovitis)
  hyperemia of sublining layer of, pathologic change in rheumatoid arthritis, 133
  hyperplasia of lining cells of, pathologic change in rheumatoid arthritis, 133
  in psoriatic and rheumatoid arthritis, 140–141
  inflammatory arthritis, 130
  malignant metastasizing, differentiation from benign synovium, 168
  malignant neoplasms of, 173–181
  neoplasm and neoplasm-like lesion, 157–186
    and arborescent lipoma, 172
    and lipoma, 172–173
    hemagioma, 172
    pigmented villonodular synovitis, 162–167

Synovium—*continued*
normal, 157–159
characteristics, 157–159
cytology, 157–159
differentiation from neoplastic cell and stroma of synovial sarcoma, 175
differentiation from synovial sarcoma, 175
primary malignant epithelioid sarcoma from, 173
rheumatoid arthritis, *136*

T cell, in systemic lupus erythematosis, 95
Talus, rheumatoid arthritis, 137
Tarsal bone
coccidioidomycosis, 52
maduromycosis, 56
Tarsus
extraarticular localized nodular synovitis, 170
synovial chondromatosis, 160
Temporomandibular joint
articular synovial chondromatosis, 307
osteoarthritis, 117
synovial chondromatosis, 160
Tendon sheaths, tumor of, 179
Tenosynovitis, 259–260
pigmented villonodular, differential diagnosis, 237
site, 259
Teratogen, tibia and fibula, 11
Teratogenic agents, thalidomide, 11
Test
anti-deoxyribonucleic acid, 93
antinuclear antibody, 93
fluorescence antinuclear antibody, 89–92
Thalidomide
embryopathy, 11
radial hemimelia, 13
tibial hemimelia, 13
Thalidomide syndrome, 11
big toe duplication, 13
critical periods, 14
malformations, 11
Thigh
aneurysmal cyst, 279
benign giant cell tumor of major long tubular bones in nonepiphyseal location, 243
idiopathic aseptic necrosis, 68
synovial sarcoma, 173
Thoracic centrum, ossification, 8
Thorax
osteomyelitis, 39
vertebra, and vertebral osteomyelitis, 45
Thrombophlebitis, mistaken for rheumatoid arthritis, 101
Thumb
defective or absent, radial hemimelia, 13
osteoarthritis, 126
subcondral pseudocyst, 119
Thymosin, deficiency of, in systemic lupus erythematosis, 95
Thyroid gland, diffuse hyperplasia of, 209
Tibia
associated with teratogen, 11
benign chrondroblastoma in nonepiphyseal location, 255
benign giant cell tumor, *239*
in Paget's disease, 250
childhood osteomyelitis, 42
chondrification, 11, 13
chondromyxoid fibroma, 288
embryology, 11
Ewing's sarcoma, 312
fibrous cortical defect, 272, *272–274*, 273
fibrous dysplasia, 209, *228*, 230
as monostotic lesion, 227
giant cell tumor, 198
hematogenous osteomyelitis, *45*
hemimelia, 11, 13, 14
ossification, 11
ossifying fibroma, *203*, 230
osteolytic lesion, 35
osteosarcoma with benign giant cell, 269
Paget's disease, 148, 250
polyostotic fibrous dysplasia, 227
reticulum cell sarcoma, 316
rheumatoid arthritis, 136
sarcoma, *36*
sarcomatous transformation of fibrous dysplasia, 230
sporotrichosis, 55
"stress fracture," 37
typhoid fever associated with osteomyelitis, 48
Toe
duplication, thalidomide syndrome, 13
extraarticular localized nodular synovitis, 168
giant cell reaction, 258
tenosynovitis, 259
unilateral duplication, 14
Tonsillar crypt, actinomycosis, 55
Tooth
actinomycosis, 55
central fibroma, 225
Trabecula
embryology, 5
Trauma
and idiopathic aseptic necrosis, 61
etiologic agent in aseptic necrosis, 75–77, 79, 80
Tropocollagen molecules
bone structure, 16, *16*
side chains, 16
Trueta, J., 41, 44
Trypanosome, in measurements of anti-deoxyribonucleic acid, 92
Tuberculosis
associated with arthritis, 98, *101*, 103
similarity to Brucella osteomyelitis, 49
symptoms like those of fungal osteomyelitis, 52
Tuberculous abscess, differentiation from ankylosing spondylitis, 105
Tubular bones
embryology, 2
endochondral ossification, 2

Tumor
analytic approach, 196–208
associated with Paget's disease, 152
sites, 152
destruction
and repair, 199–205
characteristics, 199
extent of, 199
hypotheses, 199
giant cell, *203*
human
etiology, 189–190
identification of virus-like particles of, 189–190
incidence
by age, 196–198
by sites, 198–199
malignant giant cell, differentiation from extraarticular localized nodular synovitis, 171
myelogenic, classification, 312
nonrecurrent, differentiation from recurrent tumor, 226
of soft tissue malignant giant cell, 179
radiologic diagnosis, 196–208
recurrent, differentiation from nonrecurrent tumor, 226
round cell, destruction of bone, 199, 202
small cell, terminological derivation, 312
small round cell, 312–319
and plasma cell myeloma, 312
and reticulum cell sarcoma, 312
tendon sheaths, 179
Typhoid fever
and salmonella osteomyelitis
incidence, 48
sites, 48

Ulcerative colitis, differentiation from ankylosing spondylitis, 140
Ulna
destruction of bone, *201*
early rheumatoid arthritis, 108
fibrous dysplasia, 209
rheumatoid arthritis, 100
viral osteomyelitis, 50
"Umbauzonen," in osteomalacia, 29
"Unmasking," cause of osteoarthritis, 112
Urethritis, a component of Reiter's syndrome, 141
Uveitis, associated with Reiter's syndrome, 141

Variola osteomyelitis, and arthritis, *51*
Vasculitis
panarteritis in, 138
pathologic change in rheumatoid arthritis, 138
Vertebra
actinomycosis, 55
aneurysmal cyst, 199
ankylosing spondylitis, 105, 140
Brucella osteomyelitis, 49
coccidioidomycosis, 52
embryology, 2, 7
extraarticular localized nodular synovitis, 170
fibrous dysplasia, 209
idiopathic osteoporosis, 29
lumbar, and, vertebral osteomyelitis, 45
lymphoma in, 199
myeloma in, 199
osteoarthritis, 121, 122
osteoid osteoma in, 199
osteomyelitis, 45, 46
osteophytes of osteoarthritis, 122
Paget's disease, *154*, 155
salmonella osteomyelitis, 48
sarcoma, 199
spondylitis, 140
Vertebral centra, hyaline cartilaginous rings, embryology, 2
Viral osteomylitis, 49–51
Virus
murine leukemia, RNA-related, contained in human sarcoma, 190–191
oncogenic, interspecies transmission of, 191–192
interspecies transmission of, immunology, 192
rubella, and rheumatoid synovial cells, 132
variola, in viral osteomyelitis, 50
Vitamin D
associated with osteomalacia, 32–36
associated with rickets, 29, *30*
Von Recklinghausen's neurofibromatosis
differentiated from fibrous dysplasia, 210

Whipple's disease, associated with intermittent migratory arthritis, 143
Woven bone
matrix, 22
mineral content, 22
Wrist
epithelioid sarcoma, 176
extraarticular localized nodular synovitis, 168
ganglion cyst, 171
lipoma, 173
pigmented villonodular synovitis, 165
rheumatoid arthritis, 100, 131

Xanthofibroma (*see* Extraarticular localized nodular synovitis)

Yersinia, and reactive arthritis, 133